Clinical Ophthalmology: A Practical Approach

Clinical Ophthalmology: A Practical Approach

Edited by Slade Decker

hayle
medical

New York

Hayle Medical,
750 Third Avenue, 9ᵗʰ Floor,
New York, NY 10017, USA

Visit us on the World Wide Web at:
www.haylemedical.com

ISBN: 978-1-63241-710-7

Cataloging-in-Publication Data

Clinical ophthalmology : a practical approach / edited by Slade Decker.
    p. cm.
Includes bibliographical references and index.
ISBN 978-1-63241-710-7
1. Ophthalmology. 2. Eye--Diseases. 3. Eye--Diseases--Treatment. I. Decker, Slade.
RE46 .C55 2019
617.7--dc23

Table of Contents

Preface

This book aims to highlight the current researches and provides a platform to further the scope of innovations in this area. This book is a product of the combined efforts of many researchers and scientists, after going through thorough studies and analysis from different parts of the world. The objective of this book is to provide the readers with the latest information of the field.

The field of medicine concerned with the eye, its functioning, structure, and disorders is known as ophthalmology. A specialist doctor or surgeon in this field is called an ophthalmologist. Pediatric ophthalmology is a subset of ophthalmology. It studies the diseases related to eye, visual development and vision care in children. Ocular diseases in children include conjunctivitis, strabismus, amblyopia, pediatric cataracts, pediatric glaucoma, and blocked tear ducts, among others. The inflammation of the outermost layer of the white part of the eye along with the inner surface of the eyelid is known as conjunctivitis. Acute conjunctivitis mostly occurs in the elderly, infants and school-age children. This book attempts to understand the multiple branches that fall under the discipline of ophthalmology and how such concepts have practical applications. It presents researches and studies performed by experts across the globe. Doctors, researchers and students actively engaged in this field will find this book full of crucial and unexplored concepts.

I would like to express my sincere thanks to the authors for their dedicated efforts in the completion of this book. I acknowledge the efforts of the publisher for providing constant support. Lastly, I would like to thank my family for their support in all academic endeavors.

Editor

Does rituximab improve clinical outcomes of patients with thyroid-associated ophthalmopathy?

Changjun Wang, Qingyao Ning, Kai Jin, Jiajun Xie and Juan Ye[*]

Abstract

Background: The current therapies of thyroid-associated ophthalmopathy (TAO) were still a challenging matter. In this study, we aimed to contrast the impact of before- after rituximab (RTX) therapy in the patients with TAO.

Methods: We searched the PubMed, EMBASE, and SCOPUS databases for articles published up to July 3, 2017. Fixed- or random-effects meta-analysis was used to provide pooled estimates of standard mean difference (SMD) both the primary outcome from clinical activity score (CAS), and secondary outcomes from thyrotropin receptor antibody (TRAb), proptosis, thyroid stimulating hormone (TSH), and interleukin-6 (IL-6) levels. In addition, the quality and each study was assessed using either the Newcastle Ottawa Scale (NOS) or the Cochrane Risk of Bias tool, and reliability of the meta-analytic result using the Grading of Recommendations Assessment, Development and Evaluation (GRADE).

Results: Of the 839 articles initially searched, 11 studies were finally eligible for inclusion. Subgroup analysis results showed that comparing with initial value, there was a decline in CAS at 1,3,6,12 month after RTX treatment, decreased TRAbs level at 6,12 month, proptosis improvement at least 1 month, unchanged IL-6 level at 6 month, decreased TSH level at 3 month but unchanged at 12 month. All included studies were classified as good quality.

Conclusions: The pooled data suggested that the preliminary effects of RTX treatment on TAO might be promising. However, more large-sample and high-quality studies targeting RTX use during this disease and long-term surveillance of prognosis are urgently needed.

Keywords: Inflammation, Orbit, Drugs, Eye lids, Vision

Background

Thyroid-associated ophthalmopathy (TAO) is an auto-immune inflammatory orbital disease, which usually is caused by 20–50% of patients with Graves' disease (GD) [1] and has the symptom of bilateral or unilateral eyeball protrusion, eyelid swelling, edema of periorbital tissue, and upper or lower eyelid retraction [2]. It was reported that lymphocytes B played an important role in TAO [3]. B cells could induce immune function via antigen presentation, co-stimulatory molecules expression and antibodies production. They can also be differentiated into antibody-producing plasma cells, which not only caused host defense, but also identified their own tissues, resulting in autoimmunity [4]. In addition, B cells produced cytokines that induced fbroblasts to generate glycosaminoglycan causing fluid and periorbital edema. In recent years, there have been many treatments for TAO, but adverse effects in follow-up should be cautious, such as hypertension, diabetes, stress ulcer, and osteoporosis during immunosuppressive therapies [5], retinopathy, neuropathy, and cataracts in single radiation therapy or combining with oral or intravenous steroids [6], around 20% to 25% of nonresponders after intravenous pulses of corticosteroids [7].

* Correspondence: yejuan@zju.edu.cn
Department of Ophthalmology, the Second Affiliated Hospital of Zhejiang University, College of Medicine, Hangzhou 310009, China

Rituximab (RTX) is a chimeric mouse monoclonal anti-human CD20 antibody against B-cell proliferation and maturation. RTX has been allowed since 2006 for treating rheumatoid arthritis and had a chance to become a candidate for the treatment of some other autoimmune diseases [8]. In recent years, although some case series have shown that RTX treatment in severe TAO may benefit patients, its application was restricted to case reports and uncontrolled studies, which was a lack of large-scale prospective studies and the effectiveness was still inconsistent. Therefore, we did a systematic review and aimed to check whether the CAS activity improved 1 month or more after RTX treatment for persons with TAO.

Methods

Search strategy

We conducted the systematic review according to the Preferred Reporting Items for Systematic Reviews and Meta-Analyses (PRISMA) statement [9]. To assess the evidence on this issue, a broad literature search was independently initiated by Changjun Wang and Qingyao Ning through the PubMed, EMBASE, and SCOPUS databases for articles published up to July 3, 2017 (Appendix 1). Search terms included the keyword terms using rituximab, Graves' ophthalmopathy, thyroid associated orbitopathy, thyroid eye disease. Discrepancy was finally resolved by the senior author (Juan Ye). All literatures were retrieved with no language restrictions. If detailed data were available from online reports, we applied for it directly from authors. These literatures were managed and duplicates were removed through Endnote X7 software (Changjun Wang and Qingyao Ning).

Study selection

The criteria deciding whether an article was included were as following: (1) cohort study or randomized controlled trial including RTX treatment for patients with TAO; (2) clinical data involving before-after RTX treatment would be available; (3) original articles including one or more parameters of CAS, TRAbs, proptosis, TSH, and IL-6 levels after clinical follow-up of at least 1 month. Studies would be removed if they were case reports, reviews, letters, or conference abstracts without full text.

Data extraction and quality assessment

Kai Jin and Jiajun Xie extracted these data from each eligible article: authors' names, the type of study, study period, country, age, gender, smoking status, follow-up. In this analysis, disease activity was estimated according to the seven-point CAS using Snellen chart based on the classical signs of inflammation (ocular pain, eyelid redness, eyelid swelling and fading eyesight) [10]. For each of included studies, CAS was calculated to examine the clinical improvement of these patients at the each ophthalmological visit. Instruments such as the Cochrane risk of bias tool for trials and the Newcastle-Ottawa Scale (NOS) for observational studies were also crosschecked by Changjun Wang and Kai Jin. Quality was assessed using the NOS and Cochrane and reliability of results using GRADE by Changjun Wang and Kai Jin [11, 12]. This was done in duplicate with disagreements handled by discussion with a final arbiter (Juan Ye).

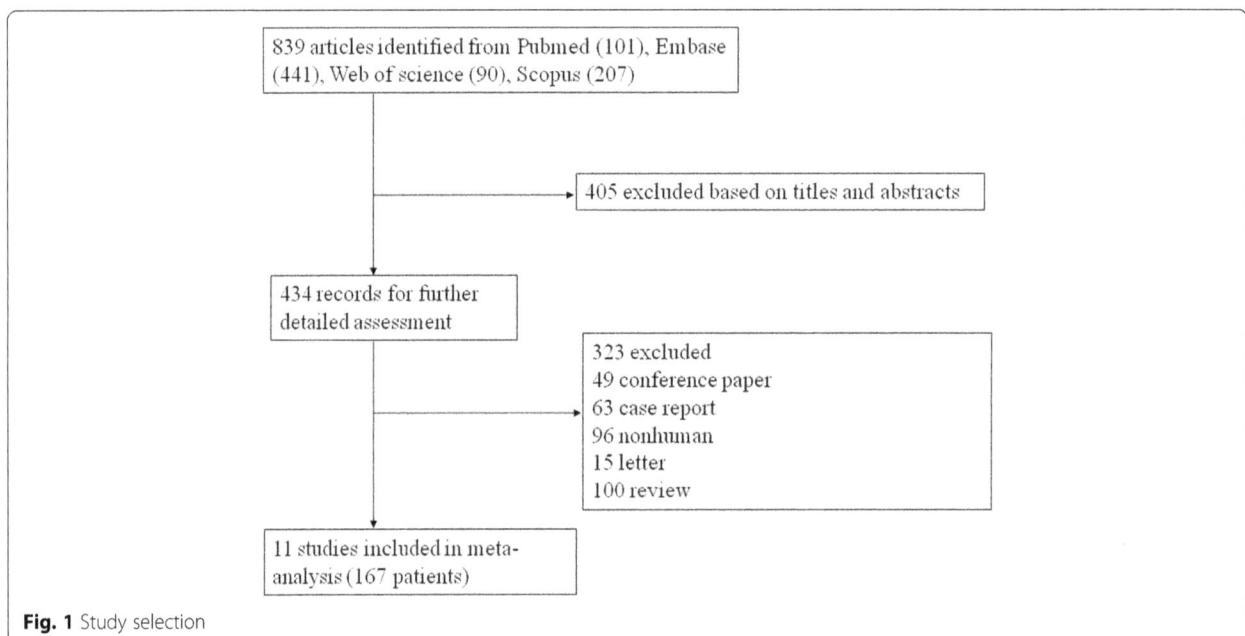

Fig. 1 Study selection

Table 1 Characteristic of the included studies in the meta-analysis

Author	Type of study	Study period	Country	Number of patients	Age (Mean ± SD) (Range)	Gender (M/F)	Smoking	Follow-up, Months (Mean ± SD)	Outcomes indexs	Complication
Salvi M et al. 2007 [14]	Cohort study	NA	Italy	9	44.8 ± 2.1 (31–51)	2/7	5	1	CAS, TRAbs, proptosis	3 nose and throat itching,mild temperature elevation
Vannucchi G et al. 2010 [17]	Cohort study	NA	Italy	10	46.6 ± 2.2 (31–54)	2/8	NA	12	TRAbs, IL-6	NA
Silkiss RZ et al. 2010 [16]	Cohort study	2007.1–2010.10	United States	12	52.1 (34–80)	5/7	4	12	CAS, TSH	No
Khanna D et al. 2010 [15]	Cohort study	2007.10.1–2009.2.1	United States	6	54.3 ± 9.1	2/4	3	7.5 ± 6.4	CAS, proptosis	1 urinary tract infection;1 hypertension;1 cardiac arrest
Mitchell AL et al. 2013 [18]	Cohort study	2008–2012	UK	9	62 (37–87)	1/8	NA	16	CAS	2 headache;1 headache and chills without pyrexia;1 mild myalgia
Savino G et al. 2013 [19]	Cohort study	NA	Italy	5	48 ± 12.1	3/2	3	18	CAS, proptosis	2 nausea and temperature elevation
Erdei A et al. 2014	Cohort study	NA	Hungary	5	47.8 ± 12.2 (31–64)	1/4	4	60	CAS, TRAbs, TSH	NA
McCoy AN et al. 2014 [21]	Cohort study	2007.10.1–?	United States	8	57 ± 6.63	3/5	4	18	CAS	NA
Stan MN et al. 2015 [23]	Randomized controlled trial	NA	United States	13	57.6 ± 12.7	4/9	2	13	CAS, TRAbs, proptosis	2 myalgias;2 skin rash and itching;1 infectious;1 vasculitis;2 optic neuropathy;1 severe lacrimation;2 gastrointestinal;
Salvi M et al. 2015 [22]	Randomized controlled trial	NA	Italy	15	51.9 ± 13.1	1/14	10	19	CAS, TRAbs, TSH, proptosis	1 orbital edema and decrease of vision;1 hypotension;1 myocardial infarction
Li J et al. 2017 [24]	Randomized controlled trial	NA	China	75	48.1 ± 10.0	25/50	15	10	CAS, proptosis, IL-6	1 flushing;9 nose and throat itching;2 dyspepsia;9 temperature elevation

NA not available

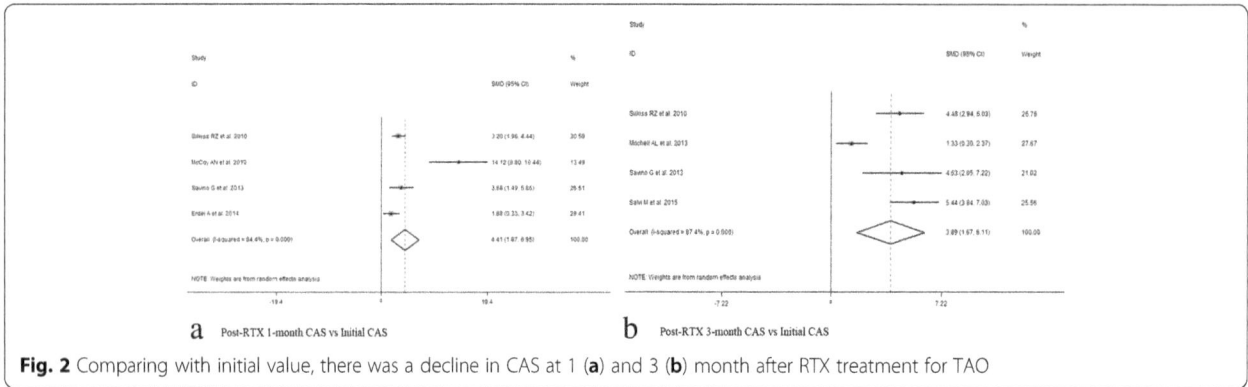

Fig. 2 Comparing with initial value, there was a decline in CAS at 1 (**a**) and 3 (**b**) month after RTX treatment for TAO

Statistical analysis

Based on the initial baseline value, the meta-analysis compared the outcome changes at different time interval (1,3,6,12 month, respectively) after RTX therapy, in view of mean CAS as the primary outcome, and mean of TRAbs, proptosis, TSH, IL-6 levels as secondary outcomes. Data were pooled and calculated their SMDs and the 95% confidence interval (CI) for each subgroup when at least two studies focused on the outcome (Additional file 1: Supplementary files). The meta-analysis was conducted by the Mantel–Haenszel method through Stata 12.0 software [13]. Statistical heterogeneity was estimated using the chi-square test (χ^2), τ^2 and I^2 statistic. Where $p < 0.05$ or $I^2 > 50\%$ appeared indicating moderate to large statistical heterogeneity, then a random-effects model was applied. We performed subgroup analysis for heterogeneity according to CAS, proptosis, TRAbs, TSH and IL-6. Otherwise, a fixed-effect model was performed. In addition, the impact of study quality on the results was evaluated by sensitivity analysis, and Egger's tests were assessed for potential publication bias.

Results

Characteristics of eligible studies in the final analysis

Our initial search found 839 citations, and after review of title and abstract, 323 studies were recruited for further full-text reading, of which 11 articles were finally available for inclusion [14–24]. The selection flow was showed in Fig. 1. In this study, the mean age of patients was from 44.8 to 62.0 years old. A total of the population consisted of 49 (29.3%) men and 118 (70.7%) women, and almost one third smoked. Nearly one half of the participants were from China (44.9%), followed by Europe (31.7%) and North America (23.4%). The mean follow-up of these studies were from 1 to 60 months. Regarding adverse events, mild temperature elevation, nose and throat itching, headache, myalgias, optic neuropathy, orbital edema and decrease of vision, dyspepsia were reported (Table 1). Methodological quality in included studies were acceptable by Newcastle-Ottawa Scale and Cochrane risk of bias tool, in which main drawbacks were the application of few blinding and random distribution, and insufficient sample size, which were reliable appraised through GRADE. Then we tried to minimize it by subgroup analysis based on cohort study and randomized controlled trial, which indicated that most of these results were stable (Additional file 2: Table S1, Additional file 3: Table S2, Additional file 4: Figure S1, Additional file 5: Figure S2).

Heterogeneity test result and subgroup analysis

In view of the initial CAS value, results indicated significant decrease at 1,3,6,12 months after subsequent RTX treatment (1 month, SMD 95% CI: 4.77 (2.77–6.77); 3 month,

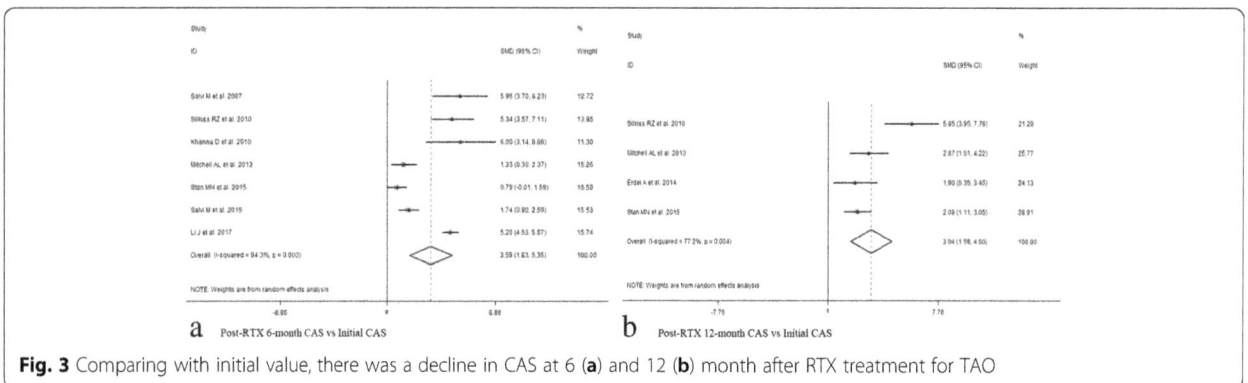

Fig. 3 Comparing with initial value, there was a decline in CAS at 6 (**a**) and 12 (**b**) month after RTX treatment for TAO

Does rituximab improve clinical outcomes of patients with thyroid-associated...

5

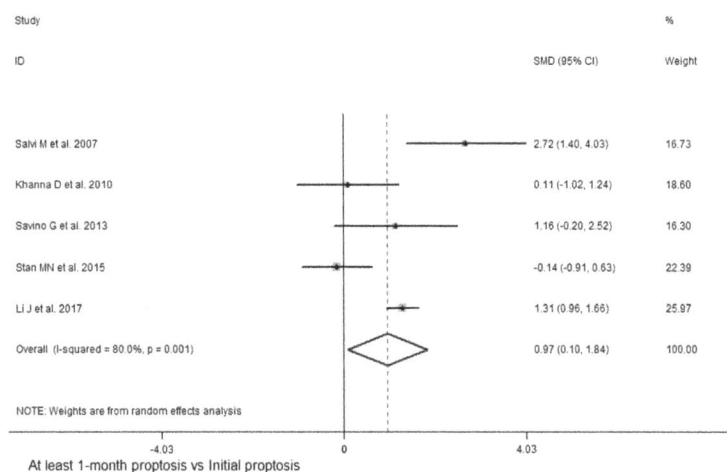

Fig. 4 Comparing with initial value, there was a decrease in proptosis at least 1 month after RTX treatment for TAO

SMD 95% CI: 3.89 (1.67–6.11); 6 month, SMD 95% CI: 3.59 (1.83–5.35); 12 month, SMD 95% CI: 3.04 (1.58–4.50)) (Figs. 2 and 3, Additional file 6: Table S3). At last month of follow-up, proptosis improvement was shown (last month of follow-up, SMD 95% CI: 0.97 (0.10–1.84)) (Fig. 4). Similarly, pooled data reported TRAbs level were both declining at 6 and 12 months (6 month, SMD 95% CI: 0.82 (0.40–1.25); 12 month, SMD 95% CI: 1.52 (0.80–2.24)) (Fig. 5). TSH level was decreased at 2 month while unchanged at 12 month (2 month, SMD 95% CI: 0.69 (0.14–1.25); 12 month, SMD 95% CI: 0.39 (– 0.74–1.52)) (Fig. 6). In addition, IL-6 level was also not see an obvious variation (6 month, SMD 95% CI: 6.47 (– 3.26–16.21)) (Fig. 7). In Additional file 6: Table S3, subgroup analysis listed heterogeneity test using I^2, in which the considerable heterogeneity ($I^2 > 75\%$) was dealt with random-effects model (CAS: 1,3,6,12 month: 84.4%, 87.4%, 94.3%,77.2%; proptosis: at least 1 month: 80%; TSH: 12 month: 76.7%; IL-6: 6 month: 99.3%).

Sensitivity analysis and publication bias
We checked the effect of each of these studies through sensitivity analyses, and all were in accordance with our main results. Egger's test suggested no publication bias was in this study (Additional file 6: Table S3).

Discussion
Thyroid-associated ophthalmopathy was the main extrathyroidal manifestation of Graves' disease. Treatment was depended on the evaluation of the activity and severity of TAO and focused on the patient's living quality. In this systematic review and meta-analysis, we showed that RTX treatment may confer a favorable improvement against TAO. The improvement of TAO remained stable during the follow-up.

Regarding CAS, which may indicate whether these patients benefit or not from RTX therapy. Pain, redness, swelling and impaired function improved in most patients at 1 month after RTX treatment, and sustained during the 12-month follow-up. As shown in a previous study, there were evident reductions from the mean baseline CAS score 5.5 to finally approximate 1.0 for weeks 4, 8, 16, 24, 36, and 52 [16]. A high CAS could help select targeting patients who will benefit from RTX treatment. The eyelids became swollen and visual acuity decreased. The serious signs and symptoms in the baseline may result from the

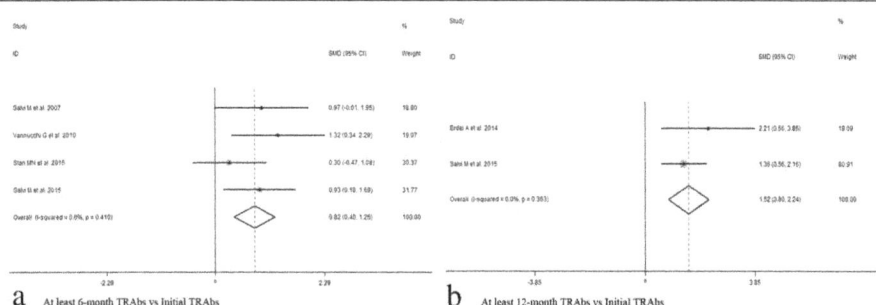

Fig. 5 Comparing with initial value, there was a reduction in TRAbs at 6 (**a**) and 12 (**b**) month after RTX treatment for TAO

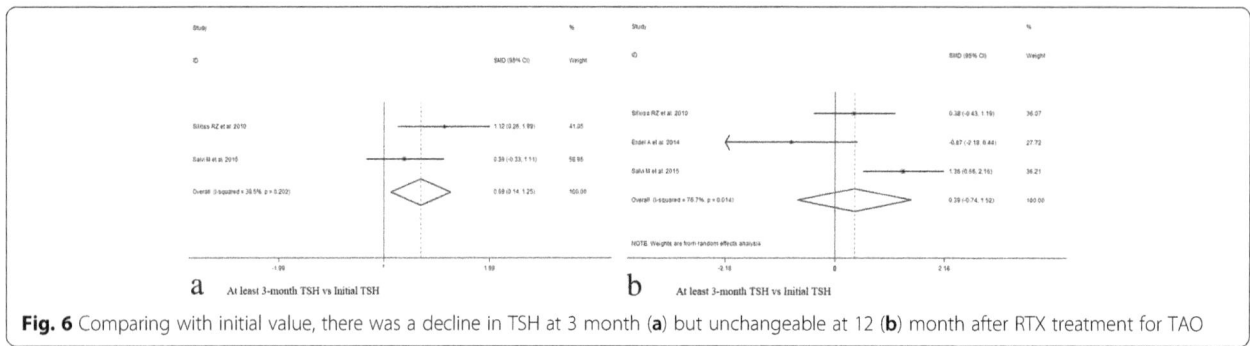

Fig. 6 Comparing with initial value, there was a decline in TSH at 3 month (**a**) but unchangeable at 12 (**b**) month after RTX treatment for TAO

inflammation caused by the autoimmune course. Orbital fibroblasts were also considered to be vital in the pathogenesis [10]. Decreased CAS in the majority of individuals meant favorable therapeutic effects. The long-term reduction in CAS scores may suggest it may depend upon the late effects of the drug in some cases.

Recently, unchangeable proptosis was visible in Khanna et al. study [15]. It should be interpreted seriously because the study was only 6 patients and uncontrolled. But in this study, RTX therapy was effective in ameliorating disease severity, as seen in the significant improvement of proptosis and soft tissue inflammation. Furthermore, previous study found that RTX associated with the consumption and resistance of mature B lymphocytes, contributing to control inflammation [25].

Besides CAS, reduction in TRAbs level was observed at 6-month and 12-month observation period after RTX use. However, it was reported that serum TRAbs levels were not changed significantly, and was slightly negatively associated with time during 75-week follow-up [14]. Vannucchi et al. found that serum TRAbs have not reduced obviously in TAO cases before 30 weeks since treatment [17]. Based on the previous limited TAO cases treated by RTX, the pooled changes in current results may because TRAb were associated significantly with TAO clinical activity [26]. During the different disease phase, participants with severe TAO have more serum TRAb levels than those with mild-moderate TAO [27]. Although it was possible to include the involvement of B cells, TRAb and cytokines, the detailed mechanism of decreased TRAb levels was still unknown [28]. In addition, the fluctuation of TSH concentration also existed in short- and long-term observation period.

There was a weakly reduced trend in IL-6, which were around the normal range. However, it was different from the prior studies [29]. IL-6 secreted by diverse cells like T and B lymphocytes, monocytes, and fibroblasts could participate in stimulating T cell, triggering immunoglobulin secretion, also have impacts in fibroblasts and macrophages in TAO [30, 31]. It was likely that blocking IL-6 might be a promising therapy in TAO. But the inapparent results in current meta-analysis could be owing to the small number of participants. Thus large-scale researches were needed in order to make reliable conclusions.

There were several limitations of our review that should be interpreted. First, we have only limited sample size to hardly explore the potential impact of other risk factors such as age, gender, smoking status, dosage of RTX. Second, the orbital variation after RTX treatment could be susceptible to the previous medication of intravenous or oral corticosteroid. Third, subgroup analysis was on the basis of aggregate data, which could mask diversity within individual level and interaction between factors.

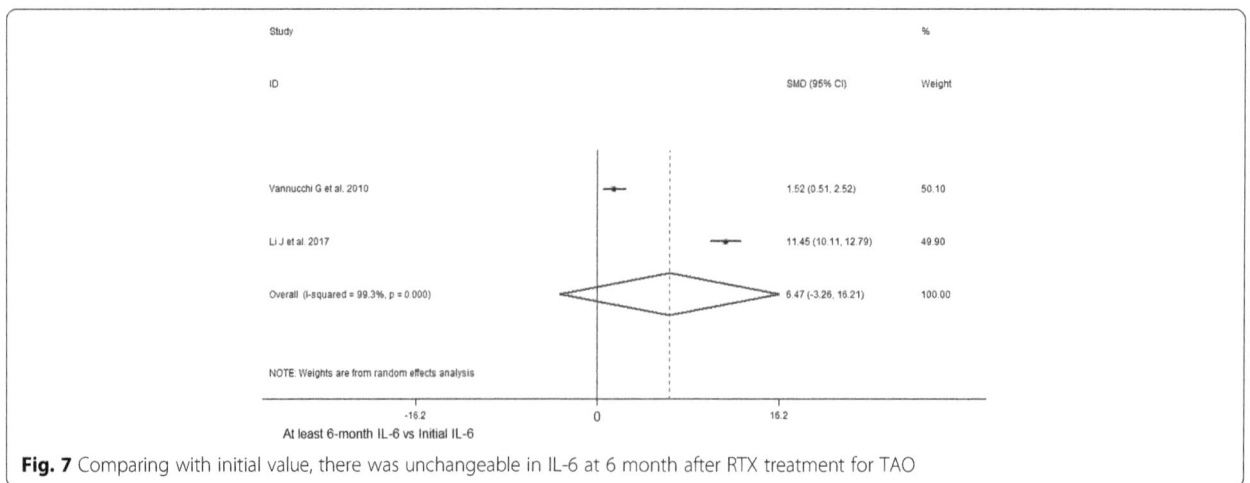

Fig. 7 Comparing with initial value, there was unchangeable in IL-6 at 6 month after RTX treatment for TAO

In spite of these, the strengths of this review were that we had a systematic search according to prespecified strategies, and tried to find additional studies. We cross-checked methodological decisions and the influence of each study through sensitivity analyses, and showed the robust results, which were similar to those previous trials, making the results more faithworthy in practice in many countries.

Conclusions

In short, our analysis of existing empirical evidences suggested that the preliminary effects of RTX treatment on TAO might be promising. We initiated the systematic review of RTX therapy of patients with TAO, which tried to fill in knowledge gaps. However, more large-sample and high-quality studies targeting RTX use during this disease and long-term surveillance of prognosis are urgently warranted.

Appendix
Search strategy:
Pubmed (1950-present)

1. (rituximab OR RTX)
2. (Graves OR thyroid)
3. (ophthalmopathy OR (eye disease))
4. 1 AND 2 AND 3
5. "rituximab"[Mesh]
6. "Graves ophthalmopathy"[Mesh]
7. 5 AND 6
8. 4 OR 7

Embase(1980-present)

1. 'rituximab':ab,ti
2. 'RTX':ab,ti
3. 1 OR 2
4. 'Graves':ab,ti
5. 'thyroid':ab,ti
6. 4 OR 5
7. 'ophthalmopathy':ab,ti
8. 'eye disease':ab,ti
9. 7 OR 8
10.3 AND 6 AND 9

Scoups

1. TITLE-ABS-KEY ("rituximab")
2. TITLE-ABS-KEY ("RTX")
3. 1 OR 2
4. TITLE-ABS-KEY ("Graves")
5. TITLE-ABS-KEY ("thyroid")
6. 4 OR 5
7. TITLE-ABS-KEY ("ophthalmopathy")

8. TITLE-ABS-KEY ("eye disease")
9. 7 OR 8
10.3 AND 6 AND 9

Abbreviations
CAS: Clinical activity score; CI: Confidence interval; GD: Graves' disease; GRADE: Grading of recommendations assessment, development and evaluation; IL-6: Interleukin-6; NOS: Newcastle-Ottawa scale; PRISMA: Preferred reporting items for systematic reviews and meta-analyses; RTX: Rituximab; SMD: Standard mean difference; TAO: Thyroid-associated ophthalmopathy; TRAb: Thyrotropin receptor antibody; TSH: Thyroid stimulating hormone

Acknowledgments
Not applicable.

Funding
Supported by grants from the Medicine and Health Science Technology Project of Zhejiang Province (2015KYA113), the Scientific Research Foundation of Traditional Chinese Medicine of Zhejiang Province (2015ZB031), the National Natural Science Foundation of China (81670888), National key research and development program (2016YFC1100403). These funding had no role in the study design, data collection and analysis, decision to publish, or preparation of the manuscript.

Authors' contributions
Study concept and design: JY. Acquisition of data: CW, QN, KJ, JX. Analysis and interpretation of data: CW, QN. Drafting of the manuscript: CW. Critical revision of the manuscript for important intellectual content: CW, JY. Statistical analysis: KJ, JX. Obtained funding: CW. Technical, or material support: KJ, JX. Study supervision: JY. All authors read and approved the final manuscript.

Competing interests
The authors state that there is no competing interests regarding the publication of this paper.

References
1. Bahn RS. Graves' ophthalmopathy. N Engl J Med. 2010;362(8):726–38.
2. Smith TJ. Pathogenesis of graves' orbitopathy: a 2010 update. J Endocrinol Investig. 2010;33(6):414–21.
3. Smith TJ, Tsai CC, Shih MJ, Tsui S, Chen B, Han R, et al. Unique attributes of orbital fibroblasts and global alterations in IGF-1 receptor signaling could explain thyroid-associated Ophthalmopathy. Thyroid Official J Am Thyroid Assoc. 2008;18(9):983.
4. Douglas RS, Naik V, Hwang CJ, Afifiyan NF, Gianoukakis AG, Sand D, et al. B cells from patients with Graves' disease aberrantly express the IGF-1 receptor: implications for disease pathogenesis. J Immunol. 2008;181(8):5768.
5. Bartalena L, Lai A, Compri E, Marcocci C, Tanda ML. Novel immunomodulating agents for graves orbitopathy. Ophthalmic Plast Reconstr Surg. 2008;24(4):251.
6. Bradley EA, Gower EW, Bradley DJ, Meyer DR, Cahill KV, Custer PL, et al. Orbital radiation for graves Ophthalmopathy : a report by the American Academy of ophthalmology. Ophthalmology. 2008;115(2):398–409.
7. Kahaly GJ, Pitz S, Hommel G, Dittmar M. Randomized, single blind trial of intravenous versus oral steroid monotherapy in Graves' orbitopathy. J Clin Endocrinol Metab. 2005;90(9):5234.
8. Anolik JH, Barnard J, Owen T, Zheng B, Kemshetti S, Looney RJ, et al. Delayed memory B cell recovery in peripheral blood and lymphoid tissue in systemic lupus erythematosus after B cell depletion therapy. Arthritis Rheum. 2007;56(9):3044.
9. Moher D, Liberati A, Tetzlaff J, Altman DG, Group TP. Preferred reporting items for systematic reviews and meta-analyses: the PRISMA statement. Revista Esp Nutr Hum Diet. 2009;18(3):889–96.

10. Mourits MP, Prummel MF, Wiersinga WM, Koornneef L. Clinical activity score as a guide in the management of patients with Graves' ophthalmopathy. Clin Endocrinol. 1997;47(1):9–14.

11. Balshem H, Helfand M, Schunemann HJ, Oxman AD, Kunz R, Brozek J, et al. GRADE guidelines: rating the quality of evidence-introduction. 2011.

12. Guyatt G, Oxman AD, Akl EA, Kunz R, Vist G, Brozek J, et al. GRADE guidelines: 1. Introduction-GRADE evidence profiles and summary of findings tables. J Clin Epidemiol. 2012;64(4):383–94.

13. Higgins J, Green SE. Cochrane Handbook for Systematic Reviews of Interventions Version 5.1.0. The Cochrane Collaboration (Eds). Naunyn-Schmiedebergs Archiv für experimentelle Pathologie und Pharmakologie. 2011;2011(14):S38.

14. Salvi M, Vannucchi G, Campi I, Currò N, Dazzi D, Simonetta S, et al. Treatment of Graves' disease and associated ophthalmopathy with the anti-CD20 monoclonal antibody rituximab: an open study. Eur J Endocrinol. 2007;156(1):33.

15. Khanna D, Chong KK, Afifiyan NF, Hwang CJ, Lee DK, Garneau HC, et al. Rituximab treatment of patients with severe, corticosteroid-resistant thyroid-associated ophthalmopathy. Ophthalmology. 2010;117(1):133–9.

16. Silkiss RZ, Reier AM, Lauer SA. Rituximab for thyroid eye disease. Ophthalmic Plast Reconstr Surg. 2010;26(5):310–4.

17. Vannucchi G, Campi I, Bonomi M, Covelli D, Dazzi D, Currò N, et al. Rituximab treatment in patients with active Graves' orbitopathy: effects on proinflammatory and humoral immune reactions. Clin Exp Immunol. 2010; 161(3):436–43.

18. Mitchell AL, Gan EH, Morris M, Johnson K, Neoh C, Dickinson AJ, et al. The effect of B cell depletion therapy on anti-TSH receptor antibodies and clinical outcome in glucocorticoid-refractory Graves' orbitopathy. Clin Endocrinol. 2013;79(3):437–42.

19. Savino G, Balia L, Colucci D, Battendieri R, Gari M, Corsello SM, et al. Intraorbital injection of rituximab: a new approach for active thyroid-associated orbitopathy, a prospective case series. Minerva Endocrinol. 2013; 38(2):173–9.

20. Erdei A, Paragh G, Kovacs P, Karanyi Z, Berenyi E, Galuska L, et al. Rapid response to and long-term effectiveness of anti-CD20 antibody in conventional therapy resistant Graves' orbitopathy: a five-year follow-up study. Autoimmunity. 2014;47(8):548–55.

21. Mccoy AN, Kim DS, Gillespie EF, Atkins SJ, Smith TJ, Douglas RS. Rituximab (Rituxan) therapy for severe thyroid-associated ophthalmopathy diminishes IGF-1R(+) T cells. J Clin Endocrinol Metab. 2014;99(7):1294–9.

22. Salvi M, Vannucchi G, Currò N, Campi I, Covelli D, Dazzi D, et al. Efficacy of B-cell targeted therapy with rituximab in patients with active moderate to severe Graves' orbitopathy: a randomized controlled study. J Clin Endocrinol Metab. 2015;100(2):422–31.

23. Stan MN, Garrity JA, Carranza Leon BG, Prabin T, Bradley EA, Bahn RS. Randomized controlled trial of rituximab in patients with Graves' orbitopathy. J Clin Endocrinol Metab. 2015;100(2):432.

24. Li J, Xiao Z, Hu X, Yun L, Xing Z, Zhang S, et al. The efficacy of Rituximab combined with 131I for ophthalmic outcomes of Graves' Ophthalmopathy patients. Pharmacology. 2017;99(3–4):144.

25. Hasselbalch HC. B-cell depletion with rituximab-a targeted therapy for Graves' disease and autoimmune thyroiditis. Immunol Lett. 2003;88(1):85–6.

26. Gerding MN, Meer JWCVD, Broenink M, Bakker O, Wiersinga WM, Prummel MF. Association of thyrotrophin receptor antibodies with the clinical features of Graves' ophthalmopathy. Clin Endocrinol. 2000;52(3):267–71.

27. Eckstein AK, Plicht M, Lax H, Neuhäuser M, Mann K, Lederbogen S, et al. Thyrotropin receptor autoantibodies are independent risk factors for Graves' ophthalmopathy and help to predict severity and outcome of the disease. J Clin Endocrinol Metab 2006;91(9):3464.

28. Minakaran N, Ezra DG. Rituximab for thyroid-associated ophthalmopathy. Cochrane Database Syst Rev. 2013;5(5):CD009226.

29. Salvi M, Vannucchi G, Beck-Peccoz P. Potential utility of rituximab for Graves' orbitopathy. J Clin Endocrinol Metab. 2013;98(11):4291–9.

30. Jyonouchi SC, Valyasevi RW, Harteneck DA, Dutton CM, Bahn RS. Interleukin-6 stimulates thyrotropin receptor expression in human orbital preadipocyte fibroblasts from patients with Graves' ophthalmopathy. Thyroid. 2001;11(10): 929–34.

31. Pérez-Moreiras JV, Alvarez-López A, Gómez EC. Treatment of active corticosteroid-resistant graves' orbitopathy. Ophthalmic Plast Reconstr Surg. 2014;30(2):162.

Expression of MyoD, insulin like growth factor binding protein, thioredoxin and p27 in secondarily overacting inferior oblique muscles with superior oblique palsy

Yeon Woong Chung[1], Jun Sub Choi[2] and Sun Young Shin[2*]

Abstract

Backgound: To identify and compare specific protein levels between overacting inferior oblique (IO) muscles in superior oblique (SO) palsy patients and normal IO muscles.

Methods: We obtained 20 IO muscle samples from SO palsy patients with IO overaction ≥ + 3 who underwent IO myectomies (IOOA group), and 20 IO samples from brain death donors whose IO had functioned normally, according to their ophthalmological chart review (control group). We used MyoD for identifying satellite cell activation, insulin-like growth factor binding protein 5 (IGFBP5) for IGF effects, thioredoxin for oxidative stress, and p27 for satellite cell activation or oxidative stress in both groups. Using immunohistochemistry and Western blot, we compared expression levels of the four proteins (MyoD, IGFBP5, thioredoxin, and p27).

Results: Levels of thioredoxin and p27 were decreased significantly in the IOOA group. MyoD and IGFBP5 levels showed no significant difference between the groups.

Conclusions: Based on these findings, the overacting IOs of patients with SO palsy had been under oxidative stress status versus normal IOs. Pathologically overacting extraocular muscles may have an increased risk of oxidative stress compared with normal extraocular muscles.

Keywords: Oxidative stress, Inferior oblique muscle overaction, Superior oblique palsy, Thioredoxin, p27

Background

Inferior oblique (IO) muscle overaction may occur as a primary condition or develop secondarily to specific events such as superior oblique (SO) palsy. When myectomies were performed to weaken the IOs, some overacting IOs were very bulky but others were of apparently normal size. A previous study using magnetic resonance imaging (MRI) demonstrated that IO belly diameter increased on upward gaze nearly equally between patients with and without inferior oblique overaction (IOOA) [1]. Bagheri et al. [2] reported that there was no detectable correlation between IOOA and muscle position or circumference. However, little is known about the molecular and microscopic differences between overacting and normal IOs.

Extraocular muscles have different metabolic and structural components compared with other skeletal muscles, both molecularly and microscopically [3]. However, both extraocular muscles and other skeletal muscles generate free radicals with repetitive contraction, which can result in cellular oxidative damage in severe or prolonged state [4–6]. Myocytes generally contain a network of antioxidant defense mechanisms to reduce the risk of oxidative damage against increased reactive oxygen species [3]. Prolonged oxidative stress can result in reduced antioxidant capacity in extraocular muscles, and a previous report revealed that the medial rectus muscles (MRM) of patients with exotropia had a redox imbalance status compared with normal MRMs [6].

* Correspondence: eyeshin@catholic.ac.kr
[2]Department of Ophthalmology & Visual Science, College of Medicine, Seoul St. Mary's Hospital, The Catholic University of Korea, Banpo-daero 222, Seocho-gu, Seoul 06591, Republic of Korea
Full list of author information is available at the end of the article

No previously reported study has compared extraocular muscles under continuously contracting conditions, as seen in IOOA due to SO palsy and normal extraocular muscles. Thus, this study was undertaken to investigate and identify any difference between pathologically overacting and normal IOs at the protein level using MyoD, IGFBP5, thioredoxin, and p27 as example proteins. The brief introductions of each protein are summarized as follows.

MyoD, which is located in a specialized niche between the myofiber sarcolemma and the the basal lamina, is an essential protein for satellite cell differentiation. Satellite cells represent 2–10% of total myonuclei [7, 8]. They are known to be. Satellite cells become activated and express the myogenic regulatory factors Myf5 and/or MyoD following injury or growth stimulus, proliferate and generate the myogenic progenitors which are needed for muscle regeneration [9–11] or become new muscle fibers. Thus, we can identify in which group the satellite cell is activated by measuring and comparing MyoD levels.

IGF is known to induce hypertrophy in cultured neonatal rat cardiomyocytes through a specific receptor [12]. IGFBP binds to IGF and regulates its half-life. Thus, IGFBP5 detected in extraocular muscles can help us to determine whether IGF has any influence on overacting or normal IOs.

Thioredoxin decreases, as an antioxidant, in an oxidative stress state [13, 14]. If IOOA is caused by oxidative stress, thioredoxin would be expected to decrease significantly in the IOOA group versus the control group.

P27 maintains or arrests the quiescent phase in the cell cycle, and decreases before cell division in stem cells like the satellite cells [15]. Recently, p27 was shown to play a role in an oxidative stress state [16, 17]. If IOOA is caused by hyperplasia or oxidative stress, a difference in p27 levels between the groups, in conjunction with a difference in MyoD or thioredoxin level, would be expected.

Methods

The IOOA group consisted of 20 IOs obtained from patients with secondary IOOA $\geq$ +3 from SO palsy. A portion of the IO (8.0 mm from the insertion) was resected during IO myectomy surgery. Approval to conduct this study was obtained from the Institutional Review Board of the Catholic Medical Center (#KC09TISI0365). Ethics, consent, permissions and approval were obtained with written documents by all participants prior to surgery. Approval to conduct and securing human tissue of this study was obtained from the institutional review board of the hospital and the study protocol adhered to the tenets of the Declaration of Helsinki. 20 normal IOs as the control

group were obtained from age-matched donor eyes of individuals within 12 h after the brain death. Ethics, consent, permissions and approval were obtained with written documents by their guardians based on each donor's intension of eyeball donation before brain death. Any subject who had history of eyelid or extraocular muscle surgery or disease, orbital diseases, and eyeball or periorbital trauma by their medical records was excluded.

All IOs were transferred to a portable tank filled with liquid nitrogen and immediately delivered from the operation room to the laboratory. Before preservation at −80 °C, portions of secured IOs were separated and proteins for analysis were extracted within 1 h from securing IOs.

We selected four proteins for investigation; MyoD, insulin-like growth factor (IGF) binding protein 5 (IGFBP5), thioredoxin, and p27.

For immunohistochemistry, we first prepared formalin-fixed, paraffin-embedded tissue sections. Then the sections were deparaffinized with xylene and transferred to 100, 95, 70, and 50% alcohols in sequence, twice each for 3 min. For blocking of non-specific binding activity, each slide was incubated in 1% bovine serum albumin at room temperature for 10 min. After removing the blocking buffer, 100 μL of appropriately diluted primary antibodies (MyoD, IGFBP5 and p27; Santa Cruz Biotechnology, Santa Cruz, CA, USA, thioredoxin; Abcam, Cambridge, London, UK) were applied to the sections on the slides and the slides were incubated in a humidified chamber at 4 °C for overnight. After washing with PBS for 30 min, secondary antibody (rhodamine-conjugated, Santa Cruz Biotechnology, Santa Cruz, CA, USA) was applied for 1 h. After washing, the sections were stained with Hoechest 33,258 (Sigma-Aldrich, St. Louis, MO, USA). Then, a cover slip was mounted on the slide glass using mounting solution. The stained tissues were observed by fluorescence microscopy (Axio imager 2, Carl Zeiss GmBH, Zena, Germany).

Western blotting was performed to compare levels of the protein, MyoD, IGFBP, thioredoxin, and p27 protein levels between the two groups. Total protein was isolated from the IOs using RIPA buffer (25 mM Tris-HCl, pH 7.4, 1% Tween 20, 0.1% SDS, 0.5% sodium deoxycholate, 10% glycerol, 150 mM NaCl, 5 mM EDTA, 1 mM PMSF, 50 mM NaF, 1 mM Na_3VO_4, and 1 μg/mL of aprotinin, leupeptin, and pepstatin) and protein concentration was determined using a BCA protein assay kit (Pierce, Rockford, IL, USA). After separating 20 μg of protein using 10% sodium dodecyl sulfate polyacrylamide gel electrophoresis, it was transferred onto polyvinylidene difluoride membranes (Amersham Life Science, Cleveland, OH, USA) with approximately 5% skim milk in

Table 1 Demographic data of the IOOA and control group

	IOOA	Control	P value*
Number of patients (number of eyes)	20 (20)	10 (20)	
Age, years (SD)	52.35 (11.43)	55.25 (9.68)	0.438
Gender (M:F)	13:7	6:4	0.282
Deviation, prism diopters (SD)	26.2 (11.8)		

*Mann-Whitney test

PBS-0.1% Tween 20 for blocking. Then, the primary antibodies (MyoD, IGFBP5 and p27; Santa Cruz Biotechnology, Santa Cruz, CA, USA, and thioredoxin; Abcam, Cambridge, London, UK) were reacted overnight in a 4 °C cold room, and the membrane was washed and reacted with horseradish peroxidase-conjugated goat anti-rabbit antibody (1:1000; Santa Cruz Biotechnology, Santa Cruz, CA, USA) and was developed with an enhanced chemiluminescence solution (Santa Cruz Biotechnology). Finally, bands on the X-ray film were quantitated by densitometry with β-actin as the protein loading control.

Using densitometry (Image Master VDS 2.0; Pharmacia Biotech Inc., San Francisco, CA, USA), we obtained the optical density of each protein band and divided them by the optical density of actin to obtain the relative optical density of each protein. The relative optical density of each protein was then compared between the IOOA and control groups.

Statistical analyses were performed using SPSS statistical software for Windows (SPSS, version 20.0, Chicago, IL, USA). Student's t-test and the Mann-Whitney U test were used to evaluate differences between groups. A P value < 0.05 was considered to indicate statistical significance.

Results

Twenty overacting IOs from 20 patients with SO palsy were obtained as the IOOA group (13 males, 7 females; mean age = 55.25 years). 20 IOs were obtained as the control group (6 males, 4 females; mean age = 55.25 years). There was no significant difference in gender or age between the two groups (Table 1).

In immunohistochemistry, few fluorescent dots representing MyoD and IGFBP5 were detected little in either groups (Fig. 1). However, many fluorescent dots for thioredoxin and p27 were detected in the control group but few dots were found out in the IOOA group (Fig. 2).

On Western blotting and densitometry analysis, the levels of MyoD and IGFBP5 did not show a statistically significant difference ($P > 0.05$). However, the levels of thioredoxin and p27 were significantly higher in the control group than in the IOOA group in optical density ($P < 0.001$, respectively; Fig. 3).

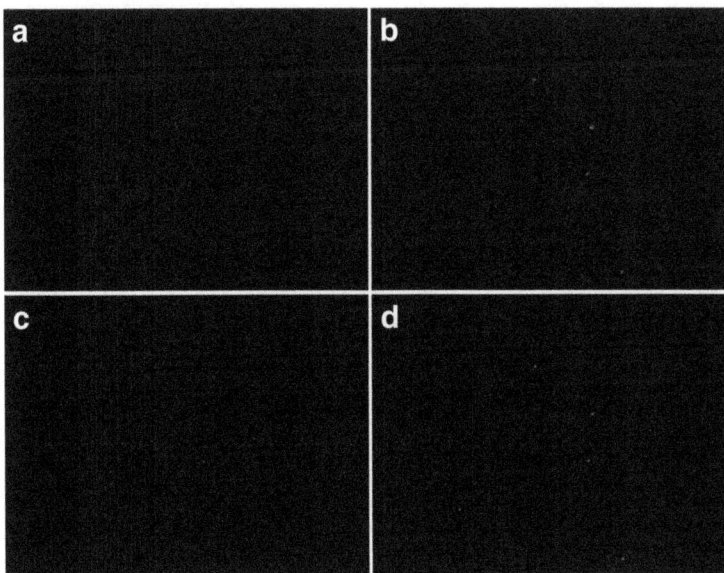

Fig. 1 Immunohistochemistry results. MyoD (**a**) inferior oblique overaction (IOOA) group, (**b**) control group, insulin-like growth factor binding protein 5 (IGFBP5) (**c**) IOOA group, (**d**) control group

Clinical Ophthalmology: A Practical Approach

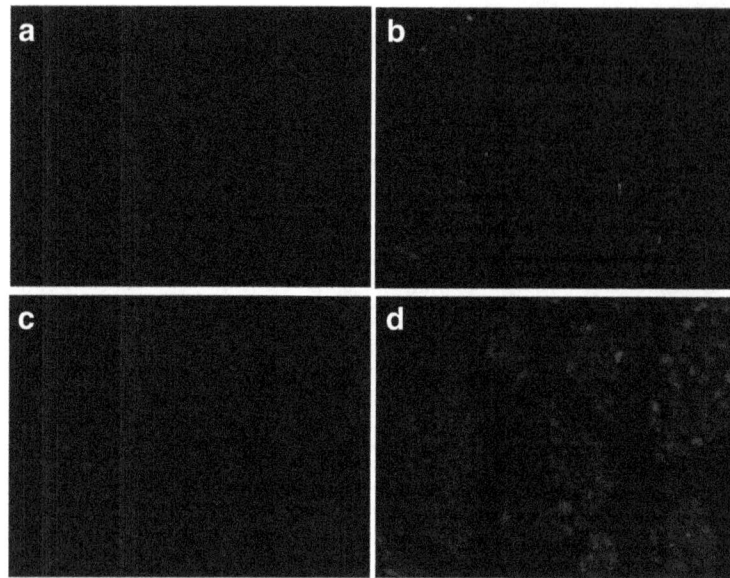

Fig. 2 Immunohistochemistry results. Thioredoxin (**a**) IOOA group, (**b**) control group, p27 (**c**) IOOA group, (**d**) control group

Discussion

Oxidative stress was defined as "a disruption of redox signaling and control" by Jones [18]. There are several methods for measuring oxidative stress in muscles and thioredoxin is a known antioxidant and an oxidative stress biomarker [14, 19]. To our knowledge, there is no previous report about thioredoxin levels in extraocular muscles. In the present study, thioredoxin was detected in the control group and was decreased significantly in the IOOA group. This indicates that thioredoxin is an antioxidant in

extraocular muscles and there was a decrease in anti-oxidative capacity in the IOOA group.

A recent study showed another role for thioredoxin, in that its downregulation resulted in the induction of apoptosis [20] and its overexpression inhibited tumor necrosis factor-alpha (TNF-α) induced apoptosis, [21] indicating an anti-apoptotic role for thioredoxin. However, in our study, the actin levels between the IOOA and the control groups did not show a significant difference, indicating that there was no significant muscle

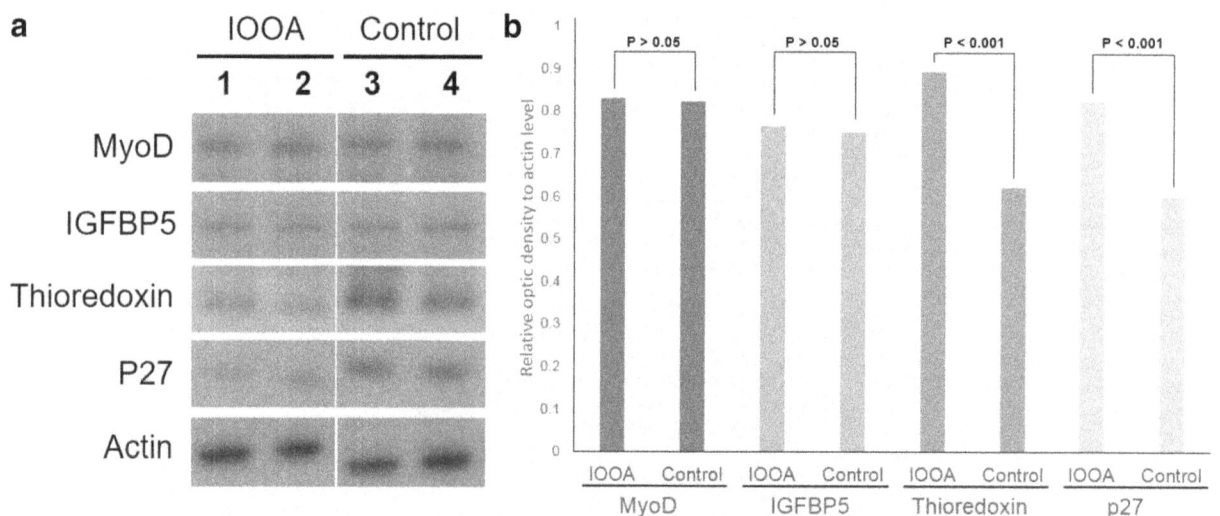

Fig. 3 Western blot analyses of MyoD, IGFBP5, thioredoxin and p27. **a** Samples in the IOOA group are in lanes 1 to 2, and those in the control group are in lanes 3 to 4. **b** Levels of each protein in the IOOA group, compared with those in the control group. MyoD and IGFBP5 showed no statistical difference between the groups. However, thioredoxin and p27 were decreased significantly in the IOOA group versus the control group

fiber loss in the IOOA group. Thus, we consider the decreased level of thioredoxin in the IOOA group to be the result of the oxidative stress.

The decrease in p27 in the IOOA group, in conjunction with the decrease in thioredoxin, may also be evidence of oxidative stress. Sherr and Roberts [16] reported that downregulation of p27 in a particular condition suggested the presence of other mechanisms in regulating p27 levels, distinguishing it from cellular apoptosis. Lesley et al. [17] revealed that hydrogen peroxide and the antioxidant delphinidin seemed to regulate intracellular levels of p27 through regulating HIF-1 levels, which were, in turn, governed by its upstream regulators, involving the PI3K/Akt/mTOR signaling pathway. These findings support the hypothesis that oxidative stress and antioxidant regulate p27 by affecting PI3K-Akt signaling pathway.

Satellite cell activation, and the effects of intrinsic IGF on the IOs, were investigated through the levels of MyoD and IGFBP5 in the groups. However, they may have no or little effect in both the overacting and normal IOs although further study are needed to confirm this.

This study had some limitations. First, the IOs obtained from the IOOA group represented only a portion of the total IO length. Thus, the antioxidant capacity in the present study may not have represented the total capacity of IOs. To overcome this limitation, we included a similar length of the IOs from donor eyes. Second, the effects of satellite cell and IGF on the secondarily overacting IOs in the initial period remain unclear. IOs in the IOOA group were collected after prolonged overaction, caused by SO underaction, for at least several years. Third, the four proteins assessed in the present study do not represent the overall state of IOs.

Conclusions

Secondarily overacting IOs in SO palsy are apparently in an oxidative stress state. In addition to our previous study that the MRMs of patients with exotropia had a redox imbalance status compared with normal MRMs, [6] extraocular muscles demanding continuous contraction may have pathological increased risk of oxidative stress compared with normal extraocular muscles.

Abbreviations
IGF: Insulin-like growth factor; IGFBP5: Insulin-like growth factor binding protein 5; IO: Inferior oblique; IOOA: Inferior oblique overaction; MRM: Medial rectus muscle; SO: Superior oblique

Acknowledgements
The English in this document has been checked by at least two professional editors, both native speakers of English. For a certificate, please see: http://www.textcheck.com/certificate/gxY3CF

Authors' contributions
YWC: Analysis and interpretation of data, draft and modification of manuscript. JSC: Experiment and data collection. SYS: Conception and design (selection of patients and proteins to be analyzed), Surgery and obtaining parts of inferior oblique muscles, final approval of manuscript. All authors read and approved the final manuscript.

Competing interests
The authors declare that they have no competing interests.

Author details
[1]Department of Ophthalmology, College of Medicine, St. Vincent's Hospital, The Catholic University of Korea, Suwon, Republic of Korea. [2]Department of Ophthalmology & Visual Science, College of Medicine, Seoul St. Mary's Hospital, The Catholic University of Korea, Banpo-daero 222, Seocho-gu, Seoul 06591, Republic of Korea.

References
1. Kono R, Demer JL. Magnetic resonance imaging of the functional anatomy of the inferior oblique muscle in superior oblique palsy. Ophthalmology. 2003;110(6):1219–29.
2. Bagheri A, Eshaghi M, Yazdani S. Relationship of inferior oblique overaction to muscle bulk and position. J AAPOS. 2009;13(3):241–4.
3. Fischer MD, Gorospe JR, Felder E, Bogdanovich S, Pedrosa-Domellof F, Ahima RS, Rubinstein NA, Hoffman EP, Khurana TS. Expression profiling reveals metabolic and structural components of extraocular muscles. Physiol Genomics. 2002;9(2):71–84.
4. Lawler JM, Cline CC, Hu Z, Coast JR. Effect of oxidative stress and acidosis on diaphragm contractile function. Am J Phys. 1997;273(2 Pt 2):R630–6.
5. Moylan JS, Reid MB. Oxidative stress, chronic disease, and muscle wasting. Muscle Nerve. 2007;35(4):411–29.
6. Jung SK, Choi JS, Shin SY. Change in the antioxidative capacity of extraocular muscles in patients with exotropia. Graefes Arch Clin Exp Ophthalmol. 2015;253(4):551–6.
7. Hawke TJ, Garry DJ. Myogenic satellite cells: physiology to molecular biology. J Appl Physiol. 2001;91(2):534–51.
8. White RB, Bierinx AS, Gnocchi VF, Zammit PS. Dynamics of muscle fibre growth during postnatal mouse development. BMC Dev Biol. 2010;10:21.
9. Stuelsatz P, Shearer A, Li Y, Muir LA, Ieronimakis N, Shen QW, Kirillova I, Yablonka-Reuveni Z. Extraocular muscle satellite cells are high performance myo-engines retaining efficient regenerative capacity in dystrophin deficiency. Dev Biol. 2015;397(1):31–44.
10. Dumont NA, Wang YX, Rudnicki MA. Intrinsic and extrinsic mechanisms regulating satellite cell function. Development. 2015;142(9):1572–81.
11. Tiidus PM, Bombardier E, Xeni J, Bestic NM, Vandenboom R, Rudnicki MA, Houston ME. Elevated catalase activity in red and white muscles of MyoD gene-inactivated mice. Biochem Mol Biol Int. 1996;39(5):1029–35.
12. Ito H, Hiroe M, Hirata Y, Tsujino M, Adachi S, Shichiri M, Koike A, Nogami A, Marumo F. Insulin-like growth factor-I induces hypertrophy with enhanced expression of muscle specific genes in cultured rat cardiomyocytes. Circulation. 1993;87(5):1715–21.
13. Barbieri E, Sestili P. Reactive oxygen species in skeletal muscle signaling. J Signal Transduc. 2012;2012:982794.
14. Whayne TF Jr, Parinandi N, Maulik N. Thioredoxins in cardiovascular disease. Can J Physiol Pharmacol. 2015;93(11):903–11.
15. Messina G, Blasi C, La Rocca SA, Pompili M, Calconi A, Grossi M. p27Kip1 acts downstream of N-cadherin-mediated cell adhesion to promote myogenesis beyond cell cycle regulation. Mol Biol Cell. 2005;16(3):1469–80.
16. Sherr CJ, Roberts JM. CDK inhibitors: positive and negative regulators of G1-phase progression. Genes Dev. 1999;13(12):1501–12.
17. Quintos L, Lee IA, Kim HJ, Lim JS, Park J, Sung MK, Seo YR, Kim JS. Significance of p27 as potential biomarker for intracellular oxidative status. Nutrit Res Practice. 2010;4(5):351–5.
18. Jones DP. Redefining oxidative stress. Antioxid Redox Signal. 2006;8(9–10):1865–79.

A quantitative analysis method for comitant exotropia using video-oculography with alternate cover

Nohae Park[1], Byunggun Park[1], Minkyung Oh[2], Sunghyuk Moon[1][*] ⓘ and Myungmi Kim[3]

Abstract

Background: The purpose of this study was to evaluate the efficacy of a quantitative analysis method for comitant exotropia using video-oculography (VOG) with alternate cover.

Methods: Thirty-four subjects with comitant exotropia were included. Two independent ophthalmologists measured the angle of ocular deviation using the alternate prism cover test (APCT). The video files and data of changes in ocular deviation during the alternate cover test were obtained using VOG. To verify the accuracy of VOG, the value obtained using VOG and the angle of a rotating model eye were compared, and a new linear equation was subsequently derived using these data. The calculated values obtained using VOG were compared with those obtained using the APCT.

Results: Rotation of the model eye and the values obtained using VOG demonstrated excellent positive correlation ($R = 1.000$; $p < 0.001$). A simple linear regression model was obtained: rotation of the model eye = $0.978 \times$ value obtained using VOG for a model eye − 0.549. The 95% limit of agreement for inter-observer variability was ±4.63 prism diopters (PD) for APCT and that for test-retest variability was ±3.56 PD for the VOG test. The results of APCT and calculated VOG test demonstrated a strong positive correlation. Bland-Altman plots revealed no overall tendency for the calculated values obtained from VOG to differ from those obtained using APCT.

Conclusions: VOG with alternate cover is a non-invasive and accurate tool for quantitatively measuring and recording ocular deviation. In particular, it is independent of the proficiency of the examiner and, can therefore, be useful in the absence of skilled personnel.

Keywords: Strabismus, Video-oculography, Ocular deviation, Alternate cover

Background

Accurate measurements are important for planning strabismus surgery. Methods available for measuring the angle of ocular deviation include the alternate prism cover test (APCT), Hirschberg test, and Krimsky test. In APCT, the subject gazes at the target with both eyes, a prism is placed in front of the uncovered eye, and an alternate cover test is performed. The angle is measured by increasing or decreasing the strength of the prism used until there is no deviation or the deviation is reversed. However, the prism must be changed several times, especially when there is an accompanying vertical strabismus. Consequently, the duration of the examination will be long in such cases and, as such, it is difficult to perform in a child who does not cooperate or gaze in accordance with instructions. In such situations, the Hirschberg and Krimsky tests are used to determine the angle of deviation. The Hirschberg test measures the distance between the corneal light reflex and the center of the pupil, and then converts it into an angle. Although it is a relatively simple method, it may not accurately measure the exact ocular deviation. The Krimsky

* Correspondence: koils79@naver.com
[1]Department of Ophthalmology, Busan Paik Hospital, Inje University College of Medicine, 75 Bokji-ro, Busanjin-gu, Busan 47392, Republic of Korea
Full list of author information is available at the end of the article

test measures the angle of ocular deviation using a prism and the corneal light reflex. For this reason, APCT measures the entire deviation, including tropic and phoric components, whereas the Krimsky tests only measure the tropic component. Both the Hirschberg and Krimsky tests require correction of angle kappa, which is largely subjective and, therefore, can lead to inter-observer errors. When the goal of surgery is to achieve orthotropia, APCT should be used whenever possible [1]. In addition, such tests may have limitations in recording eye movements themselves.

On the other hand, a scleral search coil can be used to objectively record and measure ocular deviation. This is an accurate method because it has a spatiotemporal resolution $< 1°$ and < 1 ms. However, it is difficult to wear a scleral search coil for more than 30 min because it is worn on the limbus of the cornea. Therefore, photography and video-oculography (VOG) have been proposed as methods to measure eye movements noninvasively and objectively [2–6]. VOG has demonstrated a measurement error $< 1°$ for an eye movement range $< 40°$, and a high correlation ($R^2 = 0.99$) with the scleral search coil method for both horizontal and vertical eye movements below $15°$ [6, 7]. In particular, several studies have reported measuring ocular deviation in intermittent exotropia using VOG [8–10]. To our knowledge, there has been no attempt to quantitatively measure ocular deviation using VOG with dissociation of both eyes. We believe it is important to measure ocular deviation with dissociation of both eyes, similar to APCT, for surgery. Therefore, we attempted a method of using VOG with alternate cover for non-invasive and reliable measurement of the angle of ocular deviation. Additionally, we evaluated VOG as an alternative method to standard tests to determine whether it can obviate these limitations.

Methods
This prospective study was performed at the Department of Ophthalmology, Inje University Busan Paik Hospital. All aspects of the research protocol complied with the tenets of the Declarations of Helsinki and were approved by the Institutional Review Board of Inje University Busan Paik Hospital (Busan, Korea). Written informed consent was obtained from all parents or legal guardians; children and adolescent assent forms were also provided for children 7 years of age and older.

Calibration of VOG using a model eye
A model eye with a pupil diameter of 5.5 mm and globe diameter of 26 mm was used to verify the accuracy of VOG. A protractor was attached to the center of the eyeball to verify the amount of rotation of the eyeball. Each of the two experiments was repeated four times,

and a total of eight experiments were performed. The eyeball was rotated from $0°$ to $30°$ at intervals of $2°$. The video taken of the model eye stopped for > 5 s every $2°$. The degree of rotation of the eyeball and the values obtained using VOG were compared. Based on the results of the analysis, a linear regression equation for the degree of eyeball rotation was derived. In the reliability analysis of eight repeated VOG tests for a model eye, the intra-class correlation coefficient was 1.000 (95% confidence interval [CI] 1.000 to 1.000; $p < 0.001$). The intra-class correlation coefficient between the first measurement of two independent examiners was 1.000 (95% CI 0.999 to 1.000; $p < 0.001$). The VOG demonstrated excellent agreement among all eight repeated examinations. The linear regression equation was derived from the mean value of the eight VOGs and the rotated angle of the model eye using linear regression analysis (Fig. 1).

$$\text{Rotation angle of the model eye (degrees)} = 0.978 \times \text{angle obtained using VOG (degrees)} - 0.549$$

$$\text{Calculated VOG value (prism diopters)} = \tan(\text{rotation angle of the model eye [degrees]}) \times 100$$

Participants
Thirty-four subjects with comitant exotropia who could be observed > 3 times, with a difference between distant and near deviation angle < 3 prism diopters (PD), were enrolled. All subjects underwent APCT to measure the angle of ocular deviation. On the same day, VOG (SLMED, Seoul, Korea) was performed and APCT was performed 30 min later. Subjects with incomitant strabismus, horizontal deviation > 50 PD in APCT, ocular comorbidity other than strabismus or with systemic disease, refractive errors > 6.00 diopters, those not willing to undergo VOG, children < 4 years of age, and subjects wearing spectacles during measurements were excluded.

Comparison of APCT and VOG
Two independent ophthalmologists performed APCT using a plastic prism set (Luneau SAS, Prunay LeGillon, France). The subjects were asked to fixate on a black-on-white optotype at 3 m, which subtended a visual angle of 50 min of arc (MOA), equating to a Snellen optotype of 20/200.

The VOG equipment used in the present study had a tilted semi-transparent glass through which the subject could gaze at the target with a red light with a visual angle of 50 MOA in the monitor situated at 1 m. The subject wearing the VOG goggles was instructed to look at the red light, between the two eyes, with head position kept straight so that during the examination the

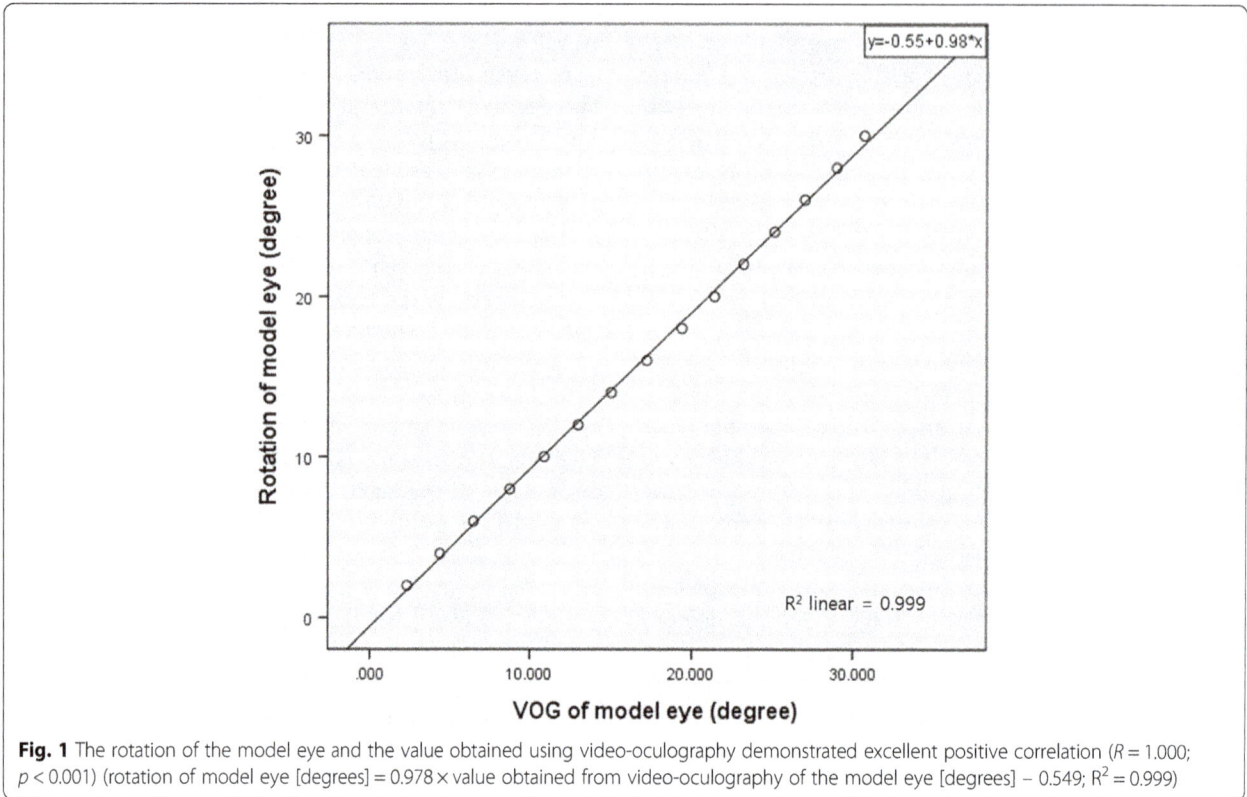

Fig. 1 The rotation of the model eye and the value obtained using video-oculography demonstrated excellent positive correlation ($R = 1.000$; $p < 0.001$) (rotation of model eye [degrees] = $0.978 \times$ value obtained from video-oculography of the model eye [degrees] $- 0.549$; $R^2 = 0.999$)

eyes were in primary position. During the first 10 s, initial binocular alignment was verified with both eyes open. Subsequently, each eye was allowed 5 s of covered time and 5 s of uncovered time, and the alternate cover test was repeated 5 times, with each eye being covered for 5 s. A 120 Hz camera was used for VOG, and the eyeball was observed to deviate during the alternate cover test; the magnitude of deviation was subsequently obtained (Fig. 2). The obtained values were expressed in degrees (°), and were substituted into the linear regression equation derived earlier using the model eye. The new angle values thus obtained were converted to PD to compare with the values obtained using APCT.

Main outcome measure

The inter-observer variability of APCT performed by two independent examiners and the inter-visit variability of four examinations by one examiner were measured.

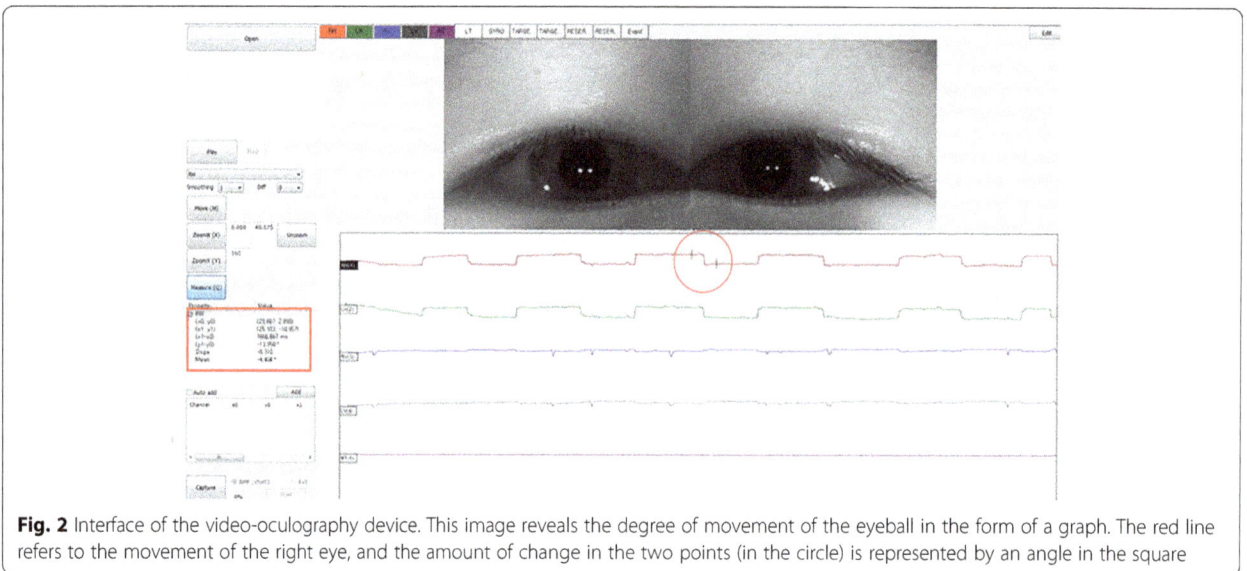

Fig. 2 Interface of the video-oculography device. This image reveals the degree of movement of the eyeball in the form of a graph. The red line refers to the movement of the right eye, and the amount of change in the two points (in the circle) is represented by an angle in the square

The VOG recorded the distance moved by the eye during re-fixation after its deviation in the alternate cover; three repeated test values were obtained and a reliability analysis was performed. The first value among the results obtained using VOG was used in the linear regression equation and subsequently compared with the value obtained using APCT.

Statistical analysis

SPSS version 18.0 (SPSS, Inc., Chicago, Illinois, USA) was used for statistical analysis. The Pearson correlation coefficient was used to determine the linear relationship between VOG and the model eye, and the linear regression equation was derived using linear regression analysis. The reliabilities of APCT and VOG were evaluated using intra-class correlation coefficient, and consistent variability between APCT and VOG was represented using a Bland-Altman plot. Correlation between the two tests was calculated using the Pearson correlation coefficient.

Results

Participants

Thirty-four subjects with comitant exotropia, of whom 22 (64.7%) were female, were included in the present study. The mean age was 13.7 ± 11.2 years (range, 5–51 years). Thirty-one of 34 subjects had uncorrected visual acuity better than 20/30 in both eyes; uncorrected visual acuity in either eye of the other three subjects was not worse than 20/70. APCT and VOG were performed in all subjects (Table 1).

Comparison of APCT and VOG

The inter-observer variability for APCT was determined using the results from two independent examiners. The Bland-Altman plot demonstrated consistent variability, except for one subject with deviation > 40 PD. The half-width of the 95% limit of agreement was ±4.63 PD (Fig. 3 [top left]). On reliability analysis, the inter-observer correlation coefficient was 0.974 (95% CI 0.947 to 0.987; $p < 0.001$).

The inter-visit reliability of the APCT was determined for 24 of 34 subjects who had been examined by one examiner > 4 times in three months; the inter-visit correlation coefficient was 0.968 (95% CI 0.941 to 0.985; $p < 0.001$). The Bland-Altman plot between the first and second APCT demonstrated consistent variability, except for two

subjects, the half-width of the 95% limit of agreement being ±5.74 PD (Fig. 3 [top right]).

Thirty-four subjects were included in the VOG test. Reliability analysis of the three VOG readings demonstrated high agreement (0.990 [95% CI 0.983 to 0.995]; $p < 0.001$), and the half-width of the 95% limit of agreement on Bland-Altman plot was ±3.56 PD (Fig. 3 [bottom]).

Of the 34 subjects, 28 (82.4%) exhibited a difference in ocular deviation of < 3 PD between VOG and APCT, and 32 (94.1%) demonstrated a difference of < 5 PD (Table 2).

The Bland-Altman plot of VOG and APCT demonstrated consistent variability, except for two subjects, the half-width of the 95% limit of agreement being ±5.05 PD (Fig. 4). Furthermore, there was also a strong positive linear relationship between the two tests ($R = 0.934$; $p < 0.001$) (Fig. 5).

Discussion

The purpose of our study was to measure the objective angle of ocular deviation using VOG with alternate cover in subjects with exotropia. The principle of the VOG device used in our study was that light was transmitted through the tilted semi-transparent glass and the subject could look at the target. As the light was being reflected, the two cameras could record the movement of the eyes without blocking the visual axes. The pupil was detected in real time, and the deviation of the eyeball was assessed by measuring the change in the reference point of the center of the pupil.

Although APCT may represent a typical test for measuring angles of deviation, the results can differ because of differences in measurements using prisms made by individual examiners. Therefore, error involved in the measurements are dependent on the skill of the examiner and the cooperation of the subject [11–13]. In particular, the Pediatric Eye Disease Investigator group [11] suggested that two skilled observers may have an error ≥ 12 PD in the measurement of esotropia exceeding 20 PD, and an error ≥ 6 PD in the measurement of 10 to 20 PD esotropia. The angle of ocular deviation measured by one observer demonstrated that the 95% limit of agreement on a measurement was ±7.3 PD for esotropia exceeding 20 PD, and ± 4.1 PD for 10–20 PD esotropia at distance. In addition, APCT could not record eye

Table 1 Mean angle of exotropia measured using alternate prism cover test and video-oculography

Value	Alternate prism cover test ($n = 34$)		Video-oculography ($n = 34$)	
	Examiner 1	Examiner 2	Average value of three test-retests	Calculated value from linear equation
Degrees	14.32 ± 3.66 (6.84–23.27)	13.84 ± 4.14 (5.71–24.23)	15.47 ± 3.91 (8.50–26.58)	14.58 ± 3.83 (7.77–25.44)
Prism diopters	25.65 ± 6.88 (12–43)	24.79 ± 7.81 (10–45)	27.81 ± 7.52 (14.95–50.02)	26.13 ± 7.28 (13.64–47.57)

Data presented as mean ± SD (range)

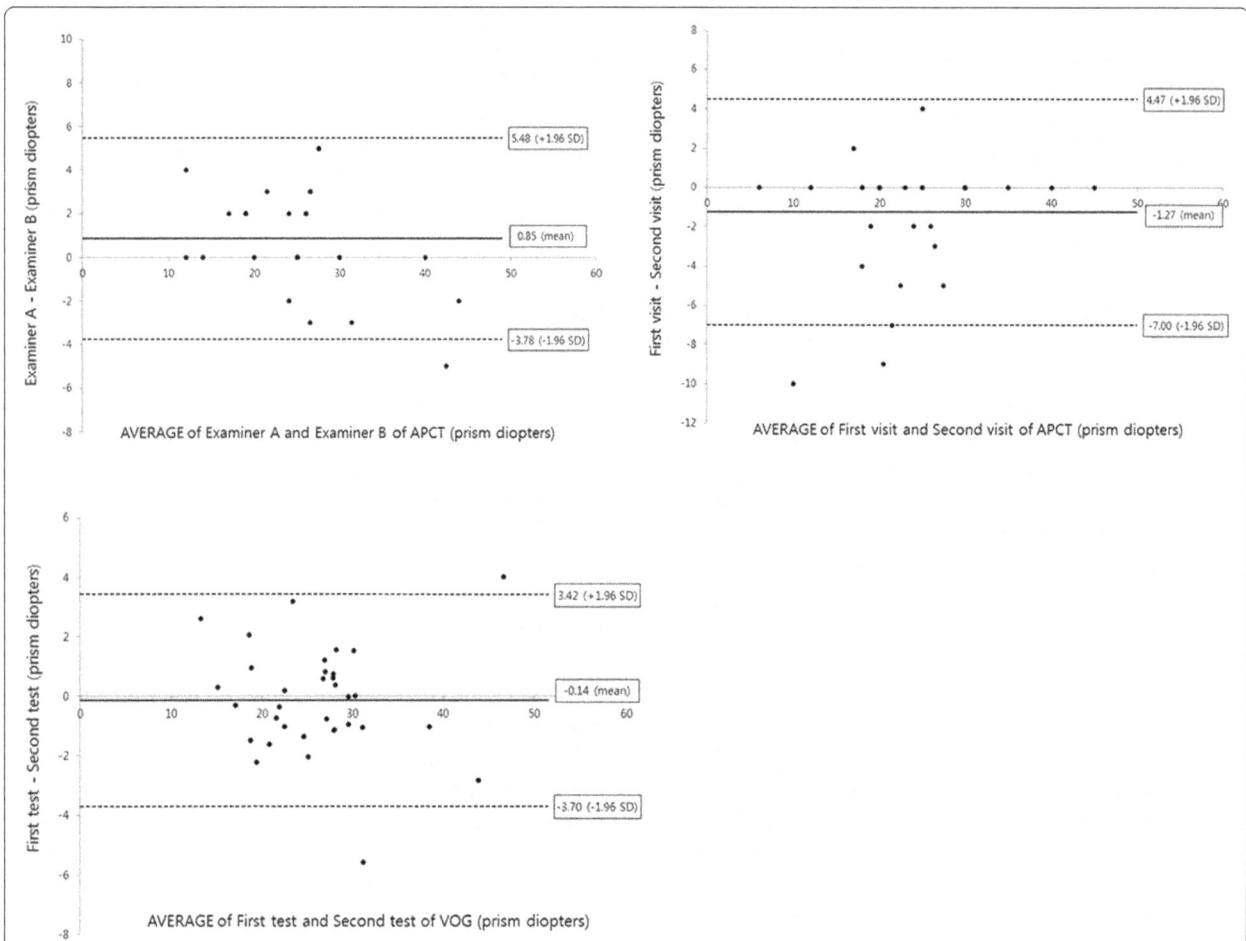

Fig. 3 Bland-Altman plots revealing interobserver variability and inter-visit variability for the alternate prism cover test (APCT) and test-retest variability for video-oculography with alternate cover. Upper and lower dotted lines represent the 95% limits of agreement. The half-width of the 95% limit of agreement measured of the interobserver variability (top left), inter-visit variability (top right) for APCT and test-retest variability (bottom) for video-oculography were 4.63 prism diopters (PD), 5.74 PD and 3.56 PD, respectively

movement itself; therefore, it depends on the record of the examiner. For this reason, methods using photography were used for measurements that are more objective. Among them, Yang et al. [2] took pictures at a distance of 1 m, and the corneal light reflex points and limbus locations were extracted from two-dimensional photographs and analyzed using a three-dimensional strabismus photo analyzer (R & DB Foundation, Seoul, Republic of Korea). The results demonstrated high correlation with the Krimsky test. This is useful to examine

Table 2 Differences between alternate prism cover test and video-oculography

Prism diopters	Subjects, n (%)
< 3	28 (82.4)
3–5	4 (11.7)
> 5	2 (5.9)
Total	34 (100)

cases of manifest strabismus. However, because this test did not dissociate the two eyes, the angle of ocular deviation would be variable according fusion of both eyes in intermittent exotropia, or changeable depending on dominant eye in incomitant strabismus. Therefore, there are restrictions to its use in intermittent exotropia and incomitant strabismus. Additionally, there are limitations in measuring the angle of ocular deviation for retinopathy of prematurity with macular dragging because the angle kappa cannot be considered. In another improvement study, the use of an infrared ray filter and an infrared camera with this method was proposed to observe the deviation angle in patients with latent strabismus [3].

An alternative for objectively measuring eye movements is to use a VOG device equipped with a camera at a sample rate of 200 to 250 Hz. In previous studies, it was reported to have high correlation with the scleral search coil in the fixation position [6, 7]. The VOG device used in our study had a frequency of 150 Hz; hence,

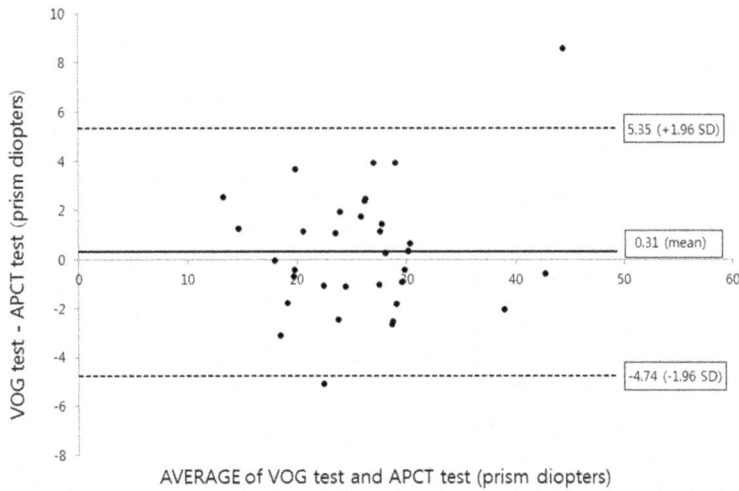

Fig. 4 Bland-Altman plot comparing the values obtained using the alternate prism cover test (APCT) and video-oculography (VOG) test. The Bland-Altman plot demonstrated consistent variability. The half-width of the 95% limit of agreement was ±5.05 prism diopters. There was no overall tendency for the values obtained using VOG to differ from those obtained using APCT

it was less accurate than the scleral search coil used to assess rapid eye movements. However, because our study was intended to measure the distance moved during an eyeball deviation, the results were not greatly influenced by camera frequency. In our study, we needed a device verification step to accurately measure the amount of eyeball rotation. The results obtained using VOG and the amount of eyeball rotation showed statistically high correlation (linear correlation coefficient = 1.000; $p < 0.001$), and a linear regression equation of the eyeball rotation angle with the angle obtained using VOG was derived. Using this equation, the degree of ocular change

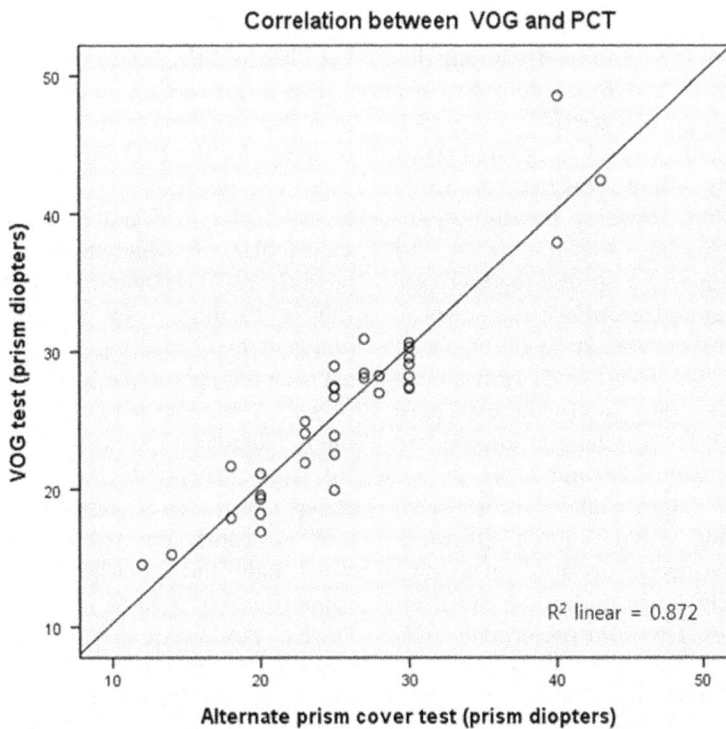

Fig. 5 Scatter plot and Pearson correlation between values calculated using video-oculography (VOG) and the values obtained using the alternate prism cover test (APCT). The values calculated from VOG demonstrated a strong correlation with the values obtained using APCT ($R = 0.934$; $p < 0.001$)

in the subject group measured using VOG was converted to actual eyeball rotation angle values. These converted values were compared with the angles of ocular deviation obtained using APCT. The Bland-Altman plot between the APCT values and the calculated VOG values showed consistent variability, except for two subjects. As for the outliers, one subject exhibited ocular deviation values of 20, 20, and 25 PD from the three APCTs, and 19.92 PD from VOG testing. In our study setting, ocular deviation was analyzed based on the last visit, and was judged to be located outside the 95% limits of agreement. The other subject had exotropia with inferior oblique overaction in both eyes. It was V-pattern exotropia with 55 PD in the upward gaze, 40 PD in the primary position, and 35 PD in the downward gaze. We presume that the upward gaze may have been the cause of the positive difference despite maintenance of head position.

The advantage of using VOG is that all eye movements can be recorded as video recordings, and the eye tracking system can record both eye movements and the angle of ocular deviation. Another advantage is the dissociation of the two eyes using alternate covering, and measurement of the distance moved by the eye by recording a video. Hence, VOG is not influenced by the angle kappa. Several studies reporting the objective measurement of strabismus were influenced by the angle kappa because their assessments were based on corneal light reflex points. In addition, the measurement of the manifest strabismus alone was performed without dissociating the two eyes [2, 5, 14–16]. In contrast, in a study measuring the angle of ocular deviation by dissociating the two eyes, Yang et al. [3] used an infrared transmission filter for dissociation and measured the ocular deviation using photographs. However, because photographs—unlike video recordings—do not reflect the continuity of time, it is different from the method used in our study in that it does not record eye movement in real time. Therefore, if we analyze the angle of ocular deviation by the method used in our study with the aid of VOG, we can analyze deviation patterns in dissociated strabismus cases and use it for screening in intermittent exotropia with good convergence. Second, it is also useful for measuring the maximum angle of ocular deviation, which is significant in intermittent exotropia. Third, it can measure the ocular deviation in a short time. It took approximately 2 min during the VOG test (1 min for wearing goggles, 1 min for performing VOG with alternate cover). Finally, because VOG can quantitatively record and compare eye movements in both eyes separately, it is possible to accurately analyze the difference between secondary and primary deviations in incomitant strabismus. This may be useful for follow-up observations. The purpose of our study was to evaluate

the accuracy of VOG and to include the inter-visit variability of a single examiner in the process of comparing and analyzing the degree of variability of APCT measurements. However, paralysis, a type of incomitant strabismus, was excluded from our study because there can be changes in ocular deviation during recovery. In the future, we will perform a comparative analysis of both eyes in cases of incomitant strabismus such as paralysis.

The first limitation of our study was that children < 4 years of age were excluded from the evaluation of the accuracy of VOG. We suspect that younger children have a lower attention span and ability to fixate well. Moreover, subjects with claustrophobia could not be assessed because the video goggles had to be worn at the time of the test. Second, subjects did not wear glasses, even if there was a refractive error, although the author found that the VOG goggle supported the use of glasses and video camera could detect the center of the pupil beyond the glasses, the results were affected by the prism effect of glasses. The aim of our study was to evaluate a method using VOG with alternate cover to measure ocular deviation in lieu of standard tests. Therefore, it was important to demonstrate the accuracy of VOG. Subjects did not wear glasses to eliminate variables caused by the prism effect. Third, the target was a red light (50 MOA) for the VOG test and a black-on-white optotype (50 MOA) for the APCT. For measuring the angle of ocular deviation, we did not use a light source as the target; instead, the visual acuity chart was used because the accommodation levels are different. If a light is used as the target, the accommodation is less than that with the acuity chart; hence, the deviation will be lesser for esotropia and vice versa for exotropia [4]. The VOG goggle is constructed from semi-transparent glass, which can degrade contrast of letter targets. The same a black-on-white optotype in VOG and APCT may be different. Surmising that red light would better attract subject attention, it was used instead of a black-on-white optotype for evaluating VOG. However, no difference between red light and a black-on-white optotype was observed. A possible reason is that subjects may perceive the red light as a red dot with higher resolution through the semi-transparent glass. In addition, a recent study using a prism cover test for far distance in intermittent exotropia reported no significant variability between light and a black-on-white optotype target [17], supporting our trial to use red light for the VOG test. Finally, the distance of the fixation target in VOG was different from that in APCT for measuring ocular deviation because the distance was set up by a meter in the software of VOG test. For reducing the variability caused the distance, we limited our study to a group of subjects with < 3 PD difference between near and far distance ocular deviation.

Conclusion

VOG with alternate cover can be used to quantitatively and non-invasively measure the angle of ocular deviation, and more reliably. Moreover, the corrected values demonstrate high agreement with APCT values. Because this test is not significantly influenced by the skill of the examiner, it can accurately measure the angle of ocular deviation, even in the absence of an expert and record of ocular deviation itself. In particular, it is highly valuable as a screening test that can detect strabismus in many patient populations.

Abbreviations
APCT: Alternate prism cover test; MOA: Min of arc; PD: Prism diopters; VOG: Video-oculography

Acknowledgments
None.

Funding
This study was supported by 2016 Inje University Busan Paik Hospital research grant.

Authors' contributions
SHM and NHP designed study, collected data, interpreted statistical analysis and drafted paper. BGP contributed to the analysis and interpretation of data at revision process. MMK aided in study design, acquisition of resources and review of the manuscript. MKO interpreted statistical analysis. All authors read and approved the final manuscript.

Competing interests
The authors declare that they have no competing interests.

Author details
[1]Department of Ophthalmology, Busan Paik Hospital, Inje University College of Medicine, 75 Bokji-ro, Busanjin-gu, Busan 47392, Republic of Korea. [2]Department of Pharmacology, Busan Paik Hospital, Inje University College of medicine, Busan, Republic of Korea. [3]Department of Ophthalmology, Yeungnam University College of Medicine, Daegu, Republic of Korea.

References
1. Choi RY, Kushner BJ. The accuracy of experienced strabismologists using the Hirschberg and Krimsky tests. Ophthalmology. 1998;105:1301–6.
2. Yang HK, Han SB, Hwang JM, Kim YJ, Jeong CB, Kim KG. Assessment of binocular alignment using the three-dimensional strabismus photo analyzer. Br J Ophthalmol. 2012;96:78–82.
3. Yang HK, Seo JM, Hwang JM, Kim KG. Automated analysis of binocular alignment using an infrared camera and selective wavelength filter. Invest Ophthalmol Vis Sci. 2013;54:2733–7.
4. von Noorden GK. Binocular vision and ocular motility: Theory and Management of Strabismus, 6. St. Louis: Mosby; 2002.
5. Quick MW, Boothe RG. A photographic technique for measuring horizontal and vertical eye alignment throughout the field of gaze. Invest Ophthalmol Vis Sci. 1992;33:234–46.
6. Houben MM, Goumans J, van der Steen J. Recording three-dimensional eye movements: scleral search coils versus video oculography. Invest Ophthalmol Vis Sci. 2006;47:179–87.
7. van der Geest JN, Frens MA. Recording eye movements with video-oculography and scleral search coils: a direct comparison of two methods. J Neurosci Methods. 2002;114:185–95.
8. Laria C, Pinero DP. Evaluation of binocular vision therapy efficacy by 3d video-oculography measurement of binocular alignment and motility. Binocul Vis Strabolog Q Simms Romano. 2013;28:136–45.
9. Hirota M, Kanda H, Endo T, Lohmann TK, Miyoshi T, Morimoto T, Fujikado T. Relationship between reading performance and saccadic disconjugacy in patients with convergence insufficiency type intermittent exotropia. Jpn J Ophthalmol. 2016;60:326–32.
10. Economides JR, Adams DL, Horton JC. Variability of ocular deviation in strabismus. JAMA Ophthalmol. 2016;134:63–9.
11. Pediatric Eye Disease Investigator Group. Interobserver reliability of the prism and alternate cover test in children with esotropia. Arch Ophthalmol. 2009;127:59–65.
12. Holmes JM, Leske DA, Hohberger GG. Defining real change in prism-cover test measurements. Am J Ophthalmol. 2008;145:381–5.
13. Hrynchak PK, Herriot C, Irving EL. Comparison of alternate cover test reliability at near in non-strabismus between experienced and novice examiners. Ophthalmic Physiol Opt. 2010;30:304–9.
14. Brodie SE. Photographic calibration of the Hirschberg test. Invest Ophthalmol Vis Sci. 1987;28:736–42.
15. Miller JM, Mellinger M, Greivenkemp J, Simons K. Videographic Hirschberg measurement of simulated strabismic deviations. Invest Ophthalmol Vis Sci. 1993;34:3220–9.
16. Hasebe S, Ohtsuki H, Tadokoro Y, Okano M, Furuse T. The reliability of a video-enhanced Hirschberg test under clinical conditions. Invest Ophthalmol Vis Sci. 1995;36:2678–85.
17. Yang HK, Hwang JM. The effect of target size and accommodation on the distant angle of deviation in intermittent exotropia. Am J Ophthalmol. 2011; 151:907–13. e901

4

Clinical outcomes of Transepithelial photorefractive keratectomy to treat low to moderate myopic astigmatism

Lei Xi[1], Chen Zhang[2] and Yanling He[3]*

Abstract

Background: To evaluate the refractive and visual outcomes of Transepithelial photorefractive keratectomy (TransPRK) in the treatment of low to moderate myopic astigmatism.

Methods: This retrospective study enrolled a total of 47 eyes that had undergone Transepithelial photorefractive keratectomy. Preoperative cylinder diopters ranged from − 0.75D to − 2.25D (mean − 1.11 ± 0.40D), and the sphere was between − 1.50D to − 5.75D. Visual outcomes and vector analysis of astigmatism that included error ratio (ER), correction ratio (CR), error of magnitude (EM) and error of angle (EA) were evaluated.

Results: At 6 months after TransPRK, all eyes had an uncorrected distance visual acuity of 20/20 or better, no eyes lost ≥2 lines of corrected distant visual acuity (CDVA), and 93.6% had residual refractive cylinder within ±0.50D of intended correction. On vector analysis, the mean correction ratio for refractive cylinder was 1.03 ± 0.30. The mean error magnitude was − 0.04 ± 0.36. The mean error of angle was 0.44° ± 7.42°and 80.9% of eyes had axis shift within ±10°. The absolute astigmatic error of magnitude was statistically significantly correlated with the intended cylinder correction ($r = 0.48$, $P < 0.01$).

Conclusions: TransPRK showed safe, effective and predictable results in the correction of low to moderate astigmatism and myopia.

Keywords: Transepithelial photorefractive keratectomy, Myopia, Astigmatism

Background

Refractive errors, such as myopia and astigmatism, are the main cause of visual impairment throughout the world. A European adult population-based study found that myopia was in 35.1% of the participants and astigmatism > 0.5 cylinder diopter (D) was in 32.3% [1]. A prevalence and characteristic of corneal astigmatism (CA) in congenital cataract patients study reported that 39.25% of subjects had CA values > 2 D [2]. Another study found that 22% had CA ≥ 1.5D or higher [3].

Surgical correction of spherical and cylindrical refractive errors has led to a decrease in complications as the improvement of recent technology. Accurate correction especially astigmatism is crucial to achieve better refractive outcomes. However, treatment of astigmatism is still a challenge. Transepithelial photorefractive keratectomy (TransPRK) is popularly chosen for its flapless feature and all-in-one step procedure. Several studies have evaluated the refractive and visual outcomes after TransPRK [4–7]. As for the correction of astigmatism, refractive surgeons are concerned more on the difference between small-incision lenticule extraction (SMILE), femtosecond lenticule extraction (FLEx) and wavefront-guided LASIK [8–11]. However, very few studies have focused on the efficacy of correcting astigmatism by TransPRK, especially in the vector method [12, 13].

The aim of this study was to evaluate the results of TransPRK in the correction of low to moderate myopic astigmatism by vector method.

* Correspondence: heyanling2002@sohu.com
[3]Department of Ophthalmology, Peking University People's Hospital, Beijing, China
Full list of author information is available at the end of the article

Methods

Patient population and study design

The retrospective study comprises 47 eyes of 36 patients with myopia (− 1.50 to − 5.75D) and astigmatism (− 0.75 to − 2.25D) [14] who received TransPRK between October 2016 and January 2017 at the department of ophthalmology of Peking University. The demographic data for the patients were in Table 1. All patients were provided written informed consent. The study protocol was in accordance with the Declaration of Helsinki and institutional review board.

All enrolled patients underwent a complete ophthalmic examination and had no ocular diseases except myopic astigmatism. Preoperative examinations included slit-lamp biomicroscopy, uncorrected distance visual acuity (UDVA), corrected distance visual acuity (CDVA), corneal topography (Optikon SpA, Rome, Italy), pentacam scheimpflug topography (Oculus, Wetzlar, Germany), manifest refraction, ultrasound pachymetry and dilated funduscopy examination. Patients with CDVA under 20/20, suspicion of keratoconus and thin cornea thickness were excluded.

Surgery

The surgery was performed by a single surgeon using the SCHWIND Amaris 500E excimer laser platform (SCHWIND eye-tech-solutions GmbH, Kleinostheim, Germany). Ablations were based on aberration-free algorithms calculated using ORK-CAM software. The ablation profile targets epithelial thickness as 55 μm centrally and 65 μm peripherally according to the population model statistics [6]. Before ablation, all patients' examinations were tested by the statistic cyclotorsion control (SCC) and dynamic cyclotorsion control (DCC) was used through the surgery. After ablation, the corneal stromal was irrigated with a cool balanced salt solution and a soft bandage contact lens was applied.

After surgery, the patients were treated with topical 0.5% levofloxacin (Cravit; Santen, Inc) eye drops four times a day for one week, 0.1% fluorometholone (Allergan, Inc) eye drops four to six times daily (tapered over 12 weeks) and preservative-free artificial tears four times daily for at least 6 months. The contact lens were removed once the epithelial closure was completed.

Table 1 Demographic Data for the Cohort of Eyes

Parameter	Mean ± SD	Age Range
Age (y)	30.69 ± 4.85	19–38
Gender		
Male (n)	33.60 ± 3.57 (10)	26–37
Female (n)	29.58 ± 4.86 (26)	19–38

SD standard deviation, *SE* spherical equivalent refraction

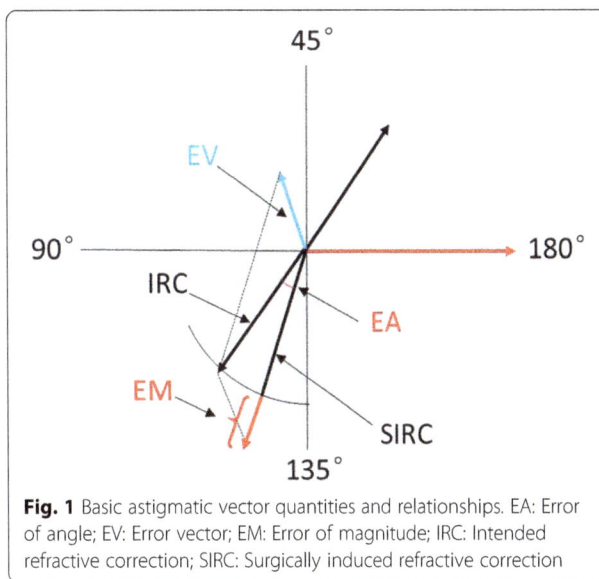

Fig. 1 Basic astigmatic vector quantities and relationships. EA: Error of angle; EV: Error vector; EM: Error of magnitude; IRC: Intended refractive correction; SIRC: Surgically induced refractive correction

Main outcome measures and vector method

The main outcomes include UDVA, CDVA, manifest refractive cylinder and sphere preoperatively and 6 months postoperatively.

Vector analysis of corneal astigmatism is based on the definitions and formulas given by Eydelman MB [15]. The vector quantities and data used in the astigmatic analysis are shown in Fig. 1 and defined as below:

The intended refractive correction (IRC) vector: the vector difference between the preoperative astigmatic correction vector and the target postoperative cylinder vector. If the target refractive state is emmetropia, the IRC vector is equal to the preoperative astigmatic correction.

Table 2 Summary statistics of refractive and visual outcomes

	Preop	6 months	
	Mean ± SD (range) [median]	Mean ± SD (range) [median]	P-value
Sphere(D)	− 3.87 ± 1.15 (−5.75 to − 1.50) [− 4.00]	0.35 ± 0.46 (− 0.50 to 1.25) [0.25]	< 0.01
Cylinder(D)	− 1.11 ± 0.40 (− 2.25 to − 0.75) [− 1.00]	− 0.33 ± 0.25 (− 1.25 to 0.00) [− 0.25]	< 0.01
MSE(D)	−4.30 ± 1.27 (− 6.38 to − 0.88) [− 4.63]	0.18 ± 0.46 (− 0.63 to 1.13) [0.13]	< 0.01
CDVA(LogMAR)	− 0.10 ± 0.07 (− 0.20 to 0.00) [− 0.10]	− 0.14 ± 0.07 (− 0.20 to 0.00) [− 0.10]	< 0.01
UDVA(LogMAR)	0.93 ± 0.28 (0.20 to 1.50) [1.00]	− 0.10 ± 0.07 (− 0.20 to 0.00) [− 0.10]	< 0.01

MSE manifest spherical equivalent; *CDVA* corrected distance visual acuity; *UDVA* uncorrected distance visual acuity

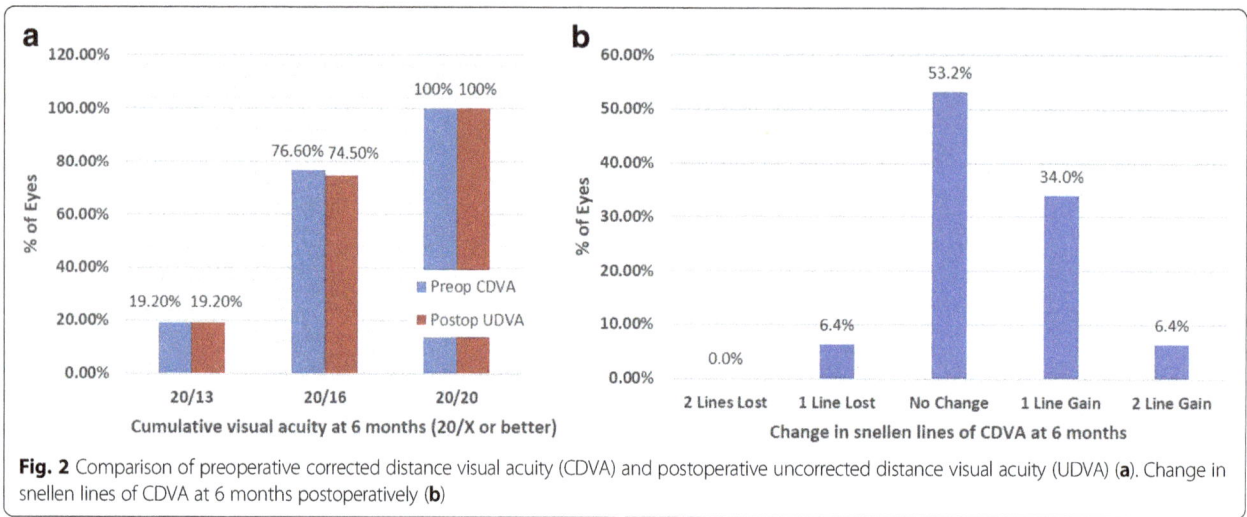

Fig. 2 Comparison of preoperative corrected distance visual acuity (CDVA) and postoperative uncorrected distance visual acuity (UDVA) (**a**). Change in snellen lines of CDVA at 6 months postoperatively (**b**)

The surgical induced refractive correction (SIRC) vector: the vector difference between the preoperative and postoperative astigmatic correction vectors. SIRC is the achieved correction.

The error vector (EV): the vector difference between the IRC and SIRC (IRC-SIRC), when the refractive target is emmetropia, the EV is equal to the postoperative astigmatic correction vector.

The error of magnitude (EM): the arithmetic difference of the magnitudes between SIRC and IRC (| IRC | - | SIRC |).

The error of angle (EA): the angular difference between the achieved treatment and the intended treatment.

The correction ratio (CR): the ratio of the achieved correction magnitude to the required correction (| SIRC | / | IRC |). If the ratio = 1, it is ideal. If > 1, it means excessive application of the treatment. If < 1, it means under correction.

Statistical analysis
Clinical data were analyzed using SPSS 20.0. Descriptive analysis with SDs for means was performed.

The distribution of the data was normality, the paired Student's t-test was used to analyze differences between preoperative and postoperative outcomes. Pearson correlation coefficient was used to analyze the correlation between the absolute EM and the intended cylinder correction. The relationship between the attempted refractive correction and achieved refractive correction was analyzed by linear regression analysis. A p-value < 0.05 was considered statistically significant.

Result
This study included 47 eyes of 36 patients treated by TransPRK. The mean patient age was 30.69 ± 4.85 years (range: 19 to 38 years). The preoperative and postoperative visual acuity (including UDAV and CDVA) and refractive outcomes such as sphere, cylinder, and spherical equivalent were summarized in Table 2. Significant improvement was observed between preoperative and 6 months postoperatively ($p < 0.01$).

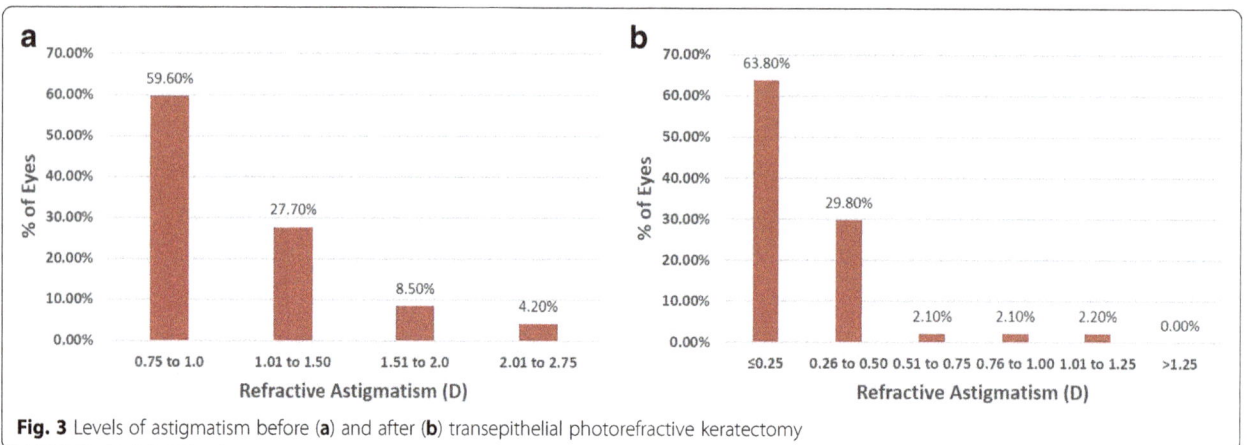

Fig. 3 Levels of astigmatism before (**a**) and after (**b**) transepithelial photorefractive keratectomy

Table 3 Summary of residual refraction

Residual magnitude	Percentage%(eyes)
0D ≤ | Sphere| ≤ 0.5D	72.3% (34)
0.5D < | Sphere| ≤ 1.0D	21.3% (10)
| Sphere|> 1.0D	6.4% (3)
0D < Cyl ≤ 0.5D	93.6% (44)
0.5D < Cyl ≤ 1D	4.3% (2)
Cyl > 1D	2.1% (1)
0D ≤ | SE | ≤ 0.5D	68.1% (32)
0.5D < | SE| ≤ 1.0D	27.7% (13)
| SE| > 1.0D	4.2% (2)

D diopter; *Cyl* cylinder; *SE* spherical equivalent

Safety and efficacy

At 6 months postoperatively, all of the eyes achieved the UCDV of 20/20 or better visual acuity. No patient lost two or more lines of CDVA. Figure 2 shows the preoperative CDVA against postoperative UDVA and there was no significant difference between the two variables ($P = 0.855$). The changes in CDVA between preoperative and 6 months postoperative were shown in Fig. 2. 53.2% (25 eyes) of eyes unchanged; 34% of eyes (16 eyes) gain one line, 6.4% of eyes (3 eyes) gain two lines and 6.4% (3 eyes) of eyes lose one line.

Refractive outcomes

The preoperative and postoperative astigmatic refraction was shown in Fig. 3. 63.8% of the eyes with residual refractive cylinder ≤0.25D. Summaries of the refractive status were in Table 3. The percentage of eyes with residual refractive cylinder ≤0.50D and ≤ 1.0D was in 93.6% (44 eyes) and 97.9% (46 eyes) respectively.

The linear regression of the scattergram was shown in Fig. 4. The achieved versus attempted spherical equivalent correction has a slop of 0.89 and the achieved versus attempted astigmatism correction has a slop of 1.09.

Vector analysis

Figure 5 shows the scattergram of cylinder preoperatively and the error of angle postoperatively. At 6 months, 51.1% of eyes with error of angle ≤5°and 80.9% of eyes ≤10°. No eye more than 20°.

Summarizes of all vector parameters were in Table 4. The correction ratio for cylinder was 1.03 ± 0.3. The mean error of angle (EA) was $0.44 \pm 7.42°$. The error of magnitude (EM) was $- 0.04 \pm 0.36D$.

Discussion

The evaluation of the myopic correction is significant in the clinic, especially in refractive surgery. TransPRK is recommended as one of the most advanced techniques for its flapless. Several previous studies have evaluated the safety, efficacy and predictability of TransPRK [4, 5, 13, 16]. All of the eyes had postoperative UDVA 20/20 or better. 63.8% of the eyes with residual refractive cylinder ≤0.25D, and 93.6% of the eyes≤0.50D. 80.9% of eyes with EA ≤ 5°. One study found that 70.4% of eyes were within ±0.25D and 87.0% of eyes were within ±0.50D of the attempted cylindrical correction at 3 months followed SMILE surgery [11]. In addition, another study achieved 79.1% of eyes within ±0.50D of intended correction of refractive cylinder [17]. The results of this study indicate that TransPRK in myopic eyes with low to moderate cylinder is safe, effective and predictable.

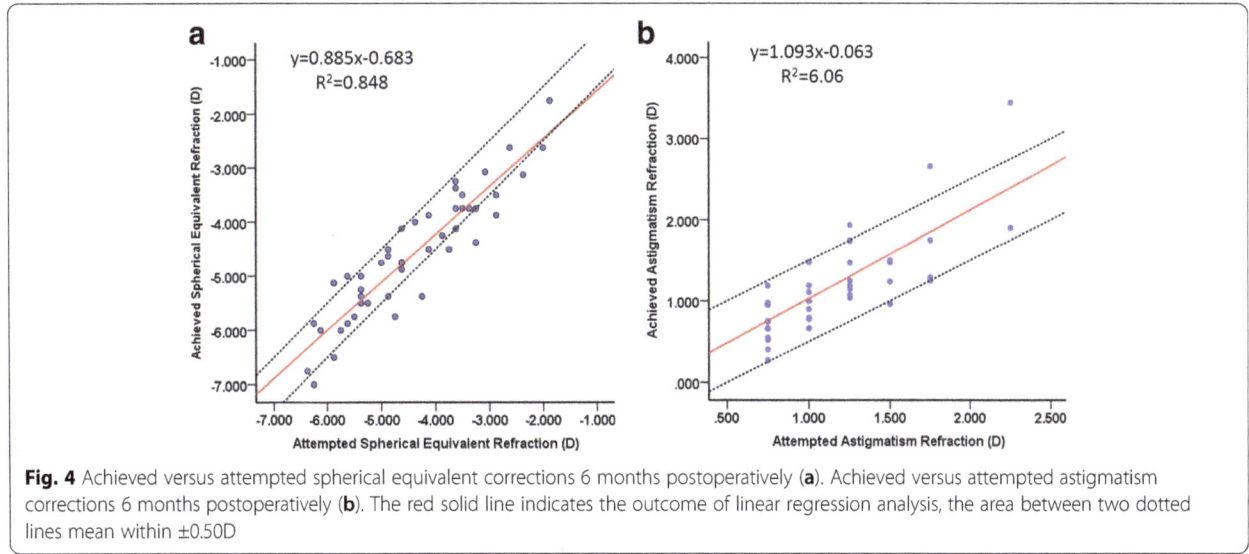

Fig. 4 Achieved versus attempted spherical equivalent corrections 6 months postoperatively (**a**). Achieved versus attempted astigmatism corrections 6 months postoperatively (**b**). The red solid line indicates the outcome of linear regression analysis, the area between two dotted lines mean within ±0.50D

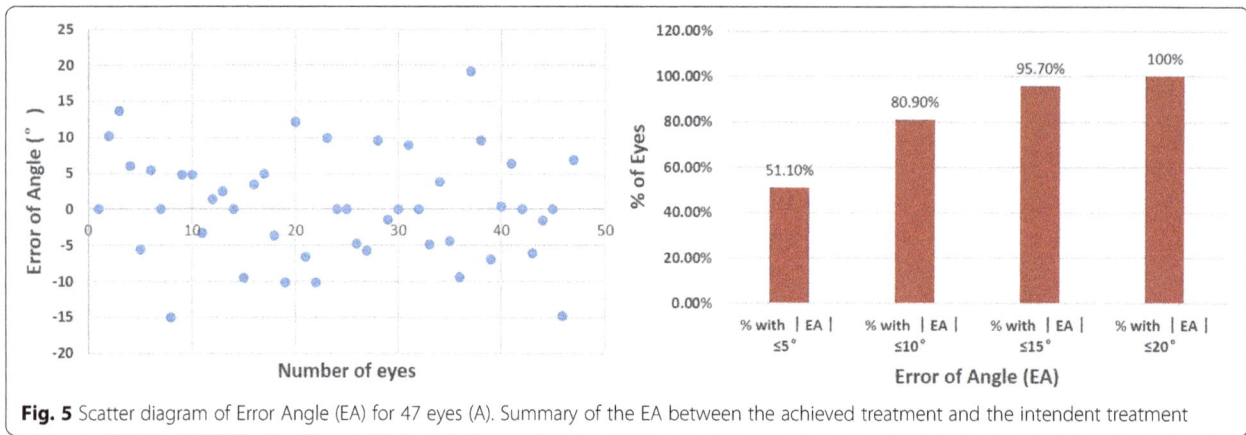

Fig. 5 Scatter diagram of Error Angle (EA) for 47 eyes (A). Summary of the EA between the achieved treatment and the intendent treatment

Other refractive surgeries had been analyzed in the correction of myopic astigmatism. It is difficult to compare because of the different degrees of refractive cylinder. Studies summarized in Table 5 [5, 8, 11, 12, 17–19] showed that we achieved favorable outcomes in comparison to the literature review. Adib et al. [5] reported that 97.26% of the eyes within ±0.50D 18 months later after the surgery of TransPRK for the correction of astigmatism. Similarly, Stojanovic et al. [12] achieved 79.1% of eyes within ±0.50D 12 months later after TransPRK. Zhang J et al. [17] found that 95.92% of eyes within ±0.50D followed SMILE surgery.

Previous studies have attempted to evaluate the refractive outcomes by the spherical equivalent (SE). It is less precise because astigmatism includes both magnitude and axis direction. For this reason, vector analysis could describe the astigmatism correctly. Very few refractive surgery results such as small-incision lenticule extraction (SMILE), femtosecond lenticule extraction (FLEx) and LASIK had been analyzed in the vector method [7, 9, 11, 18, 20]. The aim of this study is to investigate the correction of low to moderate myopic astigmatism following TransPRK in vector method, which has not been reported until now.

The vector analysis of refractive cylinder showed slight overcorrection with the correction ratio (CR, ratio of the achieved correction magnitude to the required correction) of 1.03 at 6 months postoperatively. + 9% overcorrection was observed in the linear regression of the attempted astigmatism refraction. The error of angle (EA) was anticlockwise and minimal (0.44°). Compare to other studies that use vector analysis of cylinder correction, Schallhorn et al. [7] found slight under correction of the refractive cylinder and a mean EA of − 0.45°following wavefront-guided LASIK in the treatment of moderate-to-high astigmatism. Katz et al. [21] achieved a similar CA of 1.06 to our study, and the EA of 3.60°in eyes with preoperative refractive cylinder greater than 3. 00D. Chan et al. [11] found EA of − 0.85°and 2.09°in SMILE and femtosecond-assisted LASIK respectively in the correction of low to moderate myopic astigmatism. In this study, the error ratio of cylinder correction is 0. 30, which is slightly higher than 0.13 reported by Schallhorn et al. [7]. These results indicate that TransPRK could achieve comparable results in the correction of cylinder by comparing with other surgeries. Statistic cyclotorsion control (SCC) and dynamic cyclotorsion control (DCC) may play an important role in the correction of cylinder.

The alignment is important for the refractive cylinder correction. Misalignment could result in both higher order aberrations (HOAs) and corrective performance [18, 22]. In our study, 80.9% of eyes within the error of angle (EA) ≤10°, and 95.7% within ≤15°. One study found 68.4% of eyes had EA ≤10°in a group of patients with preoperative refractive cylinder of − 0.90 ± 0.68D followed SMILE surgery [18]. Another study found 98. 4% with EA within 10°after wavefront-guided LASIK [7]. Although eye-tracking was used for every patient, the astigmatism axis could be misaligned by many factors. The cyclotorsional movements of the eyes from upright to supine position, the shift of the pupil center and the

Table 4 Vector analysis of changes in refractive cylinder

Vector parameter	Eyes (n = 47) Mean (SD)	Range
IRC (D)	1.11 (0.40)	0.75–2.25
SIRC (D)	1.15 (0.57)	0.27–3.45
ER	0.30 (0.19)	0.00–0.667
CR	1.03 (0.3)	0.36–1.59
EM (D)	−0.04 (0.36)	−1.20-0.536
EA (°)	0.44 (7.42)	−15.00-19.13

IRC intended refractive correction; *SIRC* surgically induced refractive correction; *ER* error ratio; *CR* correction ratio; *EM* error of magnitude; *EA* error of angle

Table 5 Literature studies of myopic astigmatic correction

Author (year)	Technique	Eyes (n)	Follow-up (months)	Preoperative cylinder Mean ± SD (range)	Postoperative cylinder Mean ± SD (range)	Within 0.50D (%)
Schallhorn [17] (2015)	W-LASIK	611	3	−2.76 ± 0.81 (− 2.00 to −6.00)	−0.37 ± 0.38 (− 2.00 to 0.00)	79.10%
Stojanovic [12] (2013)	TransPRK	117	12	−0.77 ± 0.65 (−4.50 to 0.00)	/	94.00%
Adib [5] (2016)	TransPRK	146	18	−1.19 ± 0.99	−0.29 ± 0.21	97.26%
Zhang J [18] (2015)	SMILE	98	12	−0.90 ± 0.68 (− 0.25 to − 2.75)	−0.20 ± 0.27	95.92%
Al-Zeraid [19] (2016)	W-LASIK	23	6	−3.22 ± 0.59 (− 2.50 to − 4.50)	−0.72 ± 0.46	39%
Ali-MA [8] (2014)	FLEx	58	6	− 0.97 ± 0.54 (− 0.5 to − 2.75)	−0.26 ± 0.37 (− 1.00 to 0.00)	86%
Chan [11] (2015)	SMILE	54	3	−1.08 ± 0.71	−0.243 ± 0.316	87%
Current study	TransPRK	47	6	−1.11 ± 0.40 (−0.75 to − 2.25)	− 0.33 ± 0.25 (− 1.25 to 0.00)	93.6%

W-LASIK wavefront-guided Laser in situ keratomileusis; *TransPRK* transepithelial photorefractive keratectomy; *SMIL* small-incision lenticule extraction; *FLEx* femtosecond lenticule extraction

large angle kappa occurred. In addition, the epithelial thickness (55 μm centrally and 65 μm periphery) estimated by the statistic of common people may lead to deep or shallow ablation of the corneal tissue. So, precise positioning center and epithelial mapping for every patient would be of great help for the precise correction of refractive cylinder.

In conclusion, the outcomes of this study suggest that TransPRK surgery is safe, effective and predictive in the treatment of low to moderate astigmatism. Based on the findings of our study, the absolute astigmatic error of magnitude was significantly correlated with the intended cylinder correction. Further investigation should be conducted to assess the treatment for correcting higher cylinder.

Conclusions

TransPRK surgery is safe, effective and predictable in the correction of low to moderate astigmatism.

Abbreviations
CA: Corneal astigmatism; CDVA: Corrected distance visual acuity; CR: Correction ratio; DCC: Dynamic cyclotorsion control; EA: Error of angle; EM: Error of magnitude; ER: Error ratio; EV: Error vector; HOAs: Higher order wavefront aberrations; IRC: Intended refractive correction; SCC: Statistic cyclotorsion control; SE: Spherical equivalent; TransPRK: Transepithelial photorefractive keratectomy; UDVA: Uncorrected distance visual acuity

Funding
This study was not supported by any research grants.

Authors' contributions
Study concept and design (YLH, LX, CZ); collection, management, analysis, and interpretation of data (LX, CZ YLH); and preparation, review, or approval of the manuscript (YLH, CZ, LX). All authors read and approved the final manuscript.

Competing interests
The authors declare that they have no competing interests.

Author details
[1]Department of Ophthalmology, Peking University International Hospital, Beijing, China. [2]Tianjin Medical University Eye hospital, Tianjin Medical University Eye Institute, School of Optometry and Ophthalmology, Tianjin, China. [3]Department of Ophthalmology, Peking University People's Hospital, Beijing, China.

References
1. Wolfram C, Höhn R, Kottler U, Wild P, Blettner M, Bühren J, et al. Prevalence of refractive errors in the European adult population: the Gutenberg health study (GHS). Br J Ophthalmol. 2014;98(7):857–61.
2. Lin D, Chen J, Liu Z, Wu X, Long E, Luo L, et al. Prevalence of Corneal Astigmatism and Anterior Segmental Biometry Characteristics BeforeSurgery in Chinese Congenital Cataract Patients. Sci Rep. 2016;6:22092.
3. Ferrer-Blasco T, Montes-Mico´ R, Peixoto-de Matos S, Gonza'lez-Mei'jome JM, Cervin¯o A. Prevalence of corneal astigmatism before cataract surgery. J Cataract Refract Surg. 2009;35:70–5.
4. Luger MH, Ewering T, Arba-Mosquera S. Myopia correction with transepithelial photorefractive keratectomy versus femtosecondLassisted laser in situ keratomileusis: one-year case-matched analysis. J Cataract Refract Surg. 2016;42(11):1579–87.
5. Adib-Moghaddam S, Soleyman-Jahi S, Salmanian B, Omidvari AH, Adili-Aghdam F, Noorizadeh F, et al. Single-step transepithelial photorefractive keratectomy in myopia and astigmatism: 18-month follow-up. J Cataract Refract Surg. 2016;42(11):1570–8.
6. Arba Mosquera S, Awwad ST. Theoretical analyses of the refractive implications of transepithelial PRK ablations. Br J Ophthalmol. 2013;97:905–11.
7. Fadlallah A, Fahed D, Khalil K, Dunia I, Menassa J, El Rami H, et al. Transepithelial photorefractive keratectomy: clinical results. J Cataract Refract Surg. 2011;37(10):1852–7.
8. Ali MA, Kobashi H, Kamiya K, Igarashi A, Miyake T, Elewa ME, et al. Comparison of astigmatic correction after femtosecond Lenticule extraction and Wavefront-guided LASIK for myopic astigmatism. J Refract Surg. 2014;30(12):806–11.
9. Kobashi H, Kamiya K, Ali MA, Igarashi A, Elewa ME, Shimizu K. Comparison of astigmatic correction after femtosecond Lenticule extraction and small-incision Lenticule extraction for myopic astigmatism. PLoS One. 2015;10(4):e0123408.
10. Zhang J, Wang Y, Chen X. Comparison of moderate- to high-astigmatism corrections using WaveFront–guided laser in situ Keratomileusis and small-incision Lenticule extraction. Cornea. 2016;35(4):523–30.
11. Chan TC, Ng AL, Cheng GP, Wang Z, Ye C, Woo VC, et al. Vector analysis of astigmatic correction after small-incision lenticule extraction and femtosecond-assisted LASIK for low to moderate myopic astigmatism. Br J Ophthalmol. 2016;100(4):553–9.
12. Stojanovic A, Chen S, Chen X, Stojanovic F, Zhang J, Zhang T, et al. One-step Transepithelial topography-guided ablation in the treatment of myopic astigmatism. PLoS One. 2013;8(6):e66618.

13. Antonios R, Abdul Fattah M, Arba Mosquera S, Abiad BH, Sleiman K, Awwad ST. Single-step transepithelial versus alcohol-assisted photorefractive keratectomy in the treatment of high myopia: a comparative evaluation over 12 months. Br J Ophthalmol. 2016;101:1106–12.

14. Richdale K, Berntsen DA, Mack CJ, Merchea MM, Barr JT. Visual acuity with spherical and toric soft contact lenses in low- to moderate-astigmatic eyes. Optom Vis Sci. 2007;84(10):969–75.

15. Eydelman MB, Drum B, Holladay J, Hilmantel G, Kezirian G, Durrie D, et al. Standardized analyses of correction of astigmatism by laser systems that reshape the cornea. J Refract Surg. 2006;22(1):81–95.

16. Kaluzny BJ, Cieslinska I, Mosquera SA, Verma S. Single-step Transepithelial PRK vs alcohol-assisted PRK in myopia and compound myopic astigmatism correction. Medicine (Baltimore). 2016;95(6):e1993.

17. Schallhorn SC, Venter JA, Hannan SJ, Hettinger KA. Clinical outcomes of wavefront-guided laser in situ keratomileusis to treat moderate-to-high astigmatism. Clin Ophthalmol. 2015;9:1291–8.

18. Zhang J, Wang Y, Wu W, Xu L, Li X, Dou R. Vector analysis of low to moderate astigmatism with small incision lenticule extraction (SMILE): results of a 1-year follow-up. BMC Ophthalmol. 2015;15:8.

19. Al-Zeraid FM, Osuagwu UL. Induced higher-order aberrations after laser in situ Keratomileusis (LASIK) performed with Wavefront-guided IntraLase femtosecond laser in moderate to high astigmatism. BMC Ophthalmol. 2016;16.29.

20. Biscevic A, Bohac M, Koncarevic M, Anticic M, Dekaris I, Patel S. Vector analysis of astigmatism before and after LASIK: a comparison of two different platforms for treatment of high astigmatism. Graefes Arch Clin Exp Ophthalmol. 2015;253(12):2325–33.

21. Katz T, Wagenfeld L, Galambos P, Darrelmann BG, Richard G, et al. LASIK versus photorefractive keratectomy for high myopic (>3 diopter) astigmatism. J Refract Surg. 2013;29(12):824–31.

22. Wang L, Koch DD. Residual higher-order aberrations caused by clinically measured cyclotorsional misalignment or decentration during wavefront-guided excimer laser corneal ablation. J Cataract Refract Surg. 2008;34(12):2057–62.

5

Heritability of myopia and its relation with *GDJ2* and *RASGRF1* genes in Lithuania

Edita Kunceviciene[1*], Margarita Sriubiene[1], Rasa Liutkeviciene[2], Ilona T. Miceikiene[1] and Alina Smalinskiene[1]

Abstract

Background: This study aimed to assess heritability of myopia in Lithuania and evaluate both genes *GJD2* (Gap Junction Protein, Delta 2) and *RASGRF1* (RAS protein-specific guanine nucleotide-releasing factor 1) relation with myopia.

Methods: In this study Lithuanian twin population aged between 18 and 40 ($n = 460$) were examined. Single-nucleotide polymorphisms of the *RASGRF1* (rs8027411) and *GJD2* (rs634990) genes were assessed by real-time polymerase chain reaction method.

Results: Intrapair correlations for spherical equivalent in all twin pairs were significantly higher in MZ twin pairs $r = 0.539$ ($p < 0.001$, 95% CI 0.353–0.684) than in DZ twin pairs $r = 0.203$ ($p < 0.01$, 95% CI 0.0633–0.442) in myopia group. Correlations for spherical equivalent in emmetropia group were not significant in MZ twin pairs $r = 0.091$ ($p > 0.05$, 95% CI -0.215-0.381) and in DZ twin pairs $r = -0.220$ ($p > 0.05$, 95% CI -0.587-0.222). The odds ratio (95% CI) were 2.7 (1.018–7.460) for combinations of genotypes of rs634990 CC and rs8027411 GT ($p = 0.046$).

Conclusions: Our studies have shown that the heritability of myopia makes 67.2% in Lithuania. Persons with combinations of genotypes rs634990 CC and rs8027411 GT have 2.7 times higher odds to have myopia.

Keywords: *RASGRF1*, *GJD2*, Twin, Myopia

Background

Refractive error is one of the priority targets of World Health Organization Vision 2020 [1]. More than 150 million people in the world are estimated to be visually impaired because of uncorrected refractive error, 8 million of them are functionally blind [2]. Myopia affects approximately one-third of adults older than 20 years in the United States, and in areas with high prevalence, specifically in urban East Asia, more than 80% of students graduating from school are myopic [3]. It is estimated that by the year 2020, 2.5 billion people - one third of the world's population will have been affected by myopia alone [4]. Worldwide, myopia affects approximately one in four individuals in western population and is the most common visual disorder [4, 5].

In Lithuania, the data on refractive errors are systematically collected, and the official statistics are published by the Lithuanian Department of Statistics. In the population of Lithuania from 2007 to 2014, the prevalence of myopia increased from 44.3 to 63.9 per 1000 population (www.sic.hi.lt).

Both genetic and environmental factors can affect development of myopia, but the exact causes are not fully understood [6]. The genetic contribution to a trait often is assessed through heritability. Heritability is the proportion of phenotypic variability in a population trait that is due to genetic differences [7]. Up to now, the heritability of myopia has not been studied in Lithuania.

Twin studies allow us to estimate the overall gene influence, and the results can show the heritability of myopia. The twin method assumes that monozygotic (MZ) twins are influenced by largely similar environmental differences as dizygotic (DZ) twins, but MZ twins share the same genes whereas DZ twins on average share only half their genes [8]. Twin method is excellent for the estimation of heritability of myopia, but it does not show the specific genes that may possibly be involved in the heritability of myopia. Thus, we chose genetic markers, in order to establish whether any of them are significantly associated with myopia.

* Correspondence: edita.kunceviciene@lsmuni.lt
[1]Institute of Biology Systems and Genetic Research, Lithuanian University of Health Sciences, 18 Tilzes St, Kaunas, Lithuania
Full list of author information is available at the end of the article

Genome-wide association studies (GWAS) for refractive error showed that single nucleotide polymorphisms (SNPs) in 15q25 and 15q14 were associated with refractive error and myopia [9]. *RASGFR1* is a gene made of 28 exons. This gene has a significant influence on development of myopia. *RASGFR1* gene encodes Ras protein-specific guanine nucleotide-releasing factor-1, which is highly expressed in the retina and neurons. Then *RASGFR1* gene proceeds to activate Ras [10, 11]. Also, RASGRF1 is a nuclear exchange factor that promotes GDP/GTP exchange on the Ras family GTPases and is related to synaptic transmission of the photoreceptor responses [12]. Muscarinic receptors and retinoic acid can regulate *RASGRF1* expression as well [11]. Some animal and human studies showed that muscarinic inhibitors prevented the development of myopia [13]. In animal models of myopia there was detected reduced synthesis of choroidal retinoic acid [14]. To date, studies of SNP rs8027411 of *RASGRF1* gene associations with high myopia in different populations have provided controversial results [6, 15–17].

The *GJD2* gene at 15q14 encodes a neuron-specific protein connexin 36 (CX36), a 36 kDa protein, which is a neuron-specific protein of a family of integral membrane proteins [18]. CX36 forms gap junction channels between adjacent membranes of neuronal cells. It is present in photoreceptors, bipolar and amacrine cells, and, by enabling intercellular transport of small molecules and ions, plays an essential role in the transmission process of the retinal electric circuitry [18, 19].

The aim of our research was to find associations between the *GJD2*, *RASGRF1* genes and myopia

Table 1 Characteristics of twin pairs, defined by zygosity

	MZ twins	DZ twins	p value
Sex, pairs			
Male	80	37	0.900[†]
Female	55	53	
Male/Female		5	
Total:	135	95	
Age, years			
Mean ± SE	24.10 ± 0.54	26.06 ± 0.93	0.379[‡]
Median	20.79	21.38	
Min, Max	18, 40	18, 40	
Spherical equivalent (D)			
OD Mean ± SE	−1.212 ± 0.102	−1.524 ± 0.196	0.667[‡]
Median	−0.75	−0.75	
Min, Max	−7.25, 0.375	−7.375, 0.49	
OS Mean ± SE	−1.112 ± 0.104	−1.449 ± 0.198	0.338[‡]
Median	−0.625	−0.75	
Min, Max	−7.25, 0.35	−6.75, 0.49	

Abbreviations: *MZ* – monozygotic twins; *DZ* - dizygotic twins, *D* diopters, *SE* Standard error, p > 0.05 – comparison between *MZ* and *DZ* twins
† p value for the chi-square test, ‡ p value for the Mann-Whitney test

development and to assess the heritability of myopia in Lithuania.

Methods
Ethics statement
Permission (Number P1–52/2005) to undertake the study was obtained from the Kaunas Regional Biomedical Research Ethics Committee. Before the study, the

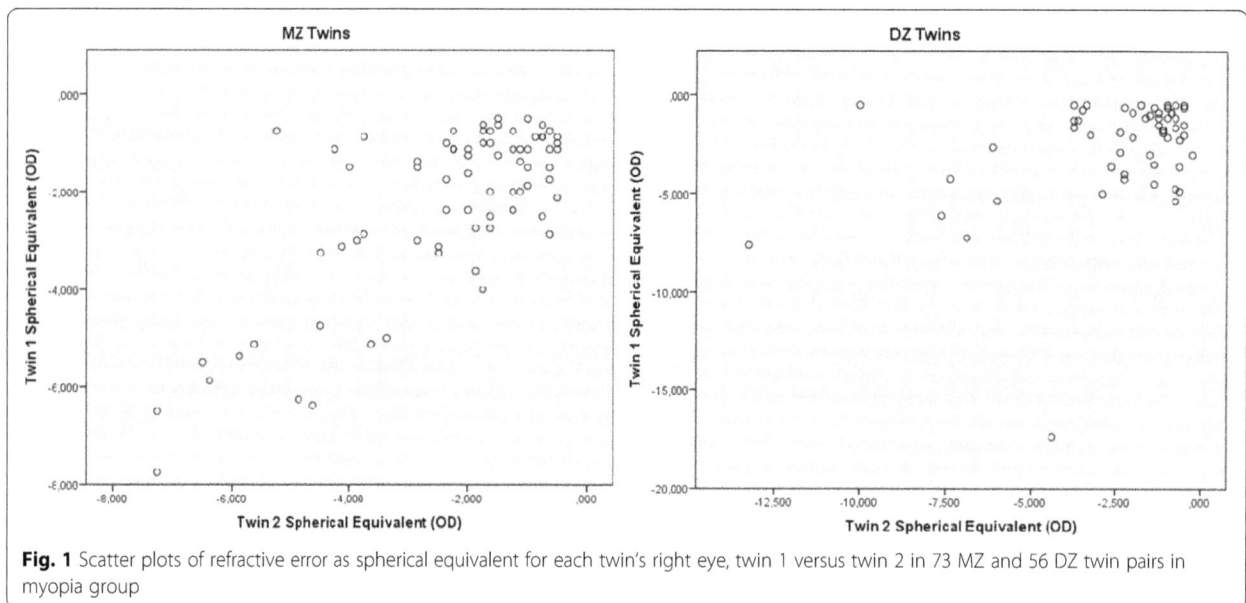

Fig. 1 Scatter plots of refractive error as spherical equivalent for each twin's right eye, twin 1 versus twin 2 in 73 MZ and 56 DZ twin pairs in myopia group

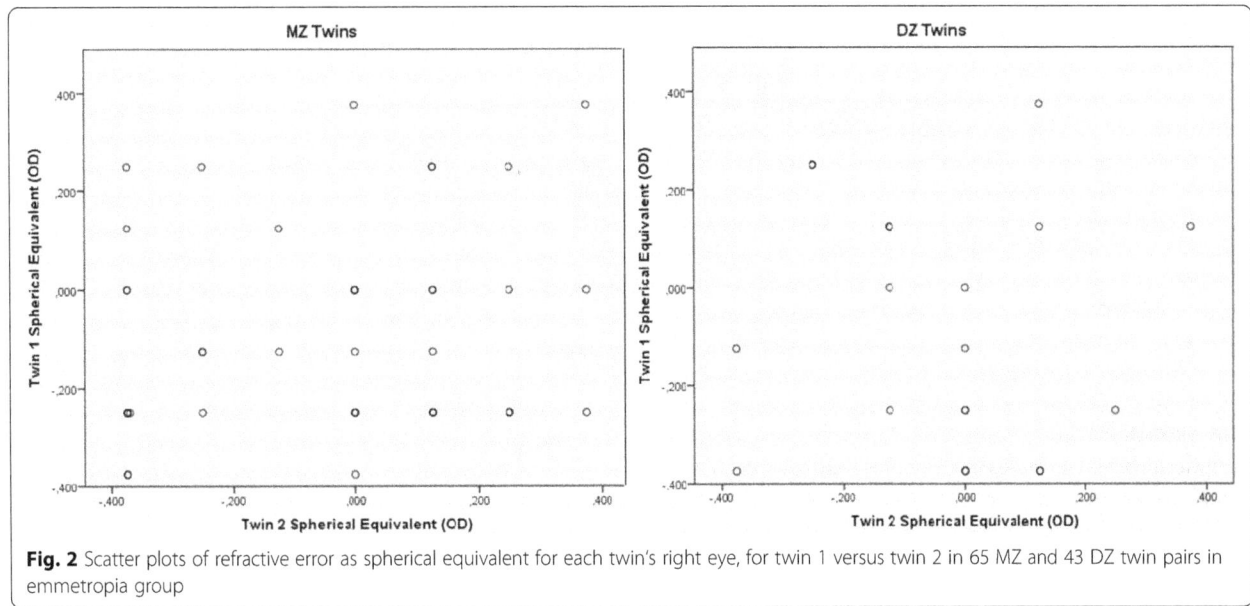

Fig. 2 Scatter plots of refractive error as spherical equivalent for each twin's right eye, for twin 1 versus twin 2 in 65 MZ and 43 DZ twin pairs in emmetropia group

procedure and purpose of the study was explained, and an informed consent was obtained from all participants.

Study samples
The twins participating in this study were from the Twin Centre of Lithuanian University of Health Sciences. The Twin Centre has registered more than 600 twin pairs who agreed to participate in various medical and genetic studies. The study was conducted in the Institute of Biological Systems and Genetics Research, Lithuanian University of Health Sciences.

Refractive error measurement
Refractive error was measured with Sol. Cyclopentolate 1% using an autorefractor (Accuref-K9001, Shin-Nippon, Japan) and calculated by the mean spherical equivalent for each of the two eyes of every individual. The mean spherical equivalent was calculated using the standard formula: spherical equivalent = sphere+(cylinder/2).

MZ and DZ twins with spherical equivalent of at least one eye > = – 0.5 D were assigned to the myopia group. Twins whose spherical equivalent was between 0.49 and – 0.49 D were included in the emmetropia group. The myopia degree was determined by the strength or optical power of a corrective lens that focuses distant images on

the retina: from – 0.5 D to – 3 D mild-degree myopia; from – 3 D to – 6.0 D medium-degree myopia; and – 6.0 D and over high-degree myopia [20, 21].

The exclusion criteria were as follows: 1) cataract, refractive surgery or other previous interventions that might have affected refractions; 2) other refractive errors; 3) refusal to participate in the research.

The inclusion criteria were as follows: 1) no ophthalmological eye disorders were found on detailed ophthalmological evaluation; 2) participation consent.

Lenses were evaluated by a slim-lamp biomicroscopy with the illumination source at a 45 degree angle and the light beam set being set to 2 mm width.

Verification of zygosity
Zygosity was determined using a DNA test. The polymerase chain reaction set (AmpFlSTR® Identifiler®, Applied Biosystems, Foster City, CA, USA) was used to amplify short tandem repeats. 15 specific DNA markers were used for comparison of genetic profiles: D8S1179, D21S11, D7S820, CSF180, D3S1358, TH01, D13S317, D16S539, D2S1338, D19S433, vWA, TROX, D18S51, D5S818, and Amelogenin. The sample's gender, age, zygosity characteristics and spherical equivalents are shown in Table 1.

Table 2 Frequency of *GJD2* and *RASGRF1* genotypes and allele (%)

SNP ID	Gene	N	Genotype Frequency			Minor allele frequency	P value
rs634990	*GJD2*	272	CC	CT	TT	C	0.1692
			56 (20.6%)	147 (54%)	69 (25.4%)	259 (47.6%)	
rs8027411	*RASGRF1*	285	GG	GT	TT	G	0.0913
			60 (21.1%)	157 (55.1%)	68 (23.8%)	277 (48.57%)	

Table 3 Pooled results of the associations between *GJD2* and myopia

Model	Genotype	Sig.	Exp(B)	95% C.I. For Exp(B) Lower	Upper
Codominant	CC	0.085	2.000	0.909	4.401
	CT	0.742	1.105	0.611	1.998
	TT	–	–	–	–
Dominant	(CC + CT) versus TT	0.390	1.284	0.727	2.268
Recessive	(CT + TT) versus CC	0.071	1.870	0.947	3.689
Overdominant	(CC + TT) versus CT	0.467	0.828	0.499	1.376
Additive	–	0.102	0.729	0.500	1.064

DNA extraction

Peripheral blood samples were collected from each individual in ethylenediaminetetraacetic (EDTA) tubes for DNA extraction. DNA was extracted from leukocytes using a reagent kit (NucleoSpin Blood L Kit; Macherey & Nagel, Düren, Germany). DNA samples from one member of each MZ pair were used for genotyping.

Genotyping

SNP of the *GJD2* gene (rs634990) were assessed using a commercial genotyping kit C_2088259_10. SNP of the *RASGRF1* gene (rs8027411) was assessed using a commercial genotyping kit C_185318_10 (Applied Biosystems, Foster City, CA, USA). The Applied Biosystems 7900HT Real-Time Polymerase Chain Reaction System was used for detecting the SNPs. The cycling program started with heating for 10 min at 95 °C, followed by 40 cycles of 15 s at 95 °C and 1 min at 60 °C. Allelic discrimination was carried out using the software of Applied Biosystems. Both SNPs (rs8027411, rs634990) were present in two previous GWASs.

Statistical analysis

The data was analysed with the statistical software package SPSS version 19.0 for Windows. Odds ratios and 95% confidence intervals were computed to assess the association between two SNPs and myopia multivariate logistic

Table 4 Pooled results of the associations between *RASGRF1* and myopia

Model	Genotype	Sig.	Exp(B)	95% C.I. For Exp(B) Lower	Upper
Codominant	GG	0.940	1.029	0.488	2.173
	GT	0.680	0.880	0.480	1.615
	TT	–	–	–	–
Dominant	(GG + GT) versus TT	0.774	0.918	0.513	1.645
Recessive	(GT + TT) versus GG	0.705	1.126	0.610	2.076
Overdominant	(GG + TT) versus GT	0.578	0.868	0.528	1.428
Additive	–	0.096	0.991	0.686	1.432

Table 5 Odds ratio of myopia according to the combinations of *GJD2* and *RASGRF1*

Myopia

Genotype GJD2 SNP ID rs634990	RASGRF1 SNP ID rs8027411	Sig.	Exp(B)	95% C.I. For Exp(B) Lower	Upper
CC	GG	0.540	0.692	0.213	2.244
CC	GT	0.046†	2.756	1.018	7.460
CC	TT	0.335	1.898	0.516	6.980
CT	GG	0.460	1.407	0.569	3.482
CT	GT	0.284	0.747	0.439	1.273
CT	TT	0.706	0.864	0.405	1.845
TT	GG	0.990	1.006	0.391	2.587
TT	GT	0.129	0.542	0.246	1.195
TT	TT	0.857	1.096	0.403	2.986

†$p < 0.05$ comparison between myopia and emmetropia combinations of genotypes

regression (Tables 3). Statistical significance was determined at a two-tailed $p = 0.05$ level. Estimate of heritability (h^2) was obtained Pearson's correlations (r) for MZ and DZ twin pairs: $h^2 = 2 \times (r_{MZ} - r_{DZ})$ [22].

Results

230 pairs of twins (135 MZ and 95 DZ) aged between 18 and 40 participated in the study, their mean age being 25.08 years (SE 0.7 years) (Table 1). The mean spherical equivalent was -1.324 ± 0.150, with a range from 0.49 D to -7.375 D. There were no significant differences between MZ and DZ twins in age and spherical equivalent of the left and right eyes.

Refractive errors for twin 1 versus twin 2 for mean of spherical equivalent are shown in figs. 1 and 2. Intrapair correlations for spherical equivalent in twin pairs were significantly higher in MZ twin pairs $r = 0.539$ ($p < 0.001$, 95% CI 0.353–0.684) than in DZ twin pairs $r = 0.203$ ($p < 0.01$, 95% CI 0.0633–0.442) in myopia group. Correlations for spherical equivalent in emmetropia group were not significant: $r = 0.091$ ($p > 0.05$, 995% CI -0.215-0.381) in MZ twin pairs and $r = -0.220$ (p > 0.05, 95% CI -0.587-0.222) in DZ twin pairs. The correlations of MZ were clearly higher compared to DZ pairs, indicating genetic effects on myopia.

We genotyped two SNPs (rs634990 and rs8027411) in 189 myopia (83 MZ and 106 DZ) and 96 emmetropia (25 MZ and 71 DZ) subjects. The results are shown in Table 2. The distribution of the two SNP genotypes matched the Hardy-Weinberg equilibrium ($p \geq 0.05$). High-degree myopia was present in 11 cases, 33 twins had medium-degree 10 and 145 twins mild-degree myopia. But we didn't find significant correlations between myopia degree and genotypes.

Table 6 Distribution of SNP rs634990 and SNP rs8027411 genotypes according to degrees of myopia

Myopia degree	N	SNP ID rs634990 N = 272			SNP ID rs8027411 N = 285			Combinations of genotypes: SNP ID rs634990 + SNP ID rs8027411								
		CC	CT	TT	GG	GT	TT	CC + GG	CC + GT	CC + TT	CT + GG	CT + GT	CT + TT	TT + GG	TT + GT	TT + TT
High	11	4	5	2	3	6	2	1	2	1	2	2	1	0	2	0
Moderate	33	7	20	6	8	17	8	2	4	1	4	10	5	2	4	0
Low	145	32	80	20	34	83	28	8	18	6	18	50	12	9	10	1
Control	96	13	42	41	15	51	30	1	8	4	8	27	7	6	16	19

5 models were used to calculate the odds ratios to have myopia separately with each gene (GJD2 or RASGRF1), results were not significant (Table 3, Table 4).

But we found significant association between the combinations of GJD2 CC and RASGRF1 GT and myopia (Table 5). The odds ratio of myopia compared to emmetropia (95% confidence intervals [CIs]) was 2.7 (1.018–7.460) for GJD2 CC and RASGRF1 GT genotypes.

The number with combinations of genotypes rs634990 CC and rs8027411 GT and myopia degrees are shown in Table 6.

Discussion

We estimated heritability of myopia according to correlations for MZ and DZ twin pairs and our study showed 67.2% heritability of myopia. Three published twin studies of refractive error have found high heritability from 84 to 86% [23], 89 to 94% [24] and 75 to 88% [25]. It is indicate that heritability in Lithuania is lower than in other Europian populations. Dirani et al. have reported that different populations have shown a wide range of heritability estimates ranging from 50 to 90% [25]. Results shown that the samples of the population and different methods may affect the estimates of heritability [25]. In our study 77% twins had mild-degree myopia, 17% - medium-degree and 6% - high-degree myopia. Meanwhile, the medium-degree myopia accounted for the largest portion in the mentioned studies of heritability in Europe.

Study showed that the gene *GJD2*, located nearest to the locus 15q14, and *RASGRF1* 15q25 are important for the transmission and processing of visual signals [23, 26]. The studies of genetic associations in some European and Japanese populations showed that common genetic variations located in *GJD2* and *RASGRF1* were associated with common myopia and refractive error [5, 11, 15].

A study of genome-wide associations (GWASs) showed associations of SNP with refractive error in 5328 individuals of the Dutch population which were not related. They found that carriers of the C allele of rs634990 have a higher risk of myopia [5]. Qiang et al. found that *RASGRF1* gene was significantly associated with high-degree myopia (risk allele T) but *GJD2* gene was not [15]. Also, results of meta-analysis, which included 2529 individuals with high-degree myopia and 3127 controls, showed that *RASGRF1* was significantly associated with high-degree myopia in Chinese and Japanese populations. However, carriers of the *RASGRF1 G* allele had a lower risk of high-degree myopia compared to carriers of the T allele (G versus T) [27]. Also, Hysi et al. found that individuals carrying TT alleles on the *RASGRF1* were significantly more likely to have myopia than those homozygous for the non-susceptibility GG alleles. We found a significant association between combinations of *GJD2* and *RASGRF1* genotypes and myopia. Our study showed that individuals with combinations of *GJD2* CC and *RASGRF1* GT genotypes were 2.7 times more likely to have myopia ($p = 0.046$). This indicates that some of our results are consistent with the previous reports. Individuals carrying CC alleles on the *GJD2* were significantly more likely to have myopia than carriers of TT alleles. But carriers of GT allele on the *RASGRF1* gene had more risk to have myopia than carriers of wild type alleles.

Conclusion

Our studies have shown that the heritability of myopia makes 66.4% in Lithuania. We detected significant associations between the combinations of *GJD2* CC and *RASGRF1* GT and odds ratio of developing myopia.

Abbreviations

D: Diopters; DZ: Dizygotic twins; GJD2: Gap Junction Protein Delta 2; MZ: Monozygotic twins; RASGRF1: RAS protein-specific guanine nucleotide-releasing factor 1; SE: Standard error

Acknowledgements

We wish to thanks all the twins who agreed to participate in this study.

Funding

Funding for the research was obtained from the Lithuanian University of Health Sciences.

Authors' contributions

EK, RL, MS analyzed the data. EK, RL wrote the manuscript. EK, AS developed the structure for the paper. AS, RL, MS made critical revisions. EK, AS, ITM approved final version. All authors approved of the final manuscript.

Competing interests

The authors declare that they have no competing interests.

Author details

[1]Institute of Biology Systems and Genetic Research, Lithuanian University of Health Sciences, 18 Tilzes St, Kaunas, Lithuania. [2]Department of Ophthalmology, Lithuanian University of Health Sciences, 2 Eiveniu St, Kaunas, Lithuania.

References

1. Dandona L, Dandona R. What is the global burden of visual impairment? BMC Med. 2006;4:6.
2. Holden BA, Fricke TR, Ho SM, et al. Global vision impairment due to uncorrected presbyopia. Arch Ophthalmol. 2008;126:1731–9.
3. Lin LL, Shih YF, Hsiao CK, Chen CJ. Prevalence of myopia in Taiwanese schoolchildren: 1983 to 2000. Ann Acad Med Singap. 2004;33:27–33.
4. Kempen JH, Mitchell P, Lee KE, et al. The prevalence of refractive errors among adults in the United States, Western Europe, and Australia. Arch Ophthalmol. 2004;122:495–505.
5. Solouki AM, Verhoeven VJ, Duijn CM, et al. A genome-wide association study identifies a susceptibility locus for refractive errors and myopia at 15q14. Nat Genet. 2010;42:897–901.
6. Hayashi H, Yamashiro K, Nakanishi H, et al. Association of 15q14 and 15q25 with high myopia in Japanese. Invest Ophthalmol Vis Sci. 2011;52:4853–8.
7. Liew SH, Elsner H, Spector TD, Hammond CJ. The first "classical" twin study? Analysis of refractive error using monozygotic and dizygotic twins published in 1922. Twin Res Hum Genet. 2005;8:198–200.
8. Luft FC. Twins in cardiovascular genetic research. Hypertension. 2001;37(2): 350–6.
9. Nakanishi H, Yamada R, Gotoh N, et al. A genome-wide association analysis identified a novel susceptible locus for pathological myopia at 11q24.1. PLoS Genet; 2009. https://doi.org/10.137/journal.pgen.1000660.
10. Zippel R, Gnesutta N, Matus-Leibovitch N, et al. Ras-grf, the activator of ras, is expressed preferentially in mature neurons of the central nervous system. Brain Res Mol Brain Res. 1997;48:140–4.
11. Hysi PG, Young TL, Mackey DA. A genome-wide association study for myopia and refractive error identifies a susceptibility locus at 15q25. Nat Genet. 2010;42:902–5.
12. Shi Y, Gong B, Chen L, et al. A genome-wide meta-analysis identifies two novel loci associated with high myopia in the Han Chinese population. Hum Mol Genet. 2013;22:2325–33.
13. Tong L, Huang XL, Koh AL, Zhang X, Tan DT, Chua WH. Atropine for the treatment of childhood myopia: effect on myopia progression after cessation of atropine. Ophthalmology. 2009;116:572–9.
14. Mertz JR, Wallman J. Choroidal retinoic acid synthesis. A possible mediator between refractive error and compensatory eye growth. Exp Eye Res. 2000; 70:519–27.
15. Qiang Y, Li W, Wang Q, et al. Association study of 15q14 and 15q25 with high myopia in the Han Chinese population. BMC Genet. 2014;15:51.
16. Zhu JY, Rong WN, Jia Q, et al. Associations of single nucleotide polymorphisms of chromosomes 15q14, 15q25 and 13q12.12 regions with high myopic eyes in hui and Han population of Chinese Ningxia area. Chin J Exp Ophthalmol. 2014;32:354–8.
17. Jiao X, Wang P, Li S, et al. Association of markers at chromosome 15q14 in Chinese patients with moderate to high myopia. Mol Vis. 2012;18:2633–46.
18. Kihara AH, Paschon V, Cardoso CM, et al. Connexin36, an essential element in the rod pathway, is highly expressed in the essentially rodless retina of Gallus gallus. J Comp Neurol. 2009;512:651–63.
19. Striedinger K, Petrasch-Parwez E, Zoidl G, et al. Loss of connexin36 increases retinal cell vulnerability to secondary cell loss. Eur J Neurosci. 2005;22:605–16.
20. Young TL, Metlapally R, Shay AE. Complex trait genetics of refractive error. Arch Ophthalmol. 2007;125:38–48.
21. Fernández-Medarde A, et al. RasGRF1 disruption causes retinal photoreception defects and associated transcriptomic alterations. J Neurochem. 2009;110:641–52.
22. Neale MC, Cardon LR. Methodology for genetic studies of twins and families. NATO ASI series. Dordrech: Kluwer; 1992.
23. Hammond CJ, Snieder H, Gilbert CE, Spector TD. Genes and environment in refractive error: the twin eye study. Invest Ophthalmol Vis Sci. 2001;42: 1232–6.
24. Lyhne N, Sjolie AK, Kyvik KO, Green A. The importance of genes and environment for ocular refraction and its determiners: a population based study among 20–45 year old twins. Br J Ophthalmol. 2001;85:1470–6.
25. Dirani M, Chamberlain M, Shekar SN, et al. Heritability of refractive error and ocular biometrics: the genes in myopia (GEM) twin study. Invest Ophthalmol Vis Sci. 2006;47:4756–61.
26. Deans MR, Volgyi B, Goodenough DA, Bloomfield SA, Paul DL. Connexin36 is essential for transmission of rod-mediated visual signals in the mammalian retina. Neuron. 2002;36(4):703–12. https://doi.org/10.1016/S0896-6273(02)01046-2.
27. Chen T, Shan G, Ma J, Zhong Y. Polymorphism in the RASGRF1 gene with high myopia: a meta-analysis. Mol Vis. 2015;21:1272–80.

6

Visual field defects and retinal nerve fiber imaging in patients with obstructive sleep apnea syndrome and in healthy controls

Paula Casas[1*] (iD), Francisco J. Ascaso[1,3], Eugenio Vicente[2], Gloria Tejero-Garcés[2], María I. Adiego[2] and José A. Cristóbal[1]

Abstract

Background: To assess the retinal sensitivity in obstructive sleep apnea hypopnea syndrome (OSAHS) patients evaluated with standard automated perimetry (SAP). And to correlate the functional SAP results with structural parameters obtained with optical coherence tomography (OCT).

Methods: This prospective, observational, case-control study consisted of 63 eyes of 63 OSAHS patients (mean age 51.7 ± 12.7 years, best corrected visual acuity $\geq 20/25$, refractive error less than three spherical or two cylindrical diopters, and intraocular pressure < 21 mmHg) who were enrolled and compared with 38 eyes of 38 age-matched controls. Peripapillary retinal nerve fiber layer (RNFL) thickness was measured by Stratus OCT and SAP sensitivities and indices were explored with Humphrey Field Analyzer perimeter. Correlations between functional and structural parameters were calculated, as well as the relationship between ophthalmologic and systemic indices in OSAHS patients.

Results: OSAHS patients showed a significant reduction of the sensitivity for superior visual field division ($p = 0.034$, t-student test). When dividing the OSAHS group in accordance with the severity of the disease, nasal peripapillary RNFL thickness was significantly lower in severe OSAHS than that in controls and mild-moderate cases ($p = 0.031$ and $p = 0.016$ respectively, Mann-Whitney U test). There were no differences between groups for SAP parameters. We found no correlation between structural and functional variables. The central visual field sensitivity of the SAP revealed a poor Pearson correlation with the apnea-hipopnea index (0.284, $p = 0.024$).

Conclusions: Retinal sensitivity show minor differences between healthy subjects and OSAHS. Functional deterioration in OSAHS patients is not easy to demonstrate with visual field examination.

Keywords: Visual field, Automated perimetry exam, Optical coherence tomography, Obstructive sleep apnea syndrome, OSAHS

Background

Obstructive sleep apnea-hypopnea syndrome (OSAHS) is a disorder characterized by brief episodes of complete or partial upper airway collapse during sleep. When those apnea-hypopnea events sum five or more events per hour, a pathological breathing status appears. Numerous ophthalmological disorders seem to be associated with OSAHS, including floppy-eyelid syndrome or central serous chorioretinopathy. Moreover, some authors suggest that certain optic nerve (ON) disorders such as papilledema, glaucoma or non-arteritic anterior ischemic optic neuropathy showed an increased incidence in the obstructive disease [1–10].

Changes in the retinal nerve fiber layer (RNFL) thickness have been reported in OSAHS by multiple authors. These alterations appear even in individuals in whom glaucomatous neuropathy has been ruled out, proposing therefore the breathing disease could be "per se" an aggressive agent for the ON [11–16].

* Correspondence: paulacasaspascual@hotmail.com
[1]Department of Ophthalmology, Hospital Clínico Universitario "Lozano Blesa", San Juan Bosco 15, ES-50009 Zaragoza, Spain
Full list of author information is available at the end of the article

Studies describing the progression of the most common neuropathy in our specialty, glaucomatous neuropathy, have contributed to establish a relationship between the functional visual impairment and the structural damage of the ON [17, 18]. Other pathologies, as sclerosis multiple, also seem to have a good agreement and correlation between abnormalities detected by standard automated perimetry (SAP) and RNFL measurements, as Cheng et al. found in eyes with optic neuritis secondary to this cause [19].

The aim of this study was to investigate whether there is a visual field (VF) functional deficit in OSAHS patients compared to healthy individuals. And to study if there is a correlation between functional variables and structural (OCT) variables in OSAHS.

Methods

Eighty OSAHS patients were consecutively recruited in the Otolaryngology Department at the Hospital Miguel Servet, in Zaragoza, Spain. All patients had a newly discovered and previously untreated mild to severe OSAHS according to clinical features and apnea–hypopnea index (AHI) greater than 4. Before OSAHS was confirmed, patients completed a questionnaire concerning epidemiological data and information about symptoms such as loud snoring, observed apnea, or excessive daytime sleepiness. The most common vascular risk factors were studied and treated if necessary.

Patients were subsequently referred for an ophthalmological examination to the Ophthalmology Department at the Hospital Clínico Lozano Blesa in Zaragoza, Spain, between December 2010 and March 2012. Patients with history of stroke with central apnea, chronic uveitis, antiglaucomatous drug usage, optic neuropathy, ocular trauma or surgeries were excluded from this study. After appropriate information, written informed consent of all subjects was obtained. The research followed the tenets of the Declaration of Helsinki, and the protocol was approved by the local Ethics Committee.

The control group included 40 age-matched healthy subjects, who were recruited among relatives and employees at the Hospital Lozano Blesa. Selection was made with Berlin questionnaire (evaluating the functional signs of OSAHS, 86% sensitivity for diagnosis and 77% specificity) [20, 21]. Epidemiological data were collected and smoking habit and vascular risk factors were treated in the same way.

All OSAHS and controls underwent a complete ophthalmologic examination, including best-corrected visual acuity (BCVA), ocular motility, slit-lamp biomicroscopy, Goldmann applanation tonometry, gonioscopy, Humphrey automated VF, and OCT examination. Values of the right eyes were selected for analysis except when they did not fulfill the inclusion criteria; in this case, left eyes were selected.

At least two reliable SAP were performed to minimize the learning effect. VFs were evaluated with a Humphrey Field Analyzer perimeter model 740i (Zeiss Humphrey Systems, Dublin, CA) by using the 24–2 SITA fast strategy, with a Goldman size III stimulus on a 31.5-apostilb background. Near addition was added to the subject's refractive correction. If fixation losses were higher than 20% or false positive or false-negative rates were higher than 15%, the test was repeated. Each perimetry was performed on different days to avoid the fatigue effect and the same experienced examiner conducted all scans.

OCT was performed with the Stratus OCT (Carl Zeiss Meditec, Dublin, CA, USA) following 1% tropicamide instillation. Only high-quality images were included. Each patient underwent scans to measure peripapillary RNFL thickness, which was automatically calculated by the fast RNFL algorithm. We considered the overall thickness and per quadrant.

Examiners were masked to the diagnosis. All participants had a BCVA of 20/30 or better, with a refractive error lower than three spherical or two cylindrical diopters. Intraocular pressure (IOP) > 21 mmHg, posterior segment pathology or patients with media opacification were excluded. Regarding VF, eyes with defects compatible with glaucoma (nasal step, paracentral or arcuate scotomas, or arcuate blind spot enlargement) with a pattern standard deviation (PSD) significantly elevated beyond the 5% level and/or a Glaucoma Hemifield Test outside normal limits were also excluded.

For comparison we used Humphrey global indices such as mean deviation (MD) and PSD, and we also calculated mean sensitivity (MS) recording each of the threshold values in decibel scale. Sector MD was calculated by averaging the deviation values on total-deviation plots for each sector. To investigate correspondence between structure and function, we used a more simplified version of the topographic map obtained by Garway-Heath [17], proposed by Cheng et al. [19]. Nevertheless, we introduced some subtle variations on Cheng's map, like the use of all sensitivity points, including the blind spot ones (Fig. 1).

Statistical analysis

Data analysis was performed by using Statistical Package for Social Sciences software (version 19.0, Chicago, IL, USA). Values were presented as mean ± standard deviation, and expressed in microns for the peripapillary RNFL thickness and in decibels for the VF sensitivities. Qualitative differences between the studied variables were assessed by using Pearson's chi-squared test.

Differences between controls and OSAHS were tested by Student's-t test when normality and equality of variances were proved. If these conditions were not satisfied, the non-parametric Mann-Whitney U test was used.

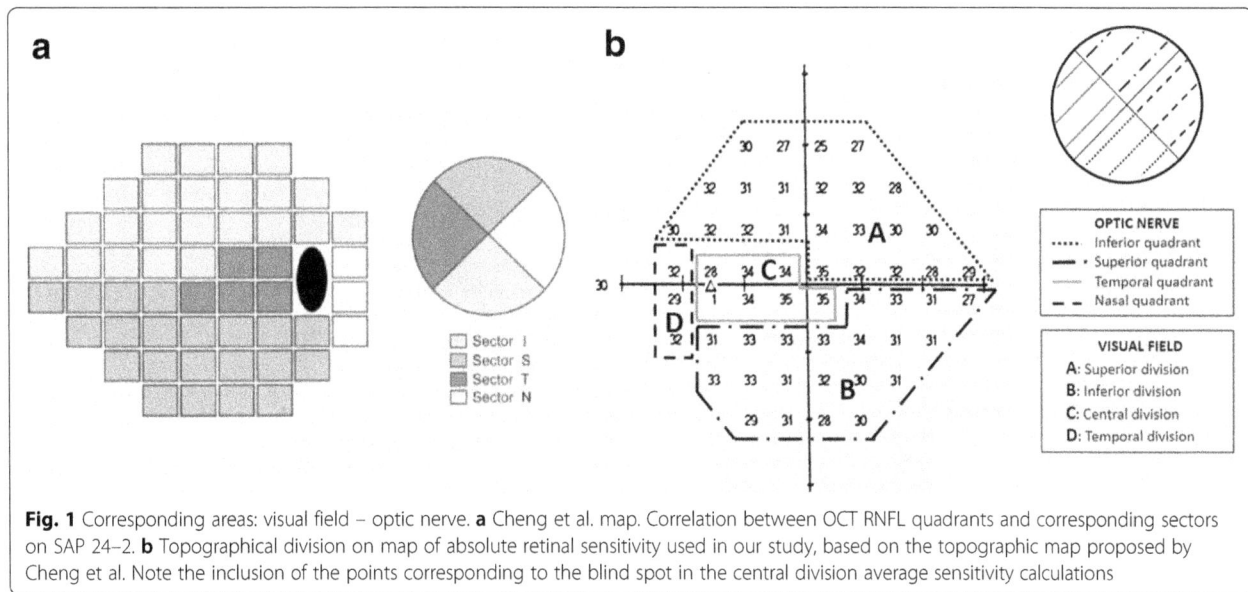

Fig. 1 Corresponding areas: visual field – optic nerve. **a** Cheng et al. map. Correlation between OCT RNFL quadrants and corresponding sectors on SAP 24–2. **b** Topographical division on map of absolute retinal sensitivity used in our study, based on the topographic map proposed by Cheng et al. Note the inclusion of the points corresponding to the blind spot in the central division average sensitivity calculations

In a second analysis, OSAHS sample was divided according to severity into two groups: those with mild-moderate OSAHS (group 1, AHI ≥5 and < 30) and those with severe OSAHS (group 2, AHI ≥30). Both groups were compared to controls. Quantitative differences between the three groups were compared by using one-way ANOVA test, once normality and homogeneity was proved with Shapiro-Wilk and Levene's tests. In the event of breach of the homogeneity and normality assumption, the non-parametric Kruskal-Wallis H test was applied. In those cases where differences had been statistically significant, two by two Scheffé comparison (after ANOVA test) or Mann-Whitney U analysis (after Kruskal-Wallis H test) were performed to know which groups were different.

The relationship between structural and functional variables were analyzed by applying linear, logarithmic, inverse, quadratic and cubic models in OSAHS and in controls separately. In addition, Pearson's correlation coefficient between AHI and VF indices in OSAHS were evaluated. A p value < 0.05 was considered statistically significant.

Results

Of 80 consecutive OSAHS who accepted to participate, 63 patients (66.9%) were included in the study (51 right eyes and 12 left eyes), whereas 36 patients (33.1%) were excluded. Twenty-nine patients had a mild-moderate OSAHS (46%), and the other 34 patients (54%) had a severe disorder.

In the control group, 40 individuals classified as "low risk subjects" by the Berlin questionnaire were examined. Two patients were excluded after exclusion criteria application, and finally the group was composed of 37 right eyes and one left eye of 38 healthy subjects.

Age showed no statistically significant difference between groups, neither when dividing the OSAHS group according to its severity. In OSAHS group, although more men than women were enrolled, we did not consider this difference because gender has no effect on RNFL thickness as previously mentioned [22]. Body mass index was not matched, and was higher in OSAHS than that in controls ($p < 0.001$). Nevertheless, no significant differences in vascular risk factors (hypertension, diabetes and dyslipidemia) and prevalence of smoking habit between cases and controls were found.

Table 1 shows the results of IOP, peripapillary RNFL thickness and VF parameters in controls and OSAHS. Differences between groups were just found in the VF superior division, sensitivity was higher in healthy subjects than in OSAHS ones. MD showed results close to the statistical significance.

Table 2 shows the results of IOP and peripapillary RNFL thickness measurements by dividing OSAHS patients according to severity. IOP showed no differences between groups. Nasal quadrant of peripapillary RNFL thickness showed a difference between categories. Thus, nasal RNFL thickness was significantly lower in severe OSAHS than that in moderate OSAHS ($p = 0.031$, Mann-Whitney U test). Moreover, nasal RNFL thickness was thinner in severe OSAHS versus controls ($p = 0.016$, Mann-Whitney U test).

Humphrey VF results showed no differences between controls and severity of OSAHS groups (Table 3). VF superior division showed a nonstatistical trend (0.08, ANOVA test). This difference was not statistically significant when we applied a multiple comparison test: $p = 0.11$ in controls versus mild-moderates; $p = 0.295$ in controls versus severes; and $p = 0.834$ in mild-moderates versus severes (Scheffé post hoc test).

Table 1 Comparison of IOP, RNFL thickness and Humphrey VF parameters between controls and OSAHS patients

Variable	CONTROLS (N = 38)	OSAHS (N = 63)	p-value
IOP	15.1 ± 2.1 [10–19]	15.7 ± 2.8 [10–22]	0.218[*]
Average RNFL	98.60 ± 10.95 [68.86–117.54]	98.79 ± 10.55 [76–125.33]	0.932[*]
RNFL superior Quadrant	119.89 ± 19.32 [69–159]	123.17 ± 16.35 [85–162]	0.385[*]
RNFL nasal Quadrant	80.08 ± 16.92 [52–126]	74.86[†] ± 15.86 [47–117]	0.128[*]
RNFL inferior Quadrant	124.21 ± 13.71 [93–160]	123.84 ± 17.29 [91–166]	0.906[*]
RNFL temporal Quadrant	70.24 ± 12.33 [47–93]	73.30 ± 13.14 [45–101]	0.241[*]
Average sensitivity	29.74 ± 1.31[†] [26.59–31.87]	29.3 ± 1.46 [23.9–32.03]	0.097[†]
VF superior division	30.05 ± 1.54 [27.04–32.91]	29.37 ± 1.56 [25.08–32.3]	0.034[*]
VF inferior division	31.13 ± 1.43[†] [27.28–32.91]	30.89 ± 1.37 [26.57–33.66]	0.211[†]
VF central division	27.59 ± 1.44 [23.28–31.14]	27.43 ± 1.83 [24–32.14]	0.406[†]
VF temporal división	30.19 ± 2.0 [25.67–33.33]	29.49[†] ± 2.75 [13–33]	0.145[†]
VFI	99.16[†] ± 0.85 [97–100]	98.97[†] ± 0.983 [96–100]	0.361[†]
MD	0.04 ± 1.13 [(− 2.78) − 1.79]	−0.389 ± 1.2 [(− 3.75) − 1.65]	0.07[*]
PSD	1.52[†] ± 0.3 [0.96–2.64]	1.61[†] ± 0.67 [0.9–5.93]	0.955[†]

IOP intraocular pressure, RNFL retinal nerve fiber layer, VF visual field, VFI visual field index, MD mean deviation, PSD pattern standard deviation, N number of eyes
[*]T-student test (p value < 0.05). Normal distribution confirmed (Shapiro-Wilk)
[†]U Mann-Whitney test. No normal distribution confirmed (Shapiro-Wilk)

Table 2 Comparison of IOP and RNFL thickness measurements between controls, mild, moderate and severe OSAHS patients

	Severity	Average ± SD [Min-Max]	Normality S-W p-value	Homogeneity Levene Test p-value	ANOVA/Kruskall W F	ANOVA/Kruskall W p-value
IOP	Control (N = 38)	15.1 ± 2.1 [10–19]	0.222	0.22	0.73	0.48[*]
	Mild-Moderate (N = 29)	15.6 ± 2.6 [11–22]	0.138			
	Severe (N = 34)	15.8 ± 3 [10–21]	0.135			
Average RNFL	Control (N = 38)	98.6 ± 10.9 [68.9–117.5]	0.617	0.78	2.13	0.12[*]
	Mild-Moderate (N = 29)	101.8 ± 10.4 [82.2–125.3]	0.651			
	Severe (N = 34)	96.3 ± 10.1 [76–118]	0.684			
RNFL superior quadrant	Control (N = 38)	119.9 ± 19.3 [69–159]	0.914	0.13	0.58	0.56[*]
	Mild-Moderate (N = 29)	124.5 ± 13.6 [85–160]	0.215			
	Severe (N = 34)	122 ± 18.4 [90–162]	0.695			
RNFL nasal quadrant	Control (N = 38)	80.1 ± 16.9 [52–126]	0.126	0.21	/	0.029[†]
	Mild-Moderate (N = 29)	79.0 ± 17.0 [47–117]	0.533			
	Severe (N = 34)	71.3 ± 14.1 [49–115]	0.05			
RNFL inferior quadrant	Control (N = 38)	124.2 ± 13.7 [93–160]	0.829	0.07	1.92	0.15[*]
	Mild-Moderate (N = 29)	128.1 ± 19.9 [91–166]	0.688			
	Severe (N = 34)	120.2 ± 13.9 [92–163]	0.398			
RNFL temporal quadrant	Control (N = 38)	70.2 ± 12.3 [47–93]	0.410	0.91	1.34	0.27[*]
	Mild-Moderate (N = 29)	75.3 ± 12.6 [51–101]	0.910			
	Severe (N = 34)	71.6 ± 13.5 [45–100]	0.272			

IOP intraocular pressure, RNFL retinal nerve fiber layer, S-W Shapiro-Wilk, Kruskall W Kruskall Wallis, N number of eyes
[*]ANOVA test
[†]Kruskal Wallis (p value < 0.05)

Table 3 Comparison of Humphrey visual field sensitivities and indices between controls, mild, moderate and severe OSAHS patients

	Severity	Average ± SD [Min - Max]	Normality S-W p-value	Homogeneity Test Levene p-value	ANOVA / Kruskall W F	ANOVA / Kruskall W p-value
Average sensitivity (dB)	Control (N = 38)	29.7 ± 1.3 [26.6–31.8]	0.04	0.61	/	0.2[†]
	Mild- Moderate (N = 29)	29.1 ± 1.6 [23.9–31.1]	0.4			
	Severe (N = 34)	29.4 ± 1.3 [26.0–32]	0.61			
VF superior division (dB)	Control (N = 38)	30.1 ± 1.5 [27–32.9]	0.158	0.83	2.49	0.08[*]
	Mild- Moderate (N = 29)	29.2 ± 1.6 [26.3–32.2]	0.7			
	Severe (N = 34)	29.5 ± 1.5 [25.1–32.3]	0.19			
VF inferior division (dB)	Control (N = 38)	31.1 ± 1.4 [27.3–33.3]	0.01	0.62	/	0.46[†]
	Mild- Moderate (N = 29)	30.9 ± 1.3 [26.6–32.9]	0.008			
	Severe (N = 34)	30.9 ± 1.4 [27.6–33.7]	0.91			
VF central division (dB)	Control (N = 38)	27.6 ± 1.4 [23.3–31.1]	0.46	0.11	0.73	0.49[*]
	Mild- Moderate (N = 29)	27.2 ± 1.6 [24.3–31.4]	0.49			
	Severe (N = 34)	27.6 ± 2.0 [24–32.1]	0.17			
VF temporal division (dB)	Control (N = 38)	30.2 ± 2 [25.7–33.3]	0.06	0.08	/	0.34[†]
	Mild- Moderate (N = 29)	29.7 ± 1.9 [26.3–33]	0.03			
	Severe (N = 34)	29.8 ± 1.7 [25.3–33]	0.33			
VFI (dB)	Control (N = 38)	99.2 ± 0.8 [97–100]	< 0.001	0.63	/	0.6[†]
	Mild- Moderate (N = 29)	98.9 ± 1.0 [96–100]	0.001			
	Severe (N = 34)	99.0 ± 0.9 [97–100]	< 0.001			
MD (dB)	Control (N = 38)	0.04 ± 1.1 [(−2.8) − 1.8]	0.08	0.92	1.66	0.19[*]
	Mild- Moderate (N = 29)	−0.4 ± 1.12 [(−2.5) − 1.6]	0.21			
	Severe (N = 34)	−0.4 ± 1.2 [(−3.8) - 1.7]	0.44			
PSD (dB)	Control (N = 38)	1.5 ± 0.3 [0.9–2.6]	0.01	0.1	/	0.97[†]
	Mild- Moderate (N = 29)	1.6 ± 0.9 [1.0–5.9]	0.002			
	Severe (N = 34)	1.6 ± 0.4 [0.9–2.8]	< 0.001			

VF visual field, VFI visual field index, MD mean deviation, PSD pattern standard deviation, S-W Shapiro-Wilk, Kruskall W Kruskall Wallis, N number of eyes
[*]ANOVA test
[†]Kruskal Wallis

A relationship between functional and structural ON parameters in both, OSAHS and controls, was not demonstrated. Table 4 shows linear, logarithmic, inverse, quadratic and cubic correlation models between linear parameters, as the thickness of peripapillary RNFL quadrants and parameters expressed in logarithmic scale such as VF sensitivities.

Only the central VF sensitivity of the SAP revealed a poor correlation with the AHI, with a Pearson's correlation coefficient of 0.284 ($p = 0.024$, Fig. 2).

Discussion

The low oxygen levels during sleep lead to the adrenergic system activation, inflammation and procoagulant mechanisms prompting to endothelial dysfunction, oxidative stress and metabolic deregulation [23]. This vascular phenomenon may compromise ON perfusion and oxygenation, ultimately leading to optic neuropathy [24, 25].

Several authors, including our own group, have published RNFL thickness variations in individuals with sleep apnea [11–16], which could be a consequence of vascular and gasometric alterations triggered by OSAHS.

Peripapillary RNFL thickness reflects neuronal axons, and would allow quantification of ganglion cell axonal loss [26]. Moreover, VF values estimates functional loss of the whole visual pathway, from retina to cortex [27]. VF maps show a correspondence with neuronal distribution of RNFL in the ON head, as Garway et al. demonstrated [17]. Therefore, theoretically, a correlation between OCT and VF parameters could be found. If this correspondence appears, both OCT and VF could be potentially used as biomarkers for neuronal degeneration in OSAHS patients.

Sensitivity of superior VF division was significantly lower in OSAHS patients than that in controls. This finding is not consistent with a significant change of inferior peripapillary RNFL thickness, which corresponds topographically

Table 4 Correlation models between structural and functional optic nerve variables in OSAHS patients

Regression model	OSAHS (N = 63)		CONTROLS (N = 38)		OSAHS (N = 63)		CONTROLS (N = 38)	
	R^2	F Test (p-value)	R^2	F Test (p-value)	R^2	F Test (p-value)	R^2	F Test (p-value)
	RNFL inferior quadrant (μm) – VF superior división (dB)				RNFL Superior quadrant (μm) – VF inferior división (dB)			
Lineal	0.042	0.106	0.04	0.226	0.054	0.068	0.002	0.777
Logarithmic	0.049	0.083	0.046	0.196	0.047	0.087	0.006	0.631
Inverse	0.054	0.066	0.052	0.169	0.04	0.117	0.014	0.484
Quadratic	0.076	0.095	0.067	0.294	0.071	0.11	0.054	0.376
Cubic	0.077	0.090	0.067	0.294	0.07	0.114	0.054	0.376
	RNFL nasal quadrant (μm) - VF temporal división (dB)				RNFL temporal quadrant (μm) - VF central división (dB)			
Lineal	0.014	0.362	0.006	0.644	0.004	0.642	0.001	0.831
Logarithmic	0.008	0.48	0.01	0.547	0.005	0.580	0.003	0.76
Inverse	0.004	0.622	0.015	0.468	0.007	0.518	0.004	0.709
Quadratic	0.045	0.25	0.048	0.421	0.012	0.691	0.045	0.447
Cubic	0.055	0.339	0.05	0.62	0.012	0.691	0.052	0.393
	Average RNFL (μm) – MD (dB)				Average RNFL (μm) - Average sensitivity (dB)			
Lineal	0.005	0,585	0.011	0.531	0.007	0.514	0.008	0.584
Logarithmic	/	/	/	/	0.008	0.489	0.01	0.557
Inverse	0.017	0.309	0.001	0.861	0.009	0.469	0.011	0.533
Quadratic	0.046	0.241	0.044	0.453	0.014	0.663	0.074	0.261
Cubic	0.061	0.291	0.046	0.658	0.014	0.66	0.075	0.255

RNFL Retinal nerve fiber layer, *MD* mean deviation, *VF* visual field. *N* number of eyes

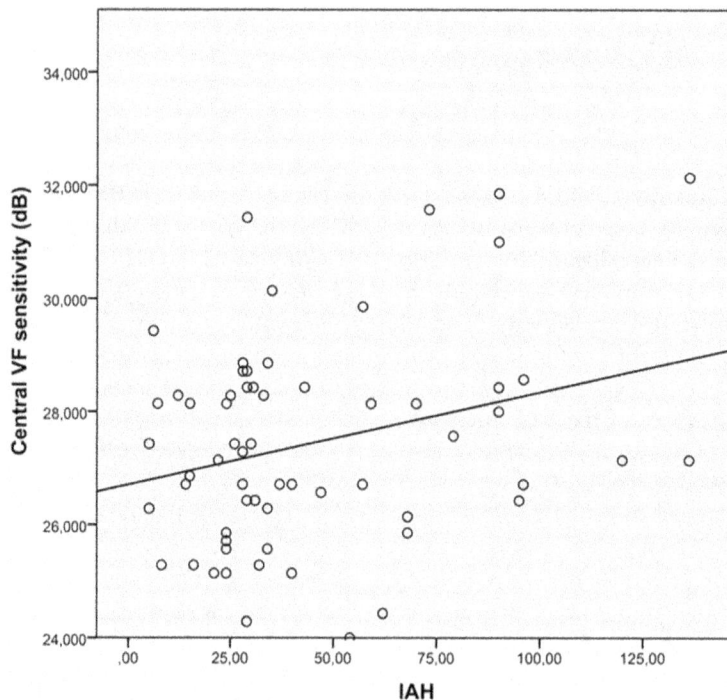

Fig. 2 Pearson's correlation coefficient (0.284, p = 0.024) between central VF sensitivity and AHI

with superior VF division and would justify the functional decline. Subtle edema secondary to vascular deregulation and increase in cerebrospinal fluid pressure [13, 28, 29] could explain the VF alterations found in our patients, and the fact that reduction in sensitivity is not associated with a decrease in RNFL thickness. As we previously suggested [14], it is possible that analysing all ranges of OSAHS severity together imply masking certain ON structural alterations. Theoretically, a first stage of edema and inflammation in mild and intermediate stages of the respiratory disease would precede an atrophy phase. We should, therefore, think that the biggest differences will be found in the most serious cases, where the decline of the RNFL will be triggered by longer exposure to hypoxia, and will be logical find higher degrees of atrophy. This fact is reflected in nasal quadrant RNFL thickness, where we found differences between severe OSAHS and the other groups. Another possible theory explaining the functional loss without structural alteration is the association of OSAHS with floppy eyelid syndrome [30–32]. A fatigue-related ptosis could reduce superior visual field acting as an artefact, as the 'normal' OCT inferior RNFL thickness confirms.

On the other hand, VF parameters showed no differences in the two by two comparisons between OSAHS groups and controls. This result contrasts with those obtained by other authors. Thus, Huseyinoglu et al. [13] found higher PSD and lower MD values in OSAHS patients comparing to controls. Xin et al. and Tsang et al. [29, 33] found affected values of MD and PSD in OSAHS comparing with controls. Nevertheless, they did not exclude any case of glaucoma and that could generate a bias in their results. Ferrandez et al. [34] found a generalized decrease in retinal sensitivity without focal defects in OSAHS. Furthermore, they reported changes in MD, PSD and VFI values with worse scores in patients with apnea. Disparities between their results and ours could be justified by different examination strategies used. We have chosen a shorter VF strategy to explore the patients since we know that "fatigue effect" could modify VF outcomes [33, 35] and is more prevalent in OSAHS patients [36–38], even when the SAP reliability criteria were kept within normal limits. We could observe a considerable difficulty to some OSAHS patients to maintain the concentration for 4 to 8 min for VF completion. Because of this, we decided to perform SITA-fast strategies in the present study, in spite of this shorter algorithm is known to improve the mean defect and to be less precise compared to SITA standard [39]. It is likely that hypersomnia, which is one of the crucial symptoms of the disease, could act as a confounding factor during VF examination, obtaining lower sensitivity rates comparing to controls, especially in longer examinations.

Regarding structure-function analysis, the absence of a common scale for both measurements, logarithmic on one side (decibels) and decimal on the other one (microns or percentages), makes it difficult to draw a parallel relationship between both examinations. There is a controversy regarding the type of association between structural and functional variables. Thus, various publications assume a linear correlation when both parameters are expressed in a linear scale, and an exponential or curvilinear relationship when one of the variables is linear whereas the other one is expressed in a logarithmic scale [40, 41]. Conversely, other authors hardly found any differences between structure-function correlations when the latter was expressed in logarithmic or linear scale [42, 43]. Based on this, our research analyses the association applying linear and non-linear models.

Special interest would have the correlation between the nasal quadrant of RNFL thickness and temporal VF division, since we found statistically significant differences for the structural parameter. Relationship between RNFL thickness quantified with Stratus OCT and VF MD was better fitted with second-order polynomials than with a linear model in patients with glaucoma [41]. These regression models describe a curvilinear relationship, suggesting that progression of VF loss, when it is expressed in MD, increases during the course of the disease. This idea is compatible with the concept of "functional reserve", i.e. there must be a significant structural damage to bring up a functional representation of the same in the VF [19, 44–47]. Therefore, the absence of correlation found in the present study may be a consequence of the perimetric exclusion criteria, by which all eyes with suggestive alterations of glaucomatous neuropathy were excluded from the analysis.

One of the strengths of our study is that we just included patients with normal IOP, normal gonioscopy, and no perimetric evidence of glaucomatous neuropathy, in order to assess a hypothetical reduction in retinal sensitivity produced exclusively by the respiratory disorder. In this way, we avoid biased results by the inclusion of glaucomatous patients, whose incidence, as we have already mentioned, is higher in patients suffering from apnea [7–10]. The main limitation of our study include the relatively small sample size, mainly when OSAHS were divided according to severity. Groups with larger number of patients could have shown some correlation between variables or more consistent conclusions.

Conclusions

In conclusion, due to the lack of association between variables and no significant differences in VF variables when dividing OSAHS patients, we cannot state that perimetry is a useful diagnostic tool to demonstrate functional deterioration in OSAHS. Moreover, future research should analyze the results obtained in patients with OSAHS prior and after effective treatment, to establish the real VF involvement in the apneic disorder.

Abbreviations

AHI: Apnea–hypopnea index; BCVA: Best-corrected visual acuity; MD: Mean deviation; MS: Mean sensitivity; OCT: Optical coherence tomography; ON: Optic nerve; OSAHS: Obstructive sleep apnea hypopnea syndrome; PSD: Pattern standard deviation; RNFL: Retinal nerve fiber layer; SAP: Standard automated perimetry; VF: Visual field

Acknowledgements

Not applicable

Funding

The authors certify that they have NO affiliations with or involvement in any organization or entity with any financial interest (such as honoraria; educational grants; participation in speakers' bureaus; membership, employment, consultancies, stock ownership, or other equity interest; and expert testimony or patent-licensing arrangements), or non-financial interest (such as personal or professional relationships, affiliations, knowledge or beliefs) in the subject matter or materials discussed in this manuscript.

Authors' contributions

PC acquired and analyzed the data. Moreover she wrote the main ideas of the work. FJA helped with the data interpretation. Moreover, he edited the final work. EV selected the OSAHS patients and acquired othorrinolaringologic data. GTG acquired the data and helped write the main ideas. MIA designed the work. JAC helped with the data interpretation. Moreover, he edited the final work. We confirm that the manuscript has been read and approved by all named authors.

Competing interests

The authors declare that they have no competing interests.

Author details

[1]Department of Ophthalmology, Hospital Clínico Universitario "Lozano Blesa", San Juan Bosco 15, ES-50009 Zaragoza, Spain. [2]Department of Otolaryngology, Hospital Universitario "Miguel Servet", Zaragoza, Spain. [3]Instituto de Investigación Sanitaria Aragón (IIS Aragón), Zaragoza, Spain.

References

1. Karger RA, White WA, Park WC, et al. Prevalence of floppy eyelid syndrome in obstructive sleep apnea-hypopnea syndrome. Ophthalmology. 2006;113: 1669–74.
2. Leroux les Jardins G, Glacet-Bernard A, Lasry S, Housset B, Coscas G, Soubrane G. Retinal vein occlusion and obstructive sleep apnea syndrome. J Fr Ophtalmol. 2009;32:420–4.
3. Jain AK, Kaines A, Schwartz S. Bilateral central serous chorioretinopathy resolving rapidly with treatment for obstructive sleep apnea. Graefes Arch Clin Exp Ophthalmol. 2010;248:1037–9.
4. Kloos P, Laube I, Thoelen. Obstructive sleep apnea in patients with central serous chorioretinopathy. Graefes Arch Clin Exp Ophthalmol. 2008;246:1225–8.
5. Purvin VA, Kawasaki A, Yee RD. Papilledema and obstructive sleep apnea syndrome. Arch Ophthalmol. 2000;118:1626–30.
6. Palombi K, Renard E, Levy P, et al. Non-arteritic anterior ischaemic optic neuropathy is nearly systematically associated with obstructive sleep apnoea. Br J Ophthalmol. 2006;90:879–82.
7. Mojon DS, Hess CW, Goldblum D, et al. High prevalence of glaucoma in patients with sleep apnea syndrome. Ophthalmology. 1999;106:1009–12.
8. Mojon DS, Hess CW, Goldblum D, Böhnke M, Körner F, Mathis J. Primary open-angle glaucoma is associated with sleep apnea syndrome. Ophthalmologica. 2000;214:115–8.
9. Bendel RE, Kaplan J, Heckman M, Fredrickson PA, Lin SC. Prevalence of glaucoma in patients with obstructive sleep apnoea—a cross-sectional case-series. Eye (Lond). 2008;22:1105–9.
10. Faridi O, Park SC, Liebmann JM, Ritch R. Glaucoma and obstructive sleep apnoea syndrome. Clin Exp Ophthalmol. 2012;40:408–19.
11. Lin PW, Friedman M, Lin HC, Chang HW, Pulver TM, Chin CH. Decreased retinal nerve fiber layer thickness in patients with obstructive sleep apnea/ hypopnea syndrome. Graefes Arch Clin Exp Ophthalmol. 2011;249:585–93.
12. Sagiv O, Fishelson-Arev T, Buckman G, et al. Retinal nerve fiber layer thickness measurements by optical coherence tomography in patients with sleep apnea syndrome. Clin Exp Ophthalmol. 2014;42:132–8.
13. Huseyinoglu N, Ekinci M, Ozben S, Buyukuysal C, Kale MY, Sanivar HS. Optic disc and retinal nerve fiber layer parameters as indicators of neurodegenerative brain changes in patients with obstructive sleep apnea syndrome. Sleep Breath. 2014;18:95–102.
14. Casas P, Ascaso FJ, Vicente E, Tejero-Garcés G, Adiego MI, Cristóbal JA. Retinal and optic nerve evaluation by optical coherence tomography in adults with obstructive sleep apnea-hypopnea syndrome (OSAHS). Graefes Arch Clin Exp Ophthalmol. 2013;251:1625–34.
15. Shiba T, Takahashi M, Sato Y, et al. Relationship between severity of obstructive sleep apnea syndrome and retinal nerve fiber layer thickness. Am J Ophthalmol. 2014;157:1202–8.
16. Kargi SH, Altin R, Koksal M, et al. Retinal nerve fibre layer measurements are reduced in patients with obstructive sleep apnoea syndrome. Eye (Lond). 2005;19:575–9.
17. Garway-Heath DF, Poinoosawmy D, Fitzke FW, Hitchings RA. Mapping the visual field to the optic disc in normal tension glaucoma eyes. Ophthalmology. 2000;107:1809–15.
18. Ferreras A, Pablo LE, Garway-Heath DF, Fogagnolo P, García-Feijoo J. Mapping standard automated perimetry to the peripapillary retinal nerve fiber layer in glaucoma. Invest Ophthalmol Vis Sci. 2008;49:3018–25.
19. Cheng H, Laron M, Schiffman JS, Tang RA, Frishman LJ. The relationship between visual field and retinal nerve fiber layer measurements in patients with multiple sclerosis. Invest Ophthalmol Vis Sci. 2007;48:5798–805.
20. Netzer NC, Stoohs RA, Netzer CM, Clark K, Strohl KP. Using the Berlin questionnaire to identify patients at risk for the sleep apnea syndrome. Ann Intern Med. 1999;131:485–91.
21. Sharma SK, Sinha S, Banga A, Pandey RM, Handa KK. Validation of the modified Berlin questionnaire to identify patients at risk for the obstructive sleep apnoea syndrome. Indian J Med Res. 2006;124:281–90.
22. Bowd C, Zangwill LM, Blumenthal EZ, et al. Imaging of the optic disc and retinal nerve fiber layer: effects of age, optic disc area, refractive error and gender. J Opt Soc Am A Opt Image Sci Vis. 2002;19:197–207.
23. Shahar E, Whitney CW, Redline S, et al. Sleep-disordered breathing and cardiovascular disease: cross sectional results of the sleep heart health study. Am J Respir Crit Care Med. 2001;163:19–25.
24. Anderson DR. Glaucoma, capillaries and pericytes. 1. Blood flow regulation. Ophthalmologica. 1996;210:257–62.
25. Karakucuk S, Goktas S, Aksu M, et al. Ocular blood flow in patients with obstructive sleep apnea syndrome (OSAS). Graefes Arch Clin Exp Ophthalmol. 2008;246:129–34.
26. Budenz DL, Anderson DR, Varma R, et al. Determinants of normal retinal nerve fiber layer thickness measured by Stratus OCT. Ophthalmology. 2007; 114:1046–52.
27. Xie K, Liu CY, Hasso AN, Crow RW. Visual field changes as an early indicator of glioblastoma multiforme progression: two cases of functional vision changes before MRI detection. Clin Ophthalmol. 2015;9:1041–7.
28. Bucci FA Jr, Krohel GB. Optic nerve swelling secondary to the obstructive sleep apnea syndrome. Am J Ophthalmol. 1988;105:428–30.
29. Xin C, Zhang W, Wang L, Yang D, Wang J. Changes of visual field and optic nerve fiber layer in patients with OSAS. Sleep Breath. 2015;19:129–34.
30. McNab AA. The eye and sleep apnea. Sleep Med Rev. 2007;11:269–76.
31. West SD, Turnbull C. Eye disorders associated with obstructive sleep apnoea. Curr Opin Pulm Med. 2016;22:595-601.
32. Leibovitch I, Selva D. Floppy eyelid syndrome: clinical features and the association with obstructive sleep apnea. Sleep Med. 2006;7:117–22.
33. Tsang CS, Chong SL, Ho CK, Li MF. Moderate to severe obstructive sleep apnoea patients is associated with a higher incidence of visual field defect. Eye. 2006;20:38–42.
34. Ferrandez B, Ferreras A, Calvo P, et al. Retinal sensitivity is reduced in patients with obstructive sleep apnea. Invest Ophthalmol Vis Sci. 2014;55: 7119–25.
35. Gonzalez de la Rosa M, Pareja A. Influence of the "fatigue effect" on the mean deviation measurement in perimetry. Eur J Ophthalmol. 1997;7:29–34.
36. Jurádo-Gámez B, Guglielmi O, Gude-Sampedro F, Buela-Casal G. Effect of CPAP therapy on job productivity and psychosocial occupational health in patients with moderate to severe sleep apnea. Sleep Breath. 2015;19:1293–9.

37. Tippin J, Sparks J, Rizzo M. Visual vigilance in drivers with obstructive sleep apnea. J Psychosom Res. 2009;67:143–51.
38. Bjornsdottir E, Keenan BT, Eysteinsdottir B, et al. Quality of life among untreated sleep apnea patients compared with the general population and changes after treatment with positive airway pressure. J Sleep Res. 2015;24: 328–38.
39. Saunders LJ, Russell RA, Crabb DP. Measurement precision in a series of visual fields acquired by the standard and fast versions of the Swedish interactive thresholding algorithm: analysis of large-scale data from clinics. JAMA Ophthalmol. 2015;133:74–80.
40. Hood DC. Relating retinal nerve fiber thickness to behavioral sensitivity in patients with glaucoma: application of a linear model. J Opt Soc Am A Opt Image Sci Vis. 2007;24:1426–30.
41. Leung CK, Chong KK, Chan WM, et al. Comparative study of retinal nerve fiber layer measurement by Stratus OCT and GDx VCC, II: structure/function regression analysis in glaucoma. Invest Ophthalmol Vis Sci. 2005;46:3702–11.
42. Nilforushan N, Nassiri N, Moghimi S, et al. Structure-function relationships between spectral-domain OCT and standard achromatic perimetry. Invest Ophthalmol Vis Sci. 2012;53:2740–8.
43. Bowd C, Zangwill LM, Medeiros FA, et al. Structure-function relationships using confocal scanning laser ophthalmoscopy, optical coherence tomography, and scanning laser polarimetry. Invest Ophthalmol Vis Sci. 2006;47:2889–95.
44. Ajtony C, Balla Z, Somoskeoy S, Kovacs B. Relationship between visual field sensitivity and retinal nerve fiber layer thickness as measured by optical coherence tomography. Invest Ophthalmol Vis Sci. 2007;48:258–63.
45. Costello F, Coupland S, Hodge W, et al. Quantifying axonal loss after optic neuritis with optical coherence tomography. Ann Neurol. 2006;59:963–9.
46. Nouri-Mahdavi K, Hoffman D, Tannenbaum DP, Law SK, Caprioli J. Identifying early glaucoma with optical coherence tomography. Am J Ophthalmol. 2004;137:228–35.
47. Bowd C, Weinreb RN, Williams JM, Zangwill LM. The retinal nerve fiber layer thickness in ocular hypertensive, normal, and glaucomatous eyes with optical coherence tomography. Arch Ophthalmol. 2000;118:22–6.

7

Usage of glaucoma-specific patient-reported outcome measures (PROMs) in the Singapore context: a qualitative scoping exercise

Owen Kim Hee[1*†], Zheng-Xian Thng[1†], Hong-Yuan Zhu[1] and Ecosse Luc Lamoureux[2]

Abstract

Background: Despite the increasing emphasis on the role of glaucoma-specific patient-reported outcome measures (PROMs) as relevant outcome measures for the impact of glaucoma and its intervention on patients' daily lives, the feasibility of implementing PROMs in the routine clinical setting in Singapore remains undefined. We aim to evaluate the comprehensibility, acceptability, and relevance of four glaucoma-specific PROMs at healthcare professionals' and patients' level in a Singapore context.

Methods: Sixteen ophthalmic healthcare professionals and 24 glaucoma patients, with average age 60 years (SD = 15), were invited from a tertiary hospital in Singapore. Semi-structured interviews were conducted to explore participants' perceptions on the content and administration of four glaucoma-specific PROMs - the Glaucoma Quality of Life-15, Glaucoma Symptom Identifier, Independent Mobility Questionnaire and Treatment Satisfaction Survey of Intra-ocular Pressure. Semi-structured interviews were hand transcribed, and analysed thematically. Each participant filled out a feasibility survey at the end of interview.

Results: 79% of glaucoma patients and 94% of glaucoma healthcare professionals felt selected PROMs relevant to patients. 63% of glaucoma patients and 50% of healthcare professionals felt that selected PROMs were sufficiently comprehensive for clinical use. 46% of glaucoma patients and 56% of healthcare professionals felt selected PROMs were user-friendly.

Conclusions: Using PROMs in the Singapore clinical setting receives promising support from both healthcare professionals and patients. The identified potential barriers tailored to Singapore clinical setting will help successful implementation of PROMs into routine clinical care.

Keywords: Glaucoma, Patient-reported outcome measures, Questionnaire

Background

Important aim of quality health care is the patient-centeredness and a focus on patient experience [1]. However, healthcare professionals have traditionally defined "successful glaucoma treatment" based on objective clinical endpoints such as lowering of intraocular pressure (IOP) and slowing or stopping visual field deterioration [2]. These clinical measures may result in more disease-centric care as opposed to more patient-centric care which requires a more holistic view of care delivery, since they only surrogate measures of an effective treatment paradigm, and cannot fully capture the actual impact of glaucoma and its treatment on patients' daily lives [3, 4], considering the chronic progressive nature of glaucoma and its potential to substantially and negatively affect patient's daily functioning [5]. Furthermore, insights into how glaucoma affects patients' lives might provide a means of tailoring treatment strategies to meet the individual's specific need [5].

* Correspondence: Owen_Hee@ttsh.com.sg

[†]Owen Kim Hee and Zheng-Xian Thng contributed equally to this work. Owen Kim Hee and Zheng-Xian Thng are co-first authors.

[1]National Healthcare Group Eye Institute, Tan Tock Seng Hospital, S308433, Singapore, Singapore

Full list of author information is available at the end of the article

The increasing realization that clinical parameters alone are inadequate to assess health outcomes has resulted in the widespread use of patient-reported outcome measures (PROMs) [6]. PROMs are a series of standardised and validated questions self-reported by patients to assess their perspectives on the impact of diseases and treatment on their own health status, well-being and functioning [6–8]. Especially disease-specific PROMs, as the gold standard for relevant endpoint measures of patients' subjective experiences, are important to clinicians as feedback on the care they have provided and for assessing the quality of care provided by healthcare services. PROMs have been widely used as effectiveness endpoints for approved drug labels in the United States [7], and outcome assessment in clinical guideline development (e.g., for pain management [9], dialysis treatment [10], and screening for prostate cancer [11]), as well as applied in the context of national audits [12], clinical governance and quality assurance [13], and integrated into routine clinical practice [14] and managing the performance of healthcare providers [15].

However in glaucoma, most attempts to measure health improvement from treatment have largely been in clinical research studies on selected population and much less frequently in routine clinical practice [16, 17]. Also, there is a plethora of PROMs with considerable heterogeneity amongst them, such as differing in terms of how the answers are scored, as well as the number, nature and the wording of the questions asked. The quality of these PROMs instruments also varies considerably in terms of their validity and reliability [16, 18]. Moreover, although most of glaucoma-specific PROMs have been constructed in accordance to basic psychometric principles [19], a conceptual framework building on patient views is absent in more than 50% of instruments [16]. The ethos of PROMs is to gauge patients' assessment on their own health status and health-associated quality of life. So arguably, the lack of patient input in the development process of these PROMs has been cited as a methodological shortcoming. An appropriate PROM should be supported by published evidence presenting that it is acceptable to patients, as well as valid, reliable, and responsive (sensitive to change) [20]. Additionally, feedback from healthcare professionals on PROMs use is also essential addition to any PROM development [21].

In Singapore, there has also been growing interest in exploring the use of PROMs in routine glaucoma care. However, most, if not all available PROMs have been developed in the context of largely western populations with different healthcare systems [16, 18]. Singapore, on the other hand, is a multi-ethnic country with a majority population of Chinese (74.2% of the resident population), with substantial Malay (13.2%), Indian minorities (9.2%) and other ethnicities (3.3%). Little is known on the use of these PROMs in a multi-ethnic Asian country like Singapore with a different healthcare system.

Hence, our study aimed to qualitatively gauge the relevance, comprehensiveness and acceptability of using four glaucoma-specific PROMs, namely: the Glaucoma Quality of Life-15 (GQL-15) [22], Glaucoma Symptom Identifier (GSI) [1], Independent Mobility Questionnaire (IMQ) [23], and Treatment Satisfaction Survey of Intra-ocular Pressure (TSS-IOP) [24], in the routine glaucoma care in the Singapore context. These four glaucoma-specific PROMs were selected based on a systematic review identifying them as the PROMs with the greatest potential for further adaptation and testing in the clinical setting [16]. To achieve our aim, we conducted a semi-structured interview with healthcare professionals and glaucoma patients about their perceptions on the content of one of four selected PROMs instrument and issues relating to the administration. A feasibility survey was performed upon the conclusion of the semi-structured interview.

Methods
This study was approved by the Institutional Review Board of Singapore National Healthcare Group.

Literature review
An extensive background literature review in PUBMED database of existing glaucoma specific "patient reported outcome measures" (PROMs) instruments was carried out in March 2014. The search terms used include "glaucoma", "quality of life", "patient reported outcome", "questionnaire", "survey", "development" and "validation". Amongst others, two systemic reviews [16, 18] analysed 33 and 27 PROMs instruments, respectively, and included details on their development and validation. Our study team took into account the authors' recommendations, availability of the full instrument in English, feasibility of actual administration during clinical practice and underwent multiple roundtable discussions before shortlisting 4 of the most promising glaucoma specific PROMs instrument for use, namely: GQL-15 [22], GSI [1], IMQ [23], and TSS-IOP [24].

Semi-structured interviews and feasibility survey
To ensure comprehensive viewpoints on the implementation of glaucoma-specific PROMs instruments in daily clinical practice were gathered, both healthcare workers involved in the care of glaucoma patients and glaucoma patients themselves took part in the semi-structured interviews. This purposive sampling process included relevant stakeholders such as consultants, optometrists, ophthalmic nurses and low vision occupational therapists. Patients were recruited to include a variety of glaucoma diagnosis types and severity. All participants were capable of giving informed consent.

These interviews were performed through trained ophthalmic healthcare professionals in English. Each participant was presented with 1 of the 4 selected PROMs instruments. A "think aloud" method was used where participants were encouraged to verbalize their views and perceptions on the items of the instrument. 'Think aloud' is one valuable cognitive interviewing technique for gaining insights into participant's cognitive processes whilst performing a task [25]. During this process, interviewers hand transcribed and verbatim these enunciated views. A topic guide developed based on literature review and clinical experience was used to guide the interview and obtain feedback on not only the content of the PROMs instrument itself but also issues relating to the administration of it. Consideration was given to the power relationship between doctors and patients, with non-doctors who were not directly involved in the patients' care assigned to conduct the interviews. At the end of the interview, participants were asked to fill out a simple 4 questions feasibility survey devised to gauge the relevance, comprehensiveness and acceptability of the usage of glaucoma specific PROMs instruments in a busy clinical setting.

Thematic analysis

Two researchers of the study team independently conducted thematic analyses of the interview results. This was followed by further roundtable discussions with the rest of the study team to refine the analysis. The themes that emerged were then assigned to domains considered important to the successful use of glaucoma specific PROMs instrument in day-to-day clinical practice. These domains were developed after extensive literature review [26], research findings and consultation with clinicians and operations staff. Subsequently, the domains were back-mapped onto the 4 PROMs instruments to gain further insight on the strengths and limitations of each individual instrument as a complement to traditional clinical assessment tools of glaucoma patients.

Results
Demographics of participants

Table 1 presents participants' demographic data. A total of 40 participants, consisting of 16 (40%) healthcare professionals and 24 (60%) glaucoma patients, took part in the semi-structured interviews. The majority of the participants was Chinese (66%), followed by and Indian (17%), Eurasian (13%), others (4%), and Malay (0%). Amongst the 16 healthcare professionals, there were four from each of the following groups: glaucoma ophthalmologists, optometrists, ophthalmic nurses and low vision occupational therapists. These were all employees of the same tertiary hospital as the study team. Of the 24 glaucoma patients, 8 each with early, moderate or severe glaucoma based on the Bascom Palmer (Hodapp-Anderson-Parrish) Glaucoma staging

Table 1 Demographic Characteristics of Patients Recruited

Age (mean ± SD)	60 ± 15 years
Gender	
Male	19 (79%)
Female	5 (21%)
Race	
Chinese	16 (66%)
Malay	0 (0%)
Indian	4 (17%)
Eurasian	3 (13%)
Others	1 (4%)
Employment status	
Fulltime	14 (58%)
Part-time	0 (0%)
Unemployed	10 (42%)
Education level	
Nil	2 (9%)
Primary	1 (4%)
Secondary	8 (33%)
Tertiary	13 (54%)
Monthly income	
Nil	12 (50%)
$1 - $4999	6 (25%)
$5000 - $9999	6 (25%)
> $10,000	0 (0%)
Glaucoma type	
POAG	15 (62%)
PACG	3 (13%)
NTG	4 (17%)
Secondary glaucoma	2 (8%)
Duration of glaucoma (mean ± SD)	7.58 ± 5.95 years
Current management	
Topical medications only	13 (54%)
Topical medications and laser	6 (25%)
Topical medications and surgery	3 (13%)
Surgery only	2 (8%)
LogMAR Visual acuity (better eye) (mean ± SD)	0.17 ± 0.3
LogMAR Visual acuity (worse eye) (mean ± SD)	0.45 ± 0.57
Mean deviation (better eye) (mean ± SD)	−7.72 ± 8.30 (dB)
Mean deviation (poor eye) (mean ± SD)	− 10.8 ± 7.84 (dB)

system. All could either read or understand English and had no other significant ocular pathology.

Thematic analysis and domain identification

A total of 286 comments were recorded from the semi-structured interviews. Of these, 139 were made by the glaucoma healthcare professionals and 147 by glaucoma patients. Following analysis, the comments were dichotomized into 2 main themes: those relating to the content of the PROMs instrument and those relating to the actual administration of the instrument. Sub-themes under content include scope of the PROMs instrument, language used, extent of localization and contextualization. Sub-themes under administration include relevance to patients and healthcare professionals, logistics and user-friendliness of the PROMs instrument form. Table 2 shows examples of patients' or healthcare professionals' comments from made that map to the aforementioned themes.

Feasibility survey results

Upon the conclusion of the semi-structured interview, all participants were presented with a simple 4 question feasibility survey. The survey questions and the results are found in Tables 3 and 4, respectively. Overall, the majority of glaucoma patients (79%) and medical professionals (94%) felt glaucoma-specific PROMs instruments had a role in the glaucoma management. Of the 5 patients who disagreed, 4 had mild glaucoma. 37% of patients and 50% of healthcare professionals felt that current PROMs instruments were not sufficiently comprehensive for clinical use. Interestingly, those who felt more had to be done for

Table 2 Narrative results of thematic analysis from Semi-structured Interviews

Main theme	Sub-theme	Narrative results	
		Patients	Healthcare professionals
Content	Scope	1. Current PROMs instruments are selectively focused and whilst providing in-depth information on i.e. symptomatology of the disease frequently neglects other important aspects like economics of treatment and psychological impact of disease.	
		1. A balance needs to be struck as to how detailed the questions should be. A significant number of PROMs questions appear repetitive and responders cannot differentiate the subtlety within.	1. PROMs instrument should also capture demographic i.e. occupation and visual requirements and comorbidity data as these factors will skew responses. 2. Not sufficient to address patient's concerns, fears and doubts.
	Language	1. Simple and specific terms should be used in the instruments to prevent confusion, increase accuracy andreduce responder fatigue.	
		1. Is there an easier word to use besides errands	1. If technical terms are unavoidable, examples or pictures can be used to improve understanding. 2. In formulating and phrasing of PROMs questions, the usage of active voice and inclusion of a temporal comparative element will enhancement comprehension and detect disease progression.
	Localization and contextualization	1. PROMs instrument should be localized to the setting it is used and allow responders to relate the questions to their daily living.	
		1. The most relevant and useful PROMs questions are those relating to disease impact on vision and how it compromises personal safety or impair daily living. 2. Playing games such as bingo or bridge…better to use local context like playing mahjong. 3. Subway should be replaced with MRT.	
Administration	Relevance	1. The instrument needs to yield tangible benefits to the patients' management i.e. in the form of follow up actions like referrals to be considered useful. 2. Not really relevant as I am doing good so no concerns. 3. As glaucoma is a symptomless disease in the early stages, PROMs instrument may not be particularly useful for patients with mild disease.	1. For a mild glaucoma patient, this may not be relevant
	Logistics	1. Time spend on the PROMs instrument should be keep to a minimum. Current questionnaires tend to be rather lengthy and unsuitable to be completed in a busy outpatient setting. 2. I need someone to read this out to me because I have very poor vision! 3. Traditional paper and pen administration may be impossible for those with advanced disease and poor vision.	
	User-friendliness	1. Font size, type and questionnaire layout is important to improve the user experience and enhance participation rates. This is especially so as responders are likely visual impaired due to disease or pharmacological dilation.	
		1. Cannot really see because of the dilation eyedrop…the fonts should be larger.	

Table 3 Glaucoma specific PROMs Feasibility Survey

1. Do you feel that such questionnaires are relevant to patients?
2. Do you feel that such questionnaires are relevant to the healthcare team?
3. Do you feel that current questionnaires are sufficiently comprehensive for clinical use?
4. Do you feel that current questionnaires are sufficiently user friendly?

the scope of existing PROMs instruments were mainly patients at the opposite ends of the disease spectrum (4 diagnosed with mild and severe glaucoma each). Current PROMs instrument fared less well in the usability area with 54% of patients and 44% of healthcare professionals suggesting a need to improve in areas of wording and phrasing (47%), questionnaire formatting (41%) and rating methods (12%).

Discussion

"Exploratory pilot work to assess comprehensibility, acceptability, relevance and answerability to the target population" is one step of a systematic 5-step approach to valid PROMs [25]. In our study, this step is taken to see if selected 4 PROMs have the pre-requisites for use in routine glaucoma care, negating the need for more extensive development work to create a novel PROM. To our knowledge, this is the first exploratory study that assesses the healthcare professionals' and glaucoma patients' perception on the content and administration of glaucoma-specific PROMs in the Singapore clinical setting.

Our results demonstrate both positive and negative aspects of glaucoma-specific PROMs for their use in the daily clinical practice. Positive aspects include the majority of healthcare professionals and patients feel that selected PROMs are relevant to patients and healthcare team. Although patients with mild glaucoma did not see the relevance of PROMs in their care, citing: "for a mild

glaucoma patient, this may not be relevant" (Table 2), it can be argued that the role of PROMs in the early stage of glaucoma may still have a role in terms of assessing the impact of treatment, such as side-effects and cost incurred from treatment.

The negative aspects in our study include barriers for glaucoma-specific PROMs in routine use. Several barriers (such as logistical, social, legal, technical, and cultural barriers) have been revealed to prevent the successful embed of PROMs into the routine clinical practice [14]. Several studies have shown the attempt to collect PRO data on a large scale in the routine eye clinic setting is disappointing [27, 28]. In our study, there are concerns expressed by the participants on the user-friendliness, comprehensiveness and logistics (Tables 2 and 4). For example, the need for brevity, and the instrument should not be too long. This has also been borne out by another study looking at the Impact of Vision Impairment questionnaire, which has the best domain coverage but is poor at assessing glaucoma patients, and may be too long for routine clinical use [27]. Our participants also feel it is impossible for patients with visual impairment to self-fill PROM questionnaire in the paper format (Table 2). Browne J et al.'s study also reflects the same concern to use VF14 to assess cataract surgery [27]. The howRu instrument is effective when conducted by telephone, which may solve the potential obstacles for the PROM questionnaire used by patients with visual impairment in routine practice [29]. It would be interesting to assess glaucoma patients' views on howRu in Singapore clinical setting in future studies.

An assessment of 11 glaucoma-specific Health-related Quality of life (HRQoL) instruments concludes that little PRO instrument covers comprehensive domains which participants are interested in [30]. Our participants also expressed a desire for a more comprehensive PROM instrument that covered more holistic issues such as

Table 4 Results of the feasibility Survey

Glaucoma specific PROMs Feasibility Survey.	Patients' response	Healthcare professionals' response
1. Do you feel that such questionnaires are relevant to patients?		
Yes	19 (79%)	15 (94%)
No	5 (21%)	1 (6%)
2. Do you feel that such questionnaires are relevant to the healthcare team?		
Yes	22 (92%)	15 (94%)
No	2 (8%)	1 (6%)
3. Do you feel that current questionnaires are sufficiently comprehensive for clinical use?		
Yes	15 (63%)	8 (50%)
No	9 (37%)	8 (50%)
4. Do you feel that current questionnaires are sufficiently user friendly?		
Yes	11 (46%)	9 (56%)
No	13 (54%)	7 (44%)

financial burden of care and psychological impact of disease (Table 2). For instance, "peace of mind" concerns between 50% [31] and 80% [32] of newly diagnosed glaucoma patients, but this item has been mentioned by little glaucoma-specific PROM instruments [27]. Participants in our study reflect the similar finding that selected PROMs did "not sufficiently address patient's concerns, fears and doubts" (Table 2). The need for inclusion of the financial impact of disease is a finding that may be unique to Singapore where patients bear a significant direct out-of-pocket burden for their care [33]. This again illustrates the need for contextual relevance when using PROMs and caution in directly "importing" PROMs that have been developed for other healthcare settings.

Our study also reveals challenges in execution that may be unique to our local context. From the outset, recruitment of willing participants proved difficult. More specifically, our recruitment is biased toward the educated participants with 54% having tertiary education (Table 1). This may be a reflection of language constraints as English was used throughout the interviews and the PROMs were all worded in English. It is noteworthy that PROMs, as a meaningful clinical routine use, must also include good generalizability to ensure that sections of the patient population are not excluded – especially the less well-educated and well-off who also tend to be more severely impacted by disease. Additionally, in our study, it is noteworthy that we recruited no Malays (Table 1), which may again reflect poor participation in this racial group due to greater comfort in using Malay as a medium of communication. Our study shows that the use of PROMs in Singapore should be available in the four main languages here, namely: English, Chinese, Tamil and Malay.

The limitations of current study should be considered. The selected PROMs may be inadequate and more work needs to be done before a large scale PROMs program can be rolled out locally. This is especially so when applied to routine care as opposed to more research-oriented settings. For a PROM to be used in the daily practice, it is important to ensure that data collection is practical and equitable, and the data produced are valid as guidelines to improve patient care and prioritize healthcare resources. Looking at the socio-demographic data from our study, it is noted that the majority participants are male (79%), while female participants is 21% (Table 1). In terms of educational status, half of participants (54%) have received the tertiary level education. There is also no Malay participant in our study. The study numbers are small to begin with and the study design qualitative in nature. However, these findings may have implications for the wider usage of PROMs in routine care. It is well-known that socioeconomic status has close correlation with the health status of an individual. Socioeconomic factors may also similarly skew response rates and response patterns such that the poorer, less educated and sicker end up being under-represented or missed altogether. In Singapore, a significant proportion of the elderly do not know English –there may be a need to have a Chinese, Indian and Malay version of the same instrument to improve generalizability. More extensive studies need to be undertaken to explore this aspect and factored into the design, not only of the instruments themselves but the logistical aspects surrounding the application of these instruments to ensure representativeness.

Despite the above limitations, we have the strength in qualitative research method-think aloud method, which is commonly used during questionnaire development to determine whether the meaning of a questionnaire item, as interpreted by the questionnaire respondent, is consistent with the questionnaire developer's intention of that item [25]. We employed this method to garner views from participants. This method has also been used to assess glaucoma patients' perceptions on the acceptability, relevance, comprehensibility and answerability of one glaucoma-specific PRO instrument - the Aberdeen glaucoma questionnaire [25].

Conclusion

As the paradigm of what constitutes successful treatment shifts, PROMs will gain in prominence, and Singapore is no exception. It is heartening to know the use of glaucoma-specific PROMs is broadly welcomed by healthcare professionals and patients here. Also, our study highlights the need for caution in directly employing PROM instruments developed in other healthcare settings and the need to "contextualise" and frame these instruments for the local socio-demographic to ensure representativeness of the data collected. The identified barriers should be necessarily considered when designing and deployment of glaucoma-specific PROM instrument.

Acknowledgements
Not available.

Authors' contributions
OKH and ZXT contributed to conception, designed the study, carried out interview, collected and analyzed data, as well as drafted manuscript. HYZ was involved in the manuscript drafting and submission. EL contributed to manuscript review. All authors read and approved the final manuscript.

Competing interests
The authors declare that they have no competing interests.

Author details
[1]National Healthcare Group Eye Institute, Tan Tock Seng Hospital, S308433, Singapore, Singapore. [2]Health Services Research, Singapore Eye Research Institute, Singapore, Singapore.

References

1.   Walt JG, Rendas-Baum R, Kosinski M, Patel V. Psychometric evaluation of the Glaucoma symptom identifier. J Glaucoma. 2011;20:148–59.
2.   Ismail R, Azuara-Blanco A, Ramsay CR. Outcome measures in Glaucoma: a systematic review of Cochrane reviews and protocols. J Glaucoma. 2015;24:533–8.
3.   Hartmann CW, Rhee DJ. The patient's journey: glaucoma. Bmj. 2006;333:738–9.
4.   Gutierrez P, Wilson MR, Johnson C, et al. Influence of glaucomatous visual field loss on health-related quality of life. Arch Ophthalmol. 1997;115:777–84.
5.   Glen FC, Crabb DP, Garway-Heath DF. The direction of research into visual disability and quality of life in glaucoma. BMC Ophthalmol England. 2011;19 https://doi.org/10.1186/1471-2415-11-19.
6.   Acquadro C, Berzon R, Dubois D, et al. Incorporating the patient's perspective into drug development and communication: an ad hoc task force report of the patient-reported outcomes (PRO) harmonization group meeting at the Food and Drug Administration, February 16, 2001. Value Health. 2003;6:522–31.
7.   Willke RJ, Burke LB, Erickson P. Measuring treatment impact: a review of patient-reported outcomes and other efficacy endpoints in approved product labels. Control Clin Trials. 2004;25:535–52.
8.   Leidy NK, Revicki DA, Geneste B. Recommendations for evaluating the validity of quality of life claims for labeling and promotion. Value Health. 1999;2:113–27.
9.   Practice guidelines for chronic pain management. A report by the American Society of Anesthesiologists Task Force on pain management, chronic pain section. Anesthesiol. 1997;86:995–1004.
10. Galla JH. Clinical practice guideline on shared decision-making in the appropriate initiation of and withdrawal from dialysis. The renal physicians association and the American Society of Nephrology. J Am Soc Nephrol. 2000;11:1340–2.
11. Lim LS, Sherin K. Screening for prostate cancer in U.S. men ACPM position statement on preventive practice. Am J Prev Med. 2008;34:164–70.
12. Williams O, Fitzpatrick R, Hajat S, et al. Mortality, morbidity, and 1-year outcomes of primary elective total hip arthroplasty. J Arthroplast. 2002;17:165–71.
13. Vallance-Owen A, Cubbin S, Warren V, Matthews B. Outcome monitoring to facilitate clinical governance; experience from a national programme in the independent sector. J Public Health (Oxf). 2004;26:187–92.
14. Nelson EC, Eftimovska E, Lind C, Hager A, Wasson JH, Lindblad S. Patient reported outcome measures in practice. Bmj. 2015;350:g7818.
15. Dawson J, Doll H, Fitzpatrick R, Jenkinson C, Carr AJ. The routine use of patient reported outcome measures in healthcare settings. BMJ. 2010;340:c186.
16. Vandenbroeck S, De Geest S, Zeyen T, Stalmans I, Dobbels F. Patient-reported outcomes (PRO's) in glaucoma: a systematic review. Eye (Lond). 2011;25:555–77.
17. Staa TP, Goldacre B, Gulliford M, et al. Pragmatic randomised trials using routine electronic health records: putting them to the test. BMJ. 2012;344:e55.
18. Che Hamzah J, Burr JM, Ramsay CR, Azuara-Blanco A, Prior M. Choosing appropriate patient-reported outcomes instrument for glaucoma research: a systematic review of vision instruments. Qual Life Res. 2011;20:1141–58.
19. Pesudovs K, Burr JM, Harley C, Elliott DB. The development, assessment, and selection of questionnaires. Optom Vis Sci. 2007;84:663–74.
20. Fitzpatrick R, Davey C, Buxton MJ, Jones DR. Evaluating patient-based outcome measures for use in clinical trials. Health Technol Assess. 1998;2(i-iv):1–74.
21. Allwood D, Hildon Z, Black N. Clinicians' views of formats of performance comparisons. J Eval Clin Pract. 2013;19:86–93.
22. Nelson P, Aspinall P, Papasouliotis O, Worton B, O'Brien C. Quality of life in glaucoma and its relationship with visual function. J Glaucoma. 2003;12:139–50.
23. Turano KA, Massof RW. Quigley HA. A self-assessment instrument designed for measuring independent mobility in RP patients: generalizability to glaucoma patients. Invest Ophthalmol Vis Sci. 2002;43:2874–81.
24. Atkinson MJ, Stewart WC, Fain JM, et al. A new measure of patient satisfaction with ocular hypotensive medications: the treatment satisfaction survey for intraocular pressure (TSS-IOP). Health Qual Life Outcomes. 2003;1:67.
25. Prior ME, Hamzah JC, Francis JJ, et al. Pre-validation methods for developing a patient reported outcome instrument. BMC Med Res Methodol. 2011;11:112.
26. Black N. Patient reported outcome measures could help transform healthcare. BMJ. 2013;346:f167.
27. Somner JE, Sii F, Bourne RR, Cross V, Burr JM, Shah P. Moving from PROMs to POEMs for glaucoma care: a qualitative scoping exercise. Invest Ophthalmol Vis Sci. 2012;53:5940–7.
28. McAlinden C, Gothwal VK, Khadka J, Wright TA, Lamoureux EL, Pesudovs K. A head-to-head comparison of 16 cataract surgery outcome questionnaires. Ophthalmol. 2011;118:2374–81.
29. Benson T, Sizmur S, Whatling J, Arikan S, McDonald D, Ingram D. Evaluation of a new short generic measure of health status: howRu. Inform Prim Care. 2010;18:89–101.
30. Severn P, Fraser S, Finch T, May C. Which quality of life score is best for glaucoma patients and why? BMC Ophthalmol. 2008;8:2.
31. Janz NK, Wren PA, Lichter PR, Musch DC, Gillespie BW, Guire KE. Quality of life in newly diagnosed glaucoma patients : the collaborative initial Glaucoma treatment study. Ophthalmol. 2001;108:887–97. discussion 898
32. Odberg T, Jakobsen JE, Hultgren SJ, Halseide R. The impact of glaucoma on the quality of life of patients in Norway. I. Results from a self-administered questionnaire. Acta Ophthalmol Scand. 2001;79:116–20.
33. Hee K, Tan DD, Zhu HY, Wong PY, Lim PH, Tan CS. Direct cost and resource consumption associated with severity of Glaucoma in Singapore. 2017. Under review.

8

Assessment of capillary dropout in the superficial retinal capillary plexus by optical coherence tomography angiography in the early stage of diabetic retinopathy

Ceying Shen*🄳, Shu Yan, Min Du, Hong Zhao, Ling Shao and Yibo Hu

Abstract

Background: To assess capillary dropout in the superficial retinal capillary plexus (SCP) by optical coherence tomography angiography (OCTA) in the early stage of diabetic retinopathy (DR).

Methods: This study was a cross-sectional observational study. Patients that underwent OCTA examinations in our hospital between November 2015 and May 2016 were included in the study. The subjects were divided into two groups: A) normal controls (41 eyes of 41 subjects) and B) the DR patients (49 eyes of 49 patients with mild non-proliferative DR (NPDR)). The retinal thickness and SCP vessel density were analyzed using built-in software in nine sections of the macular area; whole scan area; fovea; parafovea; and sub-sections of the parafovea, superior-hemi, inferior-hemi, temporal, superior, nasal, and inferior. The correlation between vessel density and retinal thickness was also analyzed.

Results: The SCP density was significantly lower ($P < 0.05$) in mild NPDR patients than in normal controls in all areas, with the exception of the fovea ($P > 0.05$). In the parafovea, superior-hemi, inferior-hemi, temporal, and nasal sectors of group B, the SCP density was negatively correlated with the corresponding retinal thickness ($P < 0.05$). Specifically, as the SCP density decreased, retinal thickness increased.

Conclusions: In the early stage of NPDR, retinal capillary dropout and retinal thickness changes can be clearly captured and analyzed by OCTA. The results confirm a negative correlation between vessel density and retinal thickness in diabetic patients. This noninvasive technique could be applied for DR detection and monitoring. Further study with a larger sample size is warranted.

Keywords: Optical coherence tomography angiography, Retinal capillary, Capillary dropout, Diabetic retinopathy, Diabetes mellitus

Background

Over the last 20 years, time domain and spectral domain optical coherence tomography (SD-OCT) has resulted in the advancement of retinal disease diagnosis [1, 2]. However, SD-OCT is limited in terms of its ability to provide retinal microvasculature information. Fundus fluorescein angiography (FFA) is currently considered the gold standard in retinal vascular network imaging for numerous retinovascular

diseases [3, 4]. A novel non-invasive technique, termed optical coherence tomography angiography (OCTA), provides imaging of the retinal vascular network as well as the retina structure, and has been introduced in clinical practice [5].

OCTA, with split spectrum amplitude decorrelation angiography (SSADA), employs motion contrast imaging to obtain high-resolution volumetric blood flow information to generate angiographic images, which does not require the injection of exogenous dyes and provides near-automatic quantification and excellent intra-visit repeatability in the measurement of macular regions [6–8]. In contrast to FFA imaging, which is two-dimensional and

* Correspondence: 516045610@qq.com
Department of Zhengzhou Second People Hospital, Ophthalmology, Zhengzhou Eye Hospital, Zhengzhou Ophthalmic Institution, Zhengzhou Hanghai Middle Road No. 90, Zhengzhou 450000, China

explores the retina only on a single plane, OCTA provides a non-invasive approach for three-dimensional (3D) retinal microcirculation imaging [9, 10]. Impressively and notably, the OCTA approach can capture superficial and deep vascular plexuses separately [11].

Vision-threatening retinovascular diseases, such as diabetic retinopathy, retinal vein occlusion, and macular telangiectasia, interfere with retinal microcirculation by modifying the foveal avascular zone (FAZ) size [12].

Therefore, in the present study we took advantage of this non-invasive technique to investigate the superficial retinal capillary plexus (SCP) of the macula in normal and diabetic subjects.

Methods

This was a cross-sectional observational study. Subjects who visited and received OCTA in the Zhengzhou Second People Hospital clinic between November 2015 and May 2016 were included, that fit within the study criteria. The study was approved by the Institutional Review Board at the Zhengzhou Second People Hospital and carried out in accordance with the tenets of the Declaration of Helsinki. Written informed consent for the study was obtained from all subjects. A total of 90 adult Chinese subjects (90 eyes) were included in the analysis. They were divided into group A (normal controls) and group B with mild non-proliferative diabetic retinopathy (NPDR), diagnosed according to the international definition of DR stages [13]. All subjects underwent comprehensive ophthalmic examination, which included a best-corrected visual acuity (BCVA) test, intraocular pressure (IOP) measurement (CT-80, Topcon Corporation, Tokyo, Japan), slit-lamp biomicroscopy, and pupil dilated fundoscopy. The DR patients underwent FFA in addition. The fundus photographs and FFA were taken by a 55 degree lens (TRC-50DX, Topcon, Tokyo, Japan) at nine fields sites; central posterior, superior, inferior, temporal, nasal, superotemporal, superonasal, inferotemporal, and inferonasal. Then, the manifestations of DR were graded based on the color fundus photos and FFA photos, according to definitions of the DR stages [13]. The inclusion criteria of the study were as follows, 1) normal controls were subjects with 20/20 BCVA or better, with spherical refraction of $\leq \pm 6.0$ D and cylinder correction of $\leq \pm 2.0$ D, normal anterior segment and fundus, normal IOP, and no diabetes mellitus; 2) DR patients were subjects that suffered from diabetes mellitus for one to ten years and a stable blood glucose level was maintained (fast blood glucose ≤ 7 mmol/L and blood glucose after meal ≤ 11 mmol/L). DR was graded as mild NPDR. The subjects had no previous history of other ocular diseases, surgery, or laser treatment and a BCVA in the 12/20 to 20/20 range. Only one eye of each subject was included in the study.

High quality images of the retinal structure and vessel network were obtained by the spectral-domain OCTA, RTVue-XR Angiovue (software version: 2015.1.0.90; Optovue, Inc., Fremont, CA, USA). The built-in software, RTVue-XR Avanti, facilitates automated scan segmentation into the SCP, deep retinal capillary plexuses (DCP), outer retina, and the choroid capillary. Measurements of SCP vessel density on en-face projections were analyzed. The reference plane for the superficial plexus was defined as the inner limiting membrane (ILM) with an offset (from the interface reference) of 3 μm to the inner plexiform layer (IPL) with an offset (from the interface reference) of 15 μm. 3D OCTA scans were acquired over 3×3 mm regions. The density occupied by vessels and microvasculature in the selected region were automatically calculated as the percentage of pixels by the built-in software. The software report included the OCT thickness (ILM-IPL and ILM-Retinal Pigment Epthelium (RPE)) and vessel density of the nine sections, i.e., whole image, fovea, parafovea, and sub-sections of the parafovea (superior-hemi, inferior-hemi, temporal, superior, nasal, and inferior; Fig. 1). The software used Early Treatment Diabetic Retinopathy Study (ETDRS) circles to generate the report. Briefly, a small round point at the center represents the fixation point; the diameter of the inner circle is 1 mm and the outer circle is 3 mm; the "whole image" means the whole area of the scan (3×3 mm); the "fovea" means the area within the 1 mm circle; and the "parafovea" means the band area from the inner circle to the outer circle; then, the parafovea band is divided into six sub-sections; superior-hemifield, inferior-hemifield, temporal, superior, inferior, and nasal. The foveal avascular zone (FAZ) was used as an anatomic landmark for locating the retinal point of fixation.

Statistical analysis

Statistical analysis was performed using a statistical software package, SPSS 19.0 (IBM-SPSS Inc. Chicago, IL, USA). Normal distribution of the data was tested. Differences in superficial vessel density between group A and group B were analyzed by the independent t-test. The correlation between the superficial vessel density and the corresponding retinal thickness was studied using Pearson correlation coefficient. The superficial vessel density and the retinal thickness were expressed as the mean ± standard deviation. $P < 0.05$ was considered as statistically significant.

Results

Group A was comprised of 41 eyes of the 41 normal controls (28 men and 13 women). The mean age of group A was 52.9 ± 8.2 years old (range, 41 to 63 years). Group B was comprised of 49 eyes of 49 subjects (21 men and 28 women) with mild NPDR. The mean age of

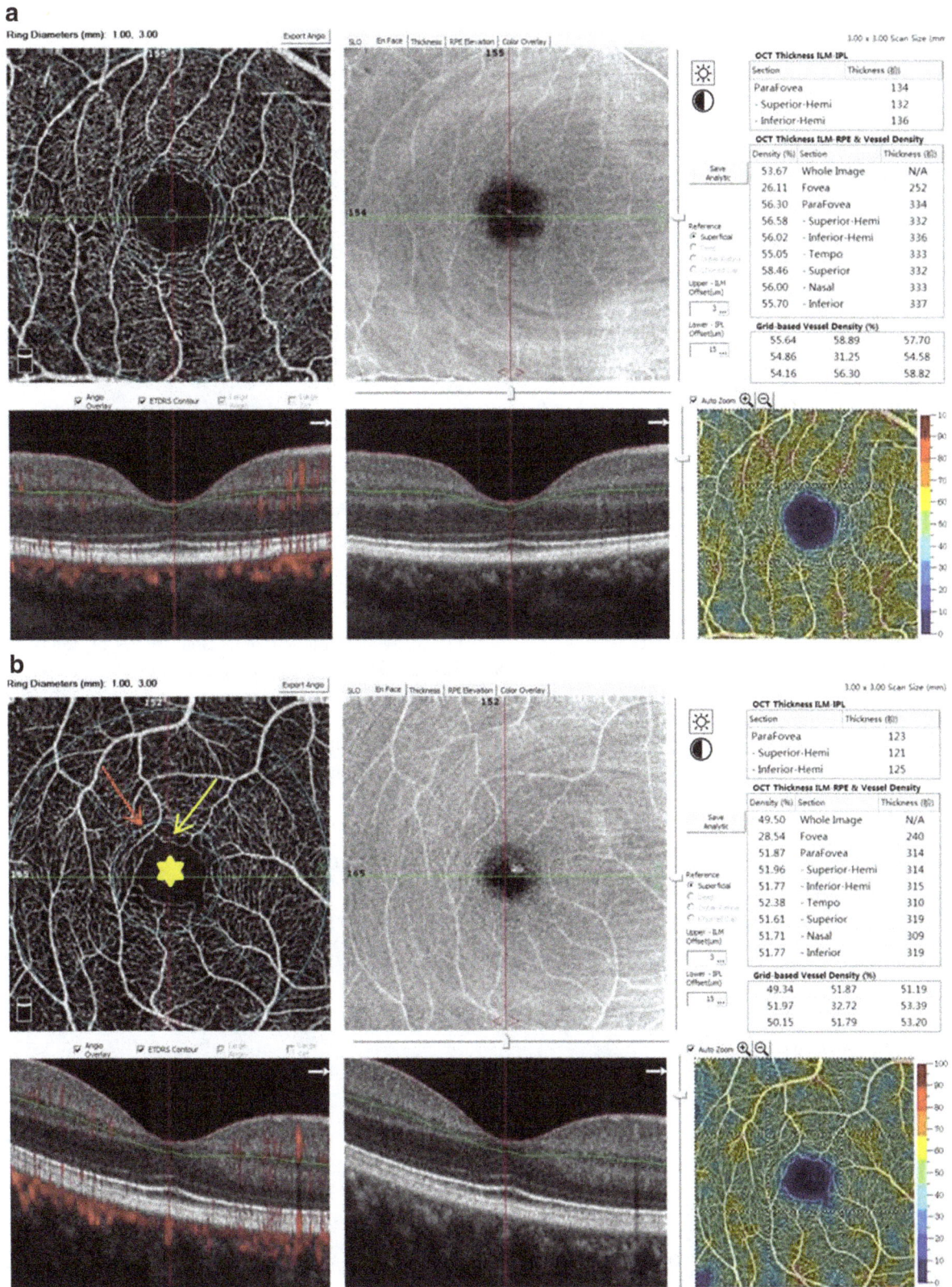

Fig. 1 (See legend on next page.)

(See figure on previous page.)
Fig. 1 OCTA images of retinal structures and vessel networks, with reports of retinal thickness and vessel density, in a normal subject and a diabetic patient (3 × 3 mm scan area). **a** The structural OCT and angiography of a normal subject did not show abnormalities and the image quality was good. **b** The structural OCT of a diabetic patient did not show abnormalities. Capillary loss (yellow arrow), morphological anomalies (red arrow), and deformed foveal avascular area (yellow star) were demonstrated in an angiography scan

group B was 56.4 ± 10.1 years (range, 41 to 70 years). There was no statistically significant difference in the mean age between the groups ($P > 0.05$).

Structural OCT imaging
The structural OCT of the normal and diabetic subjects did not show abnormalities and the image quality was good (Fig. 1a and b).

OCTA morphology
High quality images, obtained by OCTA, showed clear and organized microvascular networks in normal controls (Fig. 1a). In the diabetic group, at the superficial retinal vascular plexuses level, blood flow alterations, capillary tortuosity and dropout, vasodilation, microaneurysms, vascular remodeling, looser capillary networks with larger and sparser meshes were evident in the macula (Fig. 1b).

Superficial retinal vessel density and thickness
The 3D nature of OCTA allows for separate visualization of the retina and choroid circulation from the same volumetric scan. In healthy eyes, retinal circulation is located between the ILM and outer plexiform layer (OPL). All participants in groups A and B had adequate OCTA image quality for vessel density analysis. The data were normally distributed ($P > 0.05$).

Compared to group A, the superficial vessel density was lower by 11.61% in the whole image area, 12.90% in the parafovea, 13.13% in the superior-hemi, 12.68% in the inferior-hemi, 11.73% in the temporal, 12.96% in the superior, 13.80% in the nasal, and 13.13% in the inferior, respectively, in the diabetics (Table 1, Fig. 1). All of these differences were statistically significant ($P < 0.05$). There was no statistically significant difference between the vessel density in the fovea section between group A and group B ($P > 0.05$).

There were no statistically significant differences between the two groups, in terms of retinal thickness, in any section ($P > 0.05$; Table 1, Fig. 1).

Correlation of vessel density and retinal thickness
In group A, the vessel densities of the fovea and nasal were positively correlated with the corresponding retinal thickness (correlation coefficient = 0.689, $P < 0.05$ and 0.312, $P < 0.05$, respectively). In the parafovea, superior-hemi, inferior-hemi, temporal, and nasal sectors of group B, the SCP density had a negative correlation with the corresponding retinal thickness (correlation coefficient = -0.358, -0.359, -0.322, -0.374, -0.358, respectively, $P < 0.05$). Specifically, the lower the vessel density, the thicker the retina. For all other sections, no significant correlation could be found between the vessel density and retinal thickness in either group A or group B ($P > 0.05$).

Table 1 The superficial vessel density and the thickness of ILM-RPE in normal and diabetic subjects ($\bar{x} \pm s$)

Region	group A (n = 41)		group B (n = 49)	
	Superficial vessel density (%)	Thickness (ILM-RPE) (µm)	Superficial vessel density (%)	Thickness (ILM-RPE) (µm)
Whole image	54.10 ± 2.10	N/A	47.82 ± 4.62*	N/A
Fovea	24.48 ± 5.98	233.57 ± 17.90#	28.38 ± 5.571**	242.35 ± 26.85
Parafovea	56.60 ± 2.19	309.67 ± 12.75	49.30 ± 5.12*	313.00 ± 22.27##
-Superior-Hemi	56.66 ± 2.25	310.83 ± 13.51	49.22 ± 5.02*	313.58 ± 24.46##
-Inferior-Hemi	56.54 ± 2.29	308.45 ± 12.65	49.37 ± 5.44*	312.28 ± 21.03##
-Temporal	55.34 ± 2.24	299.19 ± 14.16	48.85 ± 5.00*	305.60 ± 22.68##
-Superior	57.70 ± 2.38	315.38 ± 13.82	50.22 ± 5.14*	317.65 ± 25.52
-Nasal	56.02 ± 2.50	313.67 ± 13.94#	48.29 ± 6.22*	314.53 ± 23.45##
-Inferior	57.35 ± 2.58	310.55 ± 12.95	49.82 ± 5.66*	314.18 ± 20.99

ILM inner limiting membrane, *RPE* retinal pigment epithelium

*$P < 0.05$. There was significant differences in vessel density in the parafovea, superior-hemi, inferior-hemi, tempo, superior, nasal, and inferior sections between group A and group B (t = 8.593, 8.871, 7.951, 7.767, 8.663, 7.542, 7.941, respectively)

**$P > 0.05$. There was no statistically significant difference between group A and group B (t = 0.079)

#$P < 0.05$. In group A, the vessel density of the fovea and nasal was positively correlated with the corresponding retinal thickness. Correlation coefficients were 0.689 and 0.312, respectively

##$P < 0.05$. In the parafovea, superior-hemi, inferior-hemi, temporal, and nasal sections of group B, the density of the superficial retinal capillary plexus had a negative correlation with the corresponding retinal thickness (correlation coefficient = -0.358, -0.359, -0.322, -0.374, -0.358, respectively)

Discussion

The results from the present study showed that the image quality obtained from the OCTA device, RTVue-XR Angiovue, was high and was sufficient for analysis using the built-in image analysis software. This technology has improved the visualization of retinal capillaries and micro-angiopathic features, and offers great potential for the study and quantification of retinal microvascular attributes such as vessel density, branching pattern, capillary tortuosity, vasodilation, microaneurysms, and vascular remodeling in both healthy and diabetic subjects [14–16]. The vessel densities of SCP and DCP were lower in diabetic eyes compared with control eyes [17]. There were reports that capillary nonperfusion occurs initially at the level of the DCP [18] and vessel density was more significantly reduced in DCP than in SCP [19]. However, our current device has its limitations and is unable to provide information accurately on the DCP, outer retina, and choroidal vessels due to the projection of the superficial retinal capillary plexus. A similar study reported that measurements of vessel density in the deep retinal layers were influenced by decorrelation tail artifacts within current technologies, and did not appear to have the same diagnostic efficacy as measurements in the superficial retinal layers [20]. Furthermore, the RTVue-XR Angiovue software (Version: 2015.1.0.90) we were using had not been upgraded to perform the analysis of deep retinal vessels and choroidal vessels. That is why the present study only focused on the SCP, where the vessel density could be analyzed accurately. However, a published report demonstrated that a projection-resolved technique detected and quantified the avascular area automatically and accurately [21]. We may apply this technique in our future studies to provide findings in DCP of the subjects at early DR stage.

We explored the correlation of capillary dropout with the corresponding retinal thickness. This analysis relies on the OCTA system providing the structural and functional information simultaneously to accurately locate the abnormalities. The correlation between vessel density and retinal thickness in the macular area of diabetics by OCTA has not been reported in the literature. The report we found was only about the thickness analysis of the retinal nerve fiber layer and ganglion cell layer, and no significant differences were disclosed between diabetics and healthy subjects [19]. In the present study, we found that during the early stage of DR, the density of the superficial retinal capillary plexus reduced significantly in all areas, when compared to normal subjects, with the exception of the fovea. Therefore, retinal capillary dropout is a very important feature observed by OCTA in the early stages of DR. However, in the present study, the retinal thickness did not show a significant difference between normal and diabetic subjects. These findings indicate that compromised circulation in the inner retinal layers during the early stages of DR could be detected before structural retinal changes, for example, edema of the retina. The results from the present study showed that the density of the superficial retinal vessels showed significant intergroup differences in all areas, with the exception of the fovea. The results of the alteration of the FAZ area were inconsistent in some reports. Our result was consistent with the reports in which no significant difference was found in FAZ area of both SCP and DCP comparing diabetic and control groups [18, 19]. However, in another report, FAZ area was greater in diabetic eyes both in the superficial and deep vascular networks [17]. The possible reasons for this interesting finding are that, 1) the fovea is the last area to undergo capillary dropout in the early stages DR, 2) most of the fovea area studied was the FAZ, where there is no vascular network; thus, significant differences could not be found when the capillary dropout was only a small amount in a study with a small sample size, 3) the size of the FAZ was highly variable in the study population [22]. A further study with a larger sample size is warranted.

In the normal controls of the present study, vessel density had a positive correlation with the corresponding retinal thickness in the fovea and nasal sections, with no apparent correlation in others. The finding is consistent with other published work [23]. However, a negative correlation between the vessel density and the corresponding retinal thickness was demonstrated in the parafovea, superior-hemi, inferior-hemi, temporal, and nasal sections of DR patients in the present study. The areas with the least retinal capillaries had the thickest retina, though there was no statistically significant difference in retinal thickness between the controls and the diabetics.

From the results of the present study, combined with the advantages of using OCTA as an imaging technique for retinal vessels and structures, e.g., equivalent to FFA to visualize perifoveal region normal retinal vasculature [24], for patients that have contraindications for FFA and indocyanine green angiography (ICGA), non-invasive, acquires volumetric scans that can be segmented to specific depths, can be obtained within seconds, provides accurate size and localization information, visualizes both the retinal and choroidal vasculature, and shows both structural and blood flow information at the same time, we recommend the application of OCTA for the detection and monitoring of DR in diabetics. Since OCTA has a limited field of view and is unable to view leakage [15], applying OCTA in the early stage of NPDR could be an alternative option to FFA.

The study population in this study was quite small, larger scale investigations are needed to further address the questions that remain unanswered to provide comprehensive guidelines in clinical practice.

Conclusion

In the early stages of NPDR, retinal capillary dropout and retinal thickness could be clearly captured and analyzed by OCTA. A negative correlation between the vessel density and the corresponding retinal thickness in diabetics was shown in the present study. During the early stages of NPDR, though the retinal thickness was not significantly different with in the healthy control and diabetic groups, the superficial retinal vessel density significantly changed in the diabetic group. This noninvasive technique could be applied by analyzing the retinal vessel density for the detection and monitoring of DR. Further study with a large sample size is warranted.

Abbreviations

BCVA: Best-corrected visual acuity; DCP: Deep retinal capillary plexuses; DR: Diabetic retinopathy; FAZ: Foveal avascular zone; FFA: Fundus fluorescent angiography; ICGA: Indocyanine green angiography; ILM: Internal limiting membrane; IOP: Intraocular pressure; NPDR: Non-proliferative diabetic retinopathy; OCTA: Optical coherence tomography angiography; OPL: Outer plexiform layer; RPE: Retinal pigment epithelium; SCP: Superficial retinal capillary plexus; SD-OCT: Spectral-domainoptical coherence tomography; SSADA: Split spectrum amplitude decorrelation angiography

Authors' contributions

Concept and design: CYS, SY and YBH; Data acquisition: CYS, SY, MD and LS; Data analysis / interpretation: CYS, SY, MD, HZ, LS and YBH; Draft the manuscript: CYS; Critical revision of the manuscript: CYS, SY, MD, HZ, LS and YBH; Supervision: HZ. All authors read and approved the final manuscript.

Competing interests

The authors declare that they have no competing interests.

References

1. Puliafito CA, Hee MR, Lin CP, et al. Imaging of macular diseases with optical coherence tomography. Ophthalmology. 1995;102:217–29.
2. Puliafito CA. Optical coherence tomography: 20 years after. Ophthalmic Surg Lasers Imaging. 2010;41(Suppl):S5.
3. Novotny HR, Alvis DL. A method of photographing fluorescence in circulating blood in the human retina. Circulation. 1961;24:82–6.
4. Laatikainen L. The fluorescein angiography revolution: a breakthrough with sustained impact. Acta Ophthalmol Scand. 2004;82:381–92.
5. Fingler J, Zawadzki RJ, Werner JS, et al. Volumetric microvascular imaging of human retina using optical coherence tomography with a novel motion contrast technique. Opt Express. 2009;17:22190–200.
6. Wei E, Jia Y, Tan O, et al. Parafoveal retinal vascular response to pattern visual stimulation assessed with OCT angiography. PLoS One. 2013;8(12):e81343.
7. Lumbroso B, Huang D, Jia Y, et al. Clinical guide to Angio-OCT "non invasive Dyeless OCT angiography". New Delhi: India: Jaypee Brothers Medical Publisher (P) Ltd 2015.
8. Jia Y, Tan O, Tokayer J, et al. Split-spectrum amplitude decorrelationangiography with optical coherence tomography. Opt Expres. 2012;20:4710–25.
9. Schwartz DM, Fingler J, Kim DY, et al. Phase-variance optical coherence tomography. A technique for noninvasive angiography. Ophthalmology. 2014;121:180–7.
10. Spaide RF, Klancnik JM Jr, Cooney MJ. Retinal vascular layers imaged byfluorescein angiography and optical coherence tomography angiography. JAMA Ophthalmol. 2015;133:45–50.
11. Savastano MC, Lumbroso B, Rispoli M. In vivo characterization of retinal vascularization morphology using optical coherence tomography angiography. Retina. 2015;35:2196–203.
12. Arend O, Wolf S, Harris A, et al. The relationship of macularmicrocirculation to visual acuity in diabetic patients. Arch Ophthalmol. 1995;113:610–4.
13. Wu L, Femandez-Loaiza P, Sauma J, et al. Classification of diabetic retinopathy and diabetic macular edema. World J Diabetes. 2013;4(6):290–4.
14. Goudot MM, Sikorav A, Semoun O, et al. Parafoveal OCT angiography features in diabetic patients without clinical diabetic retinopathy: a qualitative and quantitative analysis. J Ophthalmol.Volume. 2017; Article ID 8676091, 1-14.
15. de Carlo TE, Romano A, Waheed NK, et al. A review of optical coherence tomography angiography (OCTA). Int J Retina Vitreous. 2015;1:5.
16. Motoharu T, Masako M, Yuichi T. Delineation of capillary dropout in the deep retinal capillary plexus using optical coherence tomography angiography in apatient with Purtscher's retinopathyexhibiting normal fluorescein angiographyfindings: a case report. BMC Ophthalmol. 2016;16:113.
17. Samara WA, Shahlaee A, Adam MK, et al. Quantification of diabetic macular ischemia using optical coherence tomography angiography and its relationship with visual acuity. Ophthalmology. 2017;124(2):235–44.
18. Simonett JM, Scarinci F, Picconi F, Giorno P, De Geronimo D, Di Renzo A, et al. Early microvascular retinal changes in optical coherence tomography angiography in patients with type 1 diabetes mellitus. Acta Ophthalmol. 2017;35(Suppl 1):2353.
19. Carnevali A, Sacconi R, Corbelli E, Tomasso L, Querques L, Zerbini G, et al. Optical coherence tomography angiography analysis of retinal vascular plexuses and choriocapillaris in patients with type 1 diabetes without diabetic retinopathy. Acta Diabetol. 2017;54(7):695–702.
20. Durbin MK, et al. Quantification of retinal microvascular density in optical coherence tomographic angiography images in diabetic retinopathy. JAMA Ophthalmol. 2017;135(4):370–6.
21. Zhang M, Hwang TS, Dongye C, Wilson DJ, Huang D, Jia Y. Automated quantification of nonperfusion in three retinal plexuses using projection-resolved optical coherence tomography angiography in diabetic retinopathy. Invest Ophthal Vis Sci. 2016;57(13):5101–6.
22. Dubis AM, Hansen BR, Cooper RF, et al. Relationship between the foveal avascular zone and foveal pit Morpholog. IOVS. 2012;53(3):1628–36.
23. Yu J, Gu R, Zong Y, et al. Relationship between retinal perfusion and retinal thickness in healthy subjects: an optical coherence tomography angiography study. Invest Ophthalmol Vis Sci. 2016;57:204–10.
24. Matsunaga D, Puliafito CA, Kashani AH. OCT angiography in healthy human subjects. Ophthalmic Surg Lasers Imaging Retina. 2014;45(6):510–5.

9

Cataract surgery combined with micro-incision vitrectomy in patients with behcet's disease uveitis

Fang Fan, Zhiyang Jia, Kejun Li, Xiaobin Zhao and Qingmin Ma[*]

Abstract

Background: This study sought to report the outcomes of a combined cataract extraction, intraocular lens (IOL) insertion and micro-incision vitrectomy (MIVS) procedure for the treatment of Behcet uveitis.

Methods: This investigation involved the retrospective evaluation of a case series of patients with Behcet uveitis who underwent cataract extraction, IOL insertion and MIVS in a single surgical session at the same institution between January 2013 and November 2016. Outcome measures included visual acuity, inflammatory reaction, systemic anti-inflammatory medications, intraocular pressure (IOP) and complications.

Results: Seven eyes of seven patients with a mean age of 39.00 ± 5.54 years (range, 32 to 48 years) and a mean follow-up duration of 13.57 ± 5.83 months (range, 6 to 24 months) were studied; five patients with a history of well-controlled uveitis were included. All patients underwent cataract extraction and IOL implantation combined with MIVS. All patients received postoperative steroids, which were slowly tapered during the weeks after surgery. There were no significant complications related to the surgery. Overall, best-corrected visual acuity (BCVA) was improved from log MAR (logarithm of the minimum angle of resolution) 1.67 ± 0.67 preoperatively to log MAR 0.74 ± 0.35 postoperatively; this improvement was statistically significant ($p < 0.05$). All eyes were deemed quiet at follow-up, and no patients required the escalation of therapy for long-term uveitis control.

Conclusions: This retrospective series indicates that a procedure that combines phacoemulsification, IOL implantation and MIVS is a feasible technique for the removal of cataracts and pathologic vitreous in eyes with Behcet uveitis. This approach can restore vision without obvious complications.

Keywords: Cataract surgery, Micro-incision vitrectomy, Behcet uveitis

Background

Behcet uveitis is a common condition worldwide. This condition remains problematic because of its long course and therapeutic challenges. In combination with chronic persistent inflammation, it is also associated with a high rate of ocular complications and a high risk of permanent visual loss [1]. In certain cases, surgical treatment for Behcet uveitic eyes with cataract or posterior segment complications is inevitable. However, fear of surgery-associated intraocular inflammation has limited the clinical application of such treatment. Recently, there has been increasing progress in combined surgical techniques for cataract and pars plana vitrectomy surgeries, such as micro-incision cataract surgery combined with 23G or 25G sutureless vitrectomy (micro-incision vitrectomy (MIVS)) [2–4]. Besides, combined surgery has been complicated in eyes with uveitis [5, 6]. Thus, a procedure that combines phacoemulsification and MIVS may be a feasible treatment option in cases involving patients with Behcet uveitis accompanied by cataract and posterior segment complications.

In this study, we sought to evaluate the safety and tolerance of a procedure that combines phacoemulsification, IOL insertion and MIVS in a series of seven eyes with Behcet uveitis and to evaluate pre- and postoperative clinical factors associated with this condition.

* Correspondence: 406256595@qq.com
Department of Ophthalmology, Hebei general hospital, Shijiazhuang, Hebei 050000, People's Republic of China

Methods

Patients

We reviewed the medical records of patients suffering from Behcet uveitis who were treated in the Department of Ophthalmology of Hebei General Hospital between January 2013 and November 2016. This study adhered to the tenets set forth in the Declaration of Helsinki. Approval from the institution's ethics committee was obtained prior to conducting this study.

All patients were diagnosed with Behcet disease based on the criteria issued by the International Study Group for Behcet's Disease [7–9]. A subset of patients were receiving oral immunomodulatory therapy (cyclophosphamide and/or cyclosporine A). All patients underwent the collection of a detailed whole-body history, clinical evaluation and a comprehensive ocular examination that included the measurement of best-corrected visual acuities (BCVAs) (and conversion to the corresponding logarithm of the minimum angle of resolution (logMAR) values), slit-lamp examination, intraocular pressure (IOP) measurement, and fundus photography, if possible (FF 450plus; Carl Zeiss Meditec AG, Jena, Germany). Fluorescein angiography (FFA) and indocyanine green angiography (ICGA) were performed as required (FF 450plus; Carl Zeiss Meditec AG, Jena, Germany).Optical coherence tomography (OCT) (Cirrus HD-OCT 400, Carl Zeiss Meditec AG, Jena, Germany) and B-scan ultrasound evaluation (D0302; Meda Co., Ltd., TianJin, China) were performed during preoperative biometry, and a postoperative refraction of – 0.5 to 1.0 dioptres (D) was targeted. Whole-body examinations included determinations of typical clinical presentation, a tuberculin skin test, a chest X-ray or chest CT, a *Treponema pallidum* haemagglutination test, and serologic tests for HIV.

Surgical technique and postoperative treatment

All patients were preoperatively notified about the risks of the surgery. The combined surgical procedures were performed by one experienced surgeon. All surgical interventions were conducted under local anaesthesia. Cataract surgery was performed first. After a scleral tunnel approach was used to create microincisions (2.8 mm) in the superior sclera, lysing posterior synechiae as needed, continuous curvilinear capsulorrhexis and cortical cleaving hydrodissection were performed. Phacoaspiration was established using a bi-manual technique. If possible, a one-piece foldable hydrophobic acrylic IOL (Rayner, Rayner, UK) was inserted into either the capsule or the ciliary sulcus. A 23 G microcannular vitrectomy system was used for the MIVS procedure. All microcannulas were inserted 3.5 mm posterior to the limbus. After the first microcannula was inserted in the inferotemporal quadrant for the infusion cannula, two additional microcannulas were inserted in the superonasal and superotemporal quadrants for the light pipe and vitrectomy probe. During the vitreous surgery, the vitreous and the epiretinal membranes were removed to the greatest possible extent, and the vitreous base was clearly ablated. In all subjects, preventive capsulotomy was performed using the vitrectomy probe. If necessary, eyes were tamponaded with silicon oil, C_3F_8 or sterile air at the conclusion of the surgical procedure. For all eyes, a subtenon injection of 3 mg dexamethasone was administered at the end of the operation. Topical steroid eye drops (prednisolone acetate 1%; Alcon, USA), topical eye drops containing the non-steroidal anti-inflammatory drug pranoprofen (Santen, Japan) and a systemic steroid (prednisolone 1 mg/kg/day) were administered to all patients after surgery. Systemic corticosteroid therapy was tapered based on patients' conditions.

Patient follow-up

All patients were evaluated at 1 day, 3 days, 7 days, and 1 month after surgery. Patients were evaluated every month thereafter. Preoperative and postoperative BCVAs were measured using a Snellen visual acuity chart; spherical equivalents, anatomic outcomes and complications were also evaluated. If necessary, FFA and OCT were performed.

Statistical analysis

BCVAs were measured using a Snellen visual acuity chart and converted into logMAR values for statistical analysis. Mean values were compared using GraphPad Prism statistical software (La Jolla, CA). The threshold used for statistical significance was $p < 0.05$.

Results

This study involved a total of 7 eyes from 6 male patients and 1 female patient. The mean patient age was 39.00 ± 5.54 years (range,32 to 48 years), and the mean follow-up duration was 13.57 ± 5.83 months (range, 6 to 24 months). The duration of Behcet disease before surgery was 6.50 ± 6.32 years (range, 0.5 to 20). Clinical characteristics of the patients are summarized in Table. 1. All patients experienced systematic symptoms of Behcet disease; these symptoms included oral ulcers (all patients), genital ulcers (4 patients, 57.14%), skin lesions (2 patients, 28.57%) and arthritis (2 patients, 28.57%). All patients suffered from recurrent attacks of anterior uveitis with exacerbation of this condition over time. All subjects had a history of posterior uveitis or panuveitis. All eyes exhibited preoperative cataract. Two patients with active inflammation were treated with intravenous methylprednisolone pulse therapy before surgery. One subject exhibited combined tractional and rhegmatogenous retinal detachment and underwent tamponade with silicon oil. In 6 eyes (85.71%), IOLs were implanted during surgery, with implantation in the capsule in 5 eyes (71.43%). In 1 eye

Table 1 Patients' characteristics, sugery, vision outcomes and complications

	Patient						
	1	2	3	4	5	6	7
Age	48	36	34	39	43	32	41
Gender	female	male	male	male	male	male	male
Eye	right	right	left	right	right	left	left
Duration of BD	20	0.5	6	5	3	4	7
Indications for surgery							
Cataract	+	+	+	+	+	.+	+
PVO	+	+	+	+	+	+	+
RD	–	–	–	–	+	+	–
CME	+	–	+	–	–	–	+
Stage	active	stable	stable	stable	active	stable	stable
SystemTreatment							
Preoperative	CA + MPT	C A	–	–	CTX + MPT	–	CA
postoperative	OP	OP	OP	OP	OP	OP	OP
Surgical procedure	P + I + MIVS+C + ILMP+DA	P + I + MIVS+ C + ILMP	P + I + MIVS+ C + ILMP	P + I + MIVS+ C + ILMP	P + I + MIVS+ILMP+ C + EP + C3F8	P + MIVS+C + ILMP+ EP + SO	P + I + MIVS+ C + ILMP
Follow up months	24	12	6	12	13	18	10
BCVA							
Preoperative	0.02	0.1	0.04	0.06	0.01	LP	0.04
Postoperative							
1 M	0.12	0.5	0.12	0.4	0.08	0.02	0.2
6 M	0.15	0.5	0.12	0.5	0.1	0.02	0.2
Last visit	0.12	0.6	0.12	0.5	0.1	0.08	0.2
CME							
Preoperative	+	–	+	–	–	–	+
Postoperative 1 M	+	+	+	+	+	+	+
Postoperative 6 M	–	–	–	–	–	–	–
IOL implant							
Capsule	+	+	–	+	+	–	+
Ciliary sulcus	–	–	+	–	–	+	–
Secondary surgery	–	–	–	–	–	+	–
Complications	posterior synechiae CE	CE	posterior capsular rupture CE	–	posterior synechiae CE	Mydriasis transient rise IOP CE	–

Retinal detachment: RD Persistent vitreous opacities: PVO cystoid macular edema: CME Cyclosporine A:CA methylprednisolone pulse therapy: MPT oral prednisolone:OP Cyclophosphamide:CTX micro-incision vitrectomy: MIVS capsulotomy: C endophotocoagulation: EP silicon oil:SO disinfect air:DA internal limiting membranepeeling: ILMP corneal edema: CE

with posterior capsular rupture during surgery, an IOL was inserted into the ciliary sulcus, with sutures used for intrascleral fixation. An IOL was not implanted into 1 eye because of severe retinal detachment. In the eye tamponaded with silicon oil, the silicon oil was removed 6 months after vitrectomy, and an IOL was implanted at that time. The retina remained attached after silicone oil removal.

The patients had a mean preoperative BCVA of logMAR 1.67 ± 0.67 (range, Light Perception (LP) (logMAR 3.0) to 20/200 (logMAR 1.0)) and a mean postoperative BCVA of logMAR 0.82 ± 0.48 (range, 20/1000 (logMAR 1.70) to 20/40 (logMAR 0.30)) at 6 months after surgery. A mean postoperative BCVA of logMAR 0.74 ± 0.35 (range, 20/250(logMAR 1.10) to 20/33 (logMAR 0.22)) at last visit. For the patient with retinal detachment, the final BCVA 6 months after silicon oil removal was 20/250. Cystoid macular oedema (CME) that was preoperatively confirmed using FFA and OCT was detected in 3 eyes (42.86%). However, postoperative CME was observed in all patients. For all patients, CME was relieved at 6-month follow-up evaluations. Owing to preventive capsulotomy performed using the vitrectomy probe, no patient exhibited posterior capsule opacification during follow-up. Complications during the operation included capsular rupture in one eye (14.29%); for this eye, an IOL was implanted in the ciliary sulcus, with sutures used for intrascleral fixation. The most common complication after surgery was transient corneal oedema, which was observed in 5 eyes (71.43%) but resolved without sequelae in all patients. Significant intraocular inflammation was observed in 3 eyes (42.86%), and posterior synechiae developed to different degrees in 2 eyes (28.57%); pupillary block did not occur. The patient who received silicon oil tamponade exhibited transient postoperative IOP elevation (range, 25 to 35 mmHg) that was effectively controlled using topical treatment. However, transient postoperative ocular hypotension was detected in this patient after silicon oil removal; this condition was alleviated within 2 weeks. During follow-up, all IOLs remained in situ, and IOL decentration did not occur. In this study, no patients had recurrent attacks of uveitis, and no subjects required the escalation of baseline therapy for the long-term control of intraocular inflammation.

Discussion

Behcet disease, which presents as recurrent attacks of vasculitis involving small, medium and large blood vessels, is a multisystem disease [9]. Ocular involvement of Behcet disease with a dramatic impact on vision is typically bilateral and includes relapsing remitting panuveitis and a series of complications [10]. Reports have described the use of phacoemulsification with MIVS to treat complicated cataract and several posterior segment complications in patients with other types of chronic uveitis [6]. However, there exist only limited data on the use of combined phacoemulsification with MIVS for the management of cataract and coexisting posterior segment involvement in eyes affected by Behcet disease. The purpose of our research was to investigate an approach to treat anterior and posterior complications in eyes with Behcet uveitis.

After surgery, BCVA was improved in all eyes. Moderate uveitis control was maintained for most patients. Intraocular inflammation was observed with corneal oedema and anterior chamber inflammatory reaction; posterior synechiae developed to various extents in 2 eyes (28.57%). No eyes exhibited pupillary block. All patients developed CME 1 month after surgery; fortunately, CME had resolved by 6 months after surgery in all eyes. A possible mechanism underlying this phenomenon might be considerable intraoperative manipulation; the cataract surgery itself can disrupt the blood-aqueous barrier and produce susceptibility to CME in an eye with Behcet uveitis. However, the resolution of CME within 6 months after surgery might be attributable to the benefits of MIVS, internally limiting membrane peeling and systemic corticosteroid application. Cataract surgery is difficult in eyes with recurrent uveitis for iris depigmentation,

lack of flexibility. The incidence of capsular rupture was high. In our study, posterior capsular rupture were observed in 1 eye during surgery.

To improve long-term uveitis control, satisfactory control of inflammation for at least 3 months prior to surgery is recommended for patients with uveitis. However, there exists research suggesting that cataract surgery and vitrectomy offer a surgical approach for clearing vitreous opacities and avoiding the release from the lens of inflammatory material with high permeation during a state of persistent inflammation [11]. This study included cases in which active inflammation was treated with intravenous methylprednisolone pulse therapy before surgery; however, inflammation after surgery was not severe. Consistent with this outcome, research has indicated that systemic interferon-alpha therapy resulted in less pronounced postoperative inflammation after intraocular surgery in subjects with ocular Behcet disease [12]. Surgery might be a method for relieving persistent inflammation. Combined surgery for eyes with chronic uveitis has produced encouraging results [5, 6, 13–15]. Our findings indicated the safety and utility of our combined procedure for Behcet uveitis. Traditionally, phacoemulsification and IOL implantation are always accomplished before or after vitrectomy. This typical approach generally requires two surgeons and two operations and therefore involves relatively high costs and long hospital stays. One-stage surgery could simultaneously resolve cataract and posterior segment involvement, thereby shortening patient discomfort, reducing costs and accelerating visual recovery. Our results obtained using combined phacoemulsification, IOL implantation and MIVS in a single surgery confirm the efficiency of this technique, which has been described in previous reports [13–16]. Moreover, MIVS improves operative efficiency and is a relatively non-invasive surgery with an acceptable complication rate and mild postoperative inflammatory reactions. This procedure may be a reasonable option for eyes with Behcet uveitis that concurrently exhibit cataract and posterior changes. Such eyes are prone to serious postoperative inflammation if treated with large instruments and more surgical manipulations. A technique involving scleral tunnel phacoemulsification and IOL implantation followed by MIVS was used in our study. In our experience, this procedure has been extremely promising. A scleral tunnel can avoid corneal wound leakage during vitrectomy; furthermore, better corneal transparency can reduce the difficulty of vitrectomy. In our opinion, the technique of IOL implantation followed by MIVS is relatively easy and requires a short operation time. We used viscoelastic material when the posterior surface of an IOL was watered during gas–fluid exchange. However, whether IOL implantation was performed was dependent on the patient's condition. There were no complications during surgery. We implanted an IOL into the capsular bag to the greatest possible extent. In our study, visual acuity was improved in all patients after surgery. The longest follow-up time was 2 years. Only two patients developed obvious iris adhesion, and no secondary glaucoma or recurrence of uveitis was observed. Our study had several limitations, including an inadequate number of cases and limited follow-up time. Further investigation is needed.

Conclusions

This retrospective series indicates that a combined phacoemulsification, IOL implantation and MIVS procedure appears to improve BCVA and can be an effective and safe intervention for treating patients with Behcet uveitis with cataract and vitreoretinal complications. This technique also has beneficial effects on the long-term course of Behcet uveitis and may restore or preserve vision. However, more case series with longer follow-up periods are needed to identify the natural course of Behcet uveitis and to evaluate the outcomes of this technique.

Abbreviations

BCVA: Best-corrected visual acuity; CME: Cystoid macular edema; FFA: Fluorescein angiography; ICGA: Indocyanine green angiography; IOL: Intraocular lens; IOP: Intraocular pressure; MIVS: Micro-incision vitrectomy; OCT: Optical coherence tomography; SE: Spherical equivalents; TST: Tuberculin skin test

Acknowledgements
The authors would like to acknowledge Jie Kang, Si Min, at the Hebei general hospital, for their technical assistance on this study.

Funding
This work was supported by grants from key projects of Hebei provincial health and Family Planning Commission Award Number: ZL20140018.

Authors' contributions
Design of the Study (QMM, ZYJ); Conduct of the study (FF, KJL); Collection, management, analysis, and interpretation of the data (FF, XBZ, KJL); Preparation, review and approval of manuscript (FF, ZYJ, KJL, XBZ, QMM). All authors read and approved the final manuscript.

Competing interests
The authors declare they have no competing interests.

References

1. Mendoza-Pinto C, Garcia-Carrasco M, Jimenez-Hernandez M, Hernandez CJ, Riebeling-Navarro C, Zavala AN, et al. Etiopathogenesis of Behcet's disease. Autoimmun Rev. 2010;9(4):241–5.
2. Czajka MP, Frajdenberg A, Johansson B. Comparison of 1.8-mm incision versus 2.75-mm incision cataract surgery in combined phacoemulsification and 23-gauge vitrectomy. Acta Ophthalmol. 2016;94(5):507–13.
3. Khan BAM, Rizvi SF, Mahmood SA, Mal W, Zafar S. Visual outcome of 25-gauge microincision vitrectomy surgery in diabetic vitreous haemorrhage. Pak J Med Sci. 2015;31(5):1197–200.
4. Schonfeld CL. 23-vs 20-gauge pars plana vitrectomy in combination with bimanual microincisional cataract surgery (b-MICS) for the treatment of macular hole and cataract as a one-step procedure. Eye. 2013;27(8):952–8.
5. Murthy SI, Pappuru RR, Latha KM, Kamat S, Sangwan VS. Surgical management in patient with uveitis. Indian J Ophthalmol. 2013;61(6):284–90.
6. Soheilian M, Mirdehghan SA, Peyman GA. Sutureless combined 25-gauge vitrectomy, phacoemulsification, and posterior chamber intraocular lens implantation for management of uveitic cataract associated with posterior segment disease. Retina. 2008;28(7):941–6.
7. Kurokawa MS, Suzuki N. Behcet's disease. Clin Exp Med. 2004;4(1):10–20.
8. Marshall SE. Behcet's disease. Best Prac Res Clin Rheumatol. 2004;18(3):291–311.
9. Mendes D, Correia M, Barbedo M, Vaio T, Mota M, Goncalves O, et al. Behcet's disease - a contemporary review. J Autoimmun. 2009;32(3–4):178–88.
10. Yang PZ, Fang W, Meng QL, Ren YL, Xing L, Kijlstra A. Clinical features of Chinese patients with Behcet's disease. Ophthalmol. 2008;115(2):312–8.
11. Zierhut M, Abu El-Asrar AM, Bodaghi B, Tugal-Tutkun I. Therapy of ocular Behcet disease. Ocul Immunol Inflamm. 2014;22(1):64–76.
12. Yalcindag FN, Uzun A. Results of interferon alpha-2a therapy in patients with Behcet's disease. J Ocul Pharmacol Ther. 2012;28(4):439–43.
13. Androudi S, Praidou A, Symeonidis C, Tsironi E, Iaccheri B, Fiore T, et al. Safety and efficacy of small incision, sutureless pars plana vitrectomy for patients with posterior segment complications secondary to uveitis. Acta Ophthalmol. 2012;90(5):e409-e10.
14. Czajka MP, Frajdenberg A, Johansson B. Outcomes after combined 1.8-MM microincision cataract surgery and 23-gauge transconjunctival vitrectomy for posterior segment disease: a retrospective study. Retina. 2014;34(1):142–8.
15. Soheilian M, Ramezani A, Soheilian R. 25-gauge vitrectomy for complicated chronic endogenous/autoimmune uveitis: predictors of outcomes. Ocul Immunol Inflamm. 2013;21(2):93–101.
16. Dabour SA, Ghali MA. Outcome of surgical management for rhegmatogenous retinal detachment in Behcet's disease. BMC Ophthalmol. 2014;14:61.

10

Expression of cytokines in aqueous humor from fungal keratitis patients

Yingnan Zhang[1], Qingfeng Liang[2], Yang Liu[1], Zhiqiang Pan[1*], Christophe Baudouin[3,4], Antoine Labbé[3,4] and Qingxian Lu[5]

Abstract

Background: Although a series of reports on corneal fungal infection have been published, studies on pathogenic mechanisms and inflammation-associated cytokines remain limited. In this study, aqueous humor samples from fungal keratitis patients were collected to examine cytokine patterns and cellular profile for the pathogenesis of fungal keratitis.

Methods: The aqueous humor samples were collected from ten patients with advanced stage fungal keratitis. Eight aqueous humor samples from patients with keratoconus or corneal dystrophy were taken as control. Approximately 100 µl to 300 µl of aqueous humor in each case were obtained for examination. The aqueous humor samples were centrifuged and the cells were stained and examined under optical microscope. Bacterial and fungal cultures were performed on the aqueous humor and corneal buttons of all patients. Cytokines related to inflammation including IL-1β, IL-6, IL-8, IL-10, TNF-α, and IFN-γ were examined using multiplex bead-based Luminex liquid protein array systems.

Results: Fungus infection was confirmed in these ten patients by smear stains and/or fungal cultures. Bacterial and fungal cultures revealed negative results in all aqueous humor specimens. Polymorphonuclear leukocytes were the predominant infiltrating cells in the aqueous humor of fungal keratitis. At the advanced stages of fungal keratitis, the levels of IL-1β, IL-6, IL-8, and IFN-γ in the aqueous humor were significantly increased when compared with control ($p<0.01$). The levels of IL-10 and TNF-α also showed an ascending trend but with no statistical significance.

Conclusions: High concentration of IL-1β, IL-6, IL-8, and IFN-γ in the aqueous humor was associated with fungal keratitis.

Keywords: cytokines, aqueous humor, fungal keratitis, inflammation

Background

Corneal infection is one of the major eye diseases affecting public health worldwide [1], especially in developing countries [2]. Its increasing incidence and the difficulty associated with therapy result in severe vision problems or blindness [3]. The incidences of fungal keratitis are higher in the harvest seasons. Males and the middle-aged (41–50 years old) population are more likely to be affected by fungal keratitis. The cornea is particularly affected by fungal infections due to its susceptibility to injury and non-vascularization, resulting in lower resistance. The major pathogenic fungi are *Fusarium* species (73.3%), followed by *Aspergillus* species (12.1%) [4].

Although a series of reports on corneal fungal infection have been published including epidemiology, diagnostics, pathogenic risk factors, and treatment methods, studies on pathogenic mechanisms and inflammation-associated cytokines remain relatively limited [5, 6]. Research on the pathogenesis of fungal keratitis has been performed on animal models [7, 8] and on the tear samples of the patients with fungal keratitis [9]. However, tears are highly susceptible to environment and ophthalmic medication due to their surface location.

Clinically, we found that some fungal keratitis patients experienced hypopyon and fibrin exudation in the anterior chamber, but their corneal endothelia were clear. After deep anterior lamellar keratoplasty (DALK), the hypopyon disappeared without recurrence of infection. It has been suggested that cytokines in aqueous humor play an important role in the pathogenesis of fungal keratitis.

* Correspondence: panyj0526@163.com
[1]Beijing Tongren Eye Center, Beijing Tongren Hospital, Capital Medical University, Beijing Ophthalmology & Visual Science Key Lab, Beijing 100730, China
Full list of author information is available at the end of the article

In the present study, aqueous humor samples from fungal keratitis patients were collected to monitor the intraocular inflammatory response. Cytokine patterns and cellular profile were analyzed for pathogenesis of fungal keratitis.

Methods

Patients

This study was approved by the Medical Ethical Committee of Beijing Tongren Hospital. Before surgery, informed consents were obtained from the patients and parents/legal guardians (if the patient ≤18 years old) of all the participants after explanation of the nature and possible consequences of the study.

Ten patients of clinically diagnosed fungal keratitis and eight patients with keratoconus or corneal dystrophy who had undergone penetrating keratoplasty in Beijing Tongren Hospital from June to November of 2014 were recruited for this study.

The cases were diagnosed as fungal keratitis when fungal culture and/or scraped specimen staining were positive. Patients who did not respond to initial therapy with topical and systemic antifungal drugs were recruited. A detailed clinical and demographic history was taken and a thorough slit-lamp biomicroscopic examination was performed for all the patients. The size, depth, and margins of the ulcer were noted, along with the presence of satellite lesions and hypopyon height. The presence of an epithelial defect and pigmentation on the surface was also recorded.

Samples Collection

Before surgery, the corneal culture specimens and scrapings were taken from the base and edge of the ulcers aseptically with sterile cotton-tipped swabs and placed in transport medium. The scraped specimens were sent for inoculation in Sabouraud's dextrose agar medium for fungal culture. All the corneal scrapings were also sent for routine Gram's stain and bacterial culture in nutrient broth.

The patients received penetrating keratoplasty with general anesthesia. The donor corneas were obtained from Beijing Tongren Eye Bank. Paracentesis lancet was used to penetrate the cornea in an avascular peripheral area over a length of 1 mm. Thereafter, approximately 100 μl to 300 μl of aqueous humor was taken out of the anterior chamber without contact with intraocular structures. Each sample of aqueous humor was centrifuged for 10 min at 2000 revolutions per minute (rpm) to separate cells from fluid. Reserved 50 μl supernatants were transferred into sterile microfuge tube and stored at − 80 °C until assaying for cytokine, and the remaining supernatant was used for bacterial and fungal culture. The cell pellet was resuspended in 200 μl of phosphate buffered saline and deposited onto glass slides. After air-drying, the cells were stained with Giemsa and examined by optical microscopy. The cells were counted and morphologically classified into polymorphonuclear leukocytes (PMN), lymphocytes, and monocytes.

In all cases, the corneal buttons of patients, which were obtained at the time of penetrating keratoplasty, were sent for microbial investigations.

Microbiological Culture

The aqueous humor and cornea from all the patients were inoculated on culture medium at 28 °C with a humidity of 40% for 8–10 days. The culture medium contained Sabouraud's agar and potato glucose agar. The fungi were identified according to the characteristics of growing colonies, hyphae, and spore. In addition, the specimens of aqueous humor and cornea were inoculated on broth medium at 37 °C with a humidity of 40% for 10–14 days for bacteria identification.

Cytokines Measurement by Liquid Protein Array System

The levels of cytokines including interleukin (IL)-1β, IL-6, IL-8, IL-10, interferon-γ (IFN-γ), and tumor necrosis factor-α (TNF-α) in the aqueous humor were measured using Luminex100™ liquid protein array systems (MiraiBio, CA, US).

Statistical Analysis

Statistical analyses were performed by SPSS software (version 11.5, SPSS Inc., Chicago, Illinois, USA). The levels of each cytokine were compared by means of the data and reported as medians with minimum and maximum levels obtained for each group. The results are presented as the geometric mean concentration and the range of detectable samples (Table 2). The cytokine levels were compared between two groups with nonparametric two-sample median test. A p-value of < 0.05 was considered to be significant.

Results

Patient Cohort

The average age of patients with fungal keratitis was 49. 30 ± 17.02 years (range from 15 to 72 years old). Three patients (30%) were female and seven patients (70%) were male. Five eyes (50%) had a history of wooden foreign body or plant injury. In addition to antifungal therapy, four eyes (40%) had been treated with topical corticosteroid or corticosteroid-antibiotic combination therapy and three eyes (30%) had been treated with topical antibiotics only.

The control patients with keratoconus (87.5%) or corneal dystrophy (12.5%) received penetrating keratoplasty for visual restoration. Their average age was 24.88 ± 12.12 years (range from 11 to 50 years old). Two patients (25%) were female and six patients (75%) were male. (Table 1).

Table 1 Demographic, clinical and microbiological aspects in fungal keratitis patients and controls

No.	Gender	Age range (years old)	Diagnosis	Duration (days)	Pathogeny	Smear (fungus)	Aqueous humor culture (fungus / bacteria)		Corneal culture (fungus / bacteria)		Ulcer (mm × mm)	Hypopyon (depth, mm)
1	M	11–20	FK	7	None	+	–	–	+	–	6 × 5	2.0
2	F	51–60	FK	7	Foreign body	+	–	–	+	–	8 × 7	2.0
3	F	41–50	FK	7	None	–	–	–	+	–	5 × 4	1.0
4	F	41–50	FK	18	None	+	–	–	+	–	7 × 6	4.0
5	M	61–70	FK	30	None	+	–	–	+	–	5 × 4	1.0
6	M	41–50	FK	10	Plant Injury	+	–	–	+	–	3 × 3	0.5
7	M	41–50	FK	10	Foreign body	–	–	–	+	–	8 × 7	2.0
8	M	71–80	FK	30	Plant Injury	–	–	–	+	–	6 × 5	5.0
9	M	71–80	FK	12	None	–	–	–	+	–	5 × 4	3.0
10	M	41–50	FK	30	Plant Injury	–	–	–	+	–	4 × 3	2.0
11	F	11–20	KC				–	–	–	–		
12	F	41–50	CD				–	–	–	–		
13	M	11–20	KC				–	–	–	–		
14	M	11–20	KC				–	–	–	–		
15	M	21–30	KC				–	–	–	–		
16	M	11–20	KC				–	–	–	–		
17	M	31–40	KC				–	–	–	–		
18	M	21–30	KC				–	–	–	–		

Note: *M*: male; *F*: female; *FK*: fungal keratitis; *KC*: keratoconus; *CD*: corneal dystrophy; +, positive; –, negative

Characterization of Fungal Keratitis

Therapeutic keratoplasty had been taken since the patients did not respond to the medication treatment, with a tendency to corneal melting and perforation. The time course of disease development was ranged from 7 to 30 days, with an average of 15.89 ± 10.72 days. Epithelial defect and pigmentation on the surface, characterized as dry and pigmented ulcers with irregular and feathery margins, satellite lesions, fibrinoid aqueous reaction, and hypopyon formation, were present on the infected eyes of fungal keratitis patients. The features of ulcers are highlighted in Table 1.

Cytopathologic Examination

The PMN cell populations were the predominant infiltrated cells types in the aqueous humor samples collected from the infected eyes of fungal keratitis patients. A low percentage of lymphocytes and monocytes were also observed. The percentage of these infiltrating cells is depicted in Table 2. The difference in the pattern of infiltrating cells between fungal keratitis and the control was statistically significant ($p < 0.001$ for each population).

Microbial Investigation

The positive fungal infection rate in the keratitis patients was 50% by smear staining and 100% by corneal culture. Among ten positive cases of corneal fungal culture, strain *Fusarium spp.* was evident in six cases (60%), strain *Aspergillus spp.* was present in two cases (20%), and strain *Apospory spp.* was identified in the other two cases (20%). However, it was noteworthy that the aqueous humor cultures from both fungal keratitis and control groups showed likewise negative presentation of either fungus or bacteria.

Cytokine Profiles

The protein levels of cytokines IL-1β, IL-6, IL-8, IL-10, IFN-γ, and TNF-α were measured by Liquid Protein

Table 2 Percentage of various infiltrating cells in aqueous humor from fungal keratitis patients and controls

	% Polymorphonuclear			% Lymphocytes			% Monocytes		
	Median	Minimum	Maximum	Median	Minimum	Maximum	Median	Minimum	Maximum
FK	89.5	85.7	92.0	8.1	6.5	13.2	3.9	0.5	6.8
Control	0	0	0	0	0	0	0	0	0
p	< 0.001			< 0.001			< 0.001		

Note: *FK*: fungal keratitis

Array System. The concentration of six cytokines in the control group was used as a basal level for comparison. The cytokine levels showed remarkable difference between fungal keratitis and control group. In the aqueous humor samples of fungal keratitis group, the levels of IL-1β, IL-6, IL-8, and IFN-γ were found to be significantly increased, as compared with the control group ($P = 0.012$ for IL-1β, $P < 0.001$ for IL-6, $P < 0.001$ for IL-8, and $P = 0.001$ for IFN-γ). Although IL-10 and TNF-α levels were also elevated, they showed no statistically significant difference (Table 3).

Discussion

The aqueous humor cultures from ten fungal keratitis patients showed negative in fungal and bacterial infection, it further confirmed that a sterile reaction occurred in the aqueous humor of some fungal keratitis patients despite hypopyon. The major infiltrating cells in the aqueous humor were PMN leukocytes. Based on the animal experiments and clinical corneal histology, the PMN leukocytes in the aqueous humor are considered the major cellular basis of fungal keratitis [7, 10]. Our present results confirm this expectation. It is likely that these infiltrating cells are involved in the clearance of pathogens [11]. In contrast, no inflammatory cells were found in the control.

In the present study, we measured and analyzed the intraocular cytokine profiles in relation to fungal keratitis. During the middle-advanced stage of fungal infection, the IL-1β, IL-6, IL-8, and IFN-γ levels in the aqueous humor were significantly increased compared to non-keratitis controls.

Cytokine levels in aqueous humor have been reported as indicators of local ocular immunological processes. Increased IL-1β and IL-6 are the specific inflammatory signals for keratohelcosis and keratitis [12]. IL-1β, IL-6, and IL-8 are significantly increased in the tears of bacterial keratitis patients, along with accumulating dendritic cells [13]. In studies of animal models on the herpes simplex virus-infected keratitis, cytokines such as IL-1β, IL-6, IL-8, IL-10, IL-12, and IFN-γ were demonstrated to play a predominant role in disease development [14, 15]. In corneal epithelial cells infected with *Pseudomonas*, IL-1β functioned as the major inflammatory mediator regulating IL-6 and IL-8 expression [16]. IL-6, IL-10, and IFN-γ were elevated in acute uveitis aqueous humor. IL-10 was increased in infective uveitis compared with non-infective uveitis [17]. Cytokines IL-4, IFN-γ, and TNF-α were increased in aqueous humor in Behçet's uveitis [18, 19]. IL-6, IL-10, and IFN-γ were involved in rejection after corneal transplantation [20]. All these reports indicate that the expression of cytokines is closely related to the ocular inflammatory and immunologic reactions.

IL-1β is a proinflammatory cytokine and an important inflammation mediator. In the inflammatory reaction, it can induce synthesis of other cytokines, activation of T lymphocyte, and migration of monocyte, macrophage, and Langerhans' cells [21, 22]. In our study, a high level of IL-1β was observed in the aqueous humor samples collected from fungal keratitis patients. It is quite possible that the elevated level of IL-1β caused severe leukocyte infiltration and blood-aqueous barrier damage. IL-6 is a potential mediator of intraocular inflammation, and several evidence indicate that it plays an important multifunctional role in corneal infection and inflammation [23]. Moreover, it can activate the production of antibody and fibrous proteins, induce the production of proteins in acute inflammation, and serve as an activator of macrophage and chemotactic factors for T lymphocytes [24]. IL-6 can also be induced by other cytokines such as IL-1β, TNF-α, and IFN-γ and be released by retinal pigment epithelial cells, corneal endothelial cells, macrophage, iris, and ciliary body epithelial cells [25]. IL-8 selectively activates PMN leukocytes and T cells and imposes a chemotactic effect on neutrophilic granulocytes, which are induced to infiltrate into the inflammatory sites, thus increasing vascular permeability and activating cytokines (such as IL-1β and TNF-α) to be released. As a consequence, such inflammatory responses further lead to a continuous increase in IL-8 level and accumulation of leukocytes, which exacerbates inflammation [26, 27]. Therefore, the increased IL-8, as observed in the aqueous humor of the fungal keratitis patients, could be a primary cause for the increased PMN infiltration and the high expression level of IL-1β. IFN-γ is produced by activated lymphocytes. It can inhibit cell proliferation and prevent other cytokines from being recruited to sites of inflammation. IFN-γ is a primary cytokine involved in delayed type hypersensitivity [28]. IFN-γ in the aqueous humor of the fungal keratitis patients is secreted by the increased infiltrating lymphocytes, which, to some extent, might inhibit the inflammation severity.

IL-10 and TNF-α levels in the aqueous humor of fungal keratitis patients were higher on average than those of the control, but with no statistical differences. IL-10 is an

Table 3 Cytokine levels in aqueous humor from fungal keratitis patients and controls

Cytokine levels (pg/ml)	Fungal keratitis (n = 10)		Control (n = 8)		
	Mean (±SD)	Median	Mean (±SD)	Median	p
IL-1β	172.89 ± 45.83	121.41	7.50 ± 3.22	5.98	0.012
IL-6	6179.71 ± 1015.726	6712.84	6.22 ± 7.55	3.12	0.000
IL-8	13,003.82 ± 1803.97	13,755.86	9.61 ± 9.24	6.17	0.000
IL-10	25.32 ± 18.99	26.13	8.32 ± 0.25	8.23	0.230
TNF-α	22.82 ± 56.69	1.92	1.52 ± 2.10	0.00	0.237
IFN-γ	28.70 ± 18.93	7.91	2.32 ± 1.18	3.17	0.001

anti-inflammatory cytokine. IL-10 could represent an inhibitory factor in the T helper 1 cells response. Indeed, IL-10 takes protective effects during inflammation as an inflammatory cytokine-inhibiting factor [28, 29]. TNF-α is an important factor in connecting specific immunity and inflammatory reaction. It is mainly produced by activated monocytes and can induce monocytes to synthesize IL-1β, IL-6, and IL-8 [30].

Our subjects involved only a small number of patients, followed over a limited period of time, and the cytokines analyzed were restricted to the inflammation related cytokines. The cytokine and inflammatory cells infiltrate profiles in the aqueous humor in keratitis caused by other pathogenic microorganisms have not been reported previously. In the present study, patients with keratoconus and corneal dystrophy were selected as the negative control. Though strictly they may serve as a control for non-inflammatory ocular pathologies. Further investigations are needed to report on the roles of cytokines and other cell signal transduction factors in each stage of inflammation in fungal keratitis. Due to the diverse roles of cytokine in different signal transduction pathways and additional biological effects caused by interactions between cytokines and its productions, studies of the cytokine network are more meaningful than that of single cytokines.

Since cytokines in aqueous humor play important roles in the pathogenesis of fungal keratitis, the use of intervention strategies in related cytokines (such as blocking cytokines binding to receptors, or competitive binding to receptors using inactivated cytokine analogs and blocking their functions after binding) to achieve therapeutic goals is worthy of further investigation.

Conclusions

The present studies demonstrate that a high concentration of IL-1β, IL-6, IL-8, and IFN-γ in the aqueous humor is associated with fungal keratitis, and the infiltrating PMN leukocytes are involved in this inflammatory response. Studying the cytokine profile in the aqueous humor of fungal keratitis patients is beneficial for elucidation of pathological changes and inflammatory responses of fungal keratitis. It is anticipated that further studies in this direction will lead to innovation and development of more effective therapeutic strategies for fungal keratitis.

Abbreviations
IFN-γ: Interferon-γ; DALK: Deep anterior lamellar keratoplasty; IL: Interleukin; PMN: Polymorphonuclear leukocytes; rpm: Revolutions per minute; TNF-α: Tumor necrosis factor-α

Acknowledgements
The authors especially thank the patients and their families for taking part in this study. Thanks are due to Antoine Labbé for his help and consideration.

Funding
This work was supported by the National Natural Scientific Foundation of China: Grant No.81541105 (Y.Z.). Q.Lu is partly supported by general fund from the Research to Prevent Blindness.

Authors' contributions
Y.Z. performed the samples collection and laboratory experiment, analyzed the data, and was a major contributor in writing the manuscript. Q. Liang clinically diagnosed the patients and revised the manuscript. Y.L. performed statistical analysis. Z.P. designed the project and performed the penetrating keratoplasty surgery. C.B. and A.L. revised the manuscript. Q. Lu edited and proofread the final manuscript. All authors read and approved the final manuscript.

Competing interests
The authors declare that they have no competing interests.

Author details
[1]Beijing Tongren Eye Center, Beijing Tongren Hospital, Capital Medical University, Beijing Ophthalmology & Visual Science Key Lab, Beijing 100730, China. [2]Beijing Institute of Ophthalmology, Beijing Tongren Eye Center, Beijing Tongren Hospital, Capital Medical University, Beijing Key Laboratory of Ophthalmology and Visual Sciences, Beijing 100005, China. [3]Quinze-Vingts National Ophthalmology Hospital, Paris and Versailles Saint-Quentin-en-Yvelines University, Versailles, France. [4]INSERM, U968, Paris, F-75012, France; UPMC Univ Paris 06, UMR_S 968, Institut de la Vision, Paris F-75012, France; CNRS, UMR_7210, Paris F-75012, France, Paris, France. [5]Department of Ophthalmology and Visual Sciences, University of Louisville, 301 E. Muhammad Ali Blvd, Louisville, KY 40202, USA.

References
1. Whitcher JP, Srinivasan M, Upadhyay MP. Corneal blindness: a global perspective. Bull World Health Organ. 2001;79(3):214–21.
2. Whitcher JP, Srinivasan M. Corneal ulceration in the developing world–a silent epidemic. Br J Ophthalmol. 1997;81(8):622–3.
3. Dong X, Xie L, Shi W. Penetrating keratoplasty in management of fungal keratitis. Chin J Ophthalmol. 1994;35:386–7.
4. Xie L, Zhong W, Shi W. Spectrum of fungal keratitis in north China. Ophthalmol. 2006;113:1943–8.
5. Prajna NV, John RK, Nirmalan PK, Lalitha P, Srinivasan M. A randomised clinical trial comparing 2% econazole and 5% natamycin for the treatment of fungal keratitis. Br J Ophthalmol. 2003;87(10):1235–7.
6. Thomas PA. Current perspectives on ophthalmic mycoses. Clin Microbiol Rev. 2003;16(4):730–97.
7. Wu TG, Wilhelmus KR, Mitchell BM. Experimental keratomycosis in a mouse model. Invest Ophthalmol Vis Sci. 2003;44(1):210–6.
8. Wu TG, Keasler VV, Mitchell BM, Wilhelmus KR. Immunosuppression affects the severity of experimental Fusarium solani keratitis. J Infect Dis. 2004; 190(1):192–8.
9. Vasanthi M, Prajna NV, Lalitha P, Mahadevan K, Muthukkaruppan V. A pilot study on the infiltrating cells and cytokine levels in the tear of fungal keratitis patients. Indian J Ophthalmol. 2007;55(1):27–31.
10. Vemuganti GK, Garg P, Gopinathan U, Naduvilath TJ, John RK, Buddi R, Rao GN. Evaluation of agent and host factors in progression of mycotic keratitis: A histologic and microbiologic study of 167 corneal buttons. Ophthalmology. 2002;109(8):1538–46.
11. Thomas J, Gangappa S, Kanangat S, Rouse BT. On the essential involvement of neutrophils in the immunopathologic disease: herpetic stromal keratitis. Journal of immunology (Baltimore, Md : 1950). 1997;158(3):1383–91.
12. Becker J, Salla S, Dohmen U, Redbrake C, Reim M. Explorative study of interleukin levels in the human cornea. Graefe's archive for clinical and experimental ophthalmology = Albrecht von Graefes Archiv fur klinische und experimentelle Ophthalmologie. 1995;233(12):766–71.
13. Yamaguchi T, Calvacanti BM, Cruzat A, Qazi Y, Ishikawa S, Osuka A, Lederer J, Hamrah P. Correlation between human tear cytokine levels and cellular corneal changes in patients with bacterial keratitis by in vivo confocal microscopy. Invest Ophthalmol Vis Sci. 2014;55(11):7457–66.

14. Imanishi J. Expression of cytokines in bacterial and viral infections and their biochemical aspects. J Biochem. 2000;127(4):525–30.

15. Stumpf TH, Shimeld C, Easty DL, Hill TJ. Cytokine production in a murine model of recurrent herpetic stromal keratitis. Invest Ophthalmol Vis Sci. 2001;42(2):372–8.

16. Xue ML, Willcox MD, Lloyd A, Wakefield D, Thakur A. Regulatory role of IL-1beta in the expression of IL-6 and IL-8 in human corneal epithelial cells during Pseudomonas aeruginosa colonization. Clin Exp Ophthalmol. 2001; 29(3):171–4.

17. van Kooij B, Rothova A, Rijkers GT, de Groot-Mijnes JD. Distinct cytokine and chemokine profiles in the aqueous of patients with uveitis and cystoid macular edema. Am J Ophthalmol. 2006;142(1):192–4.

18. Hamzaoui K, Hamzaoui A, Guemira F, Bessioud M, Hamza M, Ayed K. Cytokine profile in Behcet's disease patients. Relationship with disease activity. Scand J Rheumatol. 2002;31(4):205–10.

19. Ahn JK, Yu HG, Chung H, Park YG. Intraocular cytokine environment in active Behcet uveitis. Am J Ophthalmol. 2006;142(3):429–34.

20. van Gelderen BE, Van Der Lelij A, Peek R, Broersma L, Treffers WF, Ruijter JM, van Der Gaag R. Cytokines in aqueous humour and serum before and after corneal transplantation and during rejection. Ophthalmic Res. 2000;32(4):157–64.

21. Dinarello CA. Biologic basis for interleukin-1 in disease. Blood. 1996;87(6):2095–147.

22. Rudner XL, Kernacki KA, Barrett RP, Hazlett LD. Prolonged elevation of IL-1 in Pseudomonas aeruginosa ocular infection regulates macrophage-inflammatory protein-2 production, polymorphonuclear neutrophil persistence, and corneal perforation. Journal of immunology (Baltimore, Md : 1950). 2000;164(12):6576–82.

23. Fenton RR, Molesworth-Kenyon S, Oakes JE, Lausch RN. Linkage of IL-6 with neutrophil chemoattractant expression in virus-induced ocular inflammation. Invest Ophthalmol Vis Sci. 2002;43(3):737–43.

24. Maruo N, Morita I, Shirao M, Murota S. IL-6 increases endothelial permeability in vitro. Endocrinology. 1992;131(2):710–4.

25. Noma H, Funatsu H, Yamasaki M, Tsukamoto H, Mimura T, Sone T, Jian K, Sakamoto I, Nakano K, Yamashita H, et al. Pathogenesis of macular edema with branch retinal vein occlusion and intraocular levels of vascular endothelial growth factor and interleukin-6. Am J Ophthalmol. 2005;140(2):256–61.

26. Chodosh J, Astley RA, Butler MG, Kennedy RC. Adenovirus keratitis: a role for interleukin-8. Invest Ophthalmol Vis Sci. 2000;41(3):783–9.

27. Oakes JE, Monteiro CA, Cubitt CL, Lausch RN. Induction of interleukin-8 gene expression is associated with herpes simplex virus infection of human corneal keratocytes but not human corneal epithelial cells. J Virol. 1993; 67(8):4777–84.

28. Macatonia SE, Doherty TM, Knight SC, O'Garra A. Differential effect of IL-10 on dendritic cell-induced T cell proliferation and IFN-gamma production. Journal of immunology (Baltimore, Md : 1950). 1993;150(9):3755–65.

29. Boorstein SM, Elner SG, Meyer RF, Sugar A, Strieter RM, Kunkel SL, Elner VM. Interleukin-10 inhibition of HLA-DR expression in human herpes stromal keratitis. Ophthalmology. 1994;101(9):1529–35.

30. Santos Lacomba M, Marcos Martin C, Gallardo Galera JM, Gomez Vidal MA, Collantes Estevez E, Ramirez Chamond R, Omar M. Aqueous humor and serum tumor necrosis factor-alpha in clinical uveitis. Ophthalmic Res. 2001; 33(5):251–5.

11

Interferon alpha-2a treatment for refractory Behcet uveitis in Korean patients

Ji Hwan Lee, Christopher Seungkyu Lee and Sung Chul Lee*

Abstract

Background: To evaluate therapeutic outcomes of interferon alpha-2a (IFNα2a) treatment in patients with Behcet's disease who were refractory to immunosuppressive agents.

Methods: This retrospective case series reviewed the medical records of 5 patients with refractory Behcet uveitis from January 2011 to February 2017. IFNα2a was administered at a dose of 3 million IU 3 times per week. Clinical response, relapse rate, and change of visual acuity were evaluated.

Results: The mean age of patients was 39.60 ± 9.21 years, and the median treatment duration was 6 months. Four of the 5 patients (80%) presented with responses to IFNα2a without any uveitis attack during the treatment period. The mean number of uveitis attacks/year per patient during the treatment was 0.40 ± 0.89. The mean log of the Minimum Angle of Resolution visual acuity improved from 1.44 ± 0.38 at baseline to 1.02 ± 0.58 at the final follow up.

Conclusions: IFNα2a is an effective therapy for Behcet uveitis refractory to conventional immunosuppressants in Korean patients.

Keywords: Behcet syndrome, Interferon-alpha, Therapeutics, Uveitis

Background

Behcet's disease (BD) is a chronic relapsing multisystem vasculitis mainly characterized by recurrent oral ulceration, genital ulceration, ocular lesions, and skin lesions [1]. Ocular involvement is one of the most serious complication of BD, as repeated attacks of uveitis may result in blindness [2].

Corticosteroid treatment is the mainstay in the management of acute uveitic attacks, and immunosuppressive agents such as cyclosporine and azathioprine are usually effective in long-term management [3, 4]. Interferon alpha-2a (IFNα2a) has been reported to be effective and safe in refractory cases, although the optimal regimen has not yet been established [5–13]. In this study, we aimed to evaluate the efficacy of IFNα2a in Korean patients with Behcet uveitis refractory to immunosuppressive agents.

Methods

Patients

We retrospectively reviewed the medical records of 5 patients with refractory Behcet uveitis who were treated with IFNα2a from January 2011 to February 2017. Refractory Behcet uveitis was defined as unresponsive or recurrent uveitis despite combination therapy of immunosuppressive agents and corticosteroids. Patients who were followed up for at least 3 months were included in this study. All the patients met the criteria of the International Study Group for Behcet's disease [14]. This study was approved by the institutional review board of Severance Hospital, Yonsei University College of Medicine (IRB No.4–2017-0436).

Interferon alpha-2a treatment

IFNα2a (Roferon-A®; Roche; Basel, Switzerland) was administered at a dose of 3×10^6 IU 3 times per week. All previous immunomodulatory agents were stopped the day before the initiation of IFNα2a. During IFNα2a therapy, oral corticosteroid was tapered to a low dose (5–10 mg/d prednisolone equivalent) or discontinued according to a general tapering schedule (to reduce by

* Correspondence: sunglee@yuhs.ac
Department of Ophthalmology, The Institute of Vision Research, Yonsei University College of Medicine, Yonsei-ro 50-1, Seodaemun-gu, Seoul, Republic of Korea

5 mg/day every 1–2 weeks if the dose of prednisolone is 20-40 mg/day, to reduce by 2.5 mg/day every 1–2 weeks if the dose is below 20 mg).

Assessments

All patients underwent a complete ophthalmologic examination, including best-corrected visual acuity (BCVA), slit lamp biomicroscopy, tonometry, and fundoscopy. Ancillary examinations included fluorescein angiography and optical coherence tomography. Examinations were performed weekly for 2 weeks, every 2 weeks for 1 month, and then once every month. Relapse was defined as two step increase in level of inflammation including anterior chamber cells or vitreous haze [15]. The relapse rate was calculated as attacks per year. Response to IFNα2a therapy was defined as maintenance of inactive disease without any relapse during the treatment period. The mean Log-MAR BCVA and the mean number of uveitis attacks per year at baseline and final visit were compared using Wilcoxon signed-rank test. Statistical analyses were performed using SPSS version 23.0 (IBM; Chicago, IL, USA) and a p-value< 0.05 was considered statistically significant.

Results

Patients

Demographic and clinical characteristics of patients are summarized in Table 1. The mean age of patients was 36.60 ± 9.21 years and 5 patients were male in this study.

The mean overall follow up period including the treatment period was 58.80 ± 33.48 months. All patients were Korean. Four patients (80%) presented bilateral involvement. Extraocular manifestations of BD included oral aphthous ulcers and skin lesions in all patients (100%), genital ulcer in 1 patient (20%), gastrointestinal involvement in 2 patients (40%), central nervous system involvement in 1 patient (20%), and epididymitis in 1 patient (20%). Prior to IFNα2a therapy, 3 patients received combination therapy of azathioprine, cyclosporine, or methotrexate, and 2 patients were treated with mycophenolate mofetil.

Interferon alpha-2a treatment

The median duration of IFNα2a treatment was 6 months (range 2–28 months). Four (80%) of 5 patients showed responses to IFNα2a without any uveitis attack during the treatment period (Fig. 1). The mean number of uveitis attacks per year during the treatment was 0.40 ± 0.89, which decreased from 2.16 ± 1.08 before IFNα2a therapy (p = 0.043). Four responsive patients could not discontinue IFNα2a therapy in this study. One patient (20%) received posterior subtenon triamcinolone injection during the treatment period. In 1 unresponsive patient, IFNα2a was switched to infliximab. Visual acuity improved at final visit compared with baseline in all patients. The mean log of the Minimum Angle of Resolution (logMAR) BCVA changed from 1.44 ± 0.38

Table 1 Demographic and clinical characteristics of patients with refractory Behcet uveitis

	Patient 1	Patient 2	Patient 3	Patient 4	Patient 5
Age-range at onset (years)	20–30	40–50	20–30	30–40	30–40
Duration of IFNα2a treatment (months)	6	5	28	12	2
Overall follow-up period (months)	51	27	34	72	110
Laterality	Bilateral	Unilateral	Bilateral	Bilateral	Bilateral
Anatomic classification of uveitis	Panuveitis	Panuveitis	Panuveitis	Panuveitis	Panuveitis
Extraocular manifestations of BD	Oral ulcer CNS involvement Epididymitis Arthritis Skin lesion (EN)	Oral ulcer Genital ulcer Skin lesion(EN) GI involvement	Oral ulcer Skin lesion (folliculitis) GI involvement	Oral ulcer Skin lesion (EN)	Oral ulcer Skin lesion(EN)
Previous immunosuppressive treatment	Azathioprine 100 mg/d, Methotrexate 17.5 mg weekly	Cyclosporine 200 mg/d Azathioprine 100 mg/d, Methotrexate 17.5 mg weekly	Cyclosporine 200 mg/d, Azathioprine 100 mg/d	Mycophenolate mofetil 2 g/d	Mycophenolate mofetil 2 g/d
Dose of oral corticosteroid (mg/d prednisolone equivalent), preTx→postTx	40 → 10	15 → 0	20 → 0	40 → 5	15 → 0
Relapse rate (number of uveitis attacks/year), preTx→postTx	2.13 → 2	1.64 → 0	4.00 → 0	1.80 → 0	1.22 → 0
Response to IFNα2a	No	Yes	Yes	Yes	Yes
Adverse events	Flu-like Sx Depression	Flu-like Sx	Flu-like Sx	Flu-like Sx	Flu-like Sx

BD: Behcet's disease, *CNS*: central nervous system, *EN*: erythema nodosum, *GI*: gastrointestinal, *IFNα2a*: interferon alpha-2a, *Sx*: symptoms, *Tx*: treatment

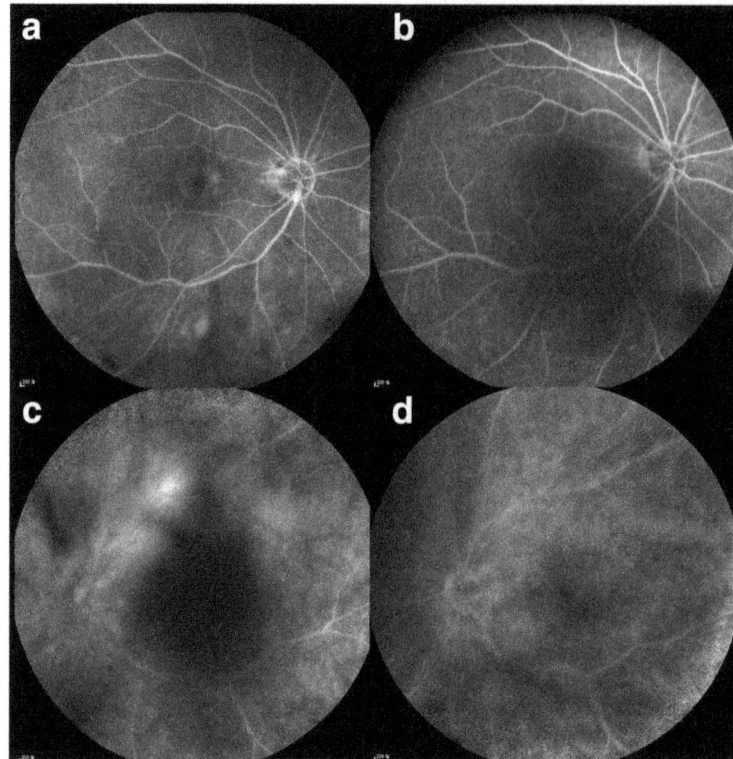

Fig. 1 Fluorescein angiographic images of patients with refractory Behcet uveitis. In patient 4, diffuse capillary leakage (**a**) decreased 6 months after interferon alpha-2a (IFNα2a) therapy (**b**). In patient 3, moderate vascluitis at the superior arcade (**c**) was significantly resolved 17 months after the initiation of IFNα2a treatment (**d**)

(Snellen equivalent 20/550) at baseline to 1.02 ± 0.58 (Snellen equivalent 20/209) at final visit ($p = 0.068$). Although the baseline BCVA was 20/200 or less in all patients (100%), the final BCVA of 20/200 or less were observed in 2 patients (40%).

Adverse events

All patients experienced flu-like symptoms at the beginning of IFNα2a treatment. One patient presented with mild depression, which was relieved by antidepressant medication. No other significant adverse effects were observed during the treatment period.

Discussion

In this study, we evaluated the efficacy of IFNα2a in patients with Behcet uveitis refractory to immunosuppressive agents. Most patients had good responses to IFNα2a. IFNα2a therapy was maintained in these patients. There were no uveitis attacks during the treatment period in the 4 patients who were responsive to IFNα2a therapy. Visual acuity improved in all patients.

Corticosteroid is the main treatment option for acute attacks of Behcet uveitis. However, its long-term use is limited because of adverse effects. Cyclosporine and azathioprine have been effectively used in Behcet uveitis

alone or combined with other immunosuppressants in severe cases [3, 4]. There are, however, some patients who are refractory to immunosuppressive agents, and biological therapies including anti-tumor necrosis factor antibody, anti-interleukin, or interferon can be considered in such cases [16, 17]. Recently, IFNα2a has been reported to be effective for the treatment of refractory Behcet uveitis [5, 7–13, 18, 19].

There is no consensus on the dose and protocol of IFNα2a therapy for Behcet uveitis. In this study, we used a lower-dose regimen of 3×10^6 IU of IFNα2a 3 times per week during the treatment period. The rate of treatment response in our series was 80%, which is similar to that in previous reports using higher doses of IFNα2a [13, 19]. A lower-dose regimen may be associated with fewer treatment-related complications. There were no severe adverse effects in the present study. In contrast, patients with leukopenia or thrombocytopenia have been reported in previous studies using higher doses of IFNα2a [18, 20]. Four responsive patients could not discontinue IFNα2a therapy in this study, which may also have been associated with the lower dose of the regimen. By comparison, 25–50% of patients may discontinue IFNα2a treatment with higher-dose regimens [11, 13].

The relapse rate of uveitis attacks significantly decreased from 2.16 ± 1.08 to 0.40 ± 0.89 after IFNα2a therapy. In the 4 patients who had responses to IFNα2a therapy, there were no uveitis attacks during the treatment period. The efficacy of IFNα2a therapy in terms of uveitis relapse was comparable to recent reports [13, 19]. We confirmed that treatment response without uveitis relapse may be achieved mostly with low-dose continuous IFNα2a therapy in Korean patients.

As refractory Behcet uveitis cases are rare, the major limitations of this study are its retrospective design and the small number of patients. We were, however, able to confirm the efficacy of IFNα2a therapy in a uniform low-dose regimen. Questions regarding the optimal dosage, treatment duration, and treatment protocol of IFNα2a therapy still remain unanswered. A prospective study would be necessary not only to determine the most effective and safest protocol, but also to compare the efficacy of IFNα2a with new biological agents currently under study.

Conclusions

IFNα2a is an effective therapeutic for Behcet uveitis refractory to other immunosuppressants in Korean patients.

Abbreviations

BCVA: best-corrected visual acuity; BD: Behcet's disease; IFNα2a: interferon alpha-2a; LogMAR: log of the minimum angle of resolution

Acknowledgements

None.

Funding

None.

Authors' contributions

Conceptualization of the study JHL and SCL Data acquisition and analysis JHL, CSL and SCL Manuscript preparation JHL and CSL Analytic revision of manuscript SCL. All authors read and approved the final manuscript.

Competing interests

The authors declare that they have no competing interests.

References

1. Sakane T, Takeno M, Suzuki N, Inaba G. Behcet's disease. N Engl J Med. 1999;341(17):1284–91.
2. Nussenblatt RB. Uveitis in Behcet's disease. Int Rev Immunol. 1997;14(1):67–79.
3. Masuda K, Nakajima A, Urayama A, Nakae K, Kogure M, Inaba G. Double-masked trial of cyclosporin versus colchicine and long-term open study of cyclosporin in Behcet's disease. Lancet Lon Engl. 1989;1(8647):1093–6.
4. Yazici H, Pazarli H, Barnes CG, Tuzun Y, Ozyazgan Y, Silman A, Serdaroglu S, Oguz V, Yurdakul S, Lovatt GE, et al. A controlled trial of azathioprine in Behcet's syndrome. N Engl J Med. 1990;322(5):281–5.
5. Wechsler B, Bodaghi B, Huong DL, Fardeau C, Amoura Z, Cassoux N, Piette JC, LeHoang P. Efficacy of interferon alfa-2a in severe and refractory uveitis associated with Behcet's disease. Ocul Immunol Inflamm. 2000;8(4):293–301.
6. Kotter I, Zierhut M, Eckstein AK, Vonthein R, Ness T, Gunaydin I, Grimbacher B, Blaschke S, Meyer-Riemann W, Peter HH, et al. Human recombinant interferon alfa-2a for the treatment of Behcet's disease with sight threatening posterior or panuveitis. Br J Ophthalmol. 2003;87(4):423–31.
7. Krause L, Altenburg A, Pleyer U, Kohler AK, Zouboulis CC, Foerster MH. Longterm visual prognosis of patients with ocular Adamantiades-Behcet's disease treated with interferon-alpha-2a. J Rheumatol. 2008;35(5):896–903.
8. Deuter CM, Zierhut M, Mohle A, Vonthein R, Stobiger N, Kotter I. Long-term remission after cessation of interferon-alpha treatment in patients with severe uveitis due to Behcet's disease. Arthritis Rheum. 2010;62(9):2796–805.
9. Sobaci G, Erdem U, Durukan AH, Erdurman C, Bayer A, Koksal S, Karagul S, Bayraktar MZ. Safety and effectiveness of interferon alpha-2a in treatment of patients with Behcet's uveitis refractory to conventional treatments. Ophthalmology. 2010;117(7):1430–5.
10. Onal S, Kazokoglu H, Koc A, Akman M, Bavbek T, Direskeneli H, Yavuz S. Long-term efficacy and safety of low-dose and dose-escalating interferon alfa-2a therapy in refractory Behcet uveitis. Arch Ophthalmol. 2011;129(3):288–94.
11. Yalcindag FN, Uzun A. Results of interferon alpha-2a therapy in patients with Behcet's disease. J Ocul Pharmacol Ther. 2012;28(4):439–43.
12. Diwo E, Gueudry J, Saadoun D, Weschler B, LeHoang P, Bodaghi B. Long-term efficacy of interferon in severe uveitis associated with Behcet disease. Ocul Immunol Inflamm. 2017;25(1):76–84.
13. Hasanreisoglu M, Cubuk MO, Ozdek S, Gurelik G, Aktas Z, Hasanreisoglu B. Interferon alpha-2a therapy in patients with refractory Behçet uveitis. Ocul Immunol Inflamm. 2017;25(1):71–5.
14. International Study Group for Becet's Disease. Critertia for diagnosis of Behcet's disease. Lancet (London, England). 1990;335(8697):1078–80.
15. Jabs DA, Nussenblatt RB, Rosenbaum JT. Standardization of uveitis nomenclature for reporting clinical data. Results of the first international workshop. Am J Ophthalmol. 2005;140(3):509–16.
16. Calvo-Rio V, Blanco R, Beltran E, Sanchez-Burson J, Mesquida M, Adan A, Hernandez MV, Hernandez Garfella M, Valls Pascual E, Martinez-Costa L, et al. Anti-TNF-alpha therapy in patients with refractory uveitis due to Behcet's disease: a 1-year follow-up study of 124 patients. Rheumatology (Oxford). 2014;53(12):2223–31.
17. Papo M, Bielefeld P, Vallet H, Seve P, Wechsler B, Cacoub P, Le Hoang P, Papo T, Bodaghi B, Saadoun D. Tocilizumab in severe and refractory non-infectious uveitis. Clin Exp Rheumatol. 2014;32(4 Suppl 84):S75–9.
18. Gueudry J, Wechsler B, Terrada C, Gendron G, Cassoux N, Fardeau C, Lehoang P, Piette JC, Bodaghi B. Long-term efficacy and safety of low-dose interferon alpha2a therapy in severe uveitis associated with Behcet disease. Am J Ophthalmol. 2008;146(6):837–44. e831
19. Park JY, Chung YR, Lee K, Song JH, Lee ES. Clinical experience of interferon alfa-2a treatment for refractory uveitis in Behcet's disease. Yonsei Med J. 2015;56(4):1158–62.
20. Tugal-Tutkun I, Guney-Tefekli E, Urgancioglu M. Results of interferon-alfa therapy in patients with Behcet uveitis. Graefes Arch Clin Exp Ophthalmol. 2006;244(12):1692–5.

12

Evaluating inner retinal dimples after inner limiting membrane removal using multimodal imaging of optical coherence tomography

Jingjing Liu, Yiye Chen, Shiyuan Wang, Xiang Zhang and Peiquan Zhao[*] (iD)

Abstract

Background: To evaluate inner retinal dimples after peeling of the inner limiting membrane (ILM) for macular holes (lamellar macular hole [LMH] and full-thickness macular hole [FTMH]) via multiple imaging modes of spectral-domain optical coherence tomography (OCT) and to assess their relationship with preoperative vitreoretinal interface conditions.

Methods: The data of 38 eyes in 35 patients who underwent surgery for LMH, and FTMH were retrospectively studied. The presence of postoperative inner retinal dimples was judged by a combination of en face OCT layer images and cross-sectional images. The demographic and clinical characteristics of eyes with and without inner retinal defects were compared to identify factors involved in the formation of the defects.

Results: Inner retinal defects were found in 26 eyes (68%) after surgery. They appeared on the en face OCT ILM layer images as multiple dark spots limited to the ILM peeling area, and corresponded to dimples or pitting of inner retinal layers on cross-sectional OCT images. In 5 cases (19%), apparent progression of inner retinal defects was observed on the en face OCT images as increasing numbers and sizes of the dark spots, which seemed to follow an eccentric growth pattern starting from the central macula. In addition, highly myopic eyes were found to be associated with the formation of more severe inner retinal defects.

Conclusions: Multiple imaging modes of en face spectral-domain OCT provide comprehensive information about the appearance of inner retinal dimples. High myopic eyes seem to develop more severe inner retinal defects after ILM peeling.

Keywords: Inner limiting membrane peeling, Inner retinal defects, Macular hole, Optical coherence tomography, Vitreoretinal interface

Background

Tadayoni et al. [1] first found inner retinal defects after epiretinal membrane (ERM) removal in 2001. They reported findings of a fundus with an appearance characterized by dark arcuate striae along the course of the optic nerve fibers, and called it dissociated optic nerve fiber layer (DONFL). To date, inner retinal defects have been reported to occur in patients after inner limiting membrane (ILM) peeling, which is performed for various indications including ERM, retinal vein occlusion, diabetic macular edema, and macular hole [2–10]. The incidence of these defects seems to be higher in cases with a macular hole (MH) [7]. To the best of our knowledge, inner retinal defects were not frequently evaluated via en face OCT imaging, which can provide not only B-scans but also en face C-scans of the different retinal layers [5, 7, 10]. On ILM layer images, we can identify inner retinal abnormalities more readily, and view their correspondence with the cross-sectional OCT images. This peculiar appearance has

* Correspondence: zhaopeiquanxh@163.com;
zhaopeiquan@xinhuamed.com.cn
Department of Ophthalmology, Xin Hua Hospital, Shanghai Jiao Tong University School of Medicine, Shanghai 200092, China

not been associated with compromised visual function to date [6, 8].

Since this discovery, inner retinal defects after ILM peeling have been associated with a DONFL appearance [1], concentric macular dark spots (CMDS) [5], and inner retinal dimpling [6]. Appropriate nomenclature for these defects is yet to be determined as their etiology remains unclear. Injury from surgical manipulation [1, 6], ILM removal [3, 4, 8], intraoperative ILM staining with dyes, and gas tamponade [9] are proposed risk factors for apparent inner retinal defects, with ILM peeling considered to be the main culprit. To date, other preoperative clinical factors related to the surgical condition have not been evaluated with respect to their relationship to the formation of inner retinal defects. Since inner retinal defects represent postoperative retinal surface changes after surgery, we assessed the preoperative vitreoretinal interface conditions (lamellar hole-associated epiretinal proliferation [LHEP]), ERM, and high myopia-associated posterior staphyloma) between eyes that developed inner retinal defects and those that did not, to identify the predisposing factors for inner retinal defect formation. LHEP is demonstrated on OCT as a thick homogenous layer of material with medium reflectivity on the epiretinal surface [11–13]. It occurs in both lamellar macular hole (LMH) and full thickness macular hole (FTMH). Unlike the conventional ERM, LHEP does not appear to have contractive properties [11]. The LHEP appearance is primarily driven by a proliferation of Müller cells onto the inner retina [13]. MHs complicated by ERM and LHEP might cause changes such as an imbalance of damaged and regenerative glial cells both before and after ILM peeling, which influences the formation of inner retinal defects. Khun [14] reported that rigidity of the ILM was responsible for the development of an MH in highly myopic eyes, and even observed the separation of the ILM from the retina within the bulging area of one eye with posterior staphyloma. Hence, the connection between ILM and the underlying retina in eyes with posterior staphyloma was assumed to be different from that in eyes without posterior staphyloma. Accordingly, the impact of ILM peeling on the inner retina was different from a chronic separation between the ILM and retina in eyes with posterior staphyloma, especially with ILM detachment. We also reviewed other general features such as age, sex, laterality, type and size of MH, and intraoperative findings (ILM peeling area, hemorrhagic spots), that may be causative factors for inner retinal defect formation.

Methods

We retrospectively reviewed the data of 138 consecutive cases of patients with MHs who underwent pars plana vitrectomy (PPV) with ILM peeling between January 2013 and October 2017. Patients who had successfully undergone PPV with ILM peeling for MHs were regularly evaluated for the postoperative macular conditions using high quality en face and B-scan imaging for at least 6 months. Patients who lacked the en face OCT images for analysis or had other notable retinal conditions that limited visual acuity, such as myopic choroidal neovascularization, diabetic retinopathy and age-related macular degeneration, were excluded from the study. Finally, 38 eyes in 35 patients were included in this study. Informed consent was obtained from all patients. The study protocol was performed in accordance with the Declaration of Helsinki, and was approved by Ethics Committee of Xin Hua Hospital affiliated to Shanghai Jiao Tong University School of Medicine.

All surgeries were carried out by the same experienced surgeon (P.Z). The surgical procedure consisted of a standard, three-port PPV, with induced posterior vitreous detachment if the posterior hyaloid was attached. The peripheral vitreous was then removed as much as possible, and the peripheral retina was checked circumferentially. Laser photocoagulation was applied to if any retinal tears or lattice were detected. ILM was removed followed by a pinch-and-peel technique in a circular manner with the end-gripping forceps under the assistance of brilliant blue G. The ILM peeling area was decided by the surgeon according to the hole's diameter. The ILM peeling area and hemorrhagic spots during ILM peeling of each patient were documented. At the end of surgery, air-fluid exchange was performed with gas tamponade by 15% perfluoropropane (C3F8). In cases where the patient presented with LHEP, the yellow tissue was not removed forcefully from the edge of the hole for fear of triggering further damage. Concomitant cataract operations were performed when a combined procedure was planned.

A preoperative and postoperative ophthalmic examination, including measurement of best corrected visual acuity (BCVA) and intraocular pressure, slit-lamp biomicroscopy, dilated fundus examination, ultrasonography and optical coherence tomography (RTVue XR100–2, Optovue Inc., Fremont, CA, USA), was performed on all the study eyes. OCT scans performed before the surgery and at 1, 3, and 6 months after surgery were analysed. The OCT scan modes included radial lines (12*9 mm), horizontal lines (12*9 mm), 3-dimensional retina (7*7 mm), and 3-dimensional Widefield Motion Correction Technology (12*9 mm). Simultaneously, reference images were obtained to observe the thickness distribution of the retina. The diameter of the FTMH was measured as the largest diameter of the 12-radial-line scan pattern centered on the MH. Patients with poor-quality en face OCT images due to poor segmentation performance (some patients with high myopic eyes) were excluded. Microperimetry was performed in 12 patients both preoperatively and postoperatively using the CenterVue MAIA (CenterVue, Padova,

Italy). The testing mode was 4–2 strategy: 37 test loci arranged in a radial pattern covering the central 6° region of the retina. The following features were recorded: age, sex, laterality of eyes, cause (s) and type of MHs, size of FTMH, presence or absence of LHEP and ERM, and posterior staphyloma associated with high myopia, anatomic outcome, and functional outcome. To distinguish inner retinal dimples from the inner retinal corrugations caused by other conditions such as ERM, en face in combination with cross-sectional OCT images were used to diagnose the presence of inner retinal dimples. All the postoperative images were evaluated by 3 individual examiners and divided into 2 groups: eyes with inner retinal dimples, and eyes without retinal dimples according to the presence of dimples (≥1) of the inner retinal layer and corresponding dark spots found on en face ILM images. The demographic and clinical features of the two groups were evaluated and compared using statistical analysis. The distribution patterns of the inner retinal defects shown on en face OCT images were analyzed.

The SPSS software, version 22.0 (SPSS, Inc., Chicago, IL), was used for all statistical analysis. The binary variables were compared using the chi-square test or Fisher's exact test, and continuous variables were compared using student's t-test and analysis of variance. Logistic regression analysis was used to analyze the risk factors in inner retinal dimple formation. Preoperative and postoperative BCVA were converted into the logarithm of the minimum angle of resolution (logMAR) for statistical analysis. Counting fingers and hand motions were replaced by a decimal visual acuity of 0.014 and 0.005, respectively, before conversion. A p value of < 0.05 was considered to indicate statistical significance.

Results

Thirty-eight eyes of 35 patients with a mean age of 61 years (range: 10–80 years) were included in this study. There were some hemorrhagic spots caused by superficial retinal capillary breakage after ILM peeling. However, no hemorrhagic spots due to direct surgical manipulation were found. Twenty-eight (80%) of the patients were women. The mean follow-up time was 8.7 months. The MH involved the right eye in 17 patients (49%), the left eye in 15 (43%), and both eyes, in 3 (9%). The preoperative diagnosis included 8 LMH (21%), and 30 FTMH (79%). The etiology of the MHs was idiopathic in 36 patients (95%), and traumatic in 2 (5%). Anatomical closure was achieved in all eyes (100%) at the last follow-up. The mean preoperative visual acuity was 1.01 logMAR, which was significantly improved to 0.63 logMAR after surgery ($p < 0.001$). Preoperative, postoperative and changes in BCVA between the two groups were not significantly different ($p = 0.693, 0.968,$ and 0.679, respectively). The mean preoperative and postoperative average sensitivity thresholds in microperimetry

were 21.70 dB and 25.10 dB, respectively ($p = 0.095$). Microperimetry was performed in 9 eyes with inner retinal dimples and in 3 eyes without inner retinal dimples. Preoperative, postoperative and changes in average sensitivity thresholds between the groups were not significantly different ($p = 0.430, 0.633,$ and 0.430, respectively).

Twenty-six eyes (68%) developed inner retinal defects, as seen on the postoperative OCT images at the last follow-up. On en face OCT ILM layer images, inner retinal defects were identified as multiple dark spots, limited to the ILM peeling area and not corresponding with the hemorrhagic areas during surgery. Preoperative en face OCT images were available for 24 eyes, and no similar appearance was found. There were 3 distribution types (Table 1): in 17 eyes (65%), the dark striae ran along the nerve fiber and spared the temporal raphe area (Fig. 1a); in 3 eyes (12%), the dark striae predominantly occurred in the papillomacular bundle area (Fig. 1d); in 6 eyes (23%), multiple dark spots were scattered about the ILM peeling area, and seemed not to run along the nerve fiber path (Fig. 1f). On cross-sectional OCT images, dimples of the inner retinal surface were discovered that corresponded to the striae, and areas with dots, representing the focal thinning of the underlying retinal nerve fiber layer (RNFL) (Fig. 1b, c, e, g, and h). The focal thinning of inner retinal layers seemed more severe in the multiple dark spots than in the other two spots (Fig. 1g, h). No similar appearances were found among the preoperative en face and B-scan OCT images. In 5 cases (19%), we observed an apparent progression, which appeared on the en face, ILM layer images, as increasing numbers and sizes of the dark spots (Fig. 2). The inner retinal defects started from the central macular and spread to the surrounding area. In 8 cases (21%), the ILM peeling area could be distinguished clearly on the en face layer images or the reference images (Fig. 2).

The associations between the development of inner retinal dimples and the demographic and clinical characteristics are summarized in Table 2. Unfortunately, we did not find any preoperative markers that predicted the development of DONFL (Table 3). The associations between the different categories of inner retinal dimples and preoperative vitreomacular interface conditions and ILM peeling area are summarized in Table 4. We found that eyes with "scattered" inner retinal defects had longer axial length and a higher incidence of posterior staphyloma.

Table 1 Number of Eyes with 3 Patterns of Inner Retinal Dimples After Inner Limiting Membrane Peeling

Categories of pattern	Number of eyes	%
1 Scattered	6	23.1%
2 Papillomacular bundle area	3	11.5%
3 Temporal raphe area-spared	17	65.4%

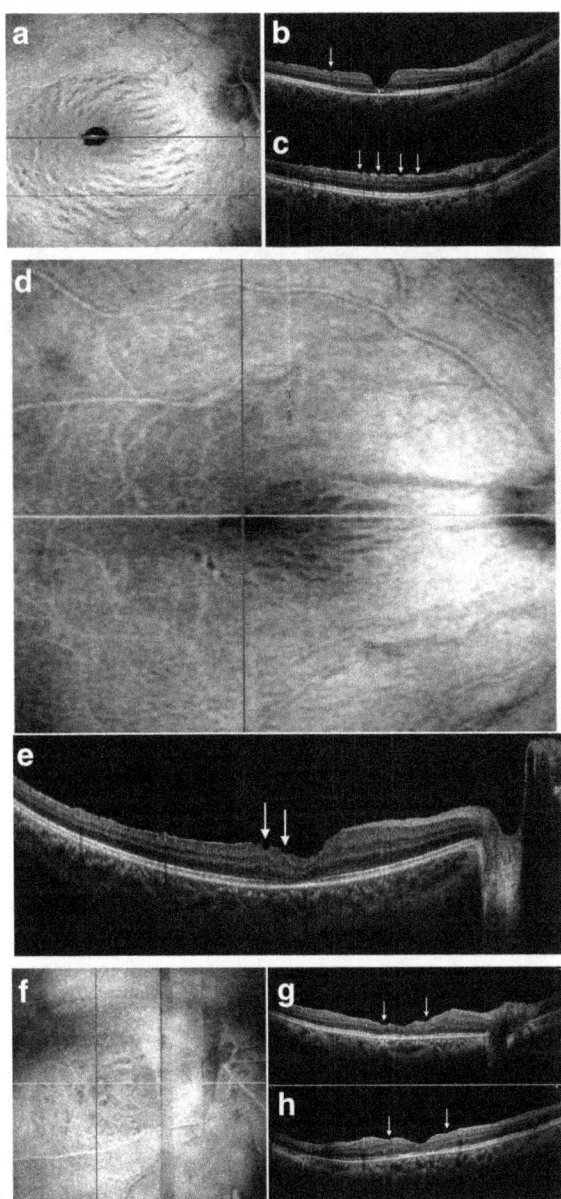

Fig. 1 Three distribution types of inner retinal defects on en face OCT ILM layer images **a** Dark striae run along the nerve fiber path and spared temporal raphe area; **b** and **c** corresponding cross-sectional OCT images show pitting of nerve fiber layer (arrows); **d** dark striae were found predominantly occurred in papillomacular bundle area; **e** corresponding B-scan OCT image shows pitting of nerve fiber layer, thinning of underlying ganglion cell layer is also noted (arrows); **f** multiple dark spots with different sizes scattered on the ILM peeling area and seem to not run along the nerve fiber path; **g** and **h** corresponding cross-sectional OCT images show significant thinning and disorganized of inner retinal layers (arrows)

Discussion

In this study, we used multiple imaging modes of spectral domain OCT to observe the inner retinal layer changes after ILM removal in patients with MHs. Inner retinal defects are frequently [1–6] seen after ILM peeling (43–100%), which was confirmed by our study (68%). On en face OCT ILM layer images, inner retinal defects can be seen as multiple dots distributed on the inner surface of the RNFLs, appearing darker than the surrounding area. On reviewing the en face OCT images, we were able to identify 3 distribution patterns of the dots: papillomacular bundle-dominated, scattered, and temporal raphe-spared. The dark dots on the ILM layer images corresponded to the dimples on the inner retinal surface noted on the cross-sectional OCT images. This is similar to the reports by Mitamura [2] and Ito [3], who found dimples in the RNFL using B-scans of OCT corresponding to each stria of the DONFL. They found that the depths of these dimples were limited to the RNFL thickness. However, we found ganglion cell layer thinning was concomitant with the dimples in some eyes, which was also found by Spaide [6]. Ganglion cell layers play a significant role in visual function. In order to determine whether retinal function was adversely influenced, we compared the BCVA and retinal average sensitivity thresholds detected by MAIA, and found no difference between the 2 groups. The outcome confirmed the findings of previous studies [1, 3, 6, 8]. However, some studies did find abnormal scotomata and reduced retinal sensitivity after surgery for MH [15, 16]. As many as 35–50% of retinal ganglion cells can be lost before a visual function deficiency is detected [17–19]. Based upon our results, we speculate that retinal ganglion cell losses occurring with inner retinal dimples may not reach the number needed to compromise visual function or our follow-up durations were not long enough to detect these changes. Another explanation was that these findings were not due to ganglion cell loss because Müller cell bodies are also located in the ganglion cell layer. Histopathologic studies [20–22] have shown that the peeled ILM contains Müller cell footplates, which would lead to Müller cell degeneration. Therefore, this may result in the thinning of the ganglion cell layer.

Müller cell footplates are reported to play a significant part in maintaining the homeostasis of the retinal milieu [23, 24]. The damaged footplate function after ILM peeling may be followed by secondary physiologic derangements of the inner retina [6]. Thus, the effects of trauma to the Müller cells, along with their regenerative growth after surgical removal of the ILM, could explain the formation of inner retinal dimples [6]. The relationships of ERM and LHEP, which are involved in the proliferation of glial cells, with inner retinal defects formation were evaluated. However, in this study, eyes with LHEP or conventional ERM in the inner retinal dimples group were not significantly different from eyes in the control group. The results suggest that the formation of inner retinal dimples may be influenced by several factors apart from Müller cells, that are yet to be explored. In addition, LHEP was found adjacent to the edges of

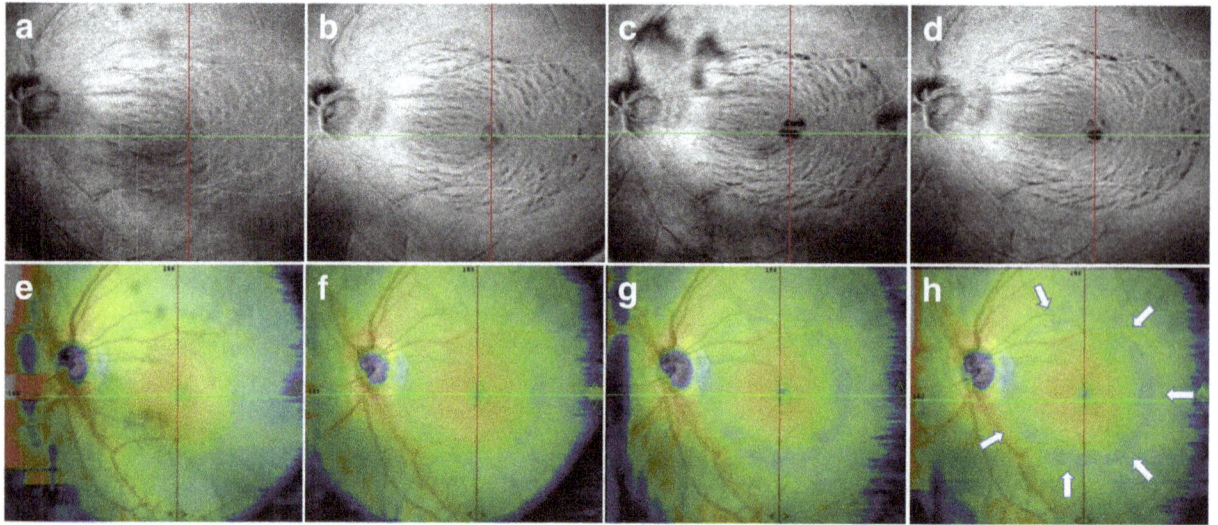

Fig. 2 En face OCT images show progression of inner retinal defects after ILM peeling **a** Inner retinal defects were found on en face OCT ILM layer image 1 month after surgery; **b** 3 months after surgery, inner retinal defects showed progression with increasing numbers of dark striae compared with the previous OCT documentation; **c** 6 months after surgery, progression of inner retinal defects was demonstrated by darker striae and some of them were even confluent with each other; **d** 15 months after surgery, inner retinal defects demonstrated similar appearance with last OCT image except for the disappearance of a previous dark spot lying superior of fovea; **e**, **f**, **g**, **h** corresponding reference images show ILM peeling area distinctly (marked by arrows)

macular holes, far away from the ILM peeling boundaries which were close to the vascular arcade in most eyes in this study. Therefore, a large portion of ILM peeling area was not covered by LHEP. Due to the small sample size of our study, the results need to be verified by further studies.

In this study, we failed to identify a relationship between inner retinal dimples formation and different vitreomacular interfaces due to high myopia in the current study. Sakimoto et al. [25] described inner retinal defects after ILM peeling in high myopic eyes and found that different ILM-retinal adhesions in different fundus areas influenced the development of inner retinal defects. However, only one eye with ILM detachment was included in our study, which had no evident inner retinal dimples observed on both OCT scans (en face and B-scan) after surgery. However, we did found that a large portion of the eyes with longer axial length and posterior staphyloma formed "scattered" inner retinal dimples. These inner retinal defects were related to significant thinning of inner retinal layers. We speculated the globe deformation of posterior staphylomas in highly myopic eyes led to different ILM retina adhesion [26, 27], thus the different type of inner retinal defects. In addition, the choroid plays an important role in offering nutrient and oxygen to the retina in the macular area [28]. Therefore, we speculate that the nerve fiber layer was susceptible to surgical manipulation in the high myopic eyes due to myopic chorioretinal atrophy [26, 29]. Further, the decreased level of neutrophic factor in high

myopic eyes [30] may compromise healing after ILM peeling in these eyes.

In 5 cases, we observed an apparent progression of inner retinal dimples, which appeared on en face ILM layer images as increasing numbers and sizes of dark dots. The inner retinal defects began in the central macular area and spread to the surrounding area. We speculated that these dynamic changes of inner retinal defects are because the retinal nerve fiber bundles surrounding the arcade which is located near the ILM peeling boundary are the thickest, and it takes some time before any changes can occur. Despite the apparent progression, the defects remained in the ILM peeling area. We believe after ILM peeling, the inner retinal may experience a continuous degeneration. However, this differs from the findings of Alkabes et al. [5] They also used en face OCT to observe these postoperative changes and believed that they were stable over time. The cause of these dynamic changes needs to be explored further.

The longest follow-up was 3 years, with no spontaneous resolution of the defects. Although we obtained B-scan OCT images through the radial and horizontal line imaging modes together, it was not feasible to observe the distribution form, and it was also difficult to analyze the dynamic changes in the inner retinal dimples on these cross-sectional OCT images. Therefore, monitoring inner retinal dimples after ILM peeling using en face and B-scan OCT imaging is far more advantageous than performing the

Table 2 Comparison of Demographic and Clinical Characteristics in Eyes With and Without Inner Retinal Dimples

	Eyes with Inner Retinal Dimples (n = 26)	Eyes without Inner Retinal Dimples (n = 12)	p
Age (years)			0.931
Mean ± SD	60.5 ± 13.7	60.9 ± 13.5	
Gender			0.453
Women	18	10	
Men	8	2	
Laterality of MH			0.734
Right	13	7	
Left	13	5	
Type of MH			0.232
LMH	4	4	
FTMH	22	8	
Size of MH (μm)			0.844
Mean size ±SD	575.55 ± 276.03	598.25 ± 278.82	
Number of MAIA			
Posterior staphyloma			1.000
Yes	3	1	
No	23	11	
LHEP			0.714
Yes	7	4	
No	19	8	
ERM			0.296
Yes	8	6	
No	18	6	
ILMP area (PD)			
Mean ± SD			
Preoperative BCVA			0.693
(logMAR)	1.03 ± 0.48	0.96 ± 0.52	
Mean ± SD			
Postoperative BCVA			0.958
(logMAR)	0.63 ± 0.27	0.63 ± 0.38	
Mean ± SD			
Preoperative Aver.ST (dB)			0.430
Mean ± SD	23.71 ± 3.52	15.67 ± 14.17	
Postoperative Aver.ST (dB)			0.633
Mean ± SD	25.42 ± 3.98	24.13 ± 3.70	

MH Macular hole, *LHEP* Lamellar hole associated epiretinal proliferation, *ERM* Epiretinal membrane, *BCVA* Best corrected visual acuity, *Aver.ST* Average sensitivity threshold

Table 3 Logistic Regression of Factors Associated with Formation of Inner Retinal Dimples after Inner Limiting Membrane Peeling

Variable	B	S.E.	Wald	Significance	Exp (B)
Age	−0.025	0.032	0.611	0.434	0.975
Sex	−1.388	1.197	1.346	0.246	0.250
Laterality	−0.615	0.850	0.523	0.470	0.541
Type	0.069	1.324	0.003	0.958	1.072
LHEP	0.154	1.063	0.021	0.885	1.167
Refraction	0.003	1.394	0.000	0.998	1.003
ERM	−1.576	1.212	1.691	0.193	0.207
Constant	5.535	7.380	0.563	0.453	253.481

individualized surgical plans in cases of failed MH closure after previous ILM peeling: enlarged peeling and insertion of ILM [31] and transplantation of lens capsular flap [32] in patients with and without enough remnant ILM, respectively. We therefore drew the conclusion that the different images obtained by various OCT imaging modes can provide detailed information about the inner retinal defects.

The primary limitations of our study include the retrospective design, the small sample size, and the short observation time. Moreover, there was not enough high myopic eyes included in this study because the poor segmentation performance in these eyes. In addition, microperimetry was only performed in a limited number of eyes, so the comparison of the average sensitivity threshold between eyes with different patterns of inner retinal defects were not conducted. Studies with prospective designs and larger sample sizes are needed to analyze the formation of inner retinal defects, and determine if they affect retinal function.

Table 4 Association between Preoperative Vitreomacular Interface Conditions and Inner Retinal Dimples Formation

Categories of pattern	1	2	3	P
AL	27.09 ± 4.47	25.09 ± 1.64	23.54 ± 1.11	0.013[a]
Posterior	3	0	0	0.015[a]
staphyloma	4	0	4	
ERM	3	0	4	0.088
LHEP				0.414
ILM peeling area (PD)				
(mean ± SD)	3.92 ± 0.49	3.67 ± 0.76	3.68 ± 0.71	0.744
BCVA improvement (mean ± SE)	0.45 ± 0.13	0.37 ± 0.15	0.17 ± 0.13	0.630

AL Axial length, *ERM* Epiretinal membrane, *LHEP* Lamellar hole associated epiretinal proliferation, *ILM* Inner limiting membrane, *PD* Papillary diameter, *BCVA* Best corrected visual acuity, *SE* Standard error
[a]Indicates a statistical significant difference between (P ≤ 0.05)

same evaluation using B-scan OCT imaging alone. On some of the reference images, we could even distinguish the ILM peeling area readily, which is difficult to find on funduscopic examination. This information could be useful in helping surgeons make

Conclusions

In conclusion, inner retinal dimples were frequently found after ILM peeling. En face OCT imaging combined with B-scan OCT imaging is highly recommended to evaluate inner retinal dimples after ILM peeling, due to the comprehensive information that these scans can provide to clinicians. High myopic eyes might develop more severe, "scattered" inner retinal defects after ILM peeling. Inner retinal dimples after surgery do not seem to compromise visual function in the short-term.

Abbreviations

BCVA: Best corrected visual acuity; DONFL: Dissociated optic nerve fiber layer; ERM: Epiretinal membrane; FTMH: Full-thickness macular hole; ILM: Innerlimiting membrane; LHEP: Lamellar hole-associated epiretinal membrane; LMH: Lamellar macular hole; logMAR: Logarithm of the minimum angle of resolution; MH: Macular hole; OCT: Optical coherence tomography; PPV: Pars plana vitrectomy

Acknowledgments

We sincerely thank all the patients and their families for their participation.

Authors' contributions

Design and conduct of the study (JL, PZ); collection, analysis and interpretation of data (JL, YC, SW, XZ); preparation of manuscript (JL); critical review and final approval of the manuscript (PZ)

Competing interests

The authors declare that they have no competing interests.

References

1. Tadayoni R, Paques M, Massin P, Mouki-Benani S, Mikol J, Gaudric A. Dissociated optic nerve fiber layer appearance of the fundus after idiopathic epiretinal membrane removal. Ophthalmology. 2001;108(12):2279–83.
2. Mitamura Y, Suzuki T, Kinoshita T, Miyano N, Tashima A, Ohtsuka K. Optical coherence tomographic findings of dissociated optic nerve fiber layer appearance. Am J Ophthalmol. 2004;137(6):1155–6.
3. Ito Y, Terasaki H, Takahashi A, Yamakoshi T, Kondo M, Nakamura M. Dissociated optic nerve fiber layer appearance after internal limiting membrane peeling for idiopathic macular holes. Ophthalmology. 2005; 112(8):1415–20.
4. Mitamura Y, Ohtsuka K. Relationship of dissociated optic nerve fiber layer appearance to internal limiting membrane peeling. Ophthalmology. 2005; 112(10):1766–70.
5. Alkabes M, Salinas C, Vitale L, Burés-Jelstrup A, Nucci P, Mateo C. En face optical coherence tomography of inner retinal defects after internal limiting membrane peeling for idiopathic macular hole. Invest Ophthalmol Vis Sci. 2011;52(11):8349–55.
6. Spaide RF. "Dissociated optic nerve fiber layer appearance" after internal limiting membrane removal is inner retinal dimpling. Retina. 2012;32(9): 1719–26.
7. Kusuhara S, Matsumiya W, Imai H, Honda S, Tsukahara Y, Negi A. Evaluating dissociated optic nerve fiber layer appearance using en face layer imaging produced by optical coherence tomography. Ophthalmologica. 2014;232(3):170–8.
8. Amouyal F, Shah SU, Pan CK, Schwartz SD, Hubschman JP. Morphologic features and evolution of inner retinal dimples on optical coherence tomography after internal limiting membrane peeling. Retina. 2014;34(10): 2096–102.
9. Park SH, Kim YJ, Lee SJ. Incidence of and risk factors for dissociated optic nerve fiber layer after epiretinal membrane surgery. Retina. 2016;36(8):1469–73.
10. Touhami S, Rousseau A, Barreau E, Troumani Y, Marcireau I, Labetoulle M, et al. En face OCT of dissociated optic nerve fiber layer (DONFL) after internal limiting membrane peeling for idiopathic macular hole. J Fr Ophthalmol. 2016;39(3):e53–5.
11. Govetto A, Dacquay Y, Farajzadeh M, Platner E, Hirabayashi K, Hosseini H, et al. Lamellar macular hole: two distinct clinical entities? Am J Ophthalmol. 2016;164:99–109.
12. Witkin AJ, Ko TH, Fujimoto JG, Schuman JS, Baumal CR, Rogers AH, et al. Redefining lamellar holes and the vitreomacular interface: an ultrahigh-resolution optical coherence tomography study. Ophthalmology. 2006; 113(3):388–97.
13. Pang CE, Spaide RF, Freund KB. Epiretinal proliferation seen in association with lamellar macular holes: a distinct clinical entity. Retina. 2014;34(8): 1513–23.
14. Kuhn F. Internal limiting membrane removal for macular detachment in highly myopic eyes. Am J Ophthalmol. 2003;135(4):547–9.
15. Haritoglou C, Ehrt O, Gass CA, Kristin N, Kampik A. Paracentral scotomata: a new finding after vitrectomy for idiopathic macular hole. Br J Ophthalmol. 2001;85(2):231–3.
16. Tadayoni R, Svorenova I, Erginay A, Gaudric A, Massin P. Decreased retinal sensitivity after internal limiting membrane peeling for macular hole surgery. Br J Ophthalmol. 2012;96(12):1513–6.
17. Quigley HA, Dunkelberger GR, Green WR. Retinal ganglion cell atrophy correlated with automated perimetry in human eyes with glaucoma. Am J Ophthalmol. 1989;107(5):453–64.
18. Kerrigan-Baumrind LA, Quigley HA, Pease ME, Kerrigan DF, Mitchell RS. Number of ganglion cells in glaucoma eyes compared with threshold visual field tests in the same persons. Invest Ophthalmol Vis Sci. 2000;41(3):741–8.
19. Harwerth RS, Carter-Dawson L, Smith EL 3rd, Barnes G, Holt WF, Crawford ML. Neural losses correlated with visual losses in clinical perimetry. Invest Ophthalmol Vis Sci. 2004;45(9):3152–60.
20. Eckardt C, Eckardt U, Groos S, Luciano L, Reale E. Removal of the internal limiting membrane in macular holes. Clin and Morpholog Findings Ophthalmol. 1997;94(8):545–51.
21. Wolf S, Schnurbusch U, Wiedemann P, Grosche J, Reichenbach A, Wolburg H. Peeling of the basal membrane in the human retina: ultrastructural effects. Ophthalmology. 2004;111(2):238–43.
22. Nakamura T, Murata T, Hisatomi T, Enaida H, Sassa Y, Ueno A, et al. Ultrastructure of the vitreoretinal interface following the removal of the internal limiting membrane using indocyanine green. Curr Eye Res. 2003; 27(6):395–9.
23. Terasaki H, Miyake Y, Nomura R, Piao CH, Hori K, Niwa T, et al. Focal macular ERGs in eyes after removal of macular ILM during macular hole surgery. Invest Ophthalmol Vis Sci. 2001;42(1):229–34.
24. Newman EA. Regional specialization of retinal glial cell membrane. Nature. 1984;309(5964):155–7.
25. Sakimoto S, Ikuno Y, Fujimoto S, Sakaguchi H, Nishida K. Characteristics of the retinal surface after internal limiting membrane peeling in highly myopic eyes. Am J Ophthalmol. 2014;158(4):762–8.
26. Curtin BJ. The posterior staphyloma of pathologic myopia. Trans Am Ophthalmol Soc. 1977;75:67–86.
27. Ohno-Matsui K. Proposed classification of posterior staphylomas based on analyses of eye shape by three-dimensional magnetic resonance imaging and wide-field fundus imaging. Ophthalmology. 2014;121(9):1798–809.
28. Kur J, Newman EA, Chan-Ling T. Cellular and physiological mechanisms underlying blood flow regulation in the retina and choroid in health and disease. Prog Retin Eye Res. 2012;31(5):377–406.
29. Ikuno Y. Overview of the complications of high myopia. Retina. 2017;37(12): 2347–51.
30. Ogata N, Imaizumi M, Miyashiro M, Arichi M, Matsuoka M, Ando A, Matsumura M. Low levels of pigment epithelium-derived factor in highly myopic eyes with chorioretinal atrophy. Am J Ophthalmol. 2005;140(5):937–9.
31. Morizane Y, Shiraga F, Kimura S, Hosokawa M, Shiode Y, Kawata T, et al. Autologous transplantation of the inner limiting membrane for refractory macular holes. Am J Ophthalmol. 2014;157(4):861–9.
32. Chen SN, Yang CM. Lens capsular flap transplantation the management of refractory macular hole from multiple etiologies. Retina. 2016;38(1):163–70.

13

TLR4 modulates inflammatory gene targets in the retina during *Bacillus cereus* endophthalmitis

Phillip S. Coburn[1]*[iD], Frederick C. Miller[2,3], Austin L. LaGrow[1], Salai Madhumathi Parkunan[1], C. Blake Randall[1], Rachel L. Staats[1] and Michelle C. Callegan[1,4,5]

Abstract

Background: Endophthalmitis is a serious intraocular infection that frequently results in significant inflammation and vision loss. Because current therapeutics are often unsuccessful in mitigating damaging inflammation during endophthalmitis, more rational targets are needed. Toll-like receptors (TLRs) recognize specific motifs on invading pathogens and initiate the innate inflammatory response. We reported that TLR4 contributes to the robust inflammation which is a hallmark of *Bacillus cereus* endophthalmitis. To identify novel, targetable host inflammatory factors in this disease, we performed microarray analysis to detect TLR4-dependent changes to the retinal transcriptome during *B. cereus* endophthalmitis.

Results: C57BL/6 J and TLR4$^{-/-}$ mouse eyes were infected with *B. cereus* and retinas were harvested at 4 h postinfection, a time representing the earliest onset of neutrophil infiltration. Genes related to acute inflammation and inflammatory cell recruitment including CXCL1 (KC), CXCL2 (MIP2-α), CXCL10 (IP-10), CCL2 (MCP1), and CCL3 (MIP1-α)) were significantly upregulated 5-fold or greater in C57BL/6 J retinas. The immune modulator IL-6, intercellular adhesion molecule ICAM1, and the inhibitor of cytokine signal transduction SOCS3 were upregulated 25-, 11-, and 10-fold, respectively, in these retinas. LIF, which is crucial for photoreceptor cell survival, was increased 6-fold. PTGS2/COX-2, which converts arachidonic acid to prostaglandin endoperoxide H2, was upregulated 9-fold. PTX3, typically produced in response to TLR engagement, was induced 15-fold. None of the aforementioned genes were upregulated in TLR4$^{-/-}$ retinas following *B. cereus* infection.

Conclusions: Our results have identified a cohort of mediators driven by TLR4 that may be important in regulating pro-inflammatory and protective pathways in the retina in response to *B. cereus* intraocular infection. This supports the prospect that blocking the activation of TLR-based pathways might serve as alternative targets for Gram-positive and Gram-negative endophthalmitis therapies in general.

Keywords: Bacterial endophthalmitis, Retinal gene expression, Toll-like receptor 4, Gram-positive intraocular infections

Background

Endophthalmitis is a serious infection of the posterior segment of the eye which occurs from introduction of microbes following a surgical procedure (post-operative endophthalmitis [POE]), a traumatic penetrating injury (post-traumatic endophthalmitis [PTE]), or bloodstream spread from an infection of a distant site in the body (endogenous endophthalmitis [EE]) [1–3]. Bacterial endophthalmitis is considered a medical emergency and often results in poor visual outcomes [4]. Much of the intraocular damage in endophthalmitis is due, in part, to the host inflammatory response [5–9]. Immediate and aggressive intervention to stop the progression of the disease is critical to salvaging vision. There is currently no universal therapeutic regimen which prevents the significant inflammation and vision loss associated with severe forms of endophthalmitis.

The Gram-positive pathogen *Bacillus cereus* is a leading cause of PTE and EE. PTE infections due to *B. cereus*

* Correspondence: phillip-coburn@ouhsc.edu
[1]Department of Ophthalmology, University of Oklahoma Health Sciences Center, DMEI PA-419, 608 Stanton L. Young Blvd, Oklahoma City, OK 73104, USA
Full list of author information is available at the end of the article

progress rapidly and result in a fulminant endophthalmitis characterized by severe intraocular inflammation, eye pain, and loss of visual acuity within hours [1–4]. Complete blindness can result in 1 or 2 days, and in nearly half of these infections, evisceration or enucleation is required to salvage healthy tissue in the orbit [10]. The severity and rapid progression of this infection has been recapitulated in a mouse model [1, 2, 6–9]. Infection of mouse eyes with as few as 100 colony-forming units (CFU) of *B. cereus* results in significant inflammation and loss of visual function within hours, similar to that observed in human infections. Because inflammation in the eye causes damage to non-regenerative neural structures, it is important to identify host factors that lead to the events that contribute to this bystander damage.

Robust inflammation in response to intraocular bacterial infection is triggered by the early recognition of cellular components via a class of pattern recognition receptors called Toll-like receptors (TLRs) that are expressed on host cells [11, 12]. Parkunan et al. recently published findings implicating the TLR4/TRIF/MYD88 axis in intraocular *B. cereus* infections [8]. *B. cereus* infected eyes of TLR4$^{-/-}$ mice had significantly less polymorphonuclear leukocytes (PMN) influx and reduced concentrations of four inflammatory mediators relative to infected eyes of C57BL/6 J wild type mice. These parameters correlated with a significant retention of retinal function. These results suggested that the inflammatory cascade in *B. cereus* endophthalmitis is initiated, in part, by TLR4 signaling through a potentially novel TLR4 ligand either expressed or induced by *B. cereus* [8].

The attenuated course of infection observed in TLR4$^{-/-}$ mice implicated downstream mediators of the TLR4 pathway as important in the robust, early response in eyes infected with *B. cereus* [8]. In the current study, we sought to identify host TLR4-dependent factors upregulated in response to *B. cereus* intraocular infection. Based on previous observations of a less severe inflammatory response in TLR4$^{-/-}$ mice [8], we hypothesized that the retinal gene expression profile would be significantly different between TLR4-deficient mice and C57BL/6 J mice following infection. Microarray analysis identified 15 genes involved in the acute inflammatory response, neutrophil recruitment, photoreceptor cell survival, and pathogen recognition and clearance that were upregulated 5-fold or greater in infected C57BL/6 J wild type mice compared to their levels in uninfected control mice (Table 1). The expression of 14 out of 15 of these genes was found to be unaltered in TLR4$^{-/-}$ mice relative to uninfected controls, indicating their dependency on TLR4 (Table 1). These genes included key mediators in neutrophil recruitment, and activation of photoreceptor survival and pathogen clearance mechanisms in response to *B. cereus* infection. These results further suggest that the TLR4 pathway

might serve as a target for new anti-inflammatory treatments critically needed to not only control the explosive inflammation seen in *B. cereus* ocular infection, but also ocular infections due to *Klebsiella pneumoniae* and other Gram negative pathogens.

Methods
Animals and ethics statement
This study was carried out in strict accordance with the recommendations in the Guide for the Care and Use of Laboratory Animals of the National Institutes of Health. The protocol was approved by the Institutional Animal Care and Use Committee of the University of Oklahoma Health Sciences Center (protocol number 16–086). Six week old C57BL/6 J (wild type) mice were acquired from the Jackson Laboratory (Catalog 000664, Bar Harbor ME) and age-matched, homozygous TLR4$^{-/-}$ mice on the C57BL/6 J background were acquired from Eric Perlman, Case Western University, with the permission of S. Akira [13]. Mice were allowed to adjust to conventional housing 2 weeks prior to injection to equilibrate their microbiota. Mice were anesthetized with a cocktail of 85 mg ketamine/kg and 14 mg xylazine/kg prior to injections of bacteria. Mice were euthanized by CO_2 inhalation.

Experimental *B. cereus* endophthalmitis
Wildtype *B. cereus* ATCC 14579 was grown to early stationary phase in BHI broth for 18 h and diluted to 100 CFU/0.5 µl for injection into the mid-vitreous of right eyes. The left eyes served as uninjected controls [5–9].

Microarray analysis of retinal gene expression
At 4 h postinfection, retinas were dissected from all eyes and were immediately frozen. Total RNAs were isolated from the frozen retinas using the Qiagen RNeasy Mini kit (Qiagen, Valenica, CA) following the manufacture's instruction with on-column DNase treatment. RNA concentrations were measured using a Nanodrop ND-1000 Spectrophotometer and RNA quality was verified with an Agilent 2100 Bioanalyzer using an RNA Nano Chip. All RNA samples displaying no visible degradation in the Bioanalyzer analysis with two sharp ribosomal peaks were deemed acceptable for further processing. Affymetrix's GeneChip IVT Express kit was used for cDNA synthesis and in vitro transcription. Affymetrix GeneChip Mouse Genome 430 2.0 Array was used in this study and the raw image was acquired by scanning the arrays using GeneChip scanner. Multiple files were generated and exported by Affymetrix's software Command console. These files were used for subsequent Bioinformatics analysis. Data analysis was performed using Partek's Genomics Suite software (Partek Inc., St. Louis, Missouri). A 5-fold change in gene expression and $p < 0.05$ threshold

Table 1 Microarray analysis of retinal genes upregulated 5-fold and higher 4 h postinfection with *B. cereus* ATCC14579

Gene symbol	Gene title	RefSeq Transcript ID	Fold-Change (C57BL6/J infected versus uninfected)	p-value	Fold-Change (TLR4$^{-/-}$ infected versus uninfected)	p-value
CXCL1	chemokine (C-X-C motif) ligand 1	NM_008176	34	0.0106	NC	NS
CXCL2	chemokine (C-X-C motif) ligand 2	NM_009140	29	0.0225	NC	NS
IL-6	interleukin 6	NM_031168	25	0.0114	NC	NS
CXCL10	chemokine (C-X-C motif) ligand 10	NM_021274	21	0.0328	NC	NS
CCL2	chemokine (C-C motif) ligand 2	NM_011333	20	0.0355	NC	NS
CCL3	chemokine (C-C motif) ligand 3	NM_011337	16	0.0006	5	0.0446
PTX3	pentraxin related gene	NM_008987	15	0.0376	NC	NS
ICAM1	intercellular adhesion molecule 1	NM_010493	11	0.0026	NC	NS
SOCS3	suppressor of cytokine signaling 3	NM_007707	10	0.0034	NC	NS
CYR61	cysteine rich protein 61	NM_010516	10	0.0116	NC	NS
MOBP	myelin-associated oligodendrocytic basic protein	NM_008614	NC	NS	10	0.0270
MBP	myelin basic protein	NM_001025245	NC	NS	10	0.0223
PTGS2	prostaglandin-endoperoxide synthase 2	NM_011198	9	0.0027	NC	NS
STEAP4	STEAP family member 4	NM_054098	6	0.0116	NC	NS
LIF	leukemia inhibitory factor	NM_008501	6	0.0055	NC	NS
CH25H	cholesterol 25-hydroxylase	NM_009890	6	0.0232	NC	NS
PLP1	proteolipid protein (myelin) 1	NM_011123	NC	NS	6	0.0236
EGR2	early growth response 2	NM_010118	5	0.0062	NC	NS

The fold changes of retinal genes in C57BL6/J mouse eyes and TLR4−/− mouse eyes after infection relative to the uninfected, contralateral eye are shown. Levels of significance were determined using ANOVA and $p < 0.05$ was considered significant
NC no change, *NS* not significant

were selected as the criteria for comparative array analyses. Arrays were performed in duplicate on independently obtained RNA samples (SeqWright Genomic Services, Houston, TX).

RNA preparation for quantitative real time PCR
At 4 h postinfection, infected and uninfected mice were euthanized and the retinal tissue harvested. Retinal tissue was placed in a 1.5 ml screw-cap tube containing 500 μl Sigma Tri reagent and 500 μl 1.0 mm glass beads (Biospec Products, Bartlesville, OK). After homogenization at 5000 rpm for 60 s, the supernatant was transferred to a sterile, nuclease free tube containing 200 μl chloroform and then mixed, incubated on ice, and centrifuged. The supernatant was added to 500 μl isopropyl alcohol and placed at -80 °C for 2 h to precipitate RNA. After centrifugation at 14,000 rpm for 20 min at 4 °C, the supernatant was discarded, the pellet washed with 500 μl 75% ethanol, and vortexed to resuspend the pellet. Following centrifugation at 12,000 rpm for 15 min at 4 °C, the supernatant was discarded and the pellet dried and then resuspended in 25 μl nuclease-free water. The concentration and purity were checked on a Nanodrop spectrophotometer and if necessary DNA contamination removed using the TURBO

DNA free kit per the manufacturer's instructions (Thermo Fisher Scientific, Waltham, MA).

Quantitative real time PCR analysis
Total RNA was isolated and an aliquot of 50 ng of RNA was subjected to qPCR using the iTaq™ Universal SYBR® Green One-Step kit (Bio-Rad, Hercules, CA), Prime-Time® qPCR primers (Integrated DNA Technologies, Inc., Coralville, Iowa) specific to the mouse genes shown in Table 2 such that each primer was present in a final concentration of 300 nM, and a Bio-Rad® CFX96 Touch™ Real-Time PCR System (Bio-Rad). Primer sequences are listed in Additional file 1: Table S2. Dissociation curves were used to assess the successful amplification of the desired product, and the threshold cycle (C_T) was used to determine relative amounts of transcripts between RNA samples from infected and uninfected eyes. Each RNA sample was normalized using an internal actin gene control. Fold increases were calculated by subtracting the C_T values of the infected samples from the C_T values of the uninfected samples. That value as a power of 2 yielded the fold increase of the transcript from the infected sample relative to the uninfected sample. Eleven genes that were identified by microarray analysis as upregulated 5-fold or greater were chosen for validation.

Table 2 Quantitative PCR confirmation of retinal gene expression 4 h postinfection with *B. cereus* ATCC14579

Gene symbol	C57BL/6 J Fold change	TLR4$^{-/-}$ Fold change
CCL2	515 ± 742	NC
IL-6	118 ± 157	NC
CXCL2	56 ± 37	NC
CCL3	47 ± 31	NC
PTX3	32 ± 36	NC
CXCL1	30 ± 23	NC
LIF	29 ± 33	NC
CXCL10	27 ± 16	NC
ICAM1	16 ± 10	NC
SOCS3	12 ± 7	NC
PTGS2	6 ± 4	NC

C57BL/6 J fold change values are relative to uninfected C57BL/6 J mice eyes, and TLR4$^{-/-}$ fold change values are relative to uninfected TLR4$^{-/-}$ mice eyes. For each gene, qPCR was performed in triplicate on two independently prepared RNA samples. Significant differences between infected and uninfected eyes were assessed using a Paired T-test, and statistical significance was defined as $p < 0.05$ *NC* no change

For each gene, qPCR was performed in triplicate on two independently prepared RNA samples. Reported fold increases of transcription represent the mean fold increase ± SD.

Statistics

Microarray analysis was performed using Partek's Genomics Suite (Partek Inc., St. Louis, Missouri) software to obtain differential gene expression data. All data were normalized using the Robust Multi-array Analysis expression statistical analysis (RMA). Analysis of variance (ANOVA) was used to compare the means of the infected versus uninfected groups. A 5-fold change in gene expression and $p < 0.05$ threshold were selected as the criteria for comparative array analyses. For analysis of the qPCR data, ΔC_T values were calculated by subtracting the CT values of the infected samples from the uninfected samples. Significant differences between the mean ΔC_T values from infected and uninfected groups were assessed by a Paired T-test using GraphPad Prism 6.05 (GraphPad Software, Inc., La Jolla CA). Statistical significance was $p < 0.05$.

Results

Identification of TLR4-dependent genes upregulated in the retina following *B. cereus* intraocular infection

Because *B. cereus* infection of the posterior segment of the eye results in a rapid and vigorous inflammatory response, we sought to identify inflammatory mediators that are expressed early in the course of *B. cereus* infection. RNA was obtained from retinas at 4 h postinfection, which represents a time prior to neutrophil infiltration of the eye. We identified 76 genes whose expression was significantly altered 2-fold or greater in infected eyes relative to control eyes (Additional file 2: Table S1, Table 1, Fig. 1a). Figure 1a depicts a volcano plot analysis of the resultant microarray data (Fig. 1a). While a 2-fold change in expression represents a common statistical cutoff value, we focused on genes whose expression changed 5-fold or more to identify genes whose expression patterns changed the most dramatically early during infection. The clinical manifestations associated with *B. cereus* ocular infection progress rapidly, therefore genes upregulated to the highest degree early during infection might represent potential treatment targets. We identified 15 genes that were upregulated 5-fold or greater in C57BL6/J mice (Table 1, Figs. 1a and 2).

To ascertain whether the expression of these genes was dependent on TLR4, we performed the same experiments described above in TLR4$^{-/-}$ mice. As shown in Fig. 1b and Table 1, none of the genes identified in wild

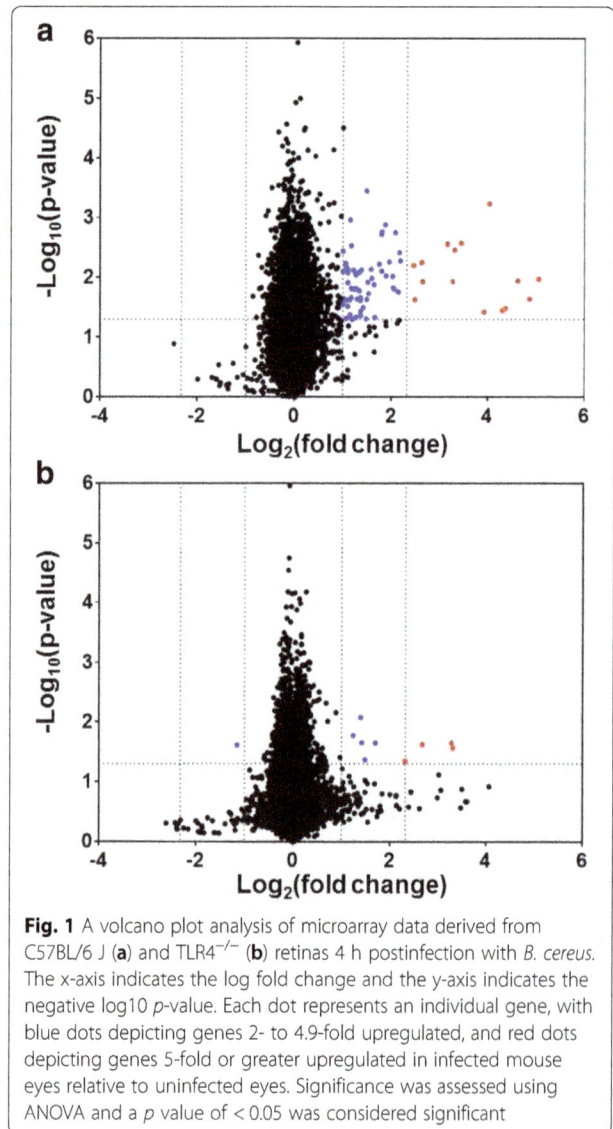

Fig. 1 A volcano plot analysis of microarray data derived from C57BL/6 J (**a**) and TLR4$^{-/-}$ (**b**) retinas 4 h postinfection with *B. cereus*. The x-axis indicates the log fold change and the y-axis indicates the negative log10 *p*-value. Each dot represents an individual gene, with blue dots depicting genes 2- to 4.9-fold upregulated, and red dots depicting genes 5-fold or greater upregulated in infected mouse eyes relative to uninfected eyes. Significance was assessed using ANOVA and a *p* value of < 0.05 was considered significant

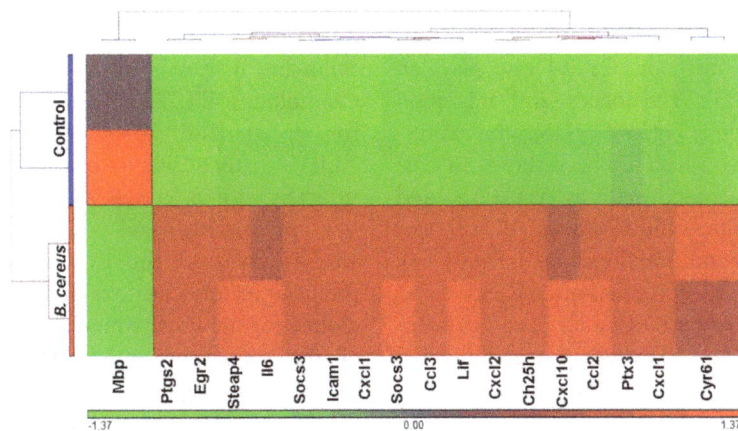

Fig. 2 Hierarchical clustering dendogram of genes upregulated 5-fold or greater in control C57BL6/J, uninfected eyes and in C57BL6/J mouse eyes 4 h following infection with *B. cereus* indicating the relatedness of upregulated genes. The horizontal color bar at the bottom of the heat map indicates that different colors in the heap map represent gradients of gene expression levels: red, up-regulated expression; green, down-regulated expression; grey, no difference in gene expression. The branch lengths on the top of the heat map indicate the correlation with which genes were joined, with longer branches indicating a lower correlation

type retinas at 4 h postinfection were significantly upregulated in TLR4$^{-/-}$ retinas, with the exception of CCL3 (upregulated 5-fold). Conversely, we observed 3 genes that were significantly upregulated in the TLR4$^{-/-}$ retinas but not upregulated in C57BL/6 J wild type mice. Myelin-associated oligodendrocytic basic protein (MOBP) and myelin basic protein (MBP) were upregulated 10-fold, and the proteolipid protein 1 (PLP1) was upregulated 6-fold at 4 h postinfection in infected TLR4$^{-/-}$ eyes (Table 1).

Upregulation of TLR4-dependent inflammatory chemokines and cytokines after *B. cereus* ocular infection

Key proinflammatory chemokines and cytokines were identified among the genes showing high level expression after *B. cereus* infection of wild type eyes. These included the inflammatory mediators chemokine (C-X-C motif) ligand 1(CXCL1) (keratinocyte chemoattractant [KC]), chemokine (C-X-C motif) ligand 2 (CXCL2) (macrophage inflammatory protein 2-alpha [MIP2-α]), chemokine (C-X-C motif) ligand 10(CXCL10) (interferon gamma-induced protein 10 [IP-10]), chemokine (C-C motif) ligand 2 (CCL2) (monocyte chemoattractant protein 1 [MCP1]), and chemokine (C-C motif) ligand 3 (CCL3) (macrophage inflammatory protein 1-alpha [MIP1-α]). These genes were all upregulated more than 16-fold by microarray analysis and are related to the acute proinflammatory response and inflammatory cell recruitment (see Additional file 3: Figure S1). The expression of CXCL1 was increased 34-fold, CXCL2 was increased 29-fold, and CXCL10 was increased 21-fold in C57BL/6 J mouse eyes when compared to uninfected control eyes. The expression of CCL2 was increased 20-fold and the expression of CCL3 was increased 16-fold.

The expression of interleukin 6 (IL-6), a powerful chemoattractant, was increased 25-fold when compared to uninfected control eyes. This group of potent, proinflammatory chemokines and cytokines were the most highly upregulated of all the significantly upregulated genes (Table 1).

Microarray analysis of the 4 h transcriptome in *B. cereus*-infected TLR4$^{-/-}$ retinas demonstrated that only 1 out of 6 of these chemokines and cytokines, CCL3, was significantly upregulated. Quantitative PCR confirmed upregulation of CXCL1, CXCL2, CXCL10, CCL2, CCL3, and IL-6 in wild type C57BL6/J mouse retinas following infection relative to uninfected mouse eyes, but no changes in expression in any of these genes in TLR4$^{-/-}$ mouse retinas 4 h after infection were observed, including CCL3 (Table 2, primer sequences are shown in Additional file 1: Table S2). There was a 30-fold change in the expression of CXCL1, a 56-fold change in CXCL2 expression, and a 27-fold change in the expression of CXCL10 when compared to uninfected control mice. Further, we demonstrated a 515-fold change in the expression of CCL2, a 47-fold change in CCL3, and a 118-fold change in IL-6 by quantitative PCR (Table 2). The only disagreement between the microarray and qPCR was in CCL3 expression.

Upregulation of TLR4-dependent mediators of neutrophil recruitment and complement activation after *B. cereus* ocular infection

Inflammatory mediators involved in neutrophil recruitment and pathogen recognition and clearance were also significantly upregulated 5-fold or greater by microarray analysis. Intercellular adhesion molecule 1 (ICAM1), an adhesin expressed on endothelium and necessary for neutrophil diapedesis [14, 15], was upregulated 11-fold

(Table 1 and Additional file 4: Figure S2). The extracellular matrix protein, cysteine rich protein 61 (CYR61), was increased 10-fold following infection. CYR61 also plays an important role in adhesion, chemotaxis and migration (Table 1 and Additional file 3: Figure S1) [16]. The expression of pentraxin 3 (PTX3), which has been shown to activate the classical complement pathway via C1q, and facilitate pathogen recognition and clearance [17, 18], was increased 15-fold (Table 1 and Additional file 3: Figure S1). Quantitative PCR confirmed upregulation of ICAM1 and PTX3 by 16- and 32-fold, respectively, after *B. cereus* infection of C57BL6/J mice (Table 2). Microarray analysis and qPCR did not detect significant changes in ICAM1, CYR61, or PTX3 transcript levels in TLR4$^{-/-}$ following infection (Tables 1 and 2), suggesting the importance of TLR4 in eliciting a neutrophil response and complement activation following *B. cereus* ocular infection.

Upregulation of TLR4-dependent inflammatory regulators after *B. cereus* ocular infection

Regulators of the inflammatory response were also found to be upregulated by greater than 5-fold following intraocular infection with *B. cereus*. The suppressor of cytokine signaling 3 (SOCS3) was upregulated 10-fold in wild type retinas following infection (Table 1 and Additional file 5: Figure S3). SOCS3 regulates signal transducer and activator of transcription 3 (STAT3) activation in response to cytokines [19]. Leukemia Inhibitory Factor (LIF), an IL-6 regulated neurocytokine was upregulated by 6-fold (Table 1 and Additional file 5: Figure S3). STEAP4 (six transmembrane epithelial antigen of prostate, family member 4), a metalloreductase that plays a role in inflammatory cytokine regulation [20], was increased by 6-fold (Table 1 and Additional file 4: Figure S2). The transcription factor early growth response 2 gene (EGR2) was upregulated 5-fold (Table 1 and Additional file 5: Figure S3). The cyclooxygenase isoenzyme (COX-2 or PTGS2) and cholesterol 25-hydroxylase (CH25H) were increased by 9- and 6-fold respectively (Table 1 and Additional file 3: Figure S1 and Additional file 5: Figure S3). Quantitative PCR confirmed the array results for SOCS3, LIF, and PTGS2 (Table 2). Significant changes in these genes were not observed following infection in TLR4$^{-/-}$ mice (Tables 1 and 2).

Discussion

B. cereus infection of the eye leads to a rapid and destructive inflammatory response that has devastating consequences for vision. TLR2 and TLR4 are key mediators of the innate immune response to bacterial pathogens during the early stages of endophthalmitis [21, 22]. TLR2 plays an important role in both *B. cereus* [21] and *S. aureus* [22] endophthalmitis. TLR4 also plays a significant role in mediating inflammation in *B. cereus* endophthalmitis [8] and, as expected, in *Klebsiella pneumoniae* endophthalmitis

[23]. Parkunan et al. [8] demonstrated an increase in TLR4 mediated chemokines and inflammatory markers following *B. cereus* intraocular infection. Levels of the chemokines CXCL1 (KC), TNF-α (tumor necrosis factor alpha), IL-6, IL-1β were significantly reduced in TLR4$^{-/-}$ mice when compared to wild type mice infected with *B. cereus* [8]. These findings corroborate our microarray and qPCR results. Our previous studies assessed the expression of a limited set of proinflammatory chemokines and cytokines and used whole globes for analysis, which did not permit identification of the source of proinflammatory mediators. Using a transcriptomics approach, we identified 15 proinflammatory and immunomodulatory TLR4-dependent genes whose expression was increased 5-fold or greater specifically in the retinas of eyes 4 h after infection with *B. cereus*. Since these genes were highly upregulated early during the course of infection, they potentially represent targetable host factors that mediate the initial response to *B. cereus* ocular infection.

In the current study, CXCL1 (KC) was the most highly upregulated gene by microarray analysis in the retinas of eyes infected with *B. cereus*. Quantitative PCR confirmed upregulation of CXCL1. Elevated CXCL1 expression was not surprising, considering its chemoattractant properties and the neutrophil burden observed in the posterior segment following infection [9]. We also observed upregulation of CXCL2 (MIP-2α), CXCL10 (IP-10), and CCL2 (MCP1) chemokines in these retinas. CXCL2 is highly homologous and shares many of the same roles in acute inflammation as CXCL1, including interaction with the CXCR2 receptor, secretion by monocytes and macrophages, and attraction of neutrophils to sites of infection and inflammation [24–26]. CXCL10 is secreted by monocytes, endothelium, and fibroblasts after IFN-γ (interferon gamma) stimulation in response to viral infection, and after LPS stimulation in response to Gram-negative infection. CXCL10 serves as a chemoattractant that recruits monocytes/macrophages, T cells, NK cells, and dendritic cells [27, 28]. Since CXCL10 production can occur as a result of stimulation by LPS through TLR4 [27], we hypothesize that the observed upregulation of CXCL10 after *B. cereus* infection may have resulted from the activation of TLR4 by novel ligand. Given that *B. cereus* is a Gram-positive bacterium and does not produce LPS, CXCL10 upregulation might occur due to the activation of TLR4 by another ligand produced or elicited by *B. cereus*. Rajamani et al. did not observe CXCL10 upregulation following intraocular infection with *S. aureus*, however inflammation in this infection is primarily driven by TLR2, and not by TLR4 [29].

IL-6 expression was upregulated 25-fold in C57BL6/J mice on the microarray analysis relative to uninfected control mice and was not upregulated in TLR4$^{-/-}$ mice relative to uninfected controls. IL-6 is both a proinflammatory chemoattractant and a modulator of inflammation via signaling that increases the expression of TNF-α and IL-1β antagonists. Rajamani et al., demonstrated that IL-6 and IL-1β were both significantly upregulated during *S. aureus* endophthalmitis and suggested that these genes were important for the response to *S. aureus* infection [29]. Parkunan reported that IL-6 levels were markedly increased at 8 and 12 h postinfection in a TLR4-dependent manner following intraocular infection with *B. cereus* [8]. In contrast to the findings of Parkunan et al., we did not detect increased levels of TNFα transcript in retinas at 4 h following infection. This suggests that the source of TNFα seen by Parkunan may not be from cells in the retina at this stage of infection, but rather from infiltrating neutrophils, given that cytokine assays were performed on homogenized whole globes [8]. Neutrophils enter the eye as early as 4 h postinfection with *B. cereus*, but do not infiltrate the retinal layers until approximately 8 h postinfection [6]. IL-6 is a pro-inflammatory mediator expressed when bacterial recognition induces inflammation via TLR4 activation. While IL-6 has also been shown to be anti-inflammatory due to its ability to induce soluble TNFα and IL-1β receptor antagonist expression [30], this is unlikely the case in our model, given that neither TNFα or IL-1β expression was altered in the retina at 4 h. The increase in IL-6 seen in our microarray analysis done at 4 h implicates IL-6's inflammatory role as a chemoattractant, while not precluding its role as a signal to downregulate TNF-α and IL-1β expression at a later time point as a means to limit inflammation thus preserving susceptible cells in the retina.

IL-6 is expressed by several cell types in the eye, including RPE cells, ganglion cells, and resident microglia [31, 32]. Others have reported that levels of IL-6 are markedly increased in the retina upon damage to the optic nerve [33], while others have reported IL-6 protects mature retinal ganglion cells from pressure-induced death [34]. In contrast, IL-6 was dispensable for an inflammatory response following *B. cereus* infection of the eye. A similar course of infection, proinflammatory mediator profile, neutrophil infiltration, and architectural changes to the retinal layers were observed in both IL-6$^{-/-}$ and C57BL/6 J eyes [9]. Redundancy due to additional gp130-dependent cytokines, such as LIF [19], which is expressed at significantly higher levels in our analysis, might explain why the inflammatory response in IL-6$^{-/-}$ mouse eyes was not significantly dampened following *B. cereus* infection. Additionally, the increased expression of IL-6 seen in this experiment might serve the dual role of helping to initiate the early inflammatory response seen in *B. cereus* endophthalmitis as well as serving to protect sensitive neuroretinal cells by limiting further inflammation and preventing apoptosis, as has been shown in glaucoma models [34].

CCL2 recruits monocytes, basophils, memory T-cells, and dendritic cells, but not neutrophils or eosinophils [35, 36], and CCL3 activates neutrophils [24]. CCL2 and CCL3 are critical to the recruitment of neutrophils in the context of keratitis [37]. In a mouse model of *Pseudomonas aeruginosa*-induced corneal infection, antibodies directed against CCL2 or CCL3 significantly reduced neutrophil infiltration into the cornea and decreased corneal damage. Both CCL2 and CCL3 were upregulated in the context of TLR4-mediated inflammation after *B. cereus* ocular infection, and their blockade might reduce neutrophil infiltration into the vitreous and decrease damage to the retina.

While the mechanisms of neutrophil infiltration into the eye during endophthalmitis are not completely understood, *S. aureus* is capable of inducing expression of E-selectin and ICAM1 on macrovascular endothelial cells in a rat model of endophthalmitis [38]. In the current study, we demonstrated that *B. cereus* infection also induces ICAM1 expression in the retina. Expression of ICAM1 is upregulated by a variety of stimuli including retinoic acid, oxidant stress, and the proinflammatory cytokines IL-1β, TNFα, and IFNγ [39]. Lipopolysaccharide (LPS) was shown to induce expression of ICAM1 in human pulmonary alveolar epithelial cells through the TLR4/c-Src/NADPH oxidase/ROS-dependent NF-κB pathway [40]. ICAM1 serves as the ligand for LFA-1 (Lymphocyte function-associated antigen 1integrin) on leukocytes [14, 15]. Leukocytes that bind to endothelium via ICAM1 / LFA-1 complex are able to initiate transmigration across the endothelial membrane [41]. The finding that ICAM1 is upregulated in wild type, but not in TLR4$^{-/-}$ eyes, correlates with our previous findings that neutrophil recruitment is decreased in TLR4$^{-/-}$ eyes following infection [8]. Interestingly, ICAM1 possesses signal-transducing functions that are associated primarily with proinflammatory pathways. Ligation of ICAM1 on the surface of endothelial cells elicits a signaling cascade resulting in production of IL-8 and RANTES (regulated on activation, normal T cell expressed and secreted) [42], as well as additional ICAM1 in a positive feedback loop [43]. Upregulation of ICAM1 early during infection and prior to PMN infiltration might indicate an additional role in signaling at this stage in addition to leukocyte trafficking.

Another gene product implicated in leukocyte migration, cysteine-rich protein 61 (CYR61), was also significantly upregulated following *B. cereus* infection. CYR61 is a modular protein that functions as a bridge between cells and the extracellular matrix, binding to integrins and to extracellular matrix proteins [16]. CYR61 is primarily involved in regulating adhesion and chemotaxis, as well as angiogenesis [16]. In contrast to the rapid and significant upregulation of CYR61 following *B. cereus* infection, Rajamani and colleagues did not observe upregulation of CYR61 until 12 h after intraocular infection with *S. aureus* [29]. This finding correlates with the delay in neutrophil influx observed in *S. aureus* endophthalmitis as compared to *B. cereus* endophthalmitis. It is likely that CYR61 is upregulated in order to mediate neutrophil invasion following *B. cereus* infection of the eye. PTX3 was also upregulated following *B. cereus* infection, and is known to be produced in response to TLR engagement [17]. PTX3 activates the classical complement pathway via C1q [18]. Therefore it could be hypothesized that PTX3 might function to activate an anti-bacterial response to *B. cereus* intraocular infection. However, it is currently unknown whether complement plays a role in *B. cereus* endophthalmitis. While complement is present in the eye [44], its absence did not alter the outcome in a mouse model of *S. aureus* endophthalmitis [45].

SOCS3 is a negative regulator of cytokine signaling induced by IL-6, IL-10, and INFγ (mediators of both the MYD88-dependent and MYD88-independent TLR pathways). SOCS3 functions to inhibit STAT3 phosphorylation and this negative regulatory function prevents excessive activation of proinflammatory genes [19]. The rapid and destructive inflammatory response observed following *B. cereus* infection suggests that SOCS3 may not adequately inhibit STAT3 phosphorylation in the cells in the retina which function as the initial responders. Wang et al. demonstrated that prolonged STAT3 activation occurs as a result of the IL-6 receptor associating with the epidermal growth factor receptor [19]. This complex is capable of STAT3 activation but is not inhibited by SOCS3. *The pathogen Mycobacterium tuberculosis* directly activates SOCS3 and therefore inhibits NF-κB/rel-mediated proinflammatory cytokine production [46], which functions to suppress the inflammatory response. It is currently unknown as to whether *B. cereus* is capable of directly activating SOCS3 in the retina, however the robust inflammatory response incited by *B. cereus* might override the inhibitory effects of SOCS3 activation.

LIF upregulation in response to *B. cereus* infection might serve to enhance the protection of the delicate, nonregenerative photoreceptors. LIF is an IL-6 regulated neurocytokine that is upregulated in Muller cells in response to retinal stress [47, 48]. Chucair-Elliott et al. demonstrated that LIF downregulates the expression of RPE65, which ultimately leads to a decrease in 11-cis-retinal, a chromophore that might be toxic in excessive amounts [49]. *B. cereus* infection may be a stressor that results in upregulation of LIF in order to protect this layer of cells in the retina. While it is unknown which cells are expressing LIF at increased levels following infection, given that Muller cells upregulate LIF in response to stress [47, 48], Muller cells might serve as at least one of the cell types that produce LIF in response to *B. cereus* infection.

Induction of PTGS2/COX-2 during infection is mediated by TLR4 and NFκB (nuclear factor kappa-light-chain-enhancer of activated B cells) [50]. This enzyme converts arachidonic acid to prostaglandin endoperoxide H2 (PGE$_2$) and is expressed during inflammation. PGE$_2$ has an immunomodulatory effect and serves to prevent the activation of neutrophils, which is an immune evasion strategy utilized by some bacterial pathogens. *Streptococcus pneumoniae* induces PGE$_2$ production by human neutrophils and prevents activation [51]. In a model of *Pseudomonas* pneumonia, lack of PTGS2/COX-2 was proven to be beneficial and resulted in increased clearance of bacteria from the lungs [52]. The mechanism for this was linked to PGE$_2$ inhibiting superoxide production by immune effectors and therefore hindering bacterial killing. PTGS2/COX-2 is usually an inflammation inducible enzyme not normally expressed in most tissues. However, PTGS2/COX-2 is constitutively expressed throughout both murine and human eyes [53], in the cornea, iris, ciliary body, and retina. Wang et al. suggested that PTGS2/COX-2 might play a protective role in eye tumorigenesis. Significant upregulation of PTGS2/COX-2 and PGE$_2$ synthesis in the retina following *B. cereus* infection might serve to modulate the function of invading neutrophils and prevent activation.

The fact that 15 genes associated with TLR4 activation were upregulated 5-fold or greater in C57BL6/J mice compared to uninfected control eyes, but were not induced in TLR4$^{-/-}$ suggests that *B. cereus* is capable of activation of TLR4. This implicates a component of *B. cereus* as a novel ligand for activating the TLR4 receptor. TLR4 typically mediates the inflammatory response to LPS in conjunction with MD2 (lymphocyte antigen 96), CD14, and MYD88 [54]. However, TLR4 has been shown to recognize additional exogenous and endogenous ligands, including respiratory syncytial virus, heat-shock proteins, fibronectin, fibrinogen, and hyaluronic acid [55–61]. Alternatively, *B. cereus* might instigate a response that results in the formation of an endogenous ligand for the TLR4 pathway. In the current study, we did not observe a transcriptional upregulation of any of the reported endogenous ligands. However, we cannot rule out the possibility that *B. cereus* infection might result in the posttranscriptional production or modification of an endogenous ligand.

The ability of *B. cereus* to activate both the TLR4 [8] and TLR2 [21] pathways might explain why *B. cereus* endophthalmitis results in an explosive inflammatory response that results in poor visual outcomes in affected patients. The early onset of TLR4-associated inflammation could play a key role in therapies designed to prevent further inflammation and damage to the sensitive and nonregenerative structures of the eye. This study identified retinal genes that were significantly upregulated early during *B. cereus* infection that might prove tractable as targets for intervention. However, inherent redundancies in these pathways and the potential for exacerbating inflammation might complicate the design of new therapeutics. Our study also presented key differences between the inflammatory mediators that are elicited by *B. cereus* and those by *S. aureus* [29] following intraocular infection. Endophthalmitis severity and outcome as result of infection with these two pathogens is starkly different, and the results of this study shed light on the differences in types and timing of inflammatory mediator production that contribute to the distinctive courses and outcomes. Given the limitations inherent to microarray analysis for assessing global gene changes, future studies confirming these results by proteomics and the analysis of the severity of *B. cereus* infections in mice specifically deficient in these pathways will be required. Future studies will evaluate the retinal and global ocular inflammatory responses over the course of *B. cereus* endophthalmitis to identify pathway-based anti-inflammatory targets, specifically, those that are regulated by TLR4, and to identify the *B. cereus* produced or induced ligand for TLR4.

Conclusions

Our results have identified key proinflammatory and immunomodulatory mediators driven by TLR4 that may be important in regulating pro-inflammatory and protective pathways in the retina in response to *B. cereus* intraocular infection. These factors were upregulated early during infection and might serve as targets for new therapies. Our results also support the prospect that blocking the activation of TLR-based pathways might serve as alternative targets for Gram-positive endophthalmitis therapies in general.

Abbreviations

IL-1β: Interleukin 1 beta; CCL2: Chemokine (C-C motif) ligand 2; CCL3: Chemokine (C-C motif) ligand 1; CFU: Colony-forming units; CH25H: Cholesterol 25-hydroxylase; COX-2 or PTGS2: Cyclooxygenase isoenzyme; C$_T$: Threshold cycle; CXCL1: Chemokine (C-X-C motif) ligand 1; CXCL10: Chemokine (C-X-C motif) ligand 10; CXCL2: Chemokine (C-X-C motif) ligand 2; CYR61: Cysteine rich protein 61; EE: Endogenous endophthalmitis; EGR2: Early growth response 2 gene; ICAM1: Intercellular adhesion molecule 1; IFN-γ: Interferon gamma; IL-6: Interleukin 6; IP-10: Interferon gamma-induced protein 10; KC: Keratinocyte chemoattractant; LFA-1: Lymphocyte function-associated antigen 1; LIF: Leukemia inhibitory factor; MBP: Myelin basic protein; MCP1: Monocyte chemoattractant protein 1; MD2: Lymphocyte antigen 96; MIP1-α: Macrophage inflammatory protein 1-alpha; MIP2-α: Macrophage inflammatory protein 2-alpha; MOBP: Myelin-associated oligodendrocytic basic protein; NFκB: Nuclear factor kappa-light-chain-enhancer of activated B cells; PGE$_2$: Prostaglandin endoperoxide H2; PLP1: Proteolipid protein 1; PMN: Polymorphonuclear leukocytes; POE: Post-operative endophthalmitis; PTE: Post-traumatic endophthalmitis; PTX3: Pentraxin 3; qPCR: Quantitative polymerase chain reaction; RANTES: Regulated on activation, normal T cell expressed and secreted; SOCS3: Suppressor of cytokine signaling 3; STAT3: Signal transducer and activator of transcription 3; STEAP4: Six transmembrane epithelial antigen of prostate, family member 4; TLR: Toll-like receptors; TNF-α: Tumor necrosis factor alpha

Acknowledgements

We thank Roger Astley, Rebekah Decosier, and Craig Land (OUHSC), and Mark Dittmar (Dean McGee Eye Institute Animal Facility) for their invaluable technical assistance. We acknowledge the OUHSC Live Animal Imaging and Analysis and Molecular Biology Core facilities for technical assistance (P30EY27125), and Seqwright Genomic Services (Pittsburg, PA) for performing the Affymetrix expression profiling. This work was presented in part at the 2015 Association for Research in Vision and Ophthalmology Annual Conference in Denver CO.

Funding

This study was funded by NIH Grant R01EY024140 (to MCC). Our research is also supported in part by NIH Grants R01EY025947 (to MCC), P30EY27125 (NIH CORE grant to Robert E. Anderson, OUHSC), a Presbyterian Health Foundation Equipment Grant (to Robert E. Anderson, OUHSC) and an unrestricted grant to the Dean A. McGee Eye Institute from Research to Prevent Blindness Inc. (https://www.rpbusa.org/rpb/?). The funders had no role in study design, data collection and analysis, decision to publish, or preparation of the manuscript.

Authors' contributions

PSC, FCM, and MCC designed the study and conducted the analyses. PSC, FCM, ALG, SMP, BR, and RS performed the experiments. PSC and FCM wrote the manuscript. All authors read and approved the final manuscript.

Competing interests

The authors declare that they have no competing interests.

Author details

[1]Department of Ophthalmology, University of Oklahoma Health Sciences Center, DMEI PA-419, 608 Stanton L. Young Blvd, Oklahoma City, OK 73104, USA. [2]Department of Family and Preventive Medicine, University of Oklahoma Health Sciences Center, Oklahoma City, Oklahoma, USA. [3]Department of Cell Biology, University of Oklahoma Health Sciences Center, Oklahoma City, Oklahoma, USA. [4]Oklahoma Center for Neuroscience, University of Oklahoma Health Sciences Center, Oklahoma City, Oklahoma, USA. [5]Department of Microbiology and Immunology, Dean McGee Eye Institute, University of Oklahoma Health Sciences Center, Oklahoma City, Oklahoma, USA.

References

1. Callegan MC, Gilmore MS, Gregory M, Ramadan RT, Wiskur BJ, Moyer AL, et al. Bacterial endophthalmitis: therapeutic challenges and host–pathogen interactions. Prog Retin Eye Res. 2007;26:189–203.
2. Callegan MC, Kane ST, Cochran DC, Gilmore MS. Molecular mechanisms of *Bacillus* endophthalmitis pathogenesis. DNA Cell Biol. 2002;21:367–73.
3. Coburn PS, Callegan MC. Endophthalmitis. In: Rumelt S, editor. Advances in ophthalmology. InTech. https://doi.org/10.5772/29130. Available from: https://www.intechopen.com/books/advances-in-ophthalmology/endophthalmitis.
4. Durand ML. Endophthalmitis. Clin Microbiol Infect. 2013;19:227–34.
5. Callegan MC, Kane ST, Cochran DC, Gilmore MS, Gominet M, Lereclus D. Relationship of *plcR*-regulated factors to *Bacillus* endophthalmitis virulence. Infect Immun. 2003;71:3116–24.
6. Ramadan RT, Ramirez R, Novosad BD, Callegan MC. Acute inflammation and loss of retinal architecture and function during experimental *Bacillus* endophthalmitis. Curr Eye Res. 2006;31:955–65.
7. Ramadan RT, Moyer AL, Callegan MC. A role for tumor necrosis factor-alpha in experimental *Bacillus cereus* endophthalmitis pathogenesis. Invest Ophthalmol Vis Sci. 2008;49:4482–9.
8. Parkunan SM, Randall CB, Coburn PS, Astley RA, Staats RL, Callegan MC. Unexpected roles for toll-like receptor 4 and TRIF in intraocular infection with gram-positive bacteria. Infect Immun. 2015;83:3926–36.

9. Parkunan SM, Randall CB, Astley RA, Furtado GC, Lira SA, Callegan MC. CXCL1, but not IL-6, significantly impacts intraocular inflammation during infection. J Leukoc Biol. 2016;100:1125–34.

10. David DB, Kirkby GR, Noble BA. Bacillus cereus endophthalmitis. Br J Ophthalmol. 1994;78:577–80.

11. Akira S, Takeda K. Toll-like receptor signalling. Nature Rev Immuno. 2004;4:499–511.

12. Kawai T, Akira S. The role of pattern-recognition receptors in innate immunity: update on toll-like receptors. Nat Immun. 2010;11:373–84.

13. Hoshino K, Takeuchi O, Kawai T, Sanjo H, Ogawa T, Takeda Y, Takeda K, Akira S. Cutting edge: toll-like receptor 4 (TLR4)-deficient mice are hyporesponsive to lipopolysaccharide: evidence for TLR4 as the Lps gene product. J Immunol. 1999;162:3749–52.

14. Rothlein R, Dustin ML, Marlin SD, Springer TA. A human intercellular adhesion molecule (ICAM-1) distinct from LFA-1. J Immunol. 1986;137:1270–4.

15. Dustin ML, Rothlein R, Bhan AK, Dinarello CA, Springer TA. Induction by IL 1 and interferon-gamma: tissue distribution, biochemistry, and function of a natural adherence molecule (ICAM-1). J Immunol. 1986;137:245–54.

16. Wiedmaier N, Müller S, Köberle M, Manncke B, Krejci J, Autenrieth IB, Bohn E. Bacteria induce CTGF and CYR61 expression in epithelial cells in a lysophosphatidic acid receptor-dependent manner. Int J Med Microbiol. 2008;298:231–43.

17. Bottazzi B, Garlanda C, Cotena A, et al. The long pentraxin PTX3 as a prototypic humoral pattern recognition receptor: interplay with cellular innate immunity. Immuno Rev. 2009;227:9–18.

18. Nauta AJ, Bottazzi B, Mantovani A, Salvatori G, Kishore U, Schwaeble WJ, Gingras AR, Tzima S, Vivanco F, Egido J, Tijsma O, Hack EC, Daha MR, Roos A. Biochemical and functional characterization of the interaction between pentraxin 3 and C1q. Eur J Immunol. 2003;33:465–73.

19. Wang Y, van Boxel-Dezaire AHH, Cheon H, Yang J, Stark GR. STAT3 activation in response to IL-6 is prolonged by the binding of IL-6 receptor to EGF receptor. Proc Natl Acad Sci. 2013;110:16975–80.

20. Scarl RT, Lawrence CM, Gordon HM, Nunemaker CS. STEAP4: its emerging role in metabolism and homeostasis of cellular iron and copper. J Endocrinol. 2017;234:R123–34.

21. Novosad BD, Astley RA, Callegan MC. Role of toll-like receptor (TLR) 2 in experimental Bacillus cereus endophthalmitis. PLoS One. 2011;6(12):e28619.

22. Talreja D, Singh PK, Kumar A. In vivo role of TLR2 and MyD88 signaling in eliciting innate immune responses in staphylococcal endophthalmitis. Invest Ophthalmol Vis Sci. 2015;56:1719–32.

23. Hunt JJ, Astley R, Wheatley N, Wang JT, Callegan MC. TLR4 contributes to the host response to Klebsiella intraocular infection. Curr Eye Res. 2014;39:790–802.

24. Wolpe SD, Sherry B, Juers D, Davatelis G, Yurt RW, Cerami A. Identification and characterization of macrophage inflammatory protein 2. Proc Nat Acad Sci. 1989;86:612–6.

25. Iida N, Grotendorst GR. Cloning and sequencing of a new gro transcript from activated human monocytes: expression in leukocytes and wound tissue. Mol Cell Biol. 1990;10:5596–9.

26. Pelus LM, Fukuda S. Peripheral blood stem cell mobilization: the CXCR2 ligand GRObeta rapidly mobilizes hematopoietic stem cells with enhanced engraftment properties. Exp Hematol. 2006;34:1010–20.

27. Dufour JH, Dziejman M, Liu MT, Leung JH, Lane TE, Luster AD. IFN-gamma-inducible protein 10 (IP-10; CXCL10)-deficient mice reveal a role for IP-10 in effector T cell generation and trafficking. J Immunol. 2002;168:3195–204.

28. Luster AD, Unkeless JC, Ravetch JV. Gamma-interferon transcriptionally regulates an early-response gene containing homology to platelet proteins. Nature. 1985;315:672–6.

29. Rajamani D, Singh PK, Rottmann BG, Singh N, Bhasin MK, Kumar A. Temporal retinal transcriptome and systems biology analysis identifies key pathways and hub genes in Staphylococcus aureus endophthalmitis. Sci Rep. 2016;6:21502.

30. Tilg H, Trehu E, Atkins MB, Dinarello CA, Mier JW. Interleukin-6 (IL-6) as an anti-inflammatory cytokine: induction of circulating IL-1 receptor antagonist and soluble tumor necrosis factor receptor p55. Blood. 1994;83:113–8.

31. Elner VM, Scales W, Elner SG, Danforth J, Kunkel SL, Strieter RM. Interleukin-6 (IL-6) gene expression and secretion by cytokine-stimulated human retinal pigment epithelial cells. Exp Eye Res. 1992;54:361–8.

32. Planck SR, Dang TT, Graves D, Tara D, Ansel JC, Rosenbaum JT. Retinal pigment epithelial cells secrete interleukin-6 in response to interleukin-1. Invest Ophthalmol Vis Sci. 1992;33:78–82.

33. Leibinger M, Müller A, Gobrecht P, Diekmann H, Andreadaki A, Fischer D. Interleukin-6 contributes to CNS axon regeneration upon inflammatory stimulation. Cell Death Dis. 2013;4:e609.

34. Sappington RM, Chan M, Calkins DJ. Interleukin-6 protects retinal ganglion cells from pressure-induced death. Invest Ophthalmol Vis Sci. 2006;47:2932–42.

35. Carr MW, Roth SJ, Luther E, Rose SS, Springer TA. Monocyte chemoattractant protein 1 acts as a T-lymphocyte chemoattractant. Proc Natl Acad Sci U S A. 1994;91:3652–6.

36. Xu LL, Warren MK, Rose WL, Gong W, Wang JM. Human recombinant monocyte chemotactic protein and other C-C chemokines bind and induce directional migration of dendritic cells in vitro. J Leukoc Biol. 1996;60:365–71.

37. Xue ML, Thakur A, Cole N, Lloyd A, Stapleton F, Wakefield D, Willcox MD. A critical role for CCL2 and CCL3 chemokines in the regulation of polymorphonuclear neutrophils recruitment during corneal infection in mice. Immunol Cell Biol. 2007;85:525–31.

38. Giese MJ, Shum DC, Rayner SA, Mondino BJ, Berliner JA. Adhesion molecule expression in a rat model of Staphylococcus aureus endophthalmitis. Invest Ophthalmol Vis Sci. 2000;41:145–53.

39. Roebuck KA, Finnegan A. Regulation of intercellular adhesion molecule-1 (CD54) gene expression. J Leukoc Biol. 1999;66:876–88.

40. Cho RL, Yang CC, Lee IT, Lin CC, Chi PL, Hsiao LD, Yang CM. Lipopolysaccharide induces ICAM-1 expression via a c-Src/NADPH oxidase/ROS-dependent NF-κB pathway in human pulmonary alveolar epithelial cells. Am J Physiol Lung Cell Mol Physiol. 2016;310(7):L639–57.

41. Yang L, Froio RM, Sciuto TE, Dvorak AM, Alon R, Luscinskas FW. ICAM-1 regulates neutrophil adhesion and transcellular migration of TNF-α-activated vascular endothelium under flow. Blood. 2005;106:584–92.

42. Blaber R, Stylianou E, Clayton A, Steadman R. Selective regulation of ICAM-1 and RANTES gene expression after ICAM-1 ligation on human renal fibroblasts. J Am Soc Nephrol. 2003;14:116–27.

43. Clayton A, Evans RA, Pettit E, Hallett M, Williams JD, Steadman R. Cellular activation through the ligation of intercellular adhesion molecule-1. J Cell Sci. 1998;111:443–53.

44. Sohn JH, Kaplan HJ, Suk HJ, Bora PS, Bora NS. Chronic low level complement activation within the eye is controlled by intraocular complement regulatory proteins. Invest Ophthalmol Vis Sci. 2000;41:3492–502.

45. Engelbert M, Gilmore MS. Fas ligand but not complement is critical for control of experimental Staphylococcus aureus Endophthalmitis. Invest Ophthalmol Vis Sci. 2005;46:2479–86.

46. Nair S, Pandey AD, Mukhopadhyay S. The PPE18 protein of Mycobacterium tuberculosis inhibits NF-κB/rel-mediated proinflammatory cytokine production by upregulating and phosphorylating suppressor of cytokine signaling 3 protein. J Immunol. 2011;186:5413–24.

47. Joly S, Lange C, Thiersch M, Samardzija M, Grimm C. Leukemia inhibitory factor extends the lifespan of injured photoreceptors in vivo. J Neurosci. 2008;28:13765–74.

48. Bürgi S, Samardzija M, Grimm C. Endogenous leukemia inhibitory factor protects photoreceptor cells against light-induced degeneration. Mol Vis. 2009;15:1631–7.

49. Chucair-Elliott AJ, Elliott MH, Wang J, Moiseyev GP, Ma JX, Politi LE, Rotstein NP, Akira S, Uematsu S, Ash JD. Leukemia inhibitory factor coordinates the down-regulation of the visual cycle in the retina and retinal-pigmented epithelium. J Biol Chem. 2012;287:24092–102.

50. Rhee SH, Hwang D. Murine TOLL-like receptor 4 confers lipopolysaccharide responsiveness as determined by activation of NF kappa B and expression of the inducible cyclooxygenase. J Biol Chem. 2000;275:34035–40.

51. Cockeran R, Steel HC, Mitchell TJ, Feldman C, Anderson R. Pneumolysin potentiates production of prostaglandin E(2) and leukotriene B(4) by human neutrophils. Infect Immun. 2001;69:3494–6.

52. Sadikot RT, Zeng H, Azim AC, Joo M, Dey SK, Breyer RM, Peebles RS, Blackwell TS, Christman JW. Bacterial clearance of Pseudomonas aeruginosa is enhanced by the inhibition of COX-2. Eur J Immunol. 2007;37:1001–9.

53. Wang J, Wu Y, Heegaard S, Kolko M. Cyclooxygenase-2 expression in the normal human eye and its expression pattern in selected eye tumours. Acta Ophthalmol. 2011;89:681 5.

54. Zhang G, Ghosh S. Toll-like receptor-mediated NF-kappaB activation: a phylogenetically conserved paradigm in innate immunity. J Clin Invest. 2001;107:13–9.

55. Smiley ST, King JA, Hancock WW. Fibrinogen stimulates macrophage chemokine secretion through toll-like receptor 4. J Immunol. 2001;167:2887–94.

56. Lee JY, Sohn KH, Rhee SH, Hwang D. Saturated fatty acids, but not unsaturated fatty acids, induce the expression of cyclooxygenase-2 mediated through toll-like receptor 4. J Biol Chem. 2001;276:16683–9.

57. Termeer C, Benedix F, Sleeman J, Fieber C, Voith U, Ahrens T, Miyake K, Freudenberg M, Galanos C, Simon JC. Oligosaccharides of Hyaluronan activate dendritic cells via toll-like receptor 4. J Exp Med. 2002;195:99–111.

58. Ohashi K, Burkart V, Flohe S, Kolb H. Cutting edge: heat shock protein 60 is a putative endogenous ligand of the toll-like receptor-4 complex. J Immunol. 2000;164:558–61.

59. Kiechl S, Lorenz E, Reindl M, Wiedermann CJ, Oberhollenzer F, Bonora E, Willeit J, Schwartz DA. Toll-like receptor 4 polymorphisms and atherogenesis. N Engl J Med. 2002;347:185–92.

60. Haeberle HA, Takizawa R, Casola A, Brasier AR, Dieterich HJ, Van Rooijen N, Gatalica Z, Garofalo RP. Respiratory syncytial virus-induced activation of nuclear factor-kappaB in the lung involves alveolar macrophages and toll-like receptor 4-dependent pathways. J Infect Dis. 2002;186:1199–206.

61. Okamura Y, Watari M, Jerud ES, Young DW, Ishizaka ST, Rose J, Chow JC, Strauss JF 3rd. The extra domain a of fibronectin activates toll-like receptor 4. J Biol Chem. 2001;276:10229–33.

14

A novel surgical technique for punctal stenosis: placement of three interrupted sutures after rectangular three-snip punctoplasty

Seong Jun Park[1], Ju Hee Noh[2], Ki Bum Park[3], Sun Young Jang[3*†] and Jong Won Lee[2*†]

Abstract

Background: We developed a novel surgical technique to treat punctal stenosis involving the placement of three interrupted sutures after rectangular three-snip punctoplasty (TSP).

Methods: Retrospective chart review of forty-eight eyes of 44 patients who underwent rectangular TSP with three interrupted sutures was performed. We investigated whether anatomical recurrences (re-stenosis) occurred during the follow-up period. The subjective symptoms of patients were surveyed.

Results: The mean patient age was 64.1 years, and the mean follow-up time was 17.4 months. The placement of three interrupted sutures after rectangular TSP afforded satisfactory outcomes. Regarding subjective symptoms, 91. 7% of the eyes (44/48) were reported as improved. Among 4 eyes determined as symptomatic failure, anatomical recurrence (re-stenosis of the punctum) was observed in only one eye. The other three (6.25%, 3/48 eyes) showed functional nasolacrimal obstruction, namely epiphora with patent tear duct.

Conclusions: Placement of three interrupted sutures after rectangular TSP to treat punctal stenosis showed promising results. Notably anatomical success rate was about 98%. Further comparisons between the novel surgical technique and conventional techniques are required.

Keywords: Punctal stenosis, Rectangular three-snip punctoplasty, Three interrupted sutures

Background

Punctal stenosis triggers epiphora in up to 94% of patients [1]. One-snip punctoplasty was first introduced by Bowman in 1853; 164 years later, the search for an optimal surgical procedure resolving punctal stenosis continues [2].

Of the various surgical techniques, three-snip punctoplasty (TSP) has been the most successful method used to enlarge a narrowed punctum [3]. There are two types of TSP, triangular TSP and rectangular TSP, reflecting the shapes of the flaps fashioned during the procedures.

Conventional triangular TSP features removal of a triangular flap created by first cutting the vertical canaliculus then the horizontal canaliculus and finally, the base of the canaliculus. Rectangular TSP (also termed posterior ampullectomy) features two snips in the vertical canaliculus and a final snip at the base, with removal of the posterior wall of the ampulla [3]. It has been suggested that sparing of the horizontal canaliculus may ensure preservation of lacrimal physiology [4]. However, this hypothesis has not been confirmed. Although rectangular TSP is associated with a slightly higher resolution rate than triangular TSP (90% vs. 83%), symptom resolution after triangular and rectangular TSP did not differ significantly [3]. Moreover, in cases of severe punctal stenosis, the punctum could not be dilated to make the two initial vertical cuts. For this reason, Kim et al. [4] introduced a new modification of rectangular TSP;

* Correspondence: ysyat01@naver.com; ophlee@naver.com
†Equal contributors
[3]Department of Ophthalmology, Soonchunhyang University Bucheon Hospital, Soonchunhyang University College of Medicine, 170 Jomaru-ro, Wonmi-gu, Bucheon 14584, Gyeonggi-do, South Korea
[2]Soo Eye Clinics, 202-13, Miadong, Kangbook-gu, Seoul 01118, South Korea
Full list of author information is available at the end of the article

rectangular four-snip punctoplasty. Four-snip puncto-plasty features one snip in the vertical canaliculus and a second horizontal cut, followed by a third vertical or horizontal cut, and finally removal of the base of the flap. In Kim et al.'s report, the anatomical success rate was 88.9% at 6 months after surgery.

In addition to advances in the surgical procedure, adjunct therapies have also been developed. These include the use of punctal plugs [5], stenting [6], prescription of mitomycin C [7], and punch punctoplasty with a Kelly punch [8]. It remains unclear whether combinations of stenting or mitomycin C with punctoplasty improve outcomes compared to those afforded by punctoplasty alone; the data are conflicting [7, 9, 10].

Here, we describe a novel surgical technique. After rectangular TSP, we placed three interrupted sutures in the posterior wall of the ampulla to maintain punctal enlargement and prevent re-approximation of the cut ends.

Methods

The study was approved by the Institutional Review Board of Soonchunhyang Bucheon Hospital, Soonchunhyang University College of Medicine, and the study protocol adhered to the tenets of the Declaration of Helsinki.

We placed three ties after rectangular TSP in 48 eyes of 44 patients with punctal stenosis treated at our eye clinics by the same experienced eye surgeon (J.W.L.) from January 2014 to December 2016. This was a non-comparative case series. Patients who had epiphora and severe lower punctal stenosis without nasolacrimal duct obstruction were included. Patients with other causes of epiphora, such as dry eye syndrome, lid laxity, entropion, and ectropion were excluded.

Surgical outcomes were evaluated both subjectively and objectively. Tear meniscus height (TMH) was measured using a slit lamp and changes in tear film volume after surgery were noted [11, 12] . Subjective symptoms of patients were surveyed as improved or not improved. We also noted all recurrences. Anatomical recurrence was assessed based on anatomic re-stenosis.

Surgical technique

Surgery was performed using an operating microscope under local anaesthesia (Fig. 1). We transconjunctivally infiltrated 2% (w/v) lidocaine (with epinephrine in a 1:100,000 weight ratio) from the posterior aspect of the eyelid into the region of the lacrimal canaliculus and punctum. A dilator or small Westcott spring scissors was used to enlarge the stenotic lacrimal punctum. A single blade of a small Westcott spring scissors was placed within the ampulla of the lacrimal canaliculus, with the remaining blade placed on the conjunctival surface of the posterior aspect of the eyelid. The first vertical snip was made at the vertical canaliculus (Fig. 1a). The second vertical snip was made from the edge of the first snip to create a flap (Fig. 1b). The final horizontal

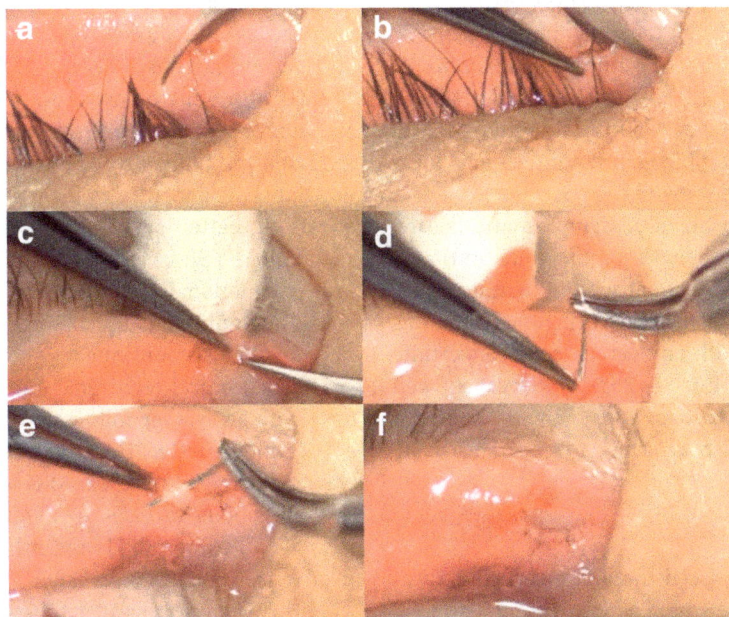

Fig. 1 Surgical procedure for the placement of three ties after rectangular three-snip punctoplasty. **a** The first vertical snip at the vertical canaliculus, (**b**) the second vertical snip made from the edge of the first snip to create a flap, (**c**) the final horizontal snip at the base, and (**d**) the three interrupted sutures being placed at the posterior wall of the ampulla after the rectangular three-snip punctoplasty. **e** For the three sutures, the inner surface of the canaliculus was slightly everted to allow sewing to the edge of the tarsal conjunctiva. **f** Immediate postoperative photograph. Note the three interrupted sutures, which are placed at the posterior wall of the ampulla

snip was made at the base (Fig. 1c). The rectangular flap was removed and three sutures were placed, in an interrupted manner, at the posterior wall of the ampulla using 10–0 nylon (Fig. 1d-f). After the suture was completed, the inner surface of the canaliculus was slightly everted to allow sewing to the edge of the tarsal conjunctiva. The sutures were removed 1 week after the surgery. Levofloxacin and fluorometholone eye drops were used q.i.d. for 1 week.

Statistical analysis

Data were analysed with the aid of the Statistical Package for the Social Sciences (SPSS) version 20.0 (SPSS INC., Chicago, IL, USA). The paired t-test was used to compare mean TMH values before and after the procedure. A p-value < 0.05 was considered to reflect statistical significance.

Results

Forty-eight eyes of 44 patients were enrolled. The mean patient age was 64.1 years. Ten patients were male and 34 were female. The average follow-up time was 17.4 months. The causes of punctal stenosis were idiopathic (35 patients), severe viral keratoconjunctivitis (six patients), ocular pemphigoid (two patients), and systematic chemotherapy (one patient).

The placement of three ties after rectangular TSP afforded both subjective and objective improvements. The surgery required 5–10 min. for one case. The patient subjective symptom survey showed that 44 eyes (91.7%) were improved, and four eyes (8.3%) remained unchanged. The mean TMH decreased from 1.4 mm (0.5–3 mm) to 0.8 mm (0.5–2 mm). The paired t-test revealed a significant difference between the pre- and postoperative TMH ($p < 0.001$). Representative photographs of pre- and postoperative punctoplasty are shown in Fig. 2.

Among four eyes determined as symptomatic failure, anatomical recurrence (restenosis of the punctum) was observed in only one eye (a patient with idiopathic punctal stenosis). Thus, the anatomical recurrence rate was about 2.1% (1/48 eyes) with an average recurrence time of 8.7 months. The other three (6.25%, 3/48eyes) showed functional nasolacrimal obstruction, namely epiphora with patent tear duct, with an average recurrence time of 5.2 months.

Discussion

In the current study, we placed three interrupted sutures in the posterior wall of the ampulla after rectangular TSP; both the subjective and objective surgical outcomes were satisfactory; 91.7% of eyes were reported improved over about 17.4 months of follow-up. TMH is significantly correlated with the volume of the tear film, of which 75–90% is contained in the tear meniscus [13–18]. We used TMH

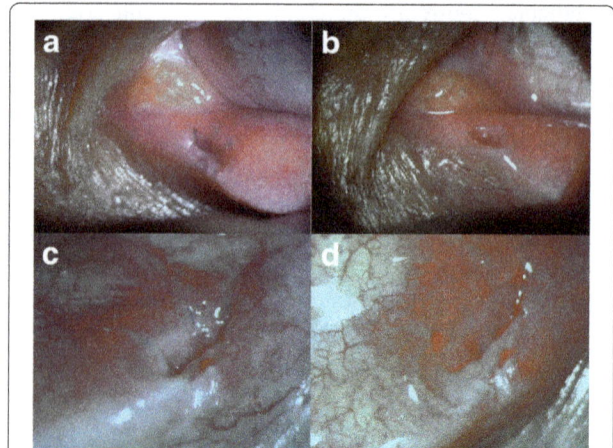

Fig. 2 Pre- and post-operative representative photographs of punctoplasty. Postoperative photographs of a 65-year-old female at (**a**) 1 week and (**b**) 1 month. Note the enlarged punctal opening. Postoperative photographs at (**c**) 1 week and (**d**) 1 month of the right lower eyelid punctum of a 63-year-old male

to measure changes in tear film volumes after surgery. The mean TMH decreased significantly ($p < 0.001$).

Punctal stenosis is the cause of 8% of all epiphora encountered in tertiary care institutions [19]. Punctoplasty is a simple surgical procedure that resolves punctal stenosis. The history of punctoplasty contains many surgical modifications and developments [2]. One-snip punctoplasty was the first modality to be introduced. Problems included deterioration of the capillarity of the lacrimal canaliculus and difficulties in re-approximation of the raw cut ends. Thus, one-snip punctoplasty was replaced by two-snip punctoplasty and TSP [2]. Currently, TSP is the most successful surgical technique used to enlarge a stenosed punctum [3]. There are two types of TSP: triangular TSP and rectangular TSP, the latter is believed to afford better symptom resolution [2, 3]. However, rectangular TSP is still associated with a high recurrence rate of functional epiphora (10.3%) [1]. Thus, efforts towards an optimal surgical procedure for resolution of punctal stenosis continue.

The anatomical recurrence rate of this study was about 2.1% with an average follow-up time of 17.4 months. Chak and Irvine reported that the anatomical recurrence rate was about 6% (3/49 eyes) after conventional rectangular TSP and about 3% (2/50 eyes) after conventional triangular TSP [3]. Ali et al. [1] recently reported an anatomical recurrence rate of 5.7% after conventional rectangular TSP; this value was similar to that of Chak and Irvine [3]. Our anatomical recurrence rate was lower and our average follow-up time was 17.4 months, which was longer compared with 8.2 months in the study of Chak and Irvine [3] and 4.2 months in the study by Ali et al. [1]. It is promising that our new technique shows a lower recurrence rate than conventional rectangular TSP of the two cited studies, despite having a longer follow-up period. In this study, the functional recurrence rate was about 6.25%, which was higher than the anatomical recurrence rate. Recently, long-term outcomes of punch punctoplasty using a Kelly punch have been reported with promising results [8]. In this report, the anatomical success was 94% and the functional success rate 92%.

Our rationale to explain the promising results of the three sutures after rectangular TSP was that the interrupted sutures helped to decrease the raw surface of the dilated punctum and making restenosis of the dilated punctum less likely.

Although the invasiveness of the new procedure still remains a concern, our new technique involving the placement of three sutures after rectangular TSP has shown promising results. Physiological preservation of the lacrimal system should be further reviewed in comparison with that provided by conventional rectangular or triangular TSP as control groups. A limitation of this study was a lack of preoperative grading of stenosed puncta.

Conclusions

Punctal stenosis commonly triggers epiphora requiring surgical intervention. Among various punctoplasty procedures, three-snip punctoplasty is the most successful surgical technique when it is necessary to enlarge the punctum in patients with punctal stenosis. In this study, we introduce a novel surgical technique involving placement of three interrupted sutures in the posterior wall of the ampulla after triangular three-snip punctoplasty. The new surgical procedure has shown promising results in punctal stenotic patients and may increase the success rate of punctoplasty.

Abbreviations
TMH: Tear meniscus height; TSP: Three-snip punctoplasty

Acknowledgements
Not applicable.

Funding
This study was supported by the Soonchunhyang University Research Fund which, however, played no role in the design or conduct of the research.

Declarations
Not applicable.

Authors' contributions
SYJ and JWL were responsible for the study conception and design, as well as the intellectual content of the paper. SJP made intellectual contributions to the text. NJH and KBP performed the chart review. JWL revised the article critically for intellectual content. All authors read and approved the final manuscript.

Competing interests
The authors declare that they have no competing interests.

Author details
[1]College of medicine, Soonchunhyang University, 204-ho, 31 Soonchunhyang-6-gil, Dongnam-gu, Cheonan 31151, Choongcheongnam-do, South Korea. [2]Soo Eye Clinics, 202-13, Miadong, Kangbook-gu, Seoul 01118, South Korea. [3]Department of Ophthalmology, Soonchunhyang University Bucheon Hospital, Soonchunhyang University College of Medicine, 170 Jomaru-ro, Wonmi-gu, Bucheon 14584, Gyeonggi-do, South Korea.

References
1. Ali MJ, Ayyar A, Naik MN. Outcomes of rectangular 3-snip punctoplasty in acquired punctal stenosis: is there a need to be minimally invasive? Eye (London, England). 2015;29(4):515–8.
2. Caesar RH, McNab AA. A brief history of punctoplasty: the 3-snip revisited. Eye (London, England). 2005;19(1):16–8.
3. Chak M, Irvine F. Rectangular 3-snip punctoplasty outcomes: preservation of the lacrimal pump in punctoplasty surgery. Ophthal Plast Reconstr Surg. 2009;25(2):134–5.
4. Kim SE, Lee SJ, Lee SY, Yoon JS. Outcomes of 4-snip punctoplasty for severe punctal stenosis: measurement of tear meniscus height by optical coherence tomography. American journal of ophthalmology. 2012;153(4): 769–73. 773.e761–762
5. Kristan RW. Treatment of lacrimal punctal stenosis with a one-snip canaliculotomy and temporary punctal plugs. Archives of ophthalmology (Chicago, Ill : 1960). 1988;106(7):878–9.
6. Kashkouli MB, Beigi B, Astbury N. Acquired external punctal stenosis: surgical management and long-term follow-up. Orbit (Amsterdam, Netherlands). 2005;24(2):73–8.
7. Ma'luf RN, Hamush NG, Awwad ST, Noureddin BN. Mitomycin C as adjunct therapy in correcting punctal stenosis. Ophthal Plast Reconstr Surg. 2002; 18(4):285–8.
8. Wong ES, Li EY, Yuen HK. Long-term outcomes of punch punctoplasty with Kelly punch and review of literature. Eye (London, England). 2017; 31(4):560–5.
9. Shahid H, Sandhu A, Keenan T, Pearson A. Factors affecting outcome of punctoplasty surgery: a review of 205 cases. Br J Ophthalmol. 2008;92(12): 1689–92.
10. Chalvatzis NT, Tzamalis AK, Mavrikakis I, Tsinopoulos I, Dimitrakos S. Self-retaining bicanaliculus stents as an adjunct to 3-snip punctoplasty in management of upper lacrimal duct stenosis: a comparison to standard 3-snip procedure. Ophthal Plast Reconstr Surg. 2013;29(2):123–7.
11. Burkat CN, Lucarelli MJ. Tear meniscus level as an indicator of nasolacrimal obstruction. Ophthalmology. 2005;112(2):344–8.
12. Roh JH, Chi MJ. Efficacy of dye disappearance test and tear meniscus height in diagnosis and postoperative assessment of nasolacrimal duct obstruction. Acta Ophthalmol. 2010;88(3):e73–7.
13. Gaffney EA, Tiffany JM, Yokoi N, Bron AJ. A mass and solute balance model for tear volume and osmolarity in the normal and the dry eye. Prog Retin Eye Res. 2010;29(1):59–78.
14. Holly FJ. Physical chemistry of the normal and disordered tear film. Trans Ophthalmol Soc U K. 1985;104(Pt 4):374–80.
15. Wang J, Aquavella J, Palakuru J, Chung S, Feng C. Relationships between central tear film thickness and tear menisci of the upper and lower eyelids. Invest Ophthalmol Vis Sci. 2006;47(10):4349–55.
16. Uchida A, Uchino M, Goto E, Hosaka E, Kasuya Y, Fukagawa K, Dogru M, Ogawa Y, Tsubota K. Noninvasive interference tear meniscometry in dry eye patients with Sjogren syndrome. Am J Ophthalmol. 2007;144(2):232–7.
17. Savini G, Barboni P, Zanini M: Tear meniscus evaluation by optical coherence tomography. Ophthalmic surgery, lasers & imaging : the official journal of the International Society for Imaging in the Eye 2006, 37(2):112–118.
18. Yokoi N, Bron AJ, Tiffany JM, Maruyama K, Komuro A, Kinoshita S: Relationship between tear volume and tear meniscus curvature. Archives of ophthalmology (Chicago, Ill : 1960) 2004, 122(9):1265–1269.
19. Mainville N, Jordan DR. Etiology of tearing: a retrospective analysis of referrals to a tertiary care oculoplastics practice. Ophthal Plast Reconstr Surg. 2011;27(3):155–7.

15

Optimal size of pterygium excision for limbal conjunctival autograft using fibrin glue in primary pterygia

Ho Sik Hwang[1], Kyong Jin Cho[2], Gabriel Rand[3], Roy S. Chuck[3] and Ji Won Kwon[4*]

Abstract

Background: In our study we describe a method that optimizes size of excision and autografting for primary pterygia along with the use of intraoperative MMC and fibrin glue. Our objective is to propose a simple, optimizedpterygium surgical technique with excellent aesthetic outcomes and low rates of recurrence and otheradverse events.

Methods: Retrospective chart review of 78 consecutive patients with stage III primary pterygia who underwent an optimal excision technique by three experienced surgeons. The technique consisted of removal of the pterygium head, excision of the pterygium body and Tenon's layer limited in proportion to the length of the head, application of intraoperative mitomycin C to the defect, harvest of superior bulbar limbal conjunctival graft, adherence of graft with fibrin glue. Outcomes included operative time, follow up period, pterygium recurrence, occurrences of incorrectly sized grafts, and other complications.

Results: All patients were followed up for more than a year. Of the 78 patients, there were 2 cases of pterygium recurrence (2.6%). There was one case of wound dehiscence secondary to small-sized donor conjunctivaand one case of over-sized donor conjunctiva, neither of which required surgical correction. There were no toxic complications associated with the use of mitomycin C.

Conclusion: Correlating the excision of the pterygium body and underlying Tenon's layer to the length of the pterygium head, along with the use intraoperative mitomycin C, limbal conjunctival autografting, and fibrin adhesionresulted in excellent outcomes with a low rate of recurrence for primary pterygia.

Keywords: Primary pterygium, Excision size, Conjunctival autograft, Mitomycin C, Fibrin adhesion

Background

Pterygium is one of the most common ocular surface diseases with a global pooled prevalence calculated at 10.2% [1]. Pterygium surgery has evolved over last 50 years with the aim of reducing post-surgical complications, primary of which is recurrence. A 2016 Cochrane meta-analysis examined the two most currently popular techniques, limbal conjunctival autografting and amniotic membrane grafting, and found conjunctival autografting superior with respect to lower 6 month recurrence rates [2]. Surgeons make use of variations of conjunctival autografting

in an effort to further reduce recurrence rates. A 2011 meta-analysis found conjunctival autografting with fibrin glue superior to sutures with respect to lower recurrence rates [3]. In addition, there have been a number of randomized control studies showing lower recurrence rates with the adjuvant use of intraoperative mitomycin C (MMC) [4–6]. In our practice we routinely make use of limbal conjunctival autografting with intraoperative MMC and fibrin glue.

The contribution of our study is that we introduce a technique that standardizes the size of excision and grafting as a function of the length of the pterygium head. The extent of excision necessary to prevent recurrence is still a matter of debate, with a spectrum of opinions ranging from simple avulsion and removal of the

* Correspondence: eyeminerva@naver.com
[4]Department of Ophthalmology, Myongji Hospital, Seonam University College of Medicine, 55 Hwasu-Ro 14, Deokyang-Gu, Goyang-Si, Gyeonggi-Do 10475, Korea
Full list of author information is available at the end of the article

pterygium head to extensive subconjunctival dissection and excision of the entire pterygium to the point of insertion [7–12]. We developed this technique because we believe that the size of excision and graft for primary pterygia should be a continuous function based on the tissue's aggressiveness as measured by the size of the pterygium head.

In our study we describe a method that optimizes size of excision and autografting for primary pterygia along with the use of intraoperative MMC and fibrin glue. Our objective is to propose a simple, optimized pterygium surgical technique with excellent aesthetic outcomes and low rates of recurrence and other adverse events.

Methods

This study is a retrospective chart review of patients having conjunctival autograft surgery for primary pterygia. We included 78 consecutive patients with primary nasal pterygia and no previous ocular surgeries or active ocular diseases. Included patients had initial visits in our hospitals from January 2014 to August 2015. This is a multicenter study performed by three experienced surgeons, the first in Myongji Hospital in Seonam University (56 eyes), the second in Dankook University Hospital (20 eyes), and the third in Chuncheon Sacred Heart Hospital in Hallym University (2 eyes). All surgeons followed an identical, predetermined surgical protocol. The presurgical factors we accounted for include age, gender, and the length of

pterygium head. All pterygia were stage III, the pterygium head between the limbus and the pupillary margin [13].

The primary outcome of this study was pterygium recurrence. Recurrence was defined as any postoperative regrowth of fibrovascular tissue crossing the corneoscleral limbus onto the clear cornea. The secondary outcome of this study was the sizing of the graft as measured by rates of wound dehiscence or oversized grafts. Other reported results include the operation time and other postoperative complications. The data was analyzed using basic statistics including percentages, ranges, means, and standard deviations. Mean values are reported with ±1 standard deviation. We adhered to the tenets of the Declaration of Helsinki. Appropriate Institutional Review Board/Ethics Committee approvals were obtained from IRB of Chuncheon Sacred Heart Hospital, Dankook University Hospital and Myongji Hospital and the need for consent was waived for this retrospective chart review study by them.

Surgical procedure

Figures 1 and 2 are composites of photographs demonstrating the surgical procedure. The maximum length from the limbus to the apex of the pterygium head was first measured (Figs. 1b and 2a). Following the same line, a point with the same distance was marked from the limbus onto the pterygium body (Fig. 1c). From this point, two symmetric curvilinear lines were marked to the superior and inferior margins of the pterygium at the level of the limbus (Fig. 1c). A 2% subconjunctival

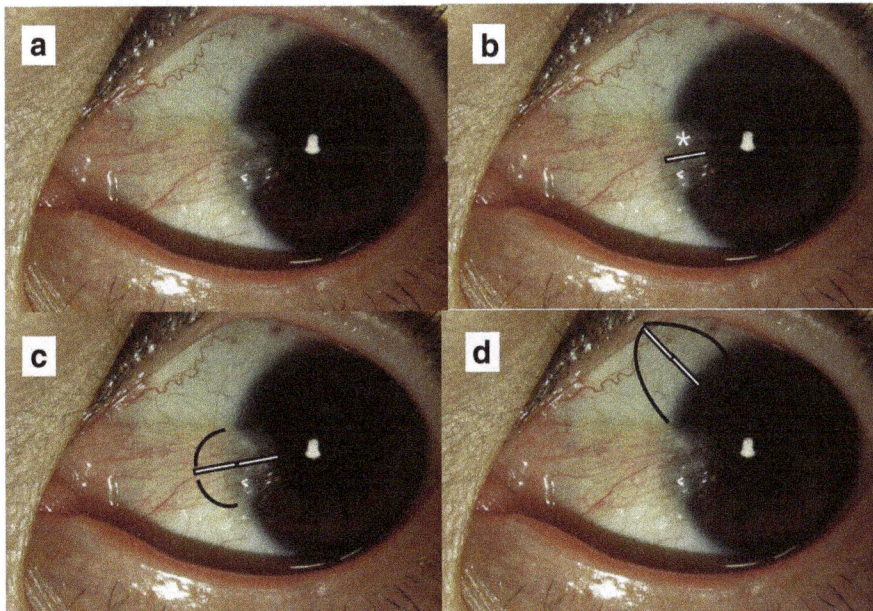

Fig. 1 The preoperative appearance of a primary pterygium (a). The length from the limbus to the apex of pterygium head (*) was measured (b). Following the same line, a point indicating the previously measured distance (*) from the limbus onto the pterygium body was marked (c). From this point, two symmetric curvilinear lines were marked from the point to the superior and inferior margins of the pterygium at the level of the limbus (c). Autograft size on the superior bulbar conjunctiva were measured and marked out (d)

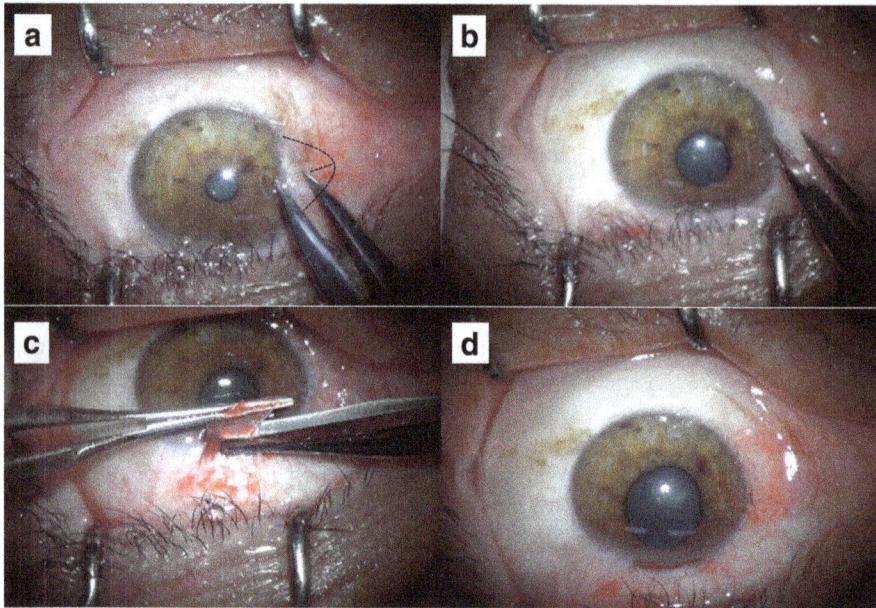

Fig. 2 The length from the limbus to the apex of the pterygium head was measured (**a**). The head was removed with a #15 blade, the body and Tenon's layer were excised with Vannas scissors, and the dimensions of the defect were measured (**b**). An autologous donor graft including limbal tissue was harvested from the superior bulbar conjunctiva (**c**). The graft was slid nasally with epithelium side down. Fibrin glue was placed on the defect and the graft is flipped epithelial side up with the limbal tissue facing the cornea (**d**)

lidocaine injection was administered at the pterygium head and body. After removing the head off the cornea with a #15 blade, the pterygium tissue within the curvlinear markings was excised along with Tenon's layer using Vannas scissors (Fig. 2b). Hemostasis was achieved with minimal electrocautery. Intraoperative 0.2 mg/ml mitomycin C soaked sponges were applied to the bare sclera for 2 min followed by vigorous irrigation with BSS (Balanced Salt Solution, Alcon, Fort Worth, TX). Using a caliper, the dimensions of the defect were measured and the donor site on the superior bulbar conjunctiva were marked out with the same dimensions (Fig. 1d). After administering a 2% lidocaine subconjunctival injection, the donor conjunctiva was harvested with Vannas scissors. The graft included limbal tissue and excluded Tenon's layer (Fig. 2c). The conjunctival autograft was secured using fibrin glue (Tisseel VH; Baxter, Vienna, Austria) as described by Koranyi et al [14]. The graft was placed with the epithelium side down on the cornea. The graft was carefully pushed to the nasal side with the limbal edge facing the wound. The two components of fibrin sealant were loaded separately in two syringes. One drop from each was placed over the recipient bed and the graft was quickly flipped over onto the pterygium defect and smoothed out (Fig. 2d). A bandage contact lens (Oasis, Johnson and Johnson: Jacksonville, FL) was placed on the cornea. Postoperatively, Moxifloxacin (Vigamox, Alcon, Fort Worth, TX) and 0.1%

Fluorometholone (Ocumetholone, Samil, Seoul, Korea) were applied four times per day for 1 month. The contact lens was removed on postoperative day 3.

The patients were followed up on postoperative days 1, 14 and at 1, 3, 6 and 12 months after surgery.

Postoperative outcome data was recorded at 12 months after the surgery. All patients were followed up to at least 12 months postoperatively to monitor for any further changes.

Results

Table 1 shows the baseline characteristics and outcomes of the 78 eyes from 78 patients (41 men and 37 women) included in this study. The mean age of the patients was 53.5 ± 14.2 (range 29–81) years. The mean length of the pterygium head was 1.9. $\pm$ 1.1 (range 0.7–5.1) mm. The mean duration of the operation was 20.9 ± 4.1 (range 15–30) minutes. The mean follow up period was 19.0 ± 4.9 (range, 14–30) months.

Figure 3 is a composite of pre- and postoperative 12 month photographs of patients having satisfactory aesthetic outcomes. In these cases there was no sign of recurrence. The donor conjunctivae were well grafted and not injected. There was neither wound dehiscence due to undersized donor conjunctivae nor irregular surface due to oversized donor conjunctivae. There were only two cases of recurrence (2.6%). There were one case of undersized and one case of oversized graft, neither of which required surgical correction (Fig. 4). The

Table 1 Demographics, Operation Time, Follow-up Period, and Complications

Number of patients	78
Number of eyes	78
Age (years)	53.5 ± 14.2
Sex (M:F)	41:37
Horizontal length of pterygium (mm)*	1.9 ± 1.1
Operation time (min)	20.9 ± 4.1
Follow up period (months)	19.0 ± 4.9
Recurrence (%)	2 (2.6)
Undersized donor conjunctiva (%)	1 (1.3)
Oversized donor conjunctiva (%)	1 (1.3)
Subconjunctival hemorrhage (%)	7 (8.9)
Granuloma (%)	1 (1.3)
Conjunctiva injection at 4 wks (%)	2 (2.6)

*From limbus to apex of pterygium

undersized graft caused wound dehiscence and the oversized graft caused an uneven surface at the wound. But, there was no problem with regard to donor size in most of cases (97.4%). The most common complication was subconjunctival hemorrhage. There were seven cases of subconjunctival hemorrhage (8.9%), all resolving within 2 weeks. There was one case of granuloma formation (1.3%). There were two cases of conjunctival injection (2.6%) resolving by 2 months. None of these adverse outcomes occurred at the donor site on the superior bulbar conjunctiva.

Discussion

The ideal pterygium surgery should use a simple technique as possible to optimize excellent aesthetics and minimize adverse outcomes. One reason our technique is simple is that we use fibrin glue instead of sutures. A meta-analysis comparing fibrin glue versus sutures in

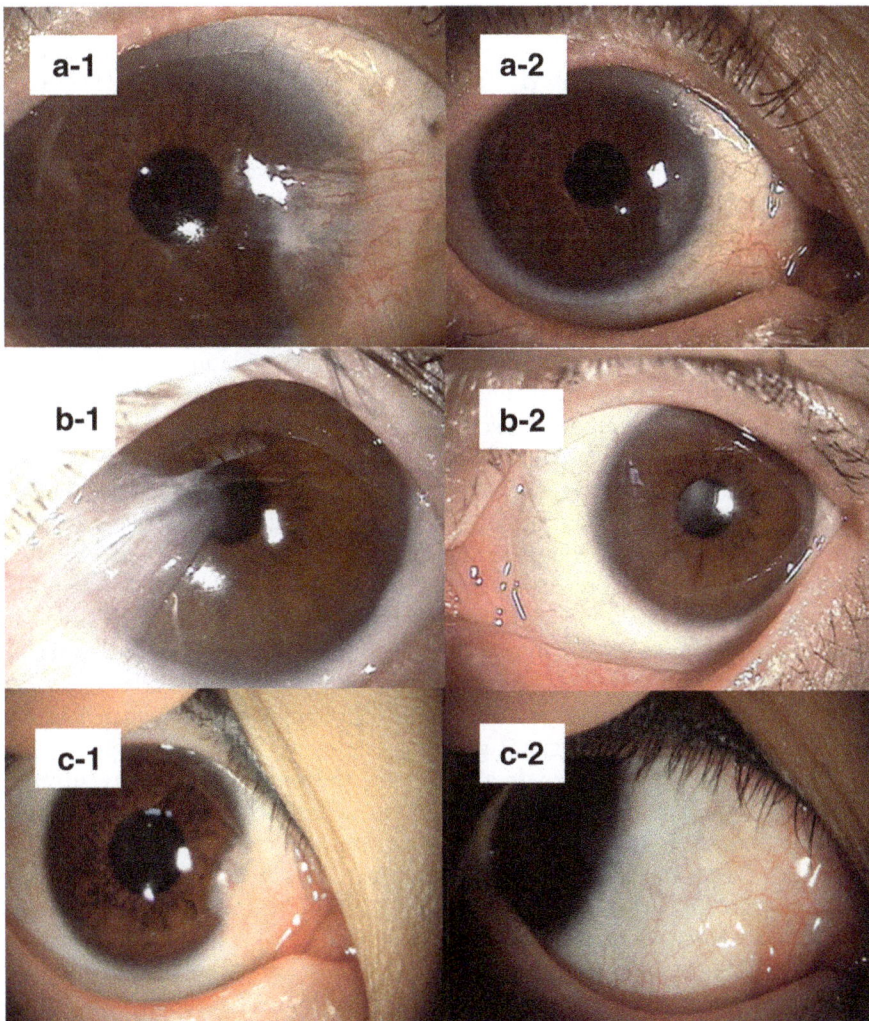

Fig. 3 A-1, B-1, and C-1 are preoperative images from three different patients. A-2, B-2, and C-2 are images of respective outcomes

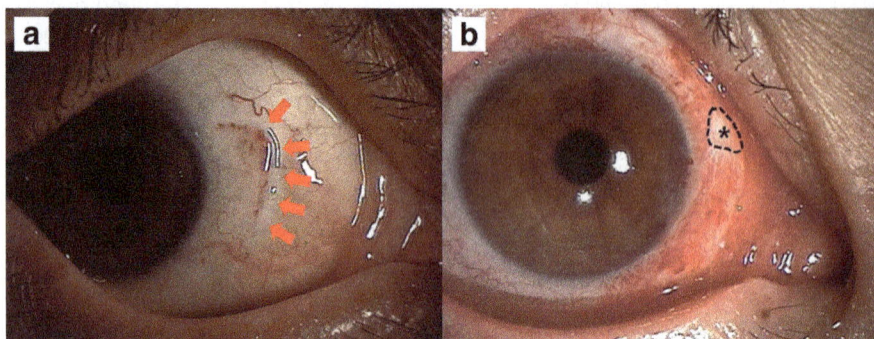

Fig. 4 Two cases of inappropriately sized grafts. A small-sized donor conjunctiva with wound dehiscence, covered with conjunctiva marked with red arrows (**a**). An oversized donor conjunctiva with extraneous tissue marked with star (**b**)

conjunctival autograft found fibrin glue was associated with shorter surgical times and a reduced recurrence rate [3]. Our mean operative time was 20.9 ± 4.1 min, comparable to other groups using fibrin glue. Ratnalingam et al. found that fibrin glue was associated with less postoperative pain [15]. The lower postoperative pain and reduced recurrence rate was hypothesized to result from less inflammation in the fibrin adhesive group. We did not use a standard measure to assess postoperative pain, but anecdotally our patients complained of very little discomfort in follow up visits.

Another simplification of our technique is that the excision is limited and does not extend to the posterior margin. At the present moment, there is no consensus regarding the optimal amount of excision that is necessary. Some argue for complete dissection and removal to the point of insertion, others argue for excision a certain distance from the limbus, and others argue for removal of just the pterygium head [7–12]. A more limited excision has a number of obvious advantages in that it should in theory require less anesthesia (subconjunctival as opposed to retro or peribulbar), shorten surgical time, and result in less postoperative pain. A major concern of limited excision techniques is the possibility of higher recurrence rates secondary to the residual pterygium left in place. It is therefore not considered a good option for more aggressive pterygia (e.g. recurrent pterygia, higher stage pterygia, etc). It is desirable to remove more pterygium tissue instead of exact length of pterygium expansion on the cornea in recurrent pterygia. For primary pterygia there is only one randomized control trial comparing recurrence rates and extent of excision with conjunctival autograft. Bazzazi et al. randomized 122 patients with primary pterygia to either conjunctival autograft with complete dissection and excision or resection of the pterygium head followed by placement of a small autograft. And they found no statistically significant difference in recurrence at 1 year [8]. Bahar et al. performed a conjunctival autograft cohort study of 161

patients with primary pterygia [7]. One group was a complete dissection and excision to the posterior margin and the other group was an excision limited to visible pterygium overlying conjunctiva. The study found no statistical difference in the total recurrence rate but found a statistically significant difference in the hazard ratio due to limited excision having earlier recurrences. With our limited excision technique for primary pterygia, we report a recurrence rate of 2.6%, a little less or comparable to recurrence rates reported for more extensive conjunctival autograft techniques on primary pterygia [16]. An additional benefit of our method is that it standardizes the geometry of the excision and graft and therefore should improve the quality of the graft fit. Of 78 cases, we only had two cases of incorrectly sized grafts, neither of which required surgical revision. Our review of the literature only showed one other method, the Stamp Technique, designed in particular to improve the fit of the graft [17].

A major difference in our technique compared to other limited excision conjunctival autograft techniques is that in ours the size of the excision is a precise function of the size of the pterygium head. The reasoning behind this approach is that in our experience pterygia with larger heads may be associated with more aggressively recurrent subtypes and therefore may benefit from relatively more extensive excision. Although we were unable to identify any studies investigating the direct association between the size of the pterygium head and recurrence rates, Tan et al. found a positive correlation between primary pterygium thickness and rate of recurrence [18]. Furthermore, Gazzard et al. found a correlation between pterygium thickness and the size of the pterygium head [19]. It therefore may follow that larger pterygium heads are associated with more aggressive subtypes and greater recurrence rates, and that these patients may benefit from more extensive excisions. There was no particular reason to select the exact length of pterygium expansion on the cornea as a measure for the excision of pterygium root. It is important that the size of the excision was a proportional to the size of the pterygium head in this study. So, it is possible to select half or double of the size of the pterygium head instead of same size.

We included the patients with only primary nasal pterygia in this study. We sometimes encountered temporal pterygia. We applied the same rule concerning the size of the excision. But it is necessary to compare the two groups (nasal versus temporal pterygia) concerning the size of the excision as a next study because the anatomy of the temporal conjunctiva is significantly different from that of the nasal conjunctiva.

A concern with any technique using MMC is toxic complications included but not limited to scleral melting, severe secondary glaucoma, and corneal edema [20, 21]. None of our cases resulted in complications associated with MMC. This may be because we used a low concentration (0.02%) on overall healthy eyes.

There are some limitations in our study. First, we did not have a control group to compare the effects of excision size, use of fibrin glue, and use of MMC. We therefore cannot analyze the effects of these different contributions had on our results. Second, our mean follow up period was 19.0 ± 4.9 months. It was once thought that 1 year follow up was sufficient to evaluate recurrence but new research has shown the risk to be continuous over the course of years [22]. Third, we measured the recurrence as a main surgical outcome, but we didn't measure the more common outcome measures of appearance, irritation and vision (refractive error). Fourth, we designed pteryium excision size according to the length of pterygium (from limbus to apex) without considering the thickness of pterygium. Fifth, this study design is not prospective but retrospective. Sixth, three surgeons were involved in this study, so the study group is relatively heterogeneous.

Conclusions

In conclusion, we proposed an optimal size of excision, intraoperative MMC and conjunctival autograft with fibrin glue in order to standardize graft sizes, simplify pterygium surgery, and reduce rates of incorrectly sized grafts. This technique showed excellent aesthetic outcomes and low rates of recurrence and other adverse events for primary pterygia.

Funding
This research was supported by a grant of the Korea Health Technology R&D Project through the Korea Health Industry Development Institute (KHIDI), funded by the Ministry of Health & Welfare, Republic of Korea (grant number: HI17C0659), Basic Science Research Program through the National Research Foundation of Korea(NRF) funded by the Ministry of Education, Republic of Korea(No. 2017R1A2A10000681) and Hallym University Research Fund (HURF-2017-59).

Authors' contributions
HHS, CKJ, GR, RC and KJW participated in the design of this study, HHS, CKJ and KJW carried out the study. HHS, CKJ, GR, RC and KJW performed the statistical analysis. HHS, CKJ, GR, RC and KJW drafted the manuscript. All authors read and approved the final manuscript.

Competing interests
Ho Sik Hwang is an associate editor and Roy S. Chuck is a section editor of of BMC Ophthalmology.

Author details
[1]Department of Ophthalmology, Chuncheon Sacred Heart Hospital, Hallym University, Chuncheon, Korea. [2]Department of Ophthalmology, Dankook University College of Medicine, Cheonan, Korea. [3]Department of Ophthalmology, Montefiore Medical Center, Bronx, New York, USA. [4]Department of Ophthalmology, Myongji Hospital, Seonam University College of Medicine, 55 Hwasu-Ro 14, Deokyang-Gu, Goyang-Si, Gyeonggi-Do 10475, Korea.

References
1. Liu L, Wu J, Geng J, et al. Geographical prevalence and risk factors for pterygium: a systematic review and meta-analysis. BMJ Open. 2013; 3(11):e003787.
2. Clearfield E, Muthappan V, Wang X, et al. Conjunctival autograft for pterygium. Cochrane Database Syst Rev. 2016;2:CD011349.
3. Pan HW, Zhong JX, Jing CX. Comparison of fibrin glue versus suture for conjunctival autografting in pterygium surgery: a meta-analysis. Ophthalmology. 2011;118:1049–54.
4. de la Hoz F, Montero JA, Alió JL, et al. Efficacy of mitomycin C associated with direct conjunctival closure and sliding conjunctival graft for pterygium surgery. Br J Ophthalmol. 2008;92:175–8.
5. Cardillo JA, Alves MR, Ambrosio LE, et al. Single intraoperative application versus postoperative mitomycin C eye drops in pterygium surgery. Ophthalmology. 1995;102:1949–52.
6. Frucht-Pery J, Raiskup F, Ilsar M, et al. Conjunctival autografting combined with low-dose mitomycin C for prevention of primary pterygium recurrence. Am J Ophthalmol. 2006;141:1044–50.
7. Bahar I, Kaiserman I, Weisbrod M, et al. Extensive versus limited pterygium excision with conjunctival autograft: outcomes and recurrence rates. Curr Eye Res. 2008;33:435–40.
8. Bazzazi N, Ramezani A, Rabiee MA. A comparative study of conjunctival autograft and minimally invasive pterygium surgery in primary pterygia. Pak J Biol Sci. 2010;13:409–12.
9. Massaoutis P, Khemka S, Ayliffe W. Clinical outcome study of a modified surgical technique for pterygium excision. Can J Ophthalmol. 2006;41:704–8.
10. John T. Pterygium excision and conjunctival minigraft: preliminary report. Eye. 2001;15:292–6.
11. Hirst LW. Recurrence and complications after 1,000 surgeries using pterygium extended removal followed by extended conjunctival transplant. Ophthalmology. 2012;119:2205–10.
12. Masters JS, Harris DJ Jr. Low recurrence rate of pterygium after excision with conjunctival Limbal autograft: a retrospective study with long-term follow-up. Cornea. 2015;34:1569–72.
13. Johnston C, Williams PB, Sheppard JD Jr. A comprehensive system for pterygium classification. Invest Ophthalmol Vis Sci. 2004;45:2940.
14. Koranyi G, Seregard S, Kopp ED. Cut and paste: a no suture, small incision approach to pterygium surgery. Br J Ophthalmol. 2004;88:911–4.
15. Ratnalingam V, Eu AL, Ng GL, et al. Fibrin adhesive is better than sutures in pterygium surgery. Cornea. 2010;29:485–9.
16. Zheng K, Cai J, Jhanji V, Chen H. Comparison of pterygium recurrence rates after limbal conjunctival autograft transplantation and other techniques: meta-analysis. Cornea. 2012;31:1422–7.
17. Hwang HS, Chul Kim E, Kim MS. A new conjunctival free flap design technique for pterygium surgery: stamp technique. Eye Contact Lens. 2016;42:171–6.
18. Tan DT, Chee SP, Dear KB, Lim AS. Effect of pterygium morphology on pterygium recurrence in a controlled trial comparing conjunctival autografting with bare sclera excision. Arch Ophthalmol. 1997;115:1235–40.
19. Gazzard G, Saw SM, Farook M, et al. Pterygium in Indonesia: prevalence, severity and risk factors. Br J Ophthalmol. 2002;86:1341–6.
20. Rubinfeld RS, Pfister RR, Stein RM, et al. Serious complications of topical mitomycin-C after pterygium surgery. Ophthalmology. 1992;99:1647–54.

16

Capture of intraocular lens optic by residual capsular opening in secondary implantation: long-term follow-up

Tian Tian[1†], Chunli Chen[2†], Haiying Jin[1], Lyu Jiao[1], Qi Zhang[1] and Peiquan Zhao[1*]

Abstract

Background: To introduce a novel surgical technique for optic capture by residual capsular opening in secondary intraocular lens (IOL) implantation and to report the outcomes of a long follow-up.

Methods: Twenty patients (20 eyes) who had received secondary IOL implantation with the optic capture technique were retrospectively reviewed. We used the residual capsular opening for capturing the optic and inserted the haptics in the sulcus during surgery. Baseline clinical characteristics and surgical outcomes, including best-corrected visual acuity (BCVA), refractive status, and IOL position were recorded. The postoperative location and stability of IOL were evaluated using the ultrasound biomicroscopy.

Results: Optic capture technique was successfully performed in all cases, including 5 cases with large area of posterior capsular opacity, 6 cases with posterior capsular tear or rupture,and 9 cases with adhesive capsules. BCVA improved from 0.60 logMAR at baseline to 0.36 logMAR at the last follow-up ($P < 0.001$). Spherical equivalent changed from 10.67 ± 4.59 D at baseline to 0.12 ± 1.35 D at 6 months postoperatively ($P < 0.001$). Centered IOLs were observed in all cases and remained captured through residual capsular opening in 19 (95%) eyes at the last follow-up. In one case, the captured optic of IOL slid into ciliary sulcus at 7 months postoperatively. No other postoperative complications were observed in any cases.

Conclusions: This optic capture technique by using residual capsule opening is an efficacious and safe technique and can achieve IOL stability in the long follow-up.

Keywords: Intraocular lens, Optic capture, Dislocation, Secondary IOL implantation

Background

Posterior chamber intraocular lens (IOL) are mostly implanted in the capsular bag. However, the status of lens capsules may not be sufficient to support IOL intracapsular bag implantation, especially during secondary procedure. Under these challenging and complicated situations, variously substituted IOL implanting techniques have been reported, including sulcus-IOL implantation, using an anterior chamber IOL, an iris-fixed IOL, and a transscleral-fixed posterior chamber IOL. However, each of these techniques has postoperative problems and complications. The major complications are postoperative IOL instability, dislocation, tilting, and pupillary capture of IOL [1–5].

Compared to these substituted IOL implanting techniques mentioned above, our optic capture technique was a simple and safe choice in cases with intact residual capsular opening during the secondary IOL implantation. The concept of our optic capture technique was derived from "the rhexis-fixed Lens" which was firstly described by Neuhann for placing the haptics in the sulcus and then capturing the IOL optic through the anterior continuous curvilinear capsulorhexis (CCC) opening [6]. The concept of optic capture technique was firstly described by Gimbel and DeBroff to maintain a clear visual axis in pediatric IOL surgery with the haptics in the capsular bag and optic through a posterior

* Correspondence: zhaopeiquan@xinhuamed.com.cn
†Equal contributors
[1]Department of Ophthalmology, Xinhua Hospital, Affiliated to Medicine School of Shanghai Jiaotong University, No. 1665, Kongjiang Road, Shanghai 200092, China
Full list of author information is available at the end of the article

curvilinear capsulorhexis opening [7]. Even the optic capture technique of IOL has been described, however, the optic capture technique are mainly used in primary pediatric or adult cataract surgery. As known, the capsule remained is different one from that at primary surgery, such as fibrosis, adherent anterior and posterior capsule, and membrane-like formation. Will the residual capsular membrane offer enough strength to capture the optic of IOL? Will the IOL achieved stability in the cases with intact residual capsular opening in the long-term? However, there existed few clinical studies to manifest the safety of optic capture technique during the secondary IOL implantation. In order to answer those questions we did the present clinical study.

Methods

Patients

This study adhered to the tenets of the Declaration of Helsinki and was approved by institution review board of Xinhua hospital affiliated to medical college, Shanghai Jiaotong University. We retrospectively reviewed 20 patients (20 eyes) who had received secondary IOL implantation with optic capture technique from April 2012 to January 2016. Surgeries were performed by one surgeon (P.Q.Z). Inclusion criteria were 1) Large area of posterior capsular opacity (PCO); severe synechia of anterior and posterior capsules; posterior capsular tear or rupture with inadequate support of capsular bag (Fig. 1). The residual capsular opening should be intact and the size should be 4.0 mm to 5.0 mm approximately. Exclusion criteria were 1) IOL can be implanted in capsular bags. 2)No enough residual capsules, which made the IOL optic capture impossible. 3) Eyes with lax zonules or zonular dehiscence. 4) Eyes with anterior megalophthalmos. 5)Axial length is longer than 28 mm.

All 20 patients had a complete ophthalmologic examination including best-corrected visual acuity (BCVA), refractive status, axial length, B-scan, intraocular pressure (IOP), endothelial cell count,slit-lamp examination, Refractive status, and dilated fundus examination pre- and postoperatively. We collected refractive status for statistical analysis at 6 months after surgery when the position of IOL and the status of anterior segment tend to be stable. BCVA was measured among 18 patients with Snellen chart and converted to logarithm of the minimum angle of resolution values (logMAR) for the statistical analysis. The remaining two patients were too young to cooperate with BCVA examination. Refractive status was measured through retinoscopy with instillation of a combination of tropicamide 1%, phenylephrine 2.5% and cyclopentolate 1%. Chloral hydrate was used in pediatric patients who were uncooperative. B scans were obtained in all 20 patients (Digital B 2000 and Ultrascan

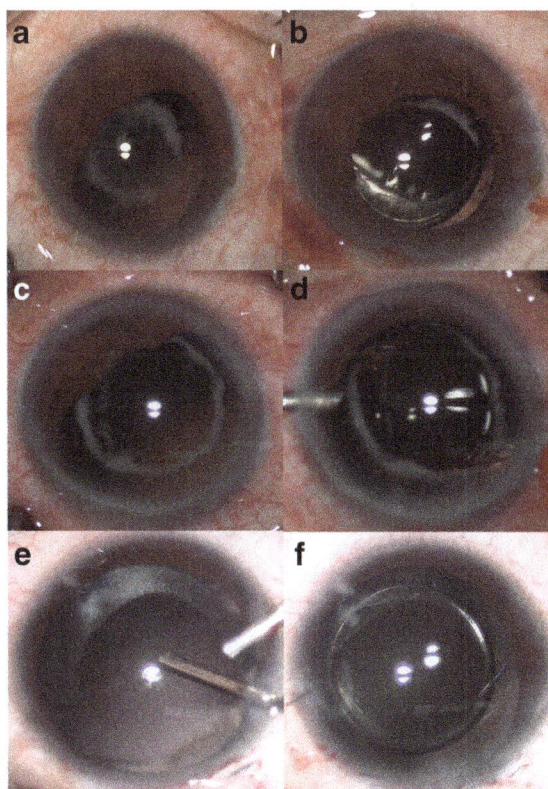

Fig. 1 Three cases underwent optic capture technique with three indications: intraoperative photos. The intraoperative photo (**a**) showed the large area of posterior capsular opacity in a 68 years old female (Case 1) with proliferative diabetic retinopathy. Optic was captured through the residual capsular opening after posterior capsule cut using vitreous cutter (**b**). The intraoperative photo (**c**) showed 360-degree synechia of capsules and posterior synechia of iris in a 61 years old male (Case 4). After managing the posterior synechia, the optic was captured through the residual capsular opening (**d**). The intraoperative photo (**e**) showed the posterior capsule tear caused by trauma in a 12-year old female (Case 2). After trimming, the posterior capsular opening was equal to the anterior capsular opening (**e**). The captured optic was centered with clear visual axis (**f**)

Imaging System; Alcon). Axial length was measured by optical biometer (Ver 5.4) (Carl Zeiss Meditec AG, Jena, Germany) or A scan (Digital B 2000 and Ultrascan Imaging System; Alcon). The capsules status was recorded according to intraoperative videos. The postoperative location and stability of IOL were evaluated by using the ultrasound biomicroscopy (UBM, Paradigm Medical Industries, Salt Lake City, UT). Corneal endothelial cell count was assessed with the EM-3000 (TOMEY, Nagoya, Japan) in patients who were older than 10 years pre- and postoperatively (6 months).

Surgical technique

After retrobulbar or general anesthesia was attained, an infusion cannula connected to a balanced salt plus solution (Alcon, Laboratories, Inc) was inserted into anterior chamber through infratemporal corneal incision. In cases with posterior capsule tear caused by trauma or inadvertent rupture in primary surgeries, the tear or rupture was converted to a circular, well-centered capsular opening as much as possible. In cases with large area of PCO, posterior capsulorhexis was performed with virtrectomy cutter. Posterior synechia of iris was meticulously dissected with assistance of viscoelastic if needed. After managing capsules properly, a foldable IOL with a 6.0 mm optic and 13.0 mm haptic diameter (Tecnis ZA9003; AMO, Santa Ana, CA) was inserted into the anterior chamber through a 2.8 mm superior clear corneal incision. Residual capsular opening should be large enough to allow the IOL optic to pass through and small enough to capture the optic. The appropriate size of residual capsular opening was 4.0–5.0 mm approximately. Then, one haptic of the IOL was inserted into the ciliary sulcus with a Sinskey hook, and then the other haptic was positioned in contralateral ciliary sulcus in the same manner. The positions of haptics should avoid the capsular defect area. After confirming the positions of the two haptics, one side of the optic was then captured through residual capsular opening, and the other side was pressed in the same manner. The successfully captured optic made an oval capsular configuration (Fig. 2). Finally, the corneoscleral incisions were closed with a single 10–0 nylonsuture if necessary.

Statistical analysis

Statistical analyses were performed using SPSS version 19 for Windows (SPSS Inc., Chicago, USA). Paired t-test was conducted in this study. P value less than 0.05 (two tails) was considered as statistical difference.

Results

Successful optic capture IOL implantation was achieved in all 20 aphakic eyes (20 patients). The mean age was 31.95 ± 26.83 years. The capsular status was collected based on the surgery video, including 5 eyes (25%) with large area of posterior capsular opacity, 6 eyes (30%) with posterior capsular tear or rupture, and 9 eyes (45%) with adhesive capsules. Fifteen eyes (75%) combined with retinal disorders. The mean follow-up was 24.51 ± 13.47 months. The details and clinical characteristics of the 20 patients were shown in Table 1.

BCVA improved from 0.60 logMAR at baseline to 0.36 logMAR at the last follow-up ($P < 0.001$). Spherical equivalent changed from 10.67 ± 4.59 D at baseline to 0.12 ± 1.35 D at 6 months postoperatively. The position of IOL remained captured through residual capsular opening in 19 (95%) eyes at the last follow-up (Fig. 3). In one case, the captured optic of IOL slid into ciliary sulcus at 7 months postoperatively (Fig. 4). The surgical outcomes were shown in Table 2. No patients had complaints of dazzle or other visual disorders. Iris synechia, anterior cells, anterior uveitis and secondary glaucoma were not observed in any cases. No other related complications were found in any case at the last follow-up.

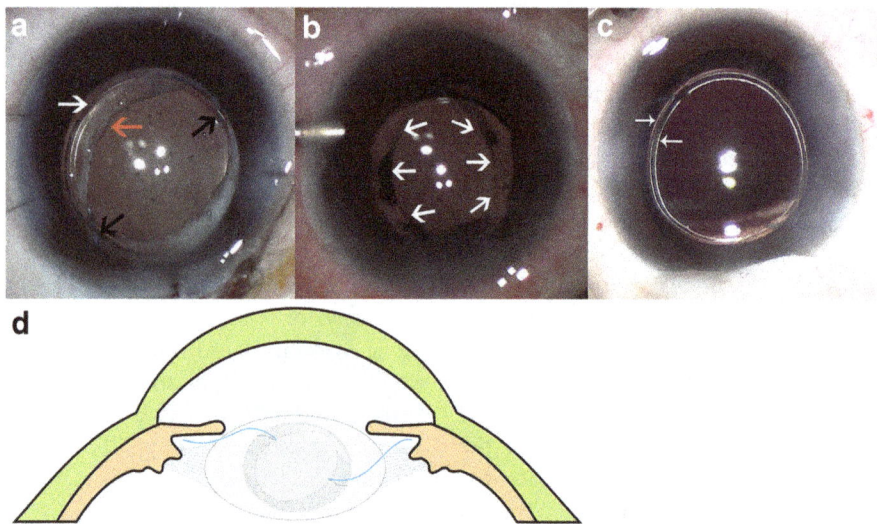

Fig. 2 Three patients who underwent IOL optic capture technique: intraoperative photos (**a**, **b** and **c**) and schematic illustration (**d**). The intraoperative photo (**a**) showed two haptics (black arrows) of IOL were inserted in the ciliary sulcus with the optic (white arrow) captured through residual capsular openings (red arrow). And the intraoperative photo (**b**) showed the successful captured optic made an oval capsular configuration (white arrows). The ideal size of capsular opening is around 4.0 mm to 5.0 mm, which should be at least 1.0 mm or 2.0 mm (white arrows) smaller than the optic diameter (**c**). The Schematic illustrations (**d**) of optic capture technique showed the optic of IOL (the edge was shown as dark gray color) captured through residual capsular opening with haptics in the ciliary sulcus

Table 1 Details and characteristics of patients who underwent secondary IOL implantation with optic capture

PT	Age (Y) / Sex	Eye	Preoperative diagnosis	History of previous operation(s)	Capsular status	BCVA pre/post	Follow-up (months)
1	68/F	OD	PDR	Phaco+PPV + C3F8	Large PCO	0.1/0.3	18
2	12/F	OD	Traumatic cataract	Lensectomy	PC tear	0.05/0.15	9
3	5/F	OD	Congenital cataract	Lensectomy+ anterior PPV	Adhesive	FC/0.1	7
4	61/M	OS	RRD	Phaco+PPV + C3F8	Adhesive	FC/0.05	26
5	1/F	OD	PHPV	Lensectomy	Large PCO	Uncooperated/ Uncooperated	6
6	35/M	OD	RRD	Lensectomy+PPV + C3F8	PC rupture	0.01/0.1	27
7	4/M	OD	Traumatic cataract	Lensectomy	Adhesive	Uncooperated/0.12	16
8	4/F	OD	Congenital cataract	Lensectomy	Adhesive	HM/FC	13
9	61/M	OS	PDR	Phaco+PPV + C3F8	Large PCO	FC/0.1	32
10	4/F	OD	PHPV; Concurrent cataract	Lensectomy	Adhesive	HM/0.12	15
11	2/M	OD	PHPV; Concurrent cataract	Lensectomy	Adhesive	Uncooperated/ Uncooperated	8
12	46/M	OD	PDR	Phaco+PPV + C3F8	Adhesive	FC/0.3	41
13	81/M	OS	Age related cataract	Phaco	PC rupture	0.08/0.20	12
14	62/F	OD	ERM; Concurrent cataract	Phaco+PPV + ILM peeling+C3F8	Large PCO	0.1/0.3	28
15	40/F	OS	RRD	Lensectomy+PPV + C3F8	PC rupture	0.3/0.8	35
16	2/F	OS	PHPV; Concurrent cataract	Lensectomy+ anterior PPV	Adhesive	Uncooperated/ Uncooperated	6
17	10/M	OS	Traumatic macular hole	Lensectomy + PPV	Adhesive	FC/0.1	18
18	53/F	OD	RRD	Phaco +PPV+ C3F8	PC rupture	FC/0.6	32
19	58/M	OS	ERM; Concurrent cataract	Phaco+PPV + C3F8	Large PCO	0.03/0.5	46
20	50/M	OS	Macular hole; Concurrent cataract	Phaco+PPV + ILM peeling+C3F8	PC rupture	FC/0.25	35

PT patient, *M* male, *F* female, *PDR* proliferative diabetic retinopathy, *RRD* rhegmatogenous retinal detachment, *PHPV* persistent hyperplasia of primary vitreous, *ERM* epiretinal retinal membrane, *PPV* pars plana vitrectomy, *PRP* panretinal photocoagulation, *ILM* internal limiting membrane, *PCO* posterior capsular opacity, *PC* posterior capsule, *BCVA* best corrected visual acuity, *Pre* preoperation, *Post* postoperation, *HM* hand motion, *FC* figure counting, *IOL* intraocular lens

Discussion

The present study described the application of optic capture technique in eyes with intact residual capsular opening during the secondary implantation. Our study demonstrated the safety and efficiency of optic capture technique; good long-term visual outcome; clinically centered IOL, and no secondary opacification of the visual axis at the mean follow-up of 23.51 months. However, the optic of IOL may slide into sulcus during the follow-up.

The situation of lens capsules may be complicated and challenging in the secondary IOL implantations, such as no adequate support of capsular bag, large area of posterior capsular opacity (PCO) and serious synechia of anterior and posterior capsules that lead no potential space for the in-the-bag IOL implantation. Until now, there is no consensus on the optimal choice of IOL implantation methods in eyes within these complicated situations of lens capsules mentioned above. In eyes with intact anterior CCC, the sulcus-fixation is

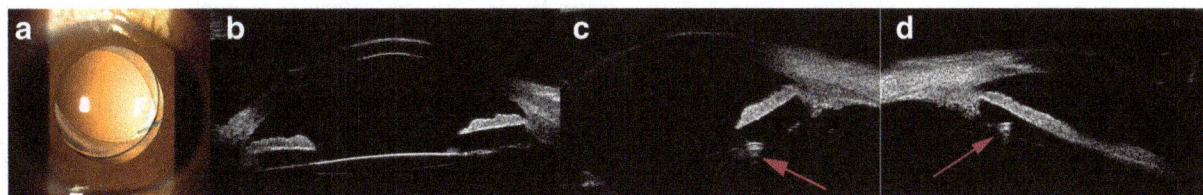

Fig. 3 A 50 years old male (Case 20), phaco and vitrectomy were performed because of macular hole. The Slit-lap photo (**a**) showed the centered IOL with optic captured through posterior capsular opening and haptics in the sulcus, at 6 months postoperatively. Ultrasound biomircoscopy (**b**, **c** and **d**) showed the optic was centered and two haptics were located at 2 o'clock and 8 o'clock, repectively

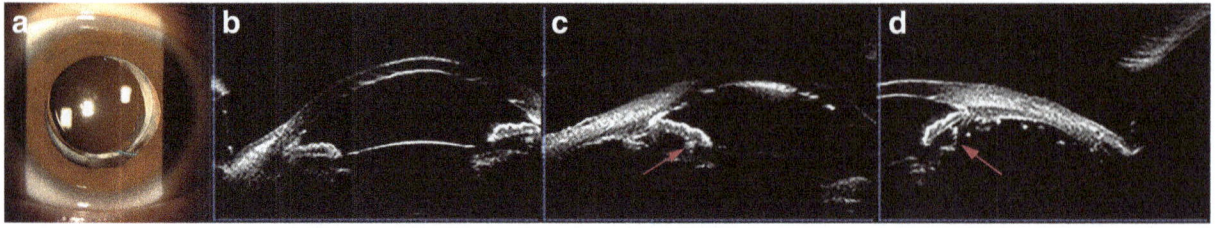

Fig. 4 A 10 years old male (Case 17), lensectomy and pans plana vitrectomy were performed because of traumatic macular hole. The Slit-lap photo (**a**) showed the centered IOL at 7 months postoperatively. However, ultrasound biomircoscopy (**b**, **c** and **d**) showed the optic and two haptics were in the sulcus. Two haptics were located at 5 o'clock and 11 o'clock, respectively

always substitute for capsular bag. However, it has been reported that the implantation of foldable IOLs into the ciliary sulcus may be related to a higher rate of decentration [5]. Besides, the incidence of pupillary capture of the sulcus-fixation IOL is raised when combined with pars planar vitrectomy and gas tamponade [8]. Moreover, the surgeon personally encountered frequent and recurrent pupillary capture of the sulcus-fixation IOL optic after phacovitrectomy. All these results demonstrated the instability of ciliary sulcus inserted IOL in eyes with posterior capsule rupture or larger PCO. Other surgeons may consider transscleral-fixed IOL, iris-fixed IOL or anterior chamber IOL in cases without adequate capsular support. Each technique has advantages and disadvantages. Several postoperative complications have been reported with these techniques, including retinal detachment, vitreous hemorrhage, endophthalmitis, IOL dislocation, and pupillary capture [4, 9]. It has been reported that pupillary capture of the

Table 2 Surgical outcomes of secondary IOL implantation with optic capture

Parameter	Mean ± SD	P value
BCVA, log MAR		< 0.001
Preoperative	0.60 ± 0.44	
Postoperative	0.36 ± 0.17	
Spherical equivalent, (D)		< 0.001
Preoperative	10.67 ± 4.59	
Postoperative	0.12 ± 1.35	
IOL position, n (%)		
Captured	19 (95%)	
Ciliary sulcus	1 (5%)	
Endothelial Cell Count		0.431
Preoperative	2326 ± 423	
Postoperative	2158 ± 389	
IOP		0.524
Preoperative	15.26 ± 3.65	
Postoperative	14.86 ± 2.82	

BCVA best corrected visual acuity, *IOL* intraocular lens, *IOP* intraocular ocular pressure

IOL optics could occurred in 7.9% to 14.3% of cases after scleral-fixated sutured posterior chamber IOL (PC IOL) implantation [3, 10]. Dong Jin Kang et al. have reported that five eyes (7.8%) had pupillary capture after transscleral IOL fixation. Other complications after transscleral fixation were vitreous hemorrhage in 5 eyes (7.8%) and IOP elevation in 8 eyes (12%) [11]. Besides, suturing of the haptics to the sclera may result in suture erosion, delayed IOL dislocation owing to suture breakage, or suture exposure-induced endophthalmitis [4, 12].

Compared to these techniques, our optic capture technique by residual capsular opening offers a tight seal of the IOL-capsule diaphragm, it helps maintain stable compartmentalization between the anterior and posterior segments of the eye and reduces the rate of postoperative IOL dislocation significantly. Besides, the optic capture procedure was simple with short learning curve. The variations of optic capture include (a) haptics in the sulcus and IOL optic capture through a CCC, (b) haptics in the sulcus and IOL optic capture through an anterior capsule opening and a posterior CCC (PCCC), (c) haptics in the capsular bag and IOL optic capture through a PCCC, (d) haptics in the capsular bag and IOL optic capture through an anterior CCC, (e) haptics in the sulcus and IOL capture through a capsular membrane opening, and (f) haptics posterior to the capsular bag and IOL capture through a capsular membrane opening [7]. In our study, the surgeon placed the haptics in the sulcus and optic captured through the residual capsular opening. To obtain successful optic capture in the secondary IOL implantation, trimming the residual capsular membranes to fit to capture the optic of IOL was the key factor. The ideal capsular opening is around 4.0 mm to 5.0 mm in primary surgery, which should be at least 1.0 mm or 2.0 mm smaller than the optic diameter but not too small [13]. In this study, we found that even the posterior capsular opening or tear was not entirely concentric, the captured optic still could achieve centered in the visual axis. It may because as long as the position of two haptics were symmetrical,the haptic-optic junction could offer a tight seal that maintain the optic centered in the visual axis. In our study, clinically centered IOLs were observed in all cases, and the optic edge was not seen through an undilated pupil at the last follow-up. In one case, however, the captured optic of IOL slid into ciliary sulcus at 7 months postoperatively. The UBM and dilated slit-lamp examination showed that the haptics and optic of IOL were in ciliary sulcus. In this case, the residual capsular opening was just approximately 1.0 mm smaller than optic diameter and completely round-shape. We hypothesized the capsular membrane became stiff after primary surgery and the size of the capsular opening was not small enough so that did not off a tight enough haptic-optic junction. Thus, we suggested the residual capsular opening should be less than 5.0 mm in cases with stiff capsular membrane during secondary IOL implantation. As the optic was still centered in the visual axis and BCVA was not impaired, the second operation was not performed to this patient.

The other advantage of optic capture technique is avoiding secondary opacification of the visual axis that may be caused by proliferation of Elschnig pearls. In our study, the surgeon placed the haptics in the sulcus and optic captured through the posterior opening, leading to apposition of anterior and posterior capsule leaflets anterior to the IOL optic. Compared to place two haptics in the capsular bag, the sulcus-placed haptics, which made a 360-degree seal of apposed capsule leaflets, avoided lens epithelial cells transdifferentiation and Elsching pearls releasing. Consequently, the rate of capsular shrinkage and visual axis opacification will be decreased significantly. In our study, capsular shrinkage and visual axis opacification were not observed in any case at the last follow-up. The BCVA improved from preoperative 0.60 ± 0.44 to postoperative 0.36 ± 0.17 logMAR. Because of primary ocular diseases, the BCVA may have a limited improvement in some cases.

The optic capture technique has limitations. It should not be performed if posterior capsular opening was quite eccentric or the size was not fit to capture the optic. Besides, the technique may not be ideal for eyes with anterior megalophthalmos. The larger capsular bags in these cases may increase the rate of IOL decentration.

Conclusions

In summary, optic capture through the residual capsular opening may be an efficacious and safe technique to achieve IOL stability in eyes with challenging capsular status during secondary IOL implantation. Attention should be paid to the cases with stiff capsular membrane when performed optic capture. Additional study with more cases and further follow-up is needed to manifest the safety and long-term efficacy before recommending the widespread application of this technique during secondary IOL implantation with challenging capsular status.

Abbreviations
BCVA: Best-corrected visual acuity; CCC: Continuous curvilinear capsulorhexis; IOL: Intraocular lens; IOP: Intraocular pressure; logMAR: Logarithm of the minimum angle of resolution values; PCO: Posterior capsular opacity; UBM: Ultrasound biomicroscopy

Acknowledgements
The authors thank the patients participated in the study. The authors also thank Professor Hui Yannian at Department of Ophthalmology, Xijing Hospital, The Fourth Military Medical University, The Eye Institute of PLA, Xi'an 710032, China.

Funding
This study was partially supported by the National Natural Science Foundation of China (No. 81271045). The funding body has no role in the design of the study and collection, analysis, and interpretation of data or in writing the manuscript.

Authors' contributions
TT and CLC have designed the study, collected and analyzed the data, wrote the manuscript. CLC, JHY, LJ and QZ assessed the patient, collected the data, check and revised the manuscript. PQZ designed the study, performed all the treatment and agreed to be accountable for all aspects of the work. All authors read and approved the final manuscript.

Competing interests
The authors declare that they have no competing interests.

Author details
[1]Department of Ophthalmology, Xinhua Hospital, Affiliated to Medicine School of Shanghai Jiaotong University, No. 1665, Kongjiang Road, Shanghai 200092, China. [2]Department of Ophthalmology, Shengli Oilfield Central Hospital, No.31, Jinan Road, Dong Ying, Shandong, China.

References
1. Ohta T, Toshida H, Murakami A. Simplified and safe method of sutureless intrascleral posterior chamber intraocular lens fixation: Y-fixation technique. J Cataract Refract Surg. 2014;40(1):2–7.
2. Yamane S, Inoue M, Arakawa A, Kadonosono K. Sutureless 27-gauge needle-guided intrascleral intraocular lens implantation with lamellar scleral dissection. Ophthalmology. 2014;121(1):61–6.
3. Bading G, Hillenkamp J, Sachs HG, Gabel VP, Framme C. Long-term safety and functional outcome of combined pars plana vitrectomy and scleral-fixated sutured posterior chamber lens implantation. Am J Ophthalmol. 2007;144(3):371–7.
4. McAllister AS, Hirst LW. Visual outcomes and complications of scleral-fixated posterior chamber intraocular lenses. J Cataract Refract Surg. 2011;37(7):1263–9.
5. Nihalani BR, Vanderveen DK. Secondary intraocular lens implantation after pediatric aphakia. J AAPOS. 2011;15(5):435–40.
6. Neuhann T (1991) The American Society of Cataract and Refractive Surgery Symposium on Cataract, IOL and Refractive Surgery: Future and past meeting perspectives, http://www.ascrs.org/future-and-past-meeting-dateslocations.pdf. Accesses 8 Apr 1991.
7. Gimbel HV, DeBroff BM. Intraocular lens optic capture. J Cataract Refract Surg. 2004;30(1):200–6.
8. Cho BJ, Yu HG. Surgical outcomes according to vitreous management after scleral fixation of posterior chamber intraocular lenses. Retina. 2014;34(10):1977–84.
9. Baykara M. Techniques of intraocular lens suspension in the absence of capsular/zonular support. Surv Ophthalmol. 2006;51(3):288. author reply
10. Johnston RL, Charteris DG, Horgan SE, Cooling RJ. Combined pars plana vitrectomy and sutured posterior chamber implant. Arch Ophthalmol. 2000;118(7):905–10.
11. Kang DJ, Kim HK. Clinical analysis of the factors contributing to pupillary optic capture after transscleral fixation of posterior chamber intraocular lens for dislocated intraocular lens. J Cataract Refract Surg. 2016;42(8):1146–50.
12. Teichmann KD, Teichmann IA. The torque and tilt gamble. J Cataract Refract Surg. 1997;23(3):413–8.
13. Lee JE, Ahn JH, Kim WS, Jea SY. Optic capture in the anterior capsulorhexis during combined cataract and vitreoretinal surgery. J Cataract Refract Surg. 2010;36(9):1449–52.

17

A comparison between topical and retrobulbar anesthesia in 27-gauge vitrectomy for vitreous floaters: a randomized controlled trial

Rong Han Wu[1], Rui Zhang[2], Zhong Lin[1*], Qi Hua Liang[1] and Nived Moonasar[3]

Abstract

Background: To compare the safety and efficacy of topical anesthesia versus retrobulbar anesthesia in 27-gauge pars plana vitrectomy (PPV) for vitreous floaters.

Methods: 30 patients with vitreous floaters were randomized into Group T (topical anesthesia, proparacaine eye drop) and Group R (retrobulbar anesthesia), and underwent 27-gauge PPV. A 5-point visual analogue pain scale (VAPS) was used to assess patients' pain experience of anesthesia and surgery procedure (during surgery, 2 h and 1 day after surgery).

Results: The VAPS of anesthesia procedure was 1.27 ± 0.59 for patients in Group R, while it was all 0 for patients in Group T ($p < 0.001$). There was no significant difference for VAPS during surgery (Group T: 1.13 ± 0.74, Group R: 0.67 ± 0.62, $p = 0.67$), 2 h (Group T: 0.80 ± 1.01, Group R: 0.67 ± 0.62, $p = 0.67$) and 1 day (Group T: 0.20 ± 0.41, Group R: 0.27 ± 0.46, $p = 0.68$) after surgery between these two groups. Only one patient (6.7%) in Group T required additional topical anesthesia during the surgery. Most of the patients reported the pain experience came from initial trocar insertion in both groups. None of the patients required post operative analgesia in both groups. No intraoperative or postoperative complications were noted in both groups.

Conclusion: This study suggested that topical anesthesia is a safe and effective anesthetic approach for patients with floaters who underwent 27-gauge PPV.

Keywords: Topical anesthesia, Retrobulbar anesthesia, 27-gauge, Pars plana vitrectomy

Background

The anesthetic methods for vitrectomy surgery include retrobulbar and peribulbar anesthesia. However, both methods have potential complications that can vary from minor to severe. For example, the complications of retrobulbar anesthesia include perforation of the ocular globe, retrobulbar hemorrhage, occlusion of the vein and/or the artery of the retina, retinal detachment, [1], subarachnoid injection, [2] intracranial diffusion, [3], cranial nerve palsies, [4], apnea and seizures [5].

Due to these potential complications, surgeons are trying to use simple and safe topical anesthesia to replace retrobulbar/peribulbar anesthesia. In a non-comparative study, Yepez et al. assessed the effect of topical anesthesia (4% lidocaine drops) combined with sedation in posterior vitrectomy procedures with various vitreoretinal diseases and found all patients had grade 1 (no) to grade 2 (mild) pain and discomfort during most of the procedure [6]. Besides, no patient required additional retrobulbar, peribulbar, or sub-Tenon's anesthesia [6]. Later, several comparative studies directly compared the effect of topical anesthesia combined with sedation, or a

* Correspondence: linzhong_@126.com
[1]The Eye Hospital, School of Ophthalmology and Optometry, Wenzhou Medical University, No. 270 West College Road, Wenzhou 325027, Zhejiang, China
Full list of author information is available at the end of the article

series of steps of topical anesthesia to the retrobulbar/peribulbar anesthesia during posterior vitrectomy procedure, and consistently found the subjective pain scores were not significantly different [7–9].

Floaters are perceived by patients as a serious medical condition that has a significant negative impact on their vision and quality of life [10, 11]. Vitrectomy surgery for vitreous floaters is widely considered more straight forward than other vitreoretinal surgeries. Regarding the vitrectomy surgery procedure for vitreous floaters, it is much simpler than other vitreoretinal surgeries, mainly reflecting in lower usage of scleral indentation, photocoagulation, and an apparently shorter duration. Especially with regard to the use of 27-gauge vitrectomy, the sclerotomy is minimally invasive, and reduces the pain of surgery to some extent. Hence, retrobulbar anesthesia seemed excessive for this kind of surgery. Here, we compared the effect of topical and retrobulbar anesthesia for 27-gauge pars plana vitrectomy (PPV) for symptomatic vitreous floaters.

Methods
Subjects
Thirty eyes of 30 patients who underwent 27-gauge PPV for systemic vitreous floaters at the Eye Hospital of Wenzhou Medical University from March 2017 to July 2017 were alternatively randomized into Group T using topical anesthesia (15 eyes) or Group R using retrobulbar anesthesia (15 eyes). Both patients and surgeon were not blind to the randomizing result, since the patients would be aware of the anesthetic method when performing anesthesia and the surgeon could distinguish from the eye movement. The randomized order was produced by Excel randomized formula in advance by one of the author (ZL). Participants was enrolled and assigned to interventions by the same doctor (ZL). The inclusion criteria of this study were: (1) age > 18 years; (2) subjective sensation of the "floaters" which disturbed his/her life moderately or severely for more than 3 months; (3) clinical examination showed the vitreous opacity crumb; (4) patients who are willing to participate in this study. The exclusion criteria were (1): patients who had vitrectomy surgery before; (2) patients who had penetrating ocular trauma before; (3) patients with mental retardation, problem with communication, dementia or other systemic diseases that could not cooperate with this surgery.

All patients were informed about the purpose and nature of the study and underwent thorough preoperative counseling on what they would experience during surgery under topical or retrobulbar anesthesia; especially, being aware of the potential complications of retrobulbar anesthesia and some pain sensation in the eye if under topical anesthesia. This study adhered to CONSORT guidelines for reporting clinical trial. A completed CONSORT checklist is available in Additional file 1. The study protocol is available in https://clinicaltrials.gov.

Comprehensive preoperative ophthalmic examinations, including a slit lamp evaluation, best-corrected visual acuity (BCVA) in LogMar, intraocular pressure (IOP), B scan, optical coherent tomography, and fundus photography, were performed for patients preoperatively, 1 day and 1 week postoperatively. The study followed the tenets of the Declaration of Helsinki and was approved by the Ethics Committee of The Eye Hospital of Wenzhou Medical University. All patients signed informed consent forms.

Surgery procedure
Before surgery, pupillary dilatation was obtained with 1% tropicamide. Retrobulbar anesthesia was achieved by injecting a 50% mixture of 2% lidocaine and 0.75% bupivacaine 4–5 ml through a 25 gauge (0.5 mm) needle. Topical anesthesia was performed by instilling 0.5% proparacaine hydrochloride (Alcaine®, Alcon, TX) 3 times (with 1 min-interval) before surgery. All retrobulbar anesthesia procedures were performed by the same doctor (ZL), while all 27-gauge PPV procedures were performed by the same surgeon (RHW). To begin the surgery, three transconjunctival sutureless 27-gauge cannulae (Constellation; Alcon Laboratories Inc., Fort Worth, TX), i.e. the inferior-temporal infusion cannula and the superior-nasal and superior-temporal operation cannulae, were made 4 mm posterior to the limbus with angled incision. Central vitreous followed by peripheral vitreous was removed with the help of a corneal contact lens. A quick scleral indentation was performed to check the extremely peripheral retina and ora serrata. Build-in laser (wavelength 532 nm) was used to perform the photocoagulation in eyes with lattice retinal degeneration or retinal break(s). At the end of the surgery, cannulae were removed and none of the eyes required suturing.

Examinations and visual analogue pain scale (VAPS)
A 5-point visual analogue pain scale (VAPS), which was the main outcomes of this study, ranged from 0 (no pain) to 4 (severe pain), was used to assess the subjective pain experience of anesthesia and surgical procedure (during surgery, 2 h and 1 day after surgery). The exact painful surgery procedure would further ask if the patient felt pain during surgery. The 5-point visual analogue scale, ranged from 0 (extremely comfortable) to 4 (unable to perform surgery), was also used to assess the surgeon's comfort and ease while performing the surgery [7–9]. Detailed information on the VAS was presented in Table 1. The detailed procedure of the pain experience during anesthesia and surgery was asked, if the patients reported a pain experience.

Table 1 Visual analogue scale for pain and surgeon's comfort

Score	Pain	Surgeon's comfort
0	No discomfort	Extremely comfortable
1	Mild discomfort	Mild movements/squeezing
2	Mild pain	Moderate discomfort (significant ocular movements/squeezing/Bells phenomenon)
3	Moderate pain	Severe discomfort hampering surgical maneuvering
4	Unbearable pain	Unable to perform surgery

Anesthesia procedure

If you felt discomfort/pain during the retrobulbar anesthesia, please choose the detailed procedure below (multiple choice).

A. topical eye drops instillation; B. needle puncture the skin; C. liquid injection; D. local pressure after injection; E. others (such as skin numbness, ptosis, lid swelling), please specify.

Surgery procedure

If you felt discomfort/pain during the surgery, please choose the detailed procedure below (multiple choice).

A. opened the lid using eye speculum; B. trocar inserted the sclera; C. vitrectomy; D. scleral indentation; E. cannula removal; F. others, please specify.

Statistical analysis

All the data used and analyzed in this study can be accessed in Additional file 2. Student's t-test or chi-square test was used for data comparison between the study groups. All statistical analysis was performed with Statistical Analysis System for Windows version 9.1.3 (SAS Inc., Cary, NC). A P value of < 0.05 was considered significant.

Results

Fifteen eyes of 15 patients were included into Group T and Group R, respectively. The mean age of the total 30 patients was 32.4 ± 11.1 (range 19 to 51) years. There

Table 2 Baseline characteristics of patients in two anesthesia groups

	Group Topical	Group Retrobulbar	P
Age (year)[1]	32.9 ± 11.8	32.1 ± 10.8	0.85
Gender (male/female)[2]	13/2	14/1	1.00
Right/left eye[2]	8/7	10/5	0.71
Duration of floaters (month)[3]	36 (12, 60)	36 (18, 120)	0.45
BCVA (LogMar)[3]	0.0 (0.04, 0.0)	0.0 (0.05, 0.0)	0.28
IOP (mmHg)[1]	13.5 ± 2.7	15.9 ± 4.2	0.08

[1]presented as mean ± standard deviation, and tested by student's t-test; [2]presented the number, and tested by Fisher Exact test; [3]presented as median and quartile range, and tested by Wilcoxon test

were 27 males (90%). The baseline characteristics of patients in these two anesthesia groups were presented in Table 2. There was no significant difference between age, gender, duration of floaters, preoperative BCVA and IOP between Group T and Group R.

The mean surgery time of Group T and Group R was 14.0 ± 3.8 (range 9.2–18.6) and 13.6 ± 4.4 (range 8.7–19.1) minutes, respectively, while no significant difference was found ($p = 0.45$). One eye in each group was performed with photocoagulation (wavelength) because of retinal degeneration. However, none of these two patients required additional pain relief. The BCVA (LogMar) at 1 day (median 0.15 vs. 0.10 $p = 0.85$) and 1 week (median 0.0 vs. 0.0 $p = 0.95$) post-op were also not significantly different between the two groups. Similar results were found for IOP (1 day 8.4 ± 4.3 vs. 9.2 ± 3.9, $p = 0.45$; 1 week: 12.8 ± 3.6 vs. 14.6 ± 5.2. $p = 0.29$).

The VAPS of anesthesia procedure was 1.27 ± 0.59 (range 0 to 2) for patients in Group R, while it was all 0 for patients in Group T ($p < 0.001$). The VAPS of surgery procedure was 1.13 ± 0.74 (range 0 to 2) and 0.67 ± 0.62 (range 0 to 2) for patients in Group T and Group R ($p = 0.14$), respectively. The VAP for surgeon's comfort during the surgery was 0.27 ± 0.59 (range 0 to 2) and 0.33 ± 0.48 (range 0 to 1) for patients in Group T and Group R ($p = 0.74$), respectively. There was also no significant difference for VAPS 2 h (Group T: 0.80 ± 1.01, range 0 to 3, Group R: 0.67 ± 0.62, range 0 to 2, $p = 0.67$) and 1 day (Group T: 0.20 ± 0.41, range 0 to 1, Group R: 0.27 ± 0.46, range 0 to 1, $p = 0.68$) after surgery between these two groups. The distributions of the VAPS and VAS for surgeon's comfort were presented in Fig. 1.

None of the patients in Group T felt discomfort or worse, while 14 patients felt discomfort or pain in Group R. Most of the patients reported that they experienced discomfort/pain when the needle punctured the skin (12/14, 85.7%), while a small proportion of patients reported a similar experience with the liquid injection (3/14, 21.4%) during the retrobulbar anesthesia. In Group T, 12 (80%) patients reported mild discomfort or worse during the surgery. Most of them reported the pain experience mainly came from initial trocar insertion (8/12, 67.7%) and use of the lid speculum (5/12, 41.7%), while a small proportion of patients reported that during scleral indentation (2/12, 16.7%), and vitrectomy procedure (1/12, 8.3%). In Group R, 9 (60%) patients reported mild discomfort or worse during the surgery. The patients reported the pain experience come from initial trocar insertion (3/9, 33.3%), use of the lid speculum (2/9, 22.2%), scleral indentation (2/9, 22.2%), vitrectomy procedure (1/9, 11.1%), and trocar removal (1/9, 11.1%). Only one patient (6.7%) in Group T required additional topical anesthesia (0.5% proparacaine hydrochloride eye drop, once) during the surgery.

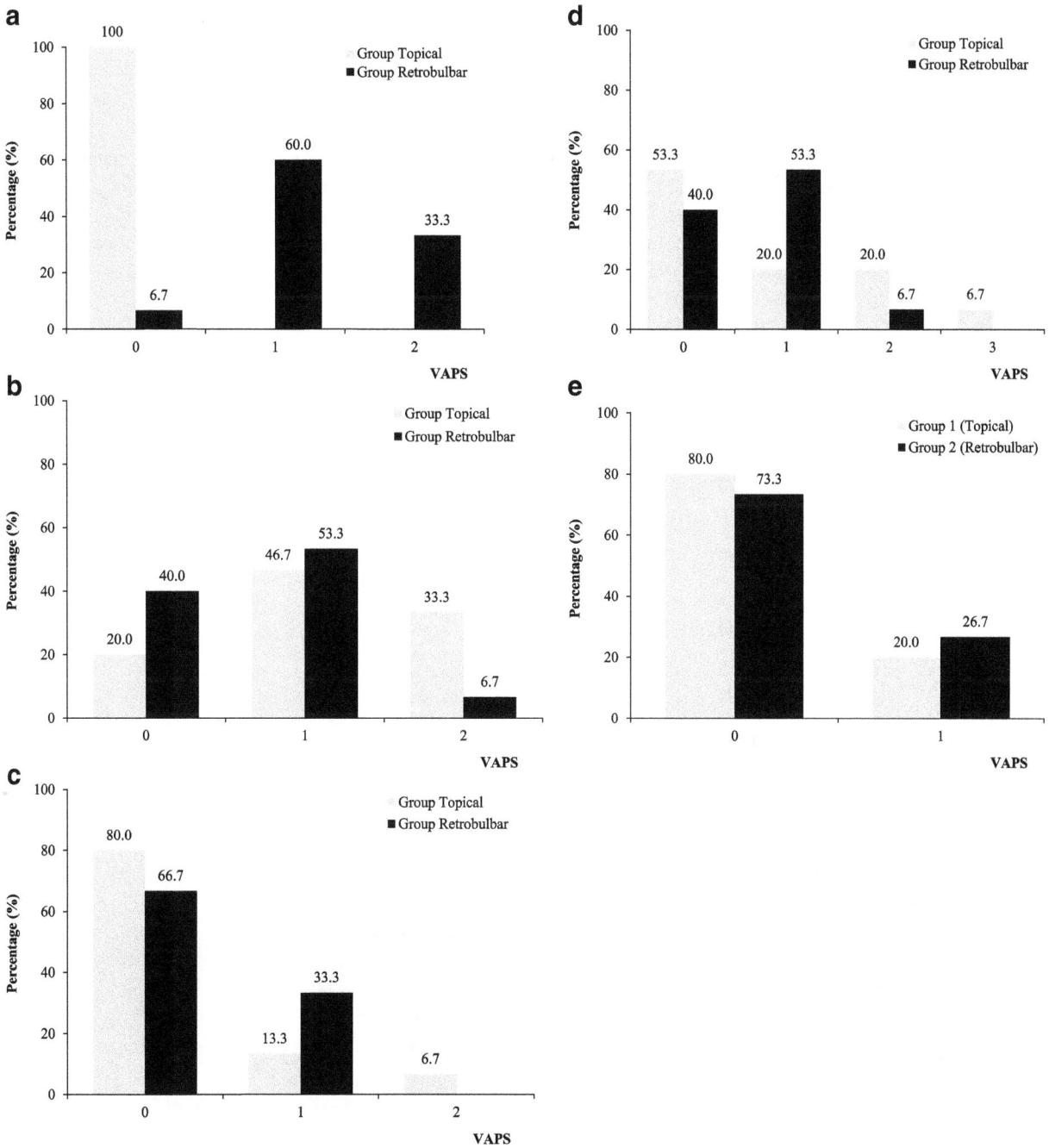

Fig. 1 a Visual Analogue Pain Scale (VAPS) during anesthesia process. **b** Visual Analogue Pain Scale (VAPS) during surgery process. **c** Visual Analogue Scale (VAS) for surgeon's comfort. **d** Visual Analogue Pain Scale (VAPS) 2 h after surgery. **e** Visual Analogue Pain Scale (VAPS) 1 day after surgery

None of the patients required post operative pain relief in both groups. No intraoperative or postoperative complications were noted in both groups.

Discussion

With development in techniques and technology, local anesthesia, including retrobulbar, peribulbar, and sub-Tenon's anesthesia, is being used for the majority of

vitreoretinal surgery. Although rare, many complications have been reported with injection anesthesia [1–5]. Topical anesthesia essentially eliminates the risk of needle-related complications associated with the injection of local anesthesia. Therefore, the safety and efficacy of the topical anesthesia have been investigated for small-gauge vitrectomy, and have been demonstrated to be safe and effective [8, 9, 12, 13]. However, to best of our knowledge, no study on the safety and efficacy of the topical anesthesia for 27-gauge PPV was reported.

There were several advantages in this study. First, this study was a randomized controlled trial, which may provide powerful evidence. Second, all of the surgeries and retrobulbar anesthesia of the study were performed by the same surgeon (RHW) and the same doctor (ZL), respectively, which may minimize the possible confounding factors, such as different pain experience during anesthesia or surgery with different techniques. Third, this study simplified the topical anesthesia procedure (only proparacaine hydrochloride eye drops for 3 times), compared to previous studies. Yepez et al. and Bahcecioglu et al. also used operative sedation for topical anesthesia patients [6, 7, 14]. Mahajan et al. used a serial topical anesthesia method, i.e., proparacaine hydrochloride drops, lignocaine gel for 1 min, another proparacaine hydrochloride infiltration with swab for 1 min [8]. Celiker et al. used proparacaine hydrochloride drops 15 min preceding surgery, and then proparacaine hydrochloride infiltration with sponges for another 15 min [9].

In this study, only eye drops were instilled for the topical anesthesia procedure, hence it was understandable that none of the patients felt uncomfortable or worse. The VAPS of surgery procedure in both groups ranged from 0 (no discomfort) to 2 (mild pain), and was not apparently different. The majority operative discomfort/pain experience reported by the patients was the trocar insertion, which was a very short period. Only one (6.7%) patient in Group T required additional topical anesthesia of eye drop, and also only one (6.7%) patient in Group T had significant eye squeezing that caused moderate discomfort for surgeon's during the surgery, which suggested that most of the patients could tolerate the pain and cooperate well during the surgery. We believe the eye squeezing or movement could be conquered by detailed preoperative and operative communication with the patient, and by an experienced surgeon. Once the vitrectomy procedure is started, the movement of the eyeball can be controlled by surgeon with intraocular instruments.

Although slightly more proportion of patients (4/15, 26.7%) in Group T felt mild pain or moderate pain than that in Group R (1/15, 6.7%) 2 h after surgery, this was not significantly different. Besides, none of the patient required analgesic after surgery, suggesting a tolerable post-operation pain. Furthermore, the post-operation pain became negligible (no worse than mild discomfort) at day 1 post operation in both groups. All the data suggested that the topical anesthesia procedure was safe and efficient for the patients with floaters who underwent 27-gauge PPV.

Besides the most important advantage of topical anesthesia, i.e., eliminating the risk of needle-related complications, this anesthesia technique also greatly reduces the preparation time, eliminates the patients' fear, has less interference to the post-operative recovery (such as lid edema, blink, eye movement, etc.), and has less surgical expenditure. The relatively small sample size and the fact that only patients with floaters were selected are some limitations to this study. For macular cases, such as macular holes and epimacular membranes, any inadvertent ocular movements might result in disastrous consequences. However, many surgeons have reported successful outcomes using topical anesthesia for such cases [6, 9, 13].

In summary, our study suggests that utilizing topical anesthesia (with only eye drops) is a safe and effective anesthesia approach for patients with floaters who underwent 27-gauge pars plana vitrectomy.

Conclusions

The topical anesthesia is a safe and effective anesthesia approach for floaters removed by 27-gauge par plana vitrectomy, and could be recommended by clinical practice.

Abbreviations
BCVA: Best-corrected visual acuity; IOP: Intraocular pressure; PPV: Pars plana vitrectomy; VAPS: Visual analogue pain scale

Acknowledgements
The authors thank Dr. Ke Lin and Yushu Xiao (The Eye Hospital of Wenzhou Medical University) for their invaluable assistance in data collection.

Authors' contributions
RHW and ZL designed the study protocol and conducted the study as a supervisor. RZ, and QHL participated in the study design. ZL and NM conducted statistical analysis, and drafted the manuscript. RHW, ZL and NM revised the manuscript. All authors read and approved the final manuscript.

Competing interests
The authors declare that they have no competing interests.

Author details
[1]The Eye Hospital, School of Ophthalmology and Optometry, Wenzhou Medical University, No. 270 West College Road, Wenzhou 325027, Zhejiang, China. [2]Liaocheng People's Hospital of Shandong Province, Liaocheng, Shandong, China. [3]Caribbean Eye Institute, Valsayn, Trinidad and Tobago.

References
1. Vestal KP, Meyers SM, Zegarra H. Retinal detachment as a complication of retrobulbar anesthesia. *Canadian journal of ophthalmology.* 1991;26(1):32–3.
2. Ahn JC, Stanley JA. Subarachnoid injection as a complication of retrobulbar anesthesia. Am J Ophthalmol. 1987;103(2):225–30.
3. Marques-Gonzalez A, Onrubia-Fuertes X, Bellver-Romero J, Seller Losada JM, Pertusa-Collado V, Barbera-Alacreu M. Intracranial diffusion. A complication of retrobulbar anesthesia. *Revista espanola de anestesiologia y reanimacion.* 1997;44(7):284–6.
4. Jackson K, Vote D. Multiple cranial nerve palsies complicating retrobulbar eye block. Anaesth Intensive Care. 1998;26(6):662–4.
5. Moorthy SS, Zaffer R, Rodriguez S, Ksiazek S, Yee RD. Apnea and seizures following retrobulbar local anesthetic injection. J Clin Anesth. 2003;15(4): 267–70.
6. Yepez J, Cedeno de Yepez J, Arevalo JF. Topical anesthesia in posterior vitrectomy. Retina. 2000;20(1):41–5.

7.   Bahcecioglu H, Unal M, Artunay O, Rasier R, Sarici A. Posterior vitrectomy
     under topical anesthesia. Canadian journal of ophthalmology Journal
     canadien d'ophtalmologie. 2007;42(2):272–7.
8.   Mahajan D, Sain S, Azad S, Arora T, Azad R. Comparison of topical
     anesthesia and peribulbar anesthesia for 23-gauge vitrectomy without
     sedation. Retina. 2013;33(7):1400–6.
9.   Celiker H, Karabas L, Sahin O. A comparison of topical or retrobulbar anesthesia
     for 23-gauge posterior vitrectomy. J Ophthalmol. 2014;2014:237028.
10. Zou H, Liu H, Xu X, Zhang X. The impact of persistent visually disabling
     vitreous floaters on health status utility values. Quality of life research : an
     international journal of quality of life aspects of treatment, care and
     rehabilitation. 2013;22(6):1507–14.
11. Webb BF, Webb JR, Schroeder MC, North CS. Prevalence of vitreous floaters
     in a community sample of smartphone users. International journal of
     ophthalmology. 2013;6(3):402–5.
12. Theocharis IP, Alexandridou A, Tomic Z. A two-year prospective study
     comparing lidocaine 2% jelly versus peribulbar anaesthesia for 25G and 23G
     sutureless vitrectomy. Graefe's archive for clinical and experimental
     ophthalmology = Albrecht von Graefes Archiv fur klinische und
     experimentelle Ophthalmologie. 2007;245(9):1253–8.
13. Tang S, Lai P, Lai M, Zou Y, Li J, Li S. Topical anesthesia in transconjunctival
     sutureless 25-gauge vitrectomy for macular-based disorders.
     Ophthalmologica Journal international d'ophtalmologie International journal
     of ophthalmology Zeitschrift fur Augenheilkunde. 2007;221(1):65–8.
14. Yepez JB, de Yepez JC, Azar-Arevalo O, Arevalo JF. Topical anesthesia with
     sedation in phacoemulsification and intraocular lens implantation
     combined with 2-port pars plana vitrectomy in 105 consecutive cases.
     Ophthalmic Surg Lasers. 2002;33(4):293–7.

18

Metabolic memory in mitochondrial oxidative damage triggers diabetic retinopathy

Zhaoge Wang, Haixia Zhao, Wenying Guan, Xin Kang, Xue Tai and Ying Shen[*]

Abstract

Background: Diabetic retinopathy (DR) is a microvascular complication induced by high blood glucose. This study was conducted to investigate the effect of metabolic memory on mitochondrial oxidative damage-induced DR.

Methods: Rat retinal endothelial cells (rRECs) were isolated from SD rats and treated with high glucose (20 mM) for various times and then cultured in normal glucose (5.6 mM) medium for 2 days. The cells were assayed for the expression of respiratory chain complexes *cytochrome c oxidase* subunit *1* (CO1) and NADPH-1 using RT-PCR, mitochondrial membrane potentials and reactive oxygen species (ROS) production using flow cytometry and apoptosis using Annexin V/PI flow cytometry.

Results: rRECs displayed like short spindles after cultured for 9–10 days and reached 100% confluency. Compared with the control grown in normal glucose (5.6 mM) medium, rRECs exposed to high glucose medium for 3, 12 and 24 h had significantly increased mRNA levels of CO1 and NAPDH-1 even after being shifted back to normal glucose medium. They also had lower mitochondrial membrane potential (89.13% vs 78.21%, $p < 0.05$), cytochrome C level (1 in control vs 0.25 after 24 h exposure to high glucose, $p < 0.05$ and higher ROS production (2.77% in control vs 9.00% after 12 h exposure to high glucose, $p < 0.05$) and apoptosis (7.15% in control vs and 29.91% after 24 h exposure to high glucose, $p < 0.05$).

Conclusion: It is likely that mitochondrial oxidative damage triggers metabolic memory via ROS overproduction, leading to diabetic retinopathy.

Keywords: Diabetic retinopathy, Metabolic memory, ROS, Mitochondria, Apoptosis

Background

Diabetic retinopathy (DR) is a microvascular complication induced by high blood glucose. It is the main cause of blindness in the working population aged 20 to 65 years old [1, 2]. Due to its the high incidence and severe complications, DR has become a priority for blindness prevention and treatment in [3, 4]. Intensive studies have been conducted to investigate DR in diabetic complications [5]. As a consequence, a special phenomenon hyperglycemic memory or metabolic memory has been discovered, which occurs when human cells have prolonged exposure to hyperglycemia conditions even after hyperglycemic control is therapeutically achieved [6, 7]. As a result, disease may continue to occur or progress after the patient's blood

glucose has been controlled for a long period of time and cells may continue to be damaged after the high glucose environment has been removed [8, 9]. For diabetic patients, metabolic memory probably is an important cause of continuing disease progress after their blood glucose is controlled.

When the balance of oxidation-antioxidation system is broken, excessive reactive oxygen species (ROS) is produced, resulting in cytotoxicity and oxidative stress. The excessive ROS is mainly produced in the mitochondrial respiratory chain [10]. Since mitochondrial DNA (mtDNA) is very close to where ROS is produced, and there is no effective DNA repair system in mtDNA as in nuclear DNA, mtDNA is very vulnerable to ROS attack. Once damaged, the expression of mitochondrial genes would be compromised, leading to reduced mitochondrial membrane potential and increased apoptosis, which

* Correspondence: 2438413496@qq.com
Center of Myopia, the Affiliated Hospital of Inner Mongolia Medical University, 1 Tongdao North Street, Hohhot 010050, China

in turn increases ROS production, and subsequently continued ROS overproduction [11]. Previous study showed that there was mtDNA oxidative damage in the retinal vessels and ROS was excessively produced in the early stage of DR [12]. Since metabolic memory is a refractory phenomenon in the progress of DR, we speculated that this vicious cycle of ROS production continuously promotes the process of metabolic memory, leading to the mtDNA oxidative damage in retinal blood vessels. In recent years, studies have shown that oxidative stress is responsible for complications of diabetes, including DR and is closely related to metabolic memory [6, 13]. Therefore, oxidative stress is likely involved in DR metabolic memory.

To better understand the effect of metabolic memory on DR with respect to mitochondrial oxidative damage, we investigated the cellular damage and functions using rat retinal endothelial cells (rRECs) by exposing the cells to high glucose to simulate metabolic memory. The work would provide insight into how mitochondrial oxidative damage triggers metabolic memory and promotes the development of DR via the excessive ROS production.

Methods
Isolation of rRECs
SD rats (purchased from Yingniurui Biotech, Wuxi, China) were sacrificed by cervical dislocation and the eyeballs were isolated. The retinas were collected, washed with the D-Hank's solution and cut into pieces of 1×1 mm in size. The tissues were incubated in 0.25% trypsin solution (Keygentec, China) at 37 °C for 30 min and filtered through a nylon sieve with 30 μm pore size. The released cells were pelleted by centrifugation at 1000 rpm for 5 min, and inoculated into culture flasks containing Dulbecco's Modified Eagle's Medium (DMEM) (HZSJQ Biotech, Hangzhou, China) with 20% fetal bovine serum (FBS, *Bio*ligo, Shanghai, China) and cultured at 37 ° C. 24 h later, the medium was refreshed and non-adherent cells were removed. One day after culture, radial cells were grown out of the vessel fragments and 3 days later the cells become visible. The cells were then passaged every 3 days and were used for experiments at the third passage. All animal experimental protocols were approved by Inner Mongolia Medical University. All animals received humane care in compliance with the 'Principles of Laboratory Animal Care' formulated by the National Society for Medical Research and the 'Guide for the Care and Use of Laboratory Animals' prepared by the Institute of Laboratory Animal Resources and published by the National Institutes of Health (NIH Publication No. 86–23, revised 1996).

Treatment of rRECs
The cells at 100% confluency were digested with 2% trypsin and suspended in DMEM containing with 20% FBS and 5.6 mM glucose. The cells were then pelleted by centrifugation at 1000 rpm for 3 min and inoculated into the DMEM medium containing normal level of glucose (5.6 mM) or high level of glucose (20 mM) for different times. The cells grown in the high-glucose medium were then transferred to normal-glucose medium to grow for another 2 days before being used for assays. The concentration and duration of glucose treatments were selected based on an early study [14, 15], where up to 30 mM glucose was used to create a hyperglycemic condition in endothelial cells.

RT-PCR
Total RNA was extracted using Trizol reagents (Invitrogen, USA) according to the manufacturer's instructions and reversely transcribed into cDNA in a total volume of 10 μl using the High Capacity cDNA Transcriptase Reverse kit (Applied Biosystems by Life Technologies, Carlsbad, California, USA) according to manufacturer's recommendations. The resulting cDNA amplified using 2 x GoldStar Taq MasterMix (CWBiotech, Beijing, China) in a total volume of 20 μl. Amplification cycling conditions were 3 min at 95 °C followed by 30 cycles, each one consisting of 10 s at 95 °C and 30 s at 50.6 °C, with a final extension of 30 S at 72 °C. RT-qPCR was performed on the 7900HT Fast Real-Time PCR system using TaqMan gene expression assays probes (Applied Biosystems). The primers used for *cytochrome c oxidase* subunit *1* (CO1) were F: GTAACTACCTACTG CCTCTG, R: CACCACCATACATCCTAA), NADPH-1 F: TGTCCAGGGTGGGTAAGA, R: TGGGAGGAATCGTG AAGT. Human glyceraldehyde-3-phosphate dehydrogenase (GADPH) was used as an internal control (primers: F: GCAAGTTCAACGGCACAG, R: CGCCAGTAGACTCC ACGAC). Samples were run in triplicate and the mean value was calculated for each case.

The data were managed using the Applied Biosystems software RQ Manager v1.2.1. Relative expression was calculated by using comparative Ct method and obtaining the fold change value ($2^{-\Delta\Delta Ct}$) according to previously described protocol [16].

Western blot analysis
After different treatments, the cells were harvested, washed twice with cold PBS and lysed with RIPA buffer that containing protease and phosphotase inhibitors cocktail (Roche, UK). The supernatants were collected after centrifugation at 12000 rpm for 20 min. The protein was applied to polyacrylamide gel electrophoresis (SDS-PAGE), transferred to a PVDF membrane, and then detected by goat anti-rat cytochrome C antibody (Abcam, USA) and goat anti-mouse horseradish peroxidase (HRP)-conjugated secondary antibodies (CWBoitech, Beijing, China) before visualization with ChemiDocXRS+ (Biorad, USA). The intensity of blot signals was quantitated using ImageQuant TL analysis software (General Electric, UK).

Analysis of mitochondrial membrane potential

Cells were harvested, washed twice with cold PBS and stained with diluted JC-1 solution (Molecular Probe by life Technology, USA) according to the manufacturer's instructions. After incubation at 37 °C in 5% CO_2, the cells were washed twice with incubation buffer and loaded to a cytometer (Bection Dikinson, USA) for analysis of mitochondrial membrane potential.

Analysis of mitochondrial ROS

Cells were harvested, washed twice with cold PBS and reacted to dichloro-dihydro-flurescein diacetate (DCFH-DA, Molecular Probes, USA) to detect mitochondria-specific ROS using MitoFLuor Red589 (MFL, Molecular Probes) according to manufacturer's instructions. The cells were analyzed on a cytometer (Bection Dikinson, USA) and the florescence was detected at an emission wavelength of 525 nm and excitation wavelength of 488 nm.

Detection of apoptosis by flow cytometry

Cells were collected and suspended in PBS, labeled with Annexin V and propidiumiodide (PI) following the manufacturer's instructions (Biosea Biotechnology, Beijing, China). Flow cytometry (Bection Dikinson, USA) was used to assess the apoptotic cells. The quantitation of apoptotic cells was calculated by CellQuest software.

Statistical analysis

All data were expressed as means ± standard derivation (s.d.) obtained from at least three independent experiments. Means were compared using the student's t-test or one-way ANOVA with the corresponding post-test. A p-value ≤ 0.05 was considered statistically significant. Statistical analyses were performed using GraphPad Prism 5.0 (GraphPad Software Inc., USA).

Results

Culture of rRECs

To obtain rREC culture, the retinal tissue was digested with collagenase and cells were isolated through filtration. One day after culture, radial cells were grown out of the vessel fragments and 3 days later the cells become visible. Seven days later the cells were long spindle-shaped and 9 days later they become short spindle-shaped. After passage, the cells were fully expended and grew faster as long spindle (Fig. 1). These cells were used for subsequent experiments.

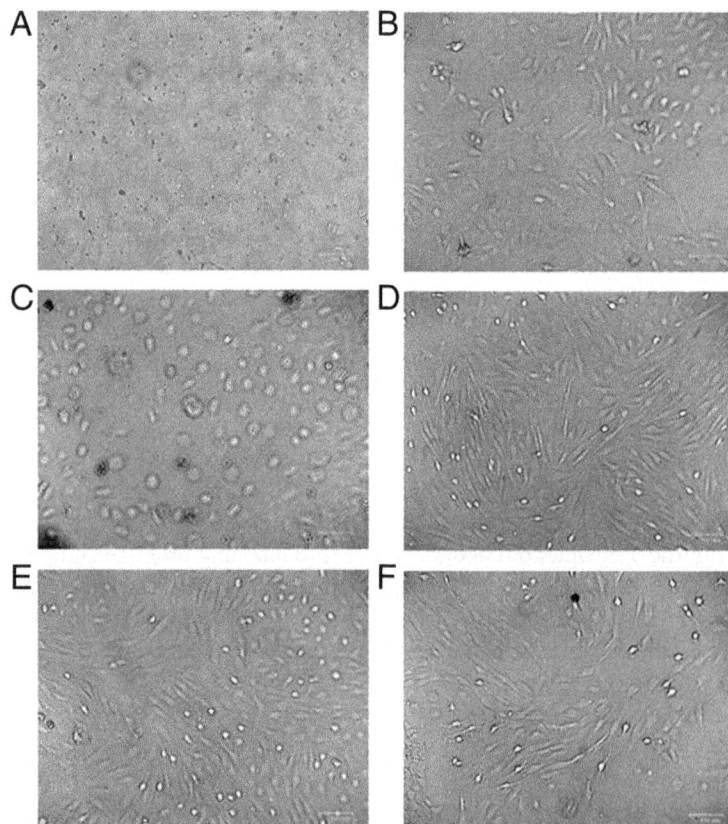

Fig. 1 Cultured rat retinal endothelial cells. **a-d**, primary cells on day 1, 3, 7 and 9; **e-f**, the first passage cells on day 1 and 5

High glucose down-regulated the transcription of CO1 and NADPH-1

We then examined the mRNA levels of CO1 and NADPH-1 in the rRECs. The results showed that compared with control cells that were grown at normal level of glucose, the expression of CO1 and NADPH-1 was gradually and significantly reduced after the cells were exposed to high-glucose from 3 to 24 h (Fig. 2). After 24 h exposure, the mRNA levels of the two genes were about half of control (Fig. 2).

High glucose down-regulated the level of cytochrome C

Similarly, compared with the control, 3 h, 12 h, and 24 h exposure to high glucose significantly down-regulated the protein expression of cytochrome C in the rRECs (Fig. 3).

High glucose reduced mitochondrial membrane potential

JC-1 dye was used as probe to measure mitochondrial membrane potential. The dye emitted green fluorescence as shown in the lower pane of Fig. 4b at lower membrane potential and did not accumulate in the mitochondrial matrix, while at higher membrane potential, it formed aggregates in the matrix and emitted red fluorescence (as shown in the upper panel of Fig. 4b). The measurements showed that when cultured in normal glucose medium, the percentage of the aggregate was 89.13%. The percentage decreased to 84.69% after the cells were exposed to 20 mM glucose for 3 h (Fig. 4a). At that time, green fluorescence was also observed (Fig. 4b). When the cells were exposed to 20 mM glucose for 12 h, they had 84.49% aggregate content with emission of green fluorescence, which was significantly lower than that of the control ($P < 0.05$). After 24 h exposure to high glucose, the percentage was even lower (78.21%, $P < 0.05$) after shifted to normal medium for 2 days as compared with control (Fig. 4a). These data suggest that high

glucose reduces mitochondrial membrane potential even after the cells are shifted to normal glucose medium.

High glucose increased ROS production

DCFH-DA ROS assays showed that the ROS was 2.77% in the control cells and increased to 6.58% after 3 h exposure to high glucose medium and further to 9.00% after 12 h exposure to high glucose ($P < 0.05$ vs control and 3 h exposure). The percentage increased to 13.63% after 24 h exposure to high glucose ($P < 0.05$ vs control and 3 h exposure) (Fig. 5).

High glucose increased apoptosis

Flow cytometry showed that the apoptosis rates increased significantly from 7.15% in the control group to 11.02, 27.39 and 29.91%, respectively, after 3, 12 and 24 h exposure to high glucose ($P < 0.05$) (Fig. 6). The increases were significantly different between the control and 3 h exposure ($P < 0.05$) or highly significantly different between the control and 24 h exposure ($P < 0.01$). Apoptosis rate after 24 h exposure was also significantly higher than after 3 h exposure ($P < 0.05$).

Discussion

This study shows that high glucose induced mitochondrial damage as revealed by reduced membrane potential, increased apoptosis and ROS production even after the cells was shifted to normal glucose condition, suggesting that there is metabolic memory in the retinal cells.

Due to low patient compliance for long-term control of blood glucose, unclear diabetic DR pathogenesis, the lack of effective medicine for early intervention and poor outcomes of laser surgery and surgical operation for later stage patients [17], it is very important to have a better understand of early mechanism involved in DR pathogenesis to develop effective strategy for the prevention and treatment of the disease [18].

Clinically, DCCT (the Diabetes Control and Complications Trials) and EDIC (Epidemiology of Diabetes Interventions and Complications) have shown that there is metabolic memory in type 2 diabetes mellitus [19, 20], which is further confirmed in UKPDS (United Kingdom Prospective Diabetes Study) [21, 22]. In diabetic rat models, retinal mitochondrial dysfunction and oxidative stress still exist even after the blood glucose level has become normal [23, 24]. In addition, metabolic memory has also been found in isolated primary retinal cells [25].

Recent studies show that mitochondrial oxidative damage and dysfunction are associated with complications of nervous system diseases, diabetic cardiomyopathy and diabetes [26]. Mitochondrial oxidative damage and dysfunction in the heart of diabetic rats reduce the activity of mitochondrial respiratory chain-related enzymes [27]. Lee et al. found that high glucose inhibited

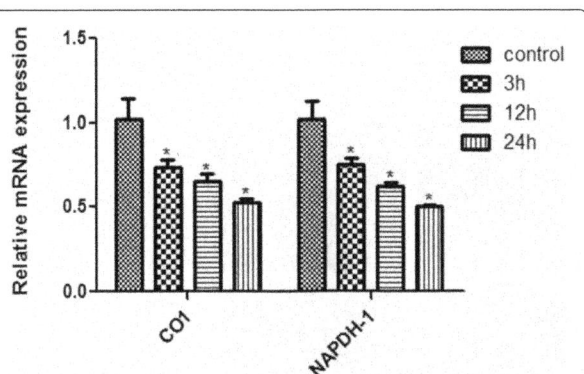

Fig. 2 Relative mRNA levels of mitochondrial complex CO1 and NAPDH-1 in rRECs after exposure to high glucose (20 mM) for different time. * denotes significant difference vs control. The bars represent std errors

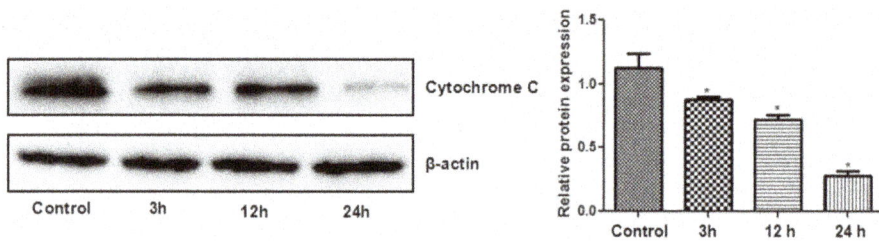

Fig. 3 Protein expression of cytochrome C in rRECs after exposure to high glucose (20 mM) for different time. Right panel: representative Western blots, left panel: relative expression levels. * denotes significant difference vs control. The bars represent std errors

the activity of mitochondrial electron transport chain complex in retinal cells and effectively promote the production of ROS and suppress the activation of NF-κB and TGF-β signaling pathways, suggesting that mitochondrial damage may result in ROS production in DR and ROS is responsible for the pathogenesis of DR [28]. Nishikawa et al. found that culturing vascular endothelial cells in high glucose medium led to ROS production and cell damage [29]. In this study we found that exposure to high glucose for 3 to 24 h resulted in time-dependent increase of ROS production as well as down-regulation of NAPDH-1 and CO-1, suggesting the high glucose could increase mitochondrial production of ROS and damage mitochondrial respiratory function. Since increase in ROS production was observed after the cells had been transferred to normal glucose condition, it is likely that the increased ROS production is due to metabolic memory.

DR is a microvascular complication of diabetes mellitus and is a microcirculation disorder. Early changes in DR include apoptosis of peripheral blood cells, microvascular occlusion, vascular leakage and microaneurysm [30]. REC is the first barrier to sense the changes in blood glucose and the main target of attack from diabetes complications. The dysfunction of REC is the common basis of microvascular complications including DR. DR pathogenesis is recognized to be associated with enhanced polyol pathway, increased glycosylated end products, activated *protein kinase C* and increased influx of glucose via hexosamine pathway [31]. The four seemly-independent pathways have been shown to be associated with a common high glucose-induced pathogenesis process - over-production of toxic mitochondrial ROS [32]. Our study also show that high glucose induced the overproduction of ROS in cultured RECs, resulting in mitochondrial oxidative damage and apoptosis.

In an early study, it was found that high glucose increased the level of 8-hydroxy-2′-deoxyguanosine after 3 h exposure of cell to high glucose, reduced mitochondrial

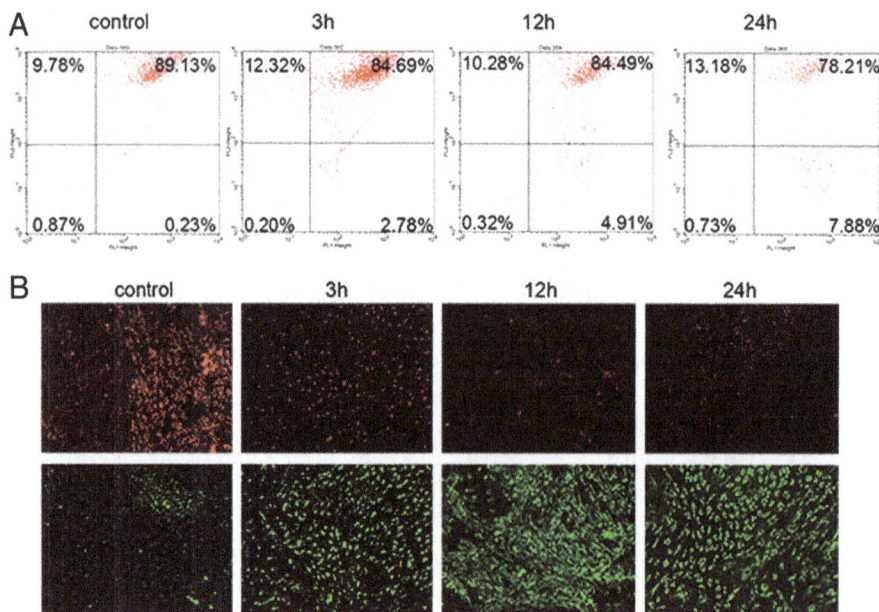

Fig. 4 Mitochondrial membrane potential of rRECs in normal glucose medium after exposure to high glucose (20 mM). **a** Flow cytometry. **b** fluorescence microscopy

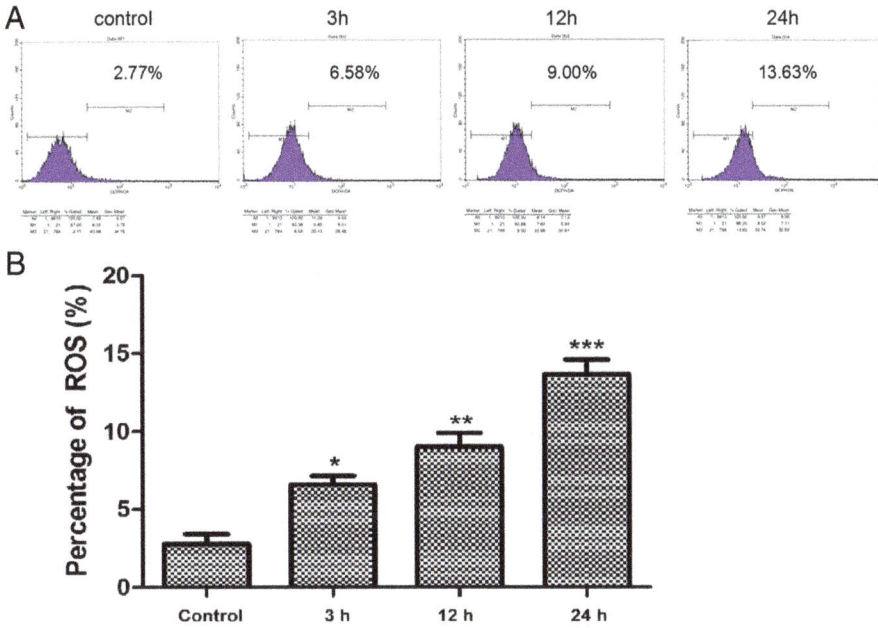

Fig. 5 Levels of mitochondrial ROS detected by flow cytometry in rRECs in normal glucose medium after exposure to high glucose (20 mM). **a** flow cytometry; **b** percentage of ROS. * and ** denotes significant or highly significant difference vs control using one-way ANOVA with statistical significance set at a level of $P < 0.05$. Post-hoc multiple comparison between the groups was performed using S-N-K method. The bars represent std errors

membrane potential and increased ROS production after 12 h exposure, and increased apoptosis after 12 h exposure [33], suggesting that there might be mtDNA oxidative damage in early stage of DR, which results in further oxidative stress. For the first time, RECs were used to investigate DR metabolic memory at DNA damage level and to define the time frame within which metabolic memory occurs. Taking together, our findings indicate that mitochondrial oxidative stress is likely an important target for improving mitochondrial function. In the further, it would be important to define the optimal timepoint to block the vicious cycle of ROS production using RNAi technology to protect mitochondria from metabolic memory as a potential therapeutic option.

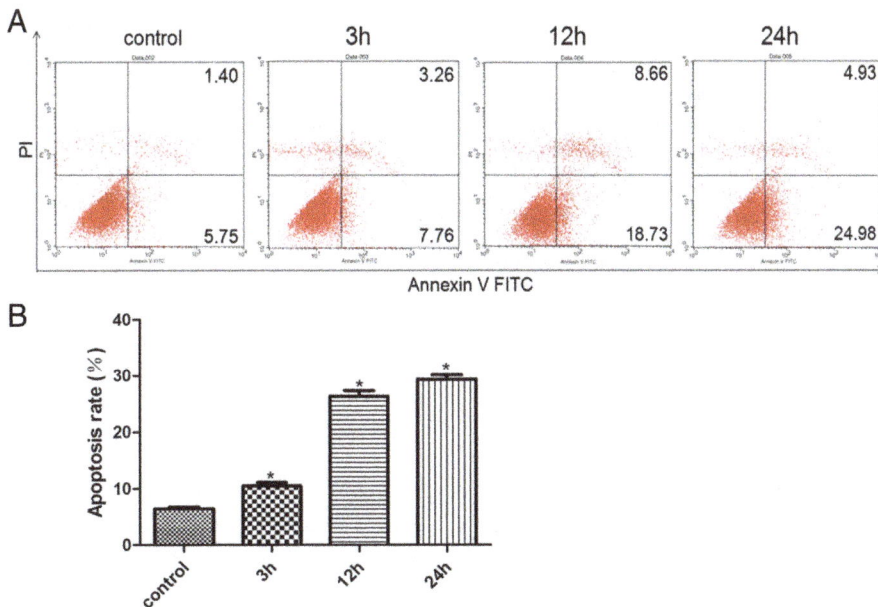

Fig. 6 Apoptosis detected by flow cytometry in rRECs in normal glucose medium after exposure to high glucose (20 mM). **a** flow cytometry; **b** apoptotic rate. * and ** denotes significant or highly significant difference vs control. The bars represent std errors

Conclusion

Our data demonstrate that mitochondrial oxidative damage is likely to trigger metabolic memory via ROS overproduction that leads to diabetic retinopathy, and may be reduced using RNAi technology to attenuate the disease.

Funding

The work was supported by Natural Science Foundation of Inner Mongolia Autonomous Region, China (grant no. 2011MS1137) and Research Funds of the Affiliated Hospital of Inner Mongolia Medical University (grant no. NYFYYB2014020).

Authors' contributions

ZW, HZ and YS designed the study. HZ, WG and XK conducted the experiments. XK and XT performed the statistical analysis. ZW, HZ, WG and YS drafted the manuscript. All authors read and approved the final manuscript.

Competing interests

The authors declare that they have no competing interests.

References

1. Weng JP, Bi Y. Epidemiological status of chronic diabetic complications in China. Chin Med J. 2015;128(24):3267–9.
2. Galetovic D, Olujic I, Znaor L, Bucan K, Karlica D, Lesin M, Susac T. The role of diabetic retinopathy in blindness and poor sight in Split-Dalmatia County 2000-2010. Acta Clin Croat. 2013;52(4):448–52.
3. Vujosevic S, Midena E. Diabetic retinopathy in Italy: epidemiology data and telemedicine screening programs. J Diabetes Res. 2016;2016:3627465.
4. Tracey ML, McHugh SM, Fitzgerald AP, Buckley CM, Canavan RJ, Kearney PM. Trends in blindness due to diabetic retinopathy among adults aged 18-69years over a decade in Ireland. Diabetes Res Clin Pract. 2016;121:1–8.
5. Alcubierre N, Rubinat E, Traveset A, Martinez-Alonso M, Hernandez M, Jurjo C, Mauricio D. A prospective cross-sectional study on quality of life and treatment satisfaction in type 2 diabetic patients with retinopathy without other major late diabetic complications. Health Qual Life Outcomes. 2014;12:131.
6. Zhang L, Chen B, Tang L. Metabolic memory: mechanisms and implications for diabetic retinopathy. Diabetes Res Clin Pract. 2012;96(3):286–93.
7. Lee C, An D, Park J. Hyperglycemic memory in metabolism and cancer. Horm Mol Biol Clin Investig. 2016;26(2):77–85.
8. Bhatt MP, Lee YJ, Jung SH, Kim YH, Hwang JY, Han ET, Park WS, Hong SH, Kim YM, Ha KS. C-peptide protects against hyperglycemic memory and vascular endothelial cell apoptosis. J Endocrinol. 2016;231(1):97–108.
9. Kowluru RA. Mitochondria damage in the pathogenesis of diabetic retinopathy and in the metabolic memory associated with its continued progression. Curr Med Chem. 2013;20(26):3226–33.
10. Kukat A, Dogan SA, Edgar D, Mourier A, Jacoby C, Maiti P, Mauer J, Becker C, Senft K, Wibom R, et al. Loss of UCP2 attenuates mitochondrial dysfunction without altering ROS production and uncoupling activity. PLoS Genet. 2014; 10(6):e1004385.
11. Wu H, Jiang C, Gan D, Liao Y, Ren H, Sun Z, Zhang M, Xu G. Different effects of low- and high-dose insulin on ROS production and VEGF expression in bovine retinal microvascular endothelial cells in the presence of high glucose. Graefes Arch Clin Exp Ophthalmol. 2011;249(9):1303–10.
12. Li SY, Fu ZJ, Lo AC. Hypoxia-induced oxidative stress in ischemic retinopathy. Oxidative Med Cell Longev. 2012;2012:426769.
13. Giacco F, Brownlee M. Oxidative stress and diabetic complications. Circ Res. 2010;107(9):1058–70.
14. Li N, Karaca M, Maechler P. Upregulation of UCP2 in beta-cells confers partial protection against both oxidative stress and glucotoxicity. Redox Biol. 2017;13:541–9.
15. Morigi M, Angioletti S, Imberti B, Donadelli R, Micheletti G, Figliuzzi M, Remuzzi A, Zoja C, Remuzzi G. Leukocyte-endothelial interaction is augmented by high glucose concentrations and hyperglycemia in a NF-kB-dependent fashion. J Clin Invest. 1998;101(9):1905 15.
16. Livak KJ, Schmittgen TD. Analysis of relative gene expression data using real-time quantitative PCR and the 2(−Delta Delta C(T)) method. Methods. 2001;25(4):402–8.
17. Santos JM, Kowluru RA. Role of mitochondria biogenesis in the metabolic memory associated with the continued progression of diabetic retinopathy and its regulation by lipoic acid. Invest Ophthalmol Vis Sci. 2011;52(12):8791–8.
18. Engerman RL, Kern TS. Progression of incipient diabetic retinopathy during good glycemic control. Diabetes. 1987;36(7):808–12.
19. Bianchi C, Del Prato S. Metabolic memory and individual treatment aims in type 2 diabetes--outcome-lessons learned from large clinical trials. Rev Diabet Stud. 2011;8(3):432–40.
20. De Felice FG, Ferreira ST. Inflammation, defective insulin signaling, and mitochondrial dysfunction as common molecular denominators connecting type 2 diabetes to Alzheimer disease. Diabetes. 2014;63(7):2262–72.
21. Pirola L, Balcerczyk A, Okabe J, El-Osta A. Epigenetic phenomena linked to diabetic complications. Nat Rev Endocrinol. 2010;6(12):665–75.
22. Ranjit Unnikrishnan I, Anjana RM, Mohan V. Importance of controlling diabetes early--the concept of metabolic memory, legacy effect and the case for early insulinisation. J Assoc Physicians India. 2011;59(Suppl):8–12.
23. Kowluru RA, Chan PS. Metabolic memory in diabetes - from in vitro oddity to in vivo problem: role of apoptosis. Brain Res Bull. 2010;81(2–3):297–302.
24. Zhong Q, Kowluru RA. Epigenetic changes in mitochondrial superoxide dismutase in the retina and the development of diabetic retinopathy. Diabetes. 2011;60(4):1304–13.
25. Zhao S, Li J, Wang N, Zheng B, Li T, Gu Q, Xu X, Zheng Z. Feno fi brate suppresses cellular metabolic memory of high glucose in diabetic retinopathy via a sirtuin 1-dependent signalling pathway. Mol Med Rep. 2015;12(4):6112–8.
26. Sharma K, Karl B, Mathew AV, Gangoiti JA, Wassel CL, Saito R, Pu M, Sharma S, You YH, Wang L, et al. Metabolomics reveals signature of mitochondrial dysfunction in diabetic kidney disease. J Am Soc Nephrol. 2013;24(11):1901–12.
27. Casalena G, Daehn I, Bottinger E. Transforming growth factor-beta, bioenergetics, and mitochondria in renal disease. Semin Nephrol. 2012; 32(3):295–303.
28. Moreira PI, Rolo AP, Sena C, Seica R, Oliveira CR, Santos MS. Insulin attenuates diabetes-related mitochondrial alterations: a comparative study. Med Chem. 2006;2(3):299–308.
29. Chacko BK, Reily C, Srivastava A, Johnson MS, Ye Y, Ulasova E, Agarwal A, Zinn KR, Murphy MP, Kalyanaraman B, et al. Prevention of diabetic nephropathy in Ins2(+/)(−)(AkitaJ) mice by the mitochondria-targeted therapy MitoQ. Biochem J. 2010;432(1):9–19.
30. Fraser-Bell S, Symes R, Vaze A. Hypertensive eye disease: a review. Clin Exp Ophthalmol. 2017;45(1):45–53.
31. Otto-Buczkowska E, Machnica L. Metabolic memory - the implications for diabetic complications. Endokrynol Pol. 2010;61(6):700–3.
32. Nishikawa T, Edelstein D, Du XL, Yamagishi S, Matsumura T, Kaneda Y, Yorek MA, Beebe D, Oates PJ, Hammes HP, et al. Normalizing mitochondrial superoxide production blocks three pathways of hyperglycaemic damage. Nature. 2000;404(6779):787–90.
33. Xie L, Zhu X, Hu Y, Li T, Gao Y, Shi Y, Tang S. Mitochondrial DNA oxidative damage triggering mitochondrial dysfunction and apoptosis in high glucose-induced HRECs. Invest Ophthalmol Vis Sci. 2008;49(9):4203–9.

19

Predicting participation of people with impaired vision in epidemiological studies

Pedro Lima Ramos[1,2], Rui Santana[3], Laura Hernandez Moreno[1], Ana Patricia Marques[3], Cristina Freitas[4], Amandio Rocha-Sousa[5,6], Antonio Filipe Macedo[1,2]* iD and The Portuguese visual impairment study group

Abstract

Background: The characteristics of the target group and the design of an epidemiologic study, in particular the recruiting methods, can influence participation. People with vision impairment have unique characteristics because those invited are often elderly and totally or partially dependent on help to complete daily activities such as travelling to study sites. Therefore, participation of people with impaired vision in studies is less predictable than predicting participation for the general population.

Methods: Participants were recruited in the context of a study of prevalence and costs of visual impairment in Portugal (PCVIP-study). Participants were recruited from 4 Portuguese public hospitals. Inclusion criteria were: acuity in the better eye from 0.5 decimal (0.30logMAR) or worse and/or visual field of less than 20 degrees. Recruitment involved sending invitation letters and follow-up phone calls. A multiple logistic regression model was used to assess determinants of participation. The J48 classifier, chi-square and Fisher's exact tests were applied to investigate the possible differences between subjects in our sample.

Results: Individual cases were divided into 3 groups: immediate, late and non-participants. A participation rate of 20% was obtained (15% immediate, 5% late). Factors positively associated with participation included years of education, annual hospital attendance, and intermediate visual acuity. Females and greater distance to the hospital were inversely associated with participation.

Conclusion: In our study, a letter followed by a phone call was efficient to recruit a significant number of participants from a larger group of people with impaired vision. However, the improvement in participation observed after the phone call might not be cost-effective. People with low levels of education and women were more difficult to recruit. These findings need to be considered to avoid studies whose results are biased by gender or socio-economic inequalities of their participants. Young subjects and those at intermediate stages of vision impairment, or equivalent conditions, may need more persuasion than other profiles.

Keywords: Study participation, Epidemiologic studies, Study design, Vision impairment, Recruitment strategies

Background

Epidemiologic studies involve collecting data from large number of individuals. However, participation rates in such studies, particularly in industrialised countries, have been falling in the past 3 or 4 decades. A study in Finland showed a decline in response rates from 84% (men) and 85% (women) in 1978 to 59% (men) and 71% (women) in 2002 [1]. High participation is necessary to ensure, for example, that the participating group is a representative sample of the population. When recruiting fails, statistical power of the results is reduced and conclusions may be distorted [2–5]. In order to produce reliable outcomes, researchers need to consider possible problems arising during the recruitment process and, if possible, control for factors that lead to reduced participation.

During recruitment general and study-specific challenges arise according with the topic and the target population. Some studies have shown that participation rates are

* Correspondence: a.macedo@ucl.ac.uk
[1]Low Vision and Visual Rehabilitation Lab, Department and Center of Physics – Optometry and Vision Science, University of Minho, Braga, Portugal
[2]Department of Medicine and Optometry, Linnaeus University, 39182 Kalmar, Sweden
Full list of author information is available at the end of the article

influenced by: education (participation increasing with the level of education [6–8]), gender (women tend to participate more than men [9–11]) and marital status (married people participating more than others [12]). Another factor that has been found to influence participation is general health, as given by the index of comorbidities [8]. There are other aspects such as age in which results are less consistent, with some studies showing that older people are more likely to participate [9, 10], whilst others found higher participation rates among young people [6]. Less commonly reported determinants include, for example, ethnicity. In a study by Patel et al. black, asian and other ethnic minorities were less likely to participate [8]. However, in addition to the characteristics of the target group, recruiting strategies can also influence rates of participation.

Previous studies have shown that researchers, when contacting prospective participants, must sound trustworthy and must take into account the motivations of the subject. Slegers and Glass recommend the use of public phone numbers and clear references stating that the study is being carried out by a public institution (when this is the case), in order to increase credibility [13]. They also recommend emphasizing that others invited have already responded to the study call and to provide open, clear and honest information from the onset (e.g. regarding monetary compensation or possible expenses). Personalised letters and reply paid envelopes are also known to improve response rates [14]. Other researchers investigated the primary reasons to take part in epidemiologic studies and concluded that participation is, amongst others, driven by moral reasons [13, 15]. In contrast, the actual effort required to participate has been identified has a barrier. Participation rates are expected to have a negative correlation with the amount of effort that participation requires [16].

The findings mentioned so far have been reported for studies in general; however, there is a lack of information about the profile of people with eye diseases and/or vision impairment (VI) who participate in epidemiological studies. Although, there is one study by Rahi et al. which investigated the engagement of families with children with VI [17]. However, this group was more interested in health service barriers for parents with children with VI [17].

Studies involving directly people with VI have unique characteristics because those invited are often elderly and totally or partially dependent on help to complete daily activities such as travelling to study sites. This makes participation more unpredictable than for many of the studies referred. The purpose of the project from where this study originates was to determine the causes of vision impairment amongst patients attending outpatient eye clinics. In parallel we also wanted to conduct a cross-sectional study about the impact of VI and other clinical and social aspects [18–21].

Our goal with this study was to determine the probability of participation as a function of personal characteristics, including severity of vision loss. We conducted a detailed investigation to distinguish between those who accepted the invitation to take part immediately from those who needed further contact before agreeing to participate. According to the "continuum of resistance" model, the more contacts a subject requires in order to take part in a study, the more similarities he/she shares with non-participants [16, 22]. The participation model was tested in our sample by comparing those that agreed to participate with non-participants.

We hypothesized that: i) the lower the acuity is the less likely participation is; ii) participation is independent of the cause of VI; iii) participation is affected by the distance residence-hospital; iv) education increases participation; v) age and gender affect participation; vi) annual hospital attendance increases participation.

To our knowledge this is the first study to investigate participation rates and its determinants in research involving people with VI. By studying participant's profiles, we hope to provide a significant contribution to the scientific community when planning studies involving people with VI and similar conditions.

Methods
Study design
The prevalence and costs of visual impairment in Portugal (PCVIP-study) was a hospital-based study whose aim was to determine, prevalence, causes and costs of VI in Portugal. The study gathered demographic, clinical, and economic information of people with VI. Participants for this report were recruited at 4 Portuguese public hospitals; patients with VI attending outpatient appointments at each of the hospitals for a period of 12 months were invited to participate in the study. The inclusion criteria were: patients with visual acuity (VA) in the better eye of 0.5 decimal (0.30logMAR) or worse and/or visual field less than 20 degrees. Cases were entered in a database by qualified and trained clinical staff. The database is online at http://www.pcdvp.org/login.php. The study protocol required inviting patients to attend an in-hospital appointment with the research team for face-to-face interviews and additional visual measurements. The study was designed considering the recommendations of the Vancouver Economic Burden of Vision Loss Group [23]. Basic demographic information was collected from administrative databases at the hospital. Information included: subject's initials, date-of-birth, gender, and place of residence ("concelho", in Portuguese, equivalent to district in many countries).

Participants

Letters were posted using the hospital mail service, the logo of the hospital was printed on the envelope and letters were sent directly to the patients' address. All documents were printed in font Arial- 16 point. The mail envelope included a letter of invitation signed by a physician from the local hospital (1 page), an information booklet (3 pages), a consent form (1 page) and a reply-paid envelope addressed to Escola Nacional de Saúde Publica, Lisboa (National School of Public Health, Lisbon). Information was printed on both sides of the paper; consent forms were printed on the reverse side of the invitation letter. In addition to information about investigators, institutions, contact details and clinicians involved in the study the letter contained a clear and isolated sentence (in Portuguese) with the instruction: *"If you agree to take part in this study, please tick the boxes in the flipside of this sheet, sign at the bottom of the page and provide a valid contact number for us to book your appointment at the hospital".*

If a response was not received within 2 weeks, a follow-up phone call was made. Calls were made by an experienced hospital staff member trained and informed about the study with instructions to ask the following questions: i) *did you receive our letter?* ii) *If yes, can I provide any further information about the study and the letter?* iii) *Would you be interested in taking part in this study?* If the person declined the invitation to participate, they were asked questions about: 1) years of education; 2) marital status; 3) annual hospital attendance.

For positive respondents, an appointment was booked at the hospital where they normally receive eye care and the same information was obtained. Those that agreed to take part in the study are defined as "participants" and those that declined after all attempts are defined as "non-participants". Those that dropped out after initially agreeing were not included in either of these categories. Participants were divided into 2 sub-grougps: "immediate participants" - those who sent the reply paid envelope with the consent form without being contacted by phone, and "late participants" - those who agreed to take part in the study only after they were contacted by telephone.

Data analysis

A database was built with information about: age, gender, distance between residence and hospital where the participant was recruited (DISTH), years of education (EDU), marital status (MST), visual acuity in the better eye (VA), annual hospital attendance (AHATTEND), cause of vision impairment (CAUSE-VI), Charlson comorbidities index (CCI). Information about causes of vision impairment and comorbidities to compute CCI was retrieved from medical records. The CCI

measures to which extent an individual is affected by comorbidities [24].

Univariate differences in participation rates according to the independent categorical variables were assessed using chi-square tests. DISTH, EDU and CCI are, unless otherwise stated, continuous variables and the remainder are categorical. Multiple logistic regression (R data analysis software, v3.2.4 for Windows) was used to determine the effect of independent variables in participation rates. The final model was built upon a database with 600 individuals and the fit quality was firstly measured also within such database. That is, the sample was both the training data and the testing data. In addition, an internal validation of this model was performed, a 10-fold cross-validation using the logistic classifier of Weka 3.8.

Results

For the current study a group of 2130 individuals were contacted by letter. Of the initial 2130 letters sent, 31 were returned to sender and 349 individuals agreed to participate immediately (17% of 2099). Of these, 49 individuals eventually dropped out of the study for health reasons or transportation difficulties (the study only covered travel expenses up to 15 euro), this resulted in 300 immediate participants (15% of 2050).

Phone calls were made to 1750 non-respondents in order to invite them to participate; 89 were unreachable by phone. From the 1661 contacted by telephone 84 (5%) agreed to take part. Therefore, the final number of participants was 384 (20%) out of 1961 that could be successful reached by letter and/or phone call.

In total, 600 individuals (260 females or 43%) with a mean age of 66 years (SD = 16.7) were included in this sample. In our analysis 325 (54%) were participants and 275 (46%) were non-participants. Non-participants analysed are a random sample of the total (1577) selected from successive cases in our list with all the required information. From the 384 participants only 325 were included in this report because the remaining 59 were waiting for the interview.

The median CCI for the entire sample was 0.6 (IQR = 1.8), amongst participants was 0.8 (IQR = 1.75), for non-participants was 0.5 (IQR = 1.5); this difference was not statistically significant (Mann-Whitney, $U = 1110$, $p = 0.45$).

The median EDU in years for the complete sample was 4 (IQR = 3), for participants was 4 (IQR = 5), for non-participants was 4 years (IQR = 1); this difference was statistically significant (Mann-Whitney, $U = 63,752$, p-value < 0.001). The number of years of education can be considered low but is expected for the age and geographical location of the participants [25].

Table 1 Summary of the distribution of 600 subjects included in the analysis. Among 600, 325 are participants [a] (immediate or late) and 275 non-participants randomly selected from 1577 total non-participants

Characteristic	n (%)	Participation YES/NO	Participation (%)	p-value (χ^2)
Gender				< 0.001
Male	339 (56.6)	225/114	66.4	
Female	261 (43.4)	100/161	38.3	
Age group				0.00535
< 20 yrs	14 (2.3)	12/2	85.7	
20 to < 30 yrs	8 (1.3)	6/2	75.0	
30 to < 40 yrs	28 (4.7)	27/1	96.4	
40 to < 50 yrs	43 (7.2)	34/9	79.1	
50 to < 60 yrs	82 (13.7)	52/30	63.4	
60 to < 70 yrs	137 (22.8)	80/57	58.4	
≥ 70 yrs	288 (48.0)	114/174	39.6	
Number of Hospital Appointments per year (AHATTEND)				< 0.001
Low - AHA (≤4×/yr)	173 (28.8)	52/121	30.1	
Medium - AHA (5 to 9×/yr)	178 (29.7)	86/92	48.3	
High – AHA (≥ 10×/yr)	249 (41.5)	187/62	75.1	
Marital Status (MST)				< 0.001
Married	261 (43.5)	110/151	42.1	
Living together	85 (14.2)	76/9	89.4	
Single	82 (13.7)	56/26	68.3	
Widow	131 (21.8)	48/83	36.6	
Divorced	41 (6.8)	35/6	85.4	
Visual Acuity- decimal scale (VA)				< 0.001
0	42 (7.0)	26/16	61.9	
0.1	80 (13.3)	51/29	63.8	
0.2	105 (17.5)	43/62	40.9	
0.3	87 (14.5)	35/52	40.2	
0.4	129 (21.5)	63/66	48.8	
0.5	157 (26.2)	107/50	68.1	
Aetiology of visual impairment (CAUSE-VI)				0.4336
Adult Macular Degeneration	76 (16.0)	31/45	40.8	
Diabetic retinopathy	191 (40.1)	110/81	57.6	
Glaucoma	60 (12.6)	26/34	43.3	
Other	149 (31.3)	81/68	54.4	
Multiple or undefined	124			

[a]Participants as mentioned here include immediate and late participants

The median DISTH (in kilometres) for the complete sample was 9.6 km (IQR = 24.2), for participants was 1 km (IQR = 15.1) and for non-participants was 19.4 km (IQR = 38.7); this difference was statistically significant (Mann-Whitney, U = 24,416, p < 0.001). Other socio-demographic and VI-related data are summarized in Tables 1 and 2.

Factors predicting participation using a logistic regression model

All the results reported in this section compare participants (the group who agreed to take part in the study after an invitation letter or letter and a follow-up phone call) with the cases of non-participants (the group of cases that declined after both contacts). We used a diagnostic test for the

Table 2 Summary of the distribution of all cases ($n = 600$) according to participation

Characteristic	Participants ($n = 325$)		Non-participants ($n = 275$) n (%)	p-value (χ^2)
	Immediate ($n = 241$) n (%)	Late ($n = 84$) n (%)		
Gender				< 0.001
Male	183 (75.9)	42 (50)	114 (41.4)	
Female	58 (24.1)	42 (50)	161 (58.6)	
Age group				0.00535
< 20 yrs	10 (4.1)	2 (2.4)	2 (0.7)	
20 to < 30 yrs	2 (0.8)	4 (4.8)	2 (0.7)	
30 to < 40 yrs	14 (5.8)	13 (15.5)	1 (0.4)	
40 to < 50 yrs	27 (11.2)	7 (8.3)	9 (3.3)	
50 to < 60 yrs	43 (17.8)	9 (10.7)	30 (10.9)	
60 to < 70 yrs	64 (26.6)	16 (19)	57 (20.7)	
≥ 70 yrs	81 (33.7)	33 (39.3)	174 (63.3)	
Number of Hospital Appointments per year				< 0.001
Low - AHA (≤4×/yr)	42 (17.4)	10 (11.9)	121 (44)	
Medium - AHA (5 to 9×/yr)	70 (29)	16 (19)	92 (33.5)	
High – AHA (≥ 10×/yr)	129 (53.6)	58 (69)	62 (22.5)	
Marital Status				< 0.001
Married	75 (31.1)	35 (41.7)	151 (54.9)	
Living together	76 (31.5)	0 (0)	9 (3.3)	
Single	35 (14.5)	21 (25)	26 (9.5)	
Widow	25 (10.4)	23 (27.3)	83 (30.2)	
Divorced	30 (12.4)	5 (6)	6 (2.1)	
Visual Acuity (decimal scale)				< 0.001
0	18 (7.5)	8 (9.5)	16 (5.8)	
0.1	28 (11.6)	23 (27.4)	29 (10.5)	
0.2	33 (13.7)	10 (11.9)	62 (22.5)	
0.3	31 (12.9)	4 (4.8)	52 (18.9)	
0.4	47 (19.5)	16 (19)	66 (24)	
0.5	84 (34.8)	23 (27.4)	50 (18.3)	
Aetiology of visual impairment(*)				0.4336
Age-related Macular Degeneration	18 (7.5)	13 (15.5)	45 (16.4)	
Diabetic retinopathy	87 (36.1)	23 (27.4)	81 (29.5)	
Glaucoma	17 (7.1)	9 (10.7)	34 (12.4)	
Other	58 (24.1)	23 (27.4)	68 (24.7)	
Multiple or undefined	124			

multicollinearity of predictors, the variance inflation factor, calculated for each predictor. The highest inflation factor was 1.67 for AHATTEND. Which means that AHATTEND was slightly correlated with the other predictors; nevertheless, this value was below the critical value of 2.5 reported in the literature as the tolerable upper limit [26].

In an initial model, with a binary dependent variable that assigned a value of 1 to "participants" and 0 to "non-participants", some variables were independent predictors of participation (see Additional file 1: Table S1).

Amongst categorical predictors we found an effect for gender (males participated more, $p < 0.001$), AHATTEND (participation for AHA-high was different from participation for AHA-low, $p < 0.001$), MST (co-habiting, single or divorced individuals were more likely to participate than married individuals, $p < 0.001$), VA (individuals with VA of 0.2 or 0.3 were less likely to participate than blind individuals, $p < 0.001$) and CAUSE- VI (individuals with diabetic retinopathy were more likely to participate than individuals with AMD, $p = 0.03$).

Amongst continuous predictors we found statistically significant effects for DISTH (participation reduced with increasing distance, $p < 0.001$) and EDU (participation increased with the number of years of education, $p < 0.001$).

The initial set of levels for each categorical variable were based on authors' experience (see Additional file 1: Table S1). For the final model, non-significant variables were removed and other levels or categories were defined as summarized in Additional file 2: Table S2. We now give an example to explain the rational. In the initial model, Additional file 1: Table S1, we observed that the effect of "Medium-AHA" in participation was not statistically different ($p = 0.075$) from the reference category "Low-AHA", therefore we merged these 2 categories and re-classified cases as "AHA-rare", Additional file 2: Table S2. Cases classified as "High-AHA" in the first model were kept separately because there was a statistically significant effect of this category in the model ($p < 0.001$). This category was renamed "AHA-frequent" to be consistent with the other category of the variable AHATTEND.

Table 3 Multivariable logistic regression model used to predict the probability of participation

Variables/Characteristic	Beta coefficient (SE)	Odds Ratio (95% CI)	p-value
Gender			< 0.001
Female vs. Male	−1.27 (0.24)	0.28 (2.23–5.71)	
Distance to clinic - km (DISTH)	−0.02 (0.004)	0.98 (1.01–1.03)	< 0.001
Education – years (EDU)	0.21 (0.04)	1.23 (1.14–1.33)	< 0.001
Annual number of hospital visits - in times-per-year (AHATTEND)			< 0.001
≥ 10×/yr vs < 10×/yr	1.64 (0.24)	5.18 (3.24–8.69)	
Marital Status (MST)			< 0.001
Living together vs. Others (married, single or widowed)	3.26 (0.46)	26.14 (10.62–64.4)	
Divorced vs. Others (married, single or widowed)	2.74 (0.56)	15.44 (5.15–46.27)	
Visual acuity (VA)			< 0.001
Intermediate (0.2–0.4) vs. extreme (0, 0.1 or 0.5)	1.10 (0.23)	3.02 (1.92–4.74)	

SE standard error, CI Confidence Interval

The variance inflation factor was recalculated for each predictor. The highest value obtained was 1.079 for MST, which means that multicollinearity can be ignored. Results for the final model are summarized in Table 3. All independent variables considered had a significant effect on the dependent variable. The deviance chi-squared goodness of fit test confirmed an excellent fit of the model to the data (p-value = 0.99).

The likelihood of participation increased if individuals were male, had AHA-frequent, had VA-extreme, if they were co-habiting or were divorced, with more EDU and less DISTH. Formula 1 and Formula 2 summarize these results:

$$\begin{aligned} Linear\ predictor = {} & -1.71-1.27\ (If\ Gender = {}^{''}female^{''}) \\ & -0.02 DISTH + 0.21 EDU \\ & +1.64\ (If\ AHATTEND = {}^{''}frequent^{''}) \\ & +3.26\ (If\ MST = {}^{''}co\text{–}habiting^{''}) \\ & +2.74\ (If\ MST = {}^{''}divorced^{''}) \\ & +1.1\ (If\ VA = {}^{''}extreme^{''}) \end{aligned}$$
(1)

$$Participation\ probability = \frac{e^{linear\ predictor}}{1 + e^{linear\ predictor}} \quad (2)$$

A 10-fold (10 iterations) cross-validation of the prediction model was performed. Before the iteration the Weka 3.8 software splits the 600 cases into 10 subsamples (60 cases each). For each iteration, during the validation process, each sample was chosen, at random, once as "testing data". The remainder 9 (540 cases) were used to generate temporary models. The 10 temporary models were then averaged to generated the final theoretical model which was tested against the real participation results for the 600 cases. The coefficients of the resulting theoretical model were very similar to those summarized in Table 3. The theoretical model classified correctly 484 out of 600 cases, with a weighted average precision of 0.809, a weighted average F-Measure of 0.808 and a weighted average ROC area of 0.872. If taken together the results of the internal validation and the deviance chi-squared goodness of fit, we can say that the model fits the real data accurately.

Table 3 provides the odds ratios (ORs) for study participation. It can be observed that, for example, the odds of a man participating in the study was 3.57 times higher than the odds of a woman.

The model expressed in Formula 1 and Formula 2 was simulated using Matlab (v2014b, Matworks inc.). The simulation allows the visualization of the probability of participation estimated by the model for extreme cases.

Table 4 Categories used to analyse differences between immediate (Ipar) and late participants (Lpar) and between late and non-participants (Npar)

AGE	AGE_1 = age less than 40 years AGE_2 = age between 40 and 69 years AGE_3 = age 70 or more years
AHATTEND	AHA-rare = number of annual hospital appointments less than 10 AHA-frequent = number of annual hospital appointments 10 or more
EDU	EDU_1 = less than 12 years of education EDU_2 = 12 or more years of education
DISTH	$DISTH_1$ = if distance residence-hospital was less than 40 Km $DISTH_2$ = if distance residence-hospital was 40 Km or more
VA	VA-extreme; includes VA of 0.0 or 0.1 or 0.5 VA-intermediate; includes VA of 0.2 or 0.3 or 0.4
MST	1 = Married; 2 = Together; 3 = Single; 4 = Widow; 5 = Divorced
GENDER	1 = Male; 2 = Female

According with the final model, the worst profile regarding the probability of participation, was being female attending the hospital 10× or less a year, married, single or widowed, with VA 0.2–0.4. The best profile was being male; attending the hospital 10× or more a year, living in a non-marital partnership, and VA ≤0.1 or 0.5. The model was implemented for these two situations as a function of the continuous variables distance residence-hospital

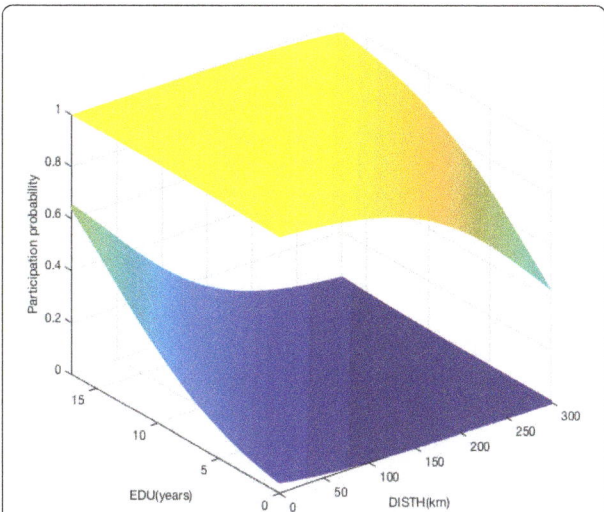

Fig. 1 Variation of the probability of participation predicted by our model according with the continuous variables DISTH and EDU. The two surfaces represent the most favourable and less favourable participation profiles defined according with the categorical variables used. The top yellow surface represents a male, with AHA-frequent, living together, with VA-extreme. The bottom blue surface represents a female, with AHA-rare, married, single or widow, with VA-intermediate

(DISTH) and education in years (EDU), the results are shown in Fig. 1.

In both cases the probability of participation increases when the distance residence-hospital decreases and education increases.

For the best profile and for distances 0-150 km, the participation probability reduces slowly. That is, the distance residence-hospital is almost irrelevant within the range 0-150 km. For distance values greater than 150 km the probability of participation decreases sharply. When living over 150 km away from the hospital, distance would be a big barrier for participation, in particular for those with less than 10 years of education.

Amongst individuals with the worst profile for participation, the distance residence-hospital had little impact for those with less than 10 years of EDU; for EDU greater than 10 years the distance residence-hospital is an important factor for participation when is below 100 km.

The group with the best profile would always have a minimum participation probability of approximately 40% and the worst profile group a maximum participation probability of approximately 60%.

Comparison between immediate participants (Ipar) and late participants (Lpar)

Here we report results of a comparison between two sub-groups of participants (participants = Ipar+Lpar). Ipar = accepted to participate when invited by letter only; Lpar = accepted to participate after letter followed by a phone call.

We found that the percentage of Lpar+Ipar was significantly higher than Ipar only (McNemar's test, $p < 0.001$). This shows that the number of participants increased significantly after the follow-up phone call. We investigated if there was a difference between Ipar and Lpar for the demographic aspects summarized in Table 4.

To build the categories defined in Table 4, first we investigated the existence of optimal cut points for the variables using the J48 classifier (Weka 3.8). The resultant decision tree is shown in Fig. 2 - in which the oval nodes represent random variables and rectangular nodes represent decisions or predictions. This classification model has a weighted average precision of 0.821, a weighted average F-Measure of 0.813 and a weighted average ROC area of 0.792. With this method we can predict, for example, that a widow man will be an immediate (Ipar) instead of a late (Lpar) participant. It also predicts that an individual that is single and has VA of 0.1 will be a Lpar instead of an Ipar.

The decision about which demographic aspects would be compared was based on 3 criteria applied according with the sequence presented here: (1) specific hypothesis

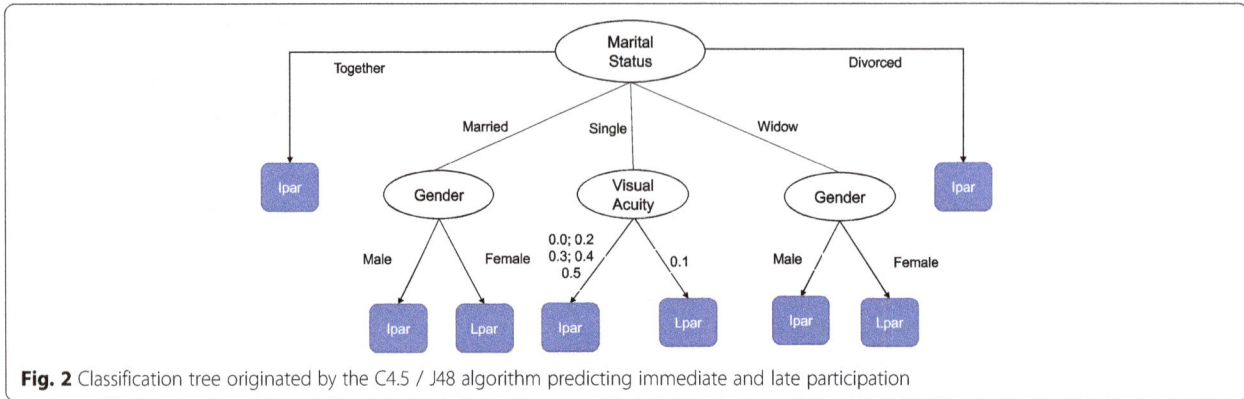

Fig. 2 Classification tree originated by the C4.5 / J48 algorithm predicting immediate and late participation

that the researchers wanted to test, (2) the cut-off points resulting from the J48 classifier analysis and (3) the number of subjects in each category.

The percentage of males in the Ipar was 76% (183 of 241) and in the Lpar was 50% (42 of 84); the distribution by gender was different in both groups (chi-square = 20.21, df = 1, $p < 0.001$).

The percentage of males in the AGE_1 group was 12% (22 of 183) amongst Ipar and 40% (17 of 42) amongst Lpar (chi-square = 19.3, df = 1, $p < 0.001$, after Bonferroni adjustment). For males with AGE_2, the percentage was 56% (102 of 183) amongst Ipar and 31% (13 of 42) amongst Lpar (chi-square = 7.3, df = 1, $p = 0.006$, after Bonferroni adjustment).

The percentage of participants with AHA-rare within the group of those who are males and AGE_2 was 46% (47 of 102) amongst Ipar and 15% (2 of 13) amongst Lpar (Fisher's exact test, $p = 0.04$).

The percentage of participants with EDU_1 within the group of those who are females, AGE_2 and AHA-frequent was 95% (18 of 19) amongst Ipar and 60% (6 of 10) amongst Lpar (Fisher's exact test, $p = 0.036$).

Comparison between late participants (Lpar) and non-participants (Npar)

Here we report an analysis comparing Lpar with Npar (Npar = those decline participation after two invitations). We wanted to investigate if the the profile of Npar and Lpar was similar. If that was true the percentage of cases in each demographic category should be similar in both sub-groups. This analysis is similar to the one performed in the previous section. The J48 classifier originated the decision tree shown in Fig. 3.

This classification model has a weighted average precision of 0.801, a weighted average F-Measure of 0.803 and a weighted average ROC area of 0.688. The classifier predicts that someone younger than 40 years that is not an Ipar will be a late participant (LPar) instead of a non-participant (NPar). The classification tree was used to define the levels summarized in Table 4. It was upon these levels that differences between Lpar and Npar were formally investigated.

The first finding was a difference in age between Lpar and Npar. The percentage of individuals with AGE_1 was 20% (17 of 84) amongst Lpar and was 2% (5 of 275)

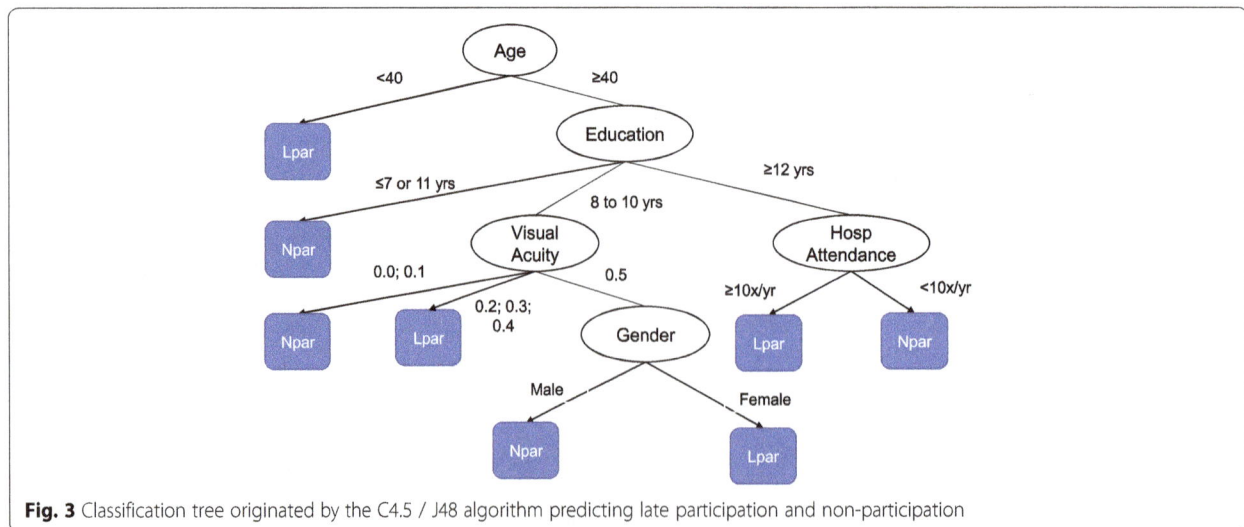

Fig. 3 Classification tree originated by the C4.5 / J48 algorithm predicting late participation and non-participation

amongst Npar (Fisher's exact test, $p < 0.001$). For those in the group AGE_3 the proportion was 39% (33 of 84) amongst Lpar and 63% (174 of 275) amongst Npar (chi-square = 12.82, df = 1, $p < 0.001$). The percentage of $DISTH_1$ subjects within the group of those who are AGE_2 was 97% (32 of 33) in Lpar and 78% (76 of 98) in Npar (Fisher's exact test, $p = 0.009$).

The percentage of individuals with EDU1 within the group AGE_2 was 73% (24 of 33) in Lpar and 98% (96 of 98) in Npar (Fisher's exact test, $p < 0.001$). The percentage of individuals with EDU_1 within the group of those who are AGE_3 was 88% (29 of 33) in Lpar and 96% (167 of 174) amongst Npar (Fisher's exact test, $p = 0.013$).

The percentage of AHA-rare subjects within the group of those who are AGE_2 was 9% (3 of 33) in the Lpar group and 45% (44 of 98) in the Npar group (Fisher's exact test, $p < 0.001$).

The percentage of individuals AGE_3 and AHA-rare was 18% (6 of 34) in the Lpar group and 45% (77 of 172) in the Npar group. (Fisher's exact test, $p = 0.004$).

The percentage of VA-extreme subjects within the group of those who are AGE_1 was 76% (13 of 17) in Lpar and 20% (1 of 5) in Npar (Fisher's exact test, $p = 0.039$). The percentage of VA-extreme subjects within the group of those who are AGE_2 was 61% (20 of 33) in Lpar and 35% (34 of 98) in Npar (chi-square = 6.84, df = 1, $p = 0.009$). The percentage of VA-extreme subjects within the group of those who are AGE_3 was 64% (21 of 33) in Lpar and 33% (58 of 174) in Npar (chi-square = 9.44, df = 1, $p = 0.002$).

Non-participants were asked to specify reasons for non-participation and the most commonly mentioned reasons were:

- *"I am too debilitated to participate"*
- *"It is far away from my home"*
- *"There are no benefits in participating"*
- *"I have no one to go with me"*

Discussion

In this study we investigated participation rates in the PCVIP study and its determinants. We obtained an overall participation rate of 20%, low participation was anticipated given that the target group of the population were people with impaired vision. Some that were willing to take part in interviews were not able to participate because travel arrangements were too expensive compared with the compensation offered by our study. Despite this, the participation rate was comparable to other studies involving participation in phone interviews in the Portuguese population [27]. Correia et al. were only able to interview 21.7% of those eligible for their study. When we analysed factors or determinants that are likely to affect participation rates in our study, we found that people at the extremes of VA (≤0.1 or less and 0.5) were more likely to participate than

those with intermediate acuities (0.2–0.4). Participation was independent of age and cause of VI but influenced by gender (males were more likely to participate). People living together or divorced were more likely to participate than those in other categories of marital status. Participation reduced with increasing traveling distances to the hospital but increased with the number of years of education. A high frequency of hospital appointments was also favourable to participation. A decision to participate was independent of the Charlson comorbidities index.

The initial hypothesis regarding the effect of acuity was partially confirmed and we were also able to confirm that the cause of VI was not a determinant of participation. Other results are in line with our initial hypotheses, specifically, we confirmed an effect of education, distance to the hospital and frequency of hospital attendance as determinants of participation in our study. Our model predicts that, for individuals with the best profile favouring participation, a minimum of 4 in 10 contacted would participate. For the worst profile, the maximum participation would be 6 out of 10. These profiles need to be considered when designing studies and planning recruitment.

Surprisingly subjects with severe vision loss, acuity 0.1 or less, were more likely to participate than those with better acuity, VA in the range 0.2–0.4. This finding seems to contradict the idea that the sustained willingness of individuals to participate can be inferred from the effort that participation requires [16]. It would be expected, from the effort perspective, that someone with a worse acuity would have more difficulties participating than someone with better acuity. A possible explanation is that individuals at more advanced stages of their conditions may perceive a greater benefit in responding to study participation than those at less advanced stages. People at more advanced may have a stronger moral drive to help others in a similar situation [28]. Another explanation for this result can be the level of adjustment to vision loss. Individuals with worse acuity might be better adjusted to vision loss whilst those in the medium range may still be in the process of adjusting and; therefore, less inclined to participate [29, 30].

The participation rate in our study was higher amongst men than women, which contrasts with some studies [9–11]. This is a result that needs further investigation but we acknowledge that this might be related to cultural factors because Correia et al. also found, in Portugal, higher participation amongst men [27]. Another result that is in contrast to other studies was the higher participation amongst subjects that were divorced or single when compared with married individuals. In a study by Sahar and colleagues married people were more likely to participate than people with other marital status [12]. We do not have a clear explanation for this result, but it could be related to the spectrum of relationships of the target group of the population.

Factors such as distance to the hospital, education or annual hospital attendance are important when planning recruitment. Individuals living further away from the hospital were less likely to participate. This result seems to be explained by the "principle of the effort" that predicts an inverse relationship between effort and participation probability [16]. In line with our results for education status, increased participation with the number of years of education has been reported in other studies [6–8]. The most likely reason for this is the ability to understand the purpose of the study and the contribution that studies can provide to the progress of knowledge. The participation odds for people visiting the hospital 10 or more times per year were higher than the participation odds of those who attend the hospital less than 10 times per year. Differences are likely to be due to the development of an acute civic awareness and/or familiarity with the hospital environment amongst those visiting the hospital more frequently.

In this study we also looked at systematic differences between immediate and late participants. This analysis provides information regarding the spectrum of individuals in which a follow-up phone call can be effective. Overall, we can say that the phone call, as others have found, seems to be important in increasing the moral obligation to participate [13, 15]. Our operators noted that a substantial number of individuals changed their minds and eventually decided to take part in the study after the importance of their participation has been emphasized. Compared with the initial letter, the follow-up call captured more women, more males younger than 40 years but fewer males within the age 40–69 years. Groups in which participation increased need more incentives or clarification than the groups that did not change in participation. Our results are in agreement with other studies showing that Lpar tend to be younger than Ipar [31, 32]. Other differences between Ipar and Lpar that we found involve very small groups with specific characteristics that seem to show only scattered combinations of patterns of participation.

By comparing late participants (Lpar) with non-participants (Npar), we investigated if the model of "continuum of resistance" was valid in our sample. According with the "continuum of resistance" model the more contacts an individual requires to participate in a study the more similar he/she is to Npar [16, 22]. However, similar to results in other studies [33, 34], we found many differences between the structure of the group of Lpar and Npar. In particular, the age distribution was different, Lpar were younger than Npar [31, 32]. Overall, there were several differences between the structure of the group Lpar and Npar which somewhat contradicts what would be expected from the model "continuum of resistance" [31–33, 35].

A limitation of our study was the lack of information concerning the economic status of the subjects that could potentially clarify some of the unexplained findings. Another aspect that we believe would strengthen our results would be the inclusion of responses from more subjects in both groups. Amongst others reasons, some non-participants were excluded from the analysis because they were unable to answer our questions by telephone (for example due to dementia, staying in nursing homes, hospitalization) or the clinical information was of poor quality (to determine, for example, the Charlson comorbidities index). Therefore, the included cases may be slightly different from the general population of interest.

Conclusion

In conclusion, participation rates in our study were influenced by gender, distance to the hospital, number of years of education, annual hospital attendance, marital status and visual acuity. There were considerable differences between immediate participants and late participants and between late participants and non-participants. Individuals with low levels of education and women were more difficult to recruit. These facts need to be taken in consideration in order to avoid studies that are biased by gender or socio-economic inequalities of the participants. Young subjects and those at intermediate stages of vision impairment, or equivalent conditions, might need more persuasion than other profiles.

Abbreviations

AGE$_1$: Age less than 40 years; AGE$_2$: age between 40 and 69 years; AGE$_3$: age 70 or more years; AHA-frequent: number of annual hospital appointments 10 or more; AHA-rare: number of annual hospital appointments less than 10; AHATTEND: annual hospital attendance; AMD: age-related macular degeneration; CAUSE-VI: cause of visual impairment; CCI: Charlson comorbidities index; DISTH: distance from the residence to the hospital; DISTH$_1$: distance residence-hospital was less than 40 km; DISTH$_2$: distance residence-hospital was 40 km or more; VA: extreme includes VA of 0.0 or 0.1 or 0.5; VA: intermediate includes VA of 0.2 or 0.3 or 0.4; EDU: number of years of education; EDU$_1$: less than 12 years of education; EDU$_2$: 12 or more years of education; Ipar: immediate participants; Lpar: late participants; MST: marital status; Npar: non-participants; PCVIP-study: Prevalence and Costs of Visual Impairment in Portugal: a hospital based study; SD: standard deviation; SE: standard error; VA: visual acuity in the better eye; VI: vision impairment

Acknowledgements

We would like to acknowledge Graham Brown and Peter Lewis for proofreading the manuscript.
The members of "The Portuguese visual impairment study group" (PORVIS group) are:

- Amandio Rocha-Sousa (i)
- Marta Silva (i)
- Sara Perestrelo (i)
- João Tavares-Ferreira (i)
- Ana Marta Oliveira (i)
- Cristina Freitas (ii)
- Keissy Sousa (ii)
- Ricardo Leite (ii)
- José C Mendes (ii)
- Andreia B Soares (ii)
- Rui C Freitas (ii)
- Pedro Reimão (iii)
- Marco Vieira (iii)
- Joel Monteiro (iii)
- Natacha Moreno (iv)
- Gary Rubin (v)
- -Ana P Marques (vi)
- Rui Santana (vi)
- Laura Moreno (vii)
- Pedro L Ramos (vii)
- Antonio F Macedo (vii)

(i)   From the Department of Surgery and Physiology; Faculty of Medicine; University of Porto and Department of Ophthalmology and Centro Hospitalar São João, Portugal
(ii) From the Department of Ophthalmology, Hospital de Braga, Portugal
(iii) From the Department of Ophthalmology, Centro Hospitalar de Alto Ave, Portugal
(iv) From the Department of Ophthalmology, Hospital Sta Maria Maior, Portugal
(v)   From the UCL-Institute of Ophthalmology, United Kingdom
(vi) From the National School of Public Health, NOVA University of Lisbon, Portugal
(vii) From the Low Vision and Visual Rehabilitation Lab, Department and Center of Physics – Optometry and Vision Science, University of Minho, Portugal and Linnaeus University, Department of Medicine and Optometry, Sweden

Funding

This study was supported by FCT (COMPETE/QREN) grant reference PTDC/DPT-EPI/0412/2012 in the context of the Prevalence and Costs of Visual Impairment in Portugal: a hospital based study (PCVIP-study). PLR is funded by FCT (COMPETE/QREN) grant reference SFRH/BD/119420/2016.

Authors' contributions

AFM, RS, CF, ARS, designed the study; PLR, LHM, APM, CF, AFM, PORVIS group collected data and PLR, LHM, APM, AFM analyzed the results; all authors participated in reporting and evaluating the results. PLR and AFM wrote the first draft of the manuscript and all authors contributed to subsequent writing. All authors approved the current version of the manuscript.

Competing interests

The authors declare that they have no competing interests.

Author details

[1]Low Vision and Visual Rehabilitation Lab, Department and Center of Physics – Optometry and Vision Science, University of Minho, Braga, Portugal. [2]Department of Medicine and Optometry, Linnaeus University, 39182 Kalmar, Sweden. [3]Centro de Investigação em Saúde Pública, Escola Nacional de Saúde Pública, Universidade NOVA de Lisboa, Lisbon, Portugal. [4]Department of Ophthalmology, Hospital de Braga, Braga, Portugal. [5]Department of Surgery and Physiology, Faculty of Medicine, University of Porto, Porto, Portugal. [6]Department of Ophthalmology, Centro Hospitalar São João, Porto, Portugal.

References

1. Tolonen H, Helakorpi S, Talala K, Helasoja V, Martelin T, Prattala R. 25-year trends and socio-demographic differences in response rates: Finnish adult health behaviour survey. Eur J Epidemiol. 2006;21(6):409–15.
2. Galea S, Tracy M. Participation rates in epidemiologic studies. Ann Epidemiol. 2007;17(9):643–53.
3. Moorman PG, Newman B, Millikan RC, Tse CK, Sandler DP. Participation rates in a case-control study: the impact of age, race, and race of interviewer. Ann Epidemiol. 1999;9(3):188–95.
4. Morton LM, Cahill J, Hartge P. Reporting participation in epidemiologic studies: a survey of practice. Am J Epidemiol. 2006;163(3):197–203.
5. Van Loon AJ, Tijhuis M, Picavet HS, Surtees PG, Ormel J. Survey non-response in the Netherlands: effects on prevalence estimates and associations. Ann Epidemiol. 2003;13(2):105–10.
6. O'Neil MJ. Estimating the nonresponse BiasDue to refusals in telephone surveys. Public Opin Q. 1979;43(2):218–32.
7. Partin MR, Malone M, Winnett M, Slater J, Bar-Cohen A, Caplan L. The impact of survey nonresponse bias on conclusions drawn from a mammography intervention trial. J Clin Epidemiol. 2003;56(9):867–73.
8. Patel MX, Doku V, Tennakoon L. Challenges in recruitment of research participants. Adv Psychiatr Treat. 2003;9(3):229–38.
9. Burg JA, Allred SL, Sapp JH 2nd. The potential for bias due to attrition in the National Exposure Registry: an examination of reasons for nonresponse, nonrespondent characteristics, and the response rate. Toxicol Ind Health. 1997;13(1):1–13.
10. Eagan TM, Eide GE, Gulsvik A, Bakke PS. Nonresponse in a community cohort study: predictors and consequences for exposure-disease associations. J Clin Epidemiol. 2002;55(8):775–81.
11. Wild TC, Cunningham J, Adlaf E. Nonresponse in a follow-up to a representative telephone survey of adult drinkers. J Stud Alcohol. 2001; 62(2):257–61.
12. Shahar E, Folsom AR, Jackson R. The effect of nonresponse on prevalence estimates for a referent population: insights from a population-based cohort study. Atherosclerosis risk in communities (ARIC) study investigators. Ann Epidemiol. 1996;6(6):498–506.
13. Slegers C, Zion D, Glass D, Kelsall H, Fritschi L, Brown N, Loff B. Why do people participate in epidemiological research? J Bioeth Inq. 2015;12(2): 227–37.
14. Edwards P, Roberts I, Clarke M, DiGuiseppi C, Pratap S, Wentz R, Kwan I. Increasing response rates to postal questionnaires: systematic review. BMJ (Clinical research ed). 2002;324(7347):1183.
15. Arfken CL, Balon R. Declining participation in research studies. Psychother Psychosom. 2011;80(6):325–8.
16. Lin IF, Schaeffer NC. Using survey participants to estimate the impact of nonparticipation. Public Opin Q. 1995;59(2):236–58.
17. Rahi JS, Manaras I, Tuomainen H, Lewando Hundt G. Health services experiences of parents of recently diagnosed visually impaired children. Br J Ophthalmol. 2005;89(2):213–8.
18. Macedo AF, Ramos PL, Hernandez-Moreno L, Cima J, Baptista AMG, Marques AP, Massof R, Santana R. Visual and health outcomes, measured with the activity inventory and the EQ-5D, in visual impairment. Acta ophthalmologica. 2017;95(8):e783–91.
19. Marques AP, Macedo AF, Perelman J, Aguiar P, Rocha-Sousa A, Santana R. Diffusion of anti-VEGF injections in the Portuguese National Health System. BMJ Open. 2015;5(11):e009006.
20. Gordon K, Crewe J, Ramos P, Macedo A, Morgan W. Capture-recapture: a method for determining the prevalence of vision impairment in the population. Clin Exp Ophthalmol. 2017;45:98.
21. Marques AP, Macedo AF, Hernandez-Moreno L, Ramos PL, Butt T, Rubin G, Santana R. The use of informal care by people with vision impairment. PLoS One. 2018;13(6):e0198631.
22. Fitzgerald R, Fuller L. I hear you knocking but you Can't come in: the effects of reluctant respondents and refusers on sample survey estimates. Sociol Methods Res. 1982;11(1):3–32.
23. Frick KD, Kymes SM, Lee PP, Matchar DB, Pezzullo ML, Rein DB, Taylor HR. The cost of visual impairment: purposes, perspectives, and guidance. Invest Ophthalmol Vis Sci. 2010;51(4):1801–5.
24. Quan H, Li B, Couris CM, Fushimi K, Graham P, Hider P, Januel JM, Sundararajan V. Updating and validating the Charlson comorbidity index and score for risk adjustment in hospital discharge abstracts using data from 6 countries. Am J Epidemiol. 2011;173(6):676–82.

25. **Portugal - Census** 2011 [http://censos.ine.pt/xportal/xmain?xpid=
     CENSOS&xpgid=censos_quadros_populacao].
26. O'Brien RM. A caution regarding rules of thumb for variance inflation factors.
     Qual Quan. 2007;41(5):673–90.
27. Correia SDP, Rolo F, Lunet N. Sampling procedures and sample
     representativeness in a national telephone survey: a Portuguese example.
     Int J Public Health. 2010;55(4):261–9.
28. Kypri K, Samaranayaka A, Connor J, Langley JD, Maclennan B. Non-response
     bias in a web-based health behaviour survey of New Zealand tertiary
     students. Prev Med. 2011;53(4–5):274–7.
29. Senra H, Barbosa F, Ferreira P, Vieira CR, Perrin PB, Rogers H, Rivera D, Leal I.
     Psychologic adjustment to irreversible vision loss in adults: a systematic
     review. Ophthalmol. 2015;122(4):851–61.
30. Senra H, Oliveira RA, Leal I. From self-awareness to self-identification with
     visual impairment: a qualitative study with working age adults at a
     rehabilitation setting. Clin Rehabil. 2011;25(12):1140–51.
31. Brogger J, Bakke P, Eide GE, Gulsvik A. Contribution of follow-up of
     nonresponders to prevalence and risk estimates: a Norwegian respiratory
     health survey. Am J Epidemiol. 2003;157(6):558–66.
32. Voigt LF, Koepsell TD, Daling JR. Characteristics of telephone survey
     respondents according to willingness to participate. Am J Epidemiol. 2003;
     157(1):66–73.
33. Friedman EM, Clusen NA, Hartzell M. Better late: Characteristics of late
     respondents to a health care survey. ASA Proc Jt Stat Meet. 2003:992–8.
34. Stinchcombe AL, Jones C, Sheatsley P. Nonresponse bias for attitude
     questions. Public Opin Q. 1981;45(3):359–75.
35. Bernick ELP D. J: improving the quality of information in mail surveys: use of
     special mailings. Soc Sci Q. 1994;75(1):212–9.

20

Application of biodegradable collagen matrix (Ologen™) implants in Dacryocystorhinostomy surgeries, a randomized clinical study

Hatem M. Marey[*], Hesham M. Elmazar, Sameh S. Mandour and Osama A. El Morsy

Abstract

Background: To introduce and evaluate the application of Ologen implants in external Dacryocystorhinostomy (DCR) Surgeries.

Methods: Prospective comparative randomized study was carried out on 60 patients coming to ophthalmology department, Menoufia University Hospitals. Patients included were suffering from primary acquired nasolacrimal duct obstruction with positive regurge test. Patients were randomly enrolled into two groups using alternating choice technique. Group A included 30 patients who had DCR surgery to treat the obstruction with Silicone tubes. Group B included 30 patients had a Dacryocystorhinostomy with Silicone tubes and Ologen implants.

Results: Success rates as regard to relief of symptomatic epiphora were 86.7% in group A and 96.7% in group B and time of dye clearance test was 4.5 ± 0.6 min in group A and 3.9 ± 0.4 min in group B with p value 0.353 &0.001 consecutively. Apart from immediate mild post operative hemorrhage that was encountered in 2 cases in group B and 1 case in group A, there were no significant complications in both groups.

Conclusion: The current study shows that application of Ologen implants in external DCR surgeries may improve symptomatic epiphora without exposing the patients to more intra-operative or post-operative complications. To the best of our knowledge, the current study is the first one to use Ologen implants in external DCR surgeries. However, the follow-up period was relatively short and the sample size is relatively small and further work is required to verify the effect of Ologen in external DCR surgeries.

Keywords: Acquired nasolacrimal duct obstruction (NLDO), Dacryocystorhinostomy (DCR), Ologen implants

Background

Dacryocystorhinostomy (DCR) is a procedure that creates an epithelium-lined tract between lacrimal sac and nasal mucosa bypassing the occluded nasolacrimal duct. The classic procedure has passed through many minor modifications; however, the basic technique still has a high success rate [1, 2]. A Silicone tube is used to keep the created fistula open specially if anterior flaps are not adequately demarcated and separated from posterior flaps.

Recurrence of symptoms may result from closure of the new tract due to excess fibrosis at the osteotomy site [3].

The Ologen™ is a relatively new material composed of lyophilized porcine atelocollagen (> 90%) and lyophilized porcine glycosaminoglycan (< 10%) with pore sizes of 10 to 300 µm. It provides a biodegradable, implantable scaffold collagen matrix. Atelocollagen (the main component) is a highly purified pepsin-treated type I collagen which has low immunogenicity, because it is free of telopeptides [4]. A telopeptide is an amino acid sequence at both N and C terminals, which is responsible for most of the collagen's antigenicity. The porous structure of Ologen™

* Correspondence: hatemmarey@yahoo.mail.com; hatemmarey@yahoo.com
Department of Ophthalmology, Menoufia Faculty of Medicine, Shebin El Kom, Menoufia, Egypt

directs fibroblasts and myoblasts to form a loose connective tissue minimizing scar formation.

Ologen has been tried as a conjunctival autograft for scleral necrosis after pterygium excision with a good results [5], and to control conjunctival fibrosis in subscleral trabeculectomy [6].

The aim of this study is to investigate the role of Ologen implants in regulating the healing process after external DCR surgery to prevent early fibrosis.

Methods

This is a prospective comparative randomized study. It was carried out at Ophthalmology Department, Menoufia University Hospitals, Egypt, in the period from Jan 2013 till Feb 2016. The study included 60 patients suffering from acquired nasolacrimal duct obstruction with positive regurgitation test. They were randomly enrolled into two groups. Group A included 30 patients who underwent DCR with Silicone tubes, and group B included 30 patients who underwent DCR with Silicone tubes and Ologen implants. Patients were allocated into either group using alternating choice technique with respect to equal match for both age and sex.

Patients included in the study were suffering from primary acquired naso lacrimal duct obstruction (NLDO) with positive regurgitation test and delayed dye clearance test more than 10 min in all cases without any previous surgery. Patients with any secondary causes for NLDO, negative regurgitation test, or history of previous surgery were excluded from the study.

After obtaining the necessary approval from the Faculty Ethics Committee of Faculty of Medicine, Menoufia University, a detailed discussion about the risk and benefits of the operation was carried out with all patients and a written consent was obtained. All measures were in accordance with the tenets of the Declaration of Helsinki.

All patients included in the study had detailed ophthalmologic examination including visual acuity, detailed eyelid examination and regurgitation test. Nasal examination was carried out by an Ear, Nose and Throat specialist to rule out nasal causes for obstruction of nasolacrimal duct (NLD) opening in the inferior meatus as deviated septum or nasal polyps. CT was done for all cases to assess the nasal cavity, anatomy of the bony lacrimal fossa and if there is anterior extension of ethmoid air cells into bony lacrimal fossa as well as to exclude malignant NLD obstruction.

Surgical technique

Patients of both groups were operated under general anesthesia with naso-tracheal intubation and packing of the oro-pharyngeal area. . All surgeries were done by the second and third authors (HFE & SSM).

A vertical small 10 mm incision line was marked on the side of the nose 11 mm from the medial canthus. The bone of the anterior lacrimal crest and the lacrimal fossa was exposed to create an adequate osteotomy to anastomose the sac and nasal mucosa. The posterior flaps of lacrimal and nasal mucosa were cut. Silicone tube was inserted and threaded through the puncti in the lacrimal passages till it appeared in the opened lacrimal sac (Fig. 1). Then, it was delivered through the nasal cavity.

In group B, Ologen™ collagen matrix (OCM, Aeon Astron Europe B.V., Leiden, and The Netherlands) 1 cm × 1 cm was placed under the anterior flaps of both the lacrimal sac and nasal mucosa . 6/0 Vicryl suture was then passed from the anterior nasal mucosal flap, through the Ologen implant underneath, to the anterior lacrimal sac flap . The suture was returned back in the opposite direction and tied over the anterior nasal mucosal flap in a mattress fashion.

In both groups, skin and muscles were sutured with 6/0 Vicryl sutures. Nasal packing was not necessary unless profuse bleeding occurs. Postoperative treatment with antibiotics for 1 week was scheduled in all cases. Silicone tubes were left in place for 6–12 weeks. Follow up period extended up to 18 months.

Post operative visits were scheduled after 1 week, 1 month, 3 months and 6 monthly thereafter. Detailed ophthalmic examination was done in these visits to evaluate patent satisfaction and absence of preoperative symptoms. Post operative complications were detected, documented and properly managed. We stressed on

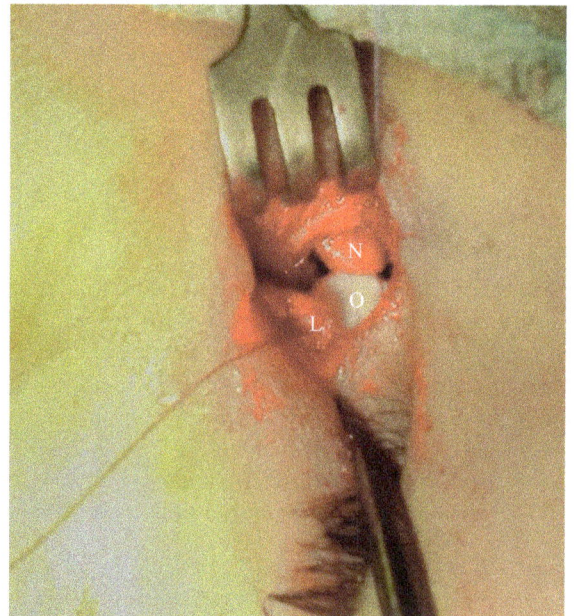

Fig. 1 Ologen implant (O) in position under the nasal mucosal flap (N) and the lacrimal sac flap (L) with stitches passing through the implant for fixation

following up the level of tear meniscus by slit lamp examination, dye clearance test, regurgitation test and patient satisfaction. Success in our study was defined as complete absence of epiphora or occasional epiphora requiring drying less than 2 times per day, 80–100% improvement in the timing of preoperative dye clearance test, negative regurgitation test, and the patient is satisfied, otherwise, it was considered as failure.

Data were collected, tabulated and analyzed by SPSS. We used t-test to compare the age, and the follow up period in Table 1, and dye clearance test in Table 3, chi square test to compare gender in Table 1, and Fischer exact test to compare hemorrhage, wound healing problems, and hypertrophic scar in Table 2, and presence of epiphora in Table 3.

Results

The study included 60 patients divided into 2 equal groups, A; included 30 cases (as a control group) and B; included 30 cases (as a case group). The mean age in group A was 51.27 ± 5.42 years and in group B was 50.53 ± 5.64 years. Females were more than males in both groups with a female: male ratio 4 to1 in group A and 11 to 4 in Group B. The follow up period extended for 12 up to 18 months with a mean of 14.87 ± 2.1 months and 15.13 ± 1.85 months for group 1 and 2 respectively. There was no statistically significant difference between the 2 groups regarding age, sex, and follow up period as shown in Table 1.

Follow up data included; post-operative hemorrhage, wound healing problems, hypertrophic cutaneous scar, dye clearance test, and postoperative epiphora.

There was no statistically significant difference regarding problems of wound healing and incidence of postoperative hypertrophic cutaneous scars. As well, there was no statistically significant difference regarding post-operative hemorrhage within first 24 h. It was encountered in 1 case in group A and in 2 cases in group B, a problem that was addressed by nasal packing and prompt control of arterial blood pressure. As shown in Table 2.

At the end of the follow up period, success rates for relief of symptomatic epiphora was (26 cases) 86.7% in group A, and (29 cases) 96.7% in group B.

Table 1 Descriptive data for both groups

Variable	Group A	Group B	p value	Test
Age				
Mean ± SD	51.27 ± 5.42	50.53 ± 5.64	p = 0.719	t test
Gender				
Male	6	8	p = 0.093	Qui Square test
Female	24	22		
Follow up period in months	14.87 ± 2.1	15.13 ± 1.85	p = 0.722	t test

Table 2 Post-operative data for both groups

Variable	Group A	Group B	p value	Test
Hemorrhage				
Present	1	2	p = 1	Fischer exact test
Absent	29	28		
Wound healing problems				
Present	2	1	p = 1	Fischer exact test
Absent	28	29		
Hypertrophic scar				
Present	1	1	p = 1	Fischer exact test
Absent	29	29		

with p value of 0.353. The time of dye clearance test has improved to 4.5 ± 0.6 min in group A and 3.9 ± 0.4 min in group B with p value 0.001, as shown in Table 3.

Discussion

External DCR is an effective procedure for managing epiphora caused by nasolacrimal duct obstruction. Its success rate is higher than endnonasal DCR. "Volume" symptoms (due to fluid retention in the lacrimal sac) can be cured in every case if there are no canalicular or eyelid abnormalities. "Flow" symptoms will improve in 95% of cases as they are affected by efficiency of canalicular conductance [7–10]. Failure of DCR is multifactorial, however, excessive fibrosis at the rhinostomy site represents a major postoperative problem [11].

Mitomycin C (MMC) has been used in lacrimal drainage surgery. A meta-analysis found that intraoperative MMC application was a safe adjuvant that could reduce the rate of closure of the rhinostomy site after primary external DCR [12]. Other controlled studies have investigated adjunctive MMC for primary or revised endoscopic DCR to augment the surgical success rate. However, the results are not completely consistent [13–15].

In the current study, Ologen™ was expected to have an effect similar to what happen when it is used in conjunctival surgeries. The porous structure of Ologen™ (during the period of its existence which extends

Table 3 Success rate, dye clearance test for both groups

Variable	Group A	Group B	p value	Test
Epiphora				
Present	4	1	p = 0.353	Fischer exact test
Absent	26	29		
Dye Clearance Test (minutes)	4.5 ± 0.6	3.9 ± 0.4	p = 0.001	t test

for 90–180 days before complete degradation) directs fibroblasts and myoblasts to form a loose connective tissue matrix during the process of wound healing which is remarkably similar to normal tissue, with less scar formation [16].

Ologen™ was used successfully to control conjunctival fibrosis in subscleral trabeculectomy in previous report [6]. Nasal mucosa is one of the highly vascular structures in the body. Hence, high incidence of fibrosis following DCR was encountered In the current study, authors tried to minimize the postoperative fibrosis of nasal mucosa by using a fibro vascular regulating substances like Ologen™. There was improvement in postoperative epiphora in the study group (96.7% success rate) as compared to control group (86.7% success rate). However, the difference between the two groups was not statistically significant and this may be attributed to the small sample size in the current study.

Wound healing problems were recorded in 2 cases in group A and 1 case in group B. As well, hypertrophic cutaneous scar was recorded in 1 case from each group. However, the hypertrophic scar was improved during follow up period. This is in agreement with Walland et al. who noticed improvements in the cosmetics of the external DCR scar with time to be almost imperceptible by 6 months postoperatively [17].

We encountered post-operative hemorrhage within first 24 h in 1 case in group A and in 2 cases in group B. This may result from the presence of Ologen implant which keeps the ostium patent and delay fibrosis. Postoperative bleeding was described in a low rate in classic DCR surgeries and could be managed with postoperative lowering of the blood pressure to normal values and by nasal packing [3].

Conclusion

To the best of our knowledge, the current study is the first to investigate the role of Ologen implantation in reducing fibrosis in external DCR. It was found to be a potentially safe and easy technique that helps improving the surgical outcomes without intra operative or post operative complications. Although, the P-value was not significant (0.3) between the non-Ologen and Ologen group, there was a difference in clinical improvement (86% vs 96% respectively). The statistically non-significant difference may be attributed to small sample size. Therefore, further work is required to verify Ologen effect on a longer follow up period and on a larger scale of cases. As well, further studies may investigate the application of Ologen without tubes which if found effective will reduce the time of surgery and eliminate the need for another intervention to remove the tubes.

Authors' contributions
HM participated in the design of the study and performed the statistical analysis, and data collection. SM participated in the design of the study, data collection, and was one of the operators. HE participated in the sequence alignment, was one of the operators, and drafted the manuscript. OE participated in the sequence alignment. All authors read and approved the final manuscript.

Competing interests
The authors declare that they have no competing interests.

References
1. Leong SC, Macewen CJ, White PS. A systematic review of outcomes after dacryocystorhinostomy in adults. Am J Rhinol Allergy. 2010;24:81–90.
2. Hurwitz JJ, Rutherford S. Computerized survey of lacrimal surgery patients. Ophthalmology. 1986;93:14–21.
3. Hurwitz JJ. The lacrimal drainage system. In: Yanoff M, Duker JS, Augsburger JJ, editors. Ophthalmology. London: Mosby; 2003. p. 761–8.
4. Stenzel K, Miyata T, Rubin A. Collagen as a biomaterial. Annu Rev Biophys Bioeng. 1974;3:231–53.
5. Cho CH, Lee SB. Biodegradable collagen matrix (Ologen™) implant and conjunctival autograft for scleral necrosis after pterygium excision: two case reports. BMC Ophthalmol. 2015;15:140.
6. Hatem MM, Sameh MS, Amin EF. Subscleral trabeculectomy with Mitomycin-C versus Ologen for treatment of glaucoma. J Ocul Pharmacol Ther. 2013;29(3):330–4.
7. Unlu HH, Toprak B, Aslan A, Guler C. Comparison of surgical outcomes in primary endoscopic dacryocystorhinostomy with and without silicone intubation. Ann Otol Rhinol Laryngol. 2002;111:704–9.
8. Hartikainen J, Grenman R, Pukka P, Seppa H. Prospective randomized comparison of external Dacryocystorhinostomy and endonasal laser dacryocystorhinostomy. Ophthalmology. 1998;105:1106–13.
9. Tarbet KJ, Custer PL. External dacryocystorhinostomy. Surgical success, patient satisfaction, and economic cost. Ophthalmology. 1995;102:1065–70.
10. Emmerich KH, Busse H, Meyer-Rüsenberg HW, H rstensmeyer CG. External dacryocystorhinostomy: indications, method, complications and results. Orbit. 1997;16:25–9.
11. Allen KM, Berlin AJ, Levine HL. Intranasal endoscopic analysis of dacrocystorhinostomy failure. Ophthal Plast Reconstr Surg. 1988;4:143–5.
12. Feng YF, Yu JG, Shi JL, Huang JH, Sun YL, et al. A meta-analysis of primary external dacryocystorhinostomy with and without mitomycin C. Ophthalmic Epidemiol. 2012;19:364–70.
13. Mudhol RR, Zingade ND, Mudhol RS, Das A. Endoscopic ostium assessment following Endonasal Dacryocystorhinostomy with Mitomycin C application. Al Ameen J Med Sci. 2012;5:320–4.
14. Prasannaraj T, Kumar BY, Narasimhan I, Shivaprakash KV. Significance of adjunctive mitomycin C in endoscopic dacryocystorhinostomy. Am J Otolaryngol. 2012;33:47–50.
15. Tirakunwichcha S, Aeumjaturapat S, Sinprajakphon S. Efficacy of mitomycin C in endonasal endoscopic dacryocystorhinostomy. Laryngoscope. 2011;121:433–6.
16. Cillino S, Di Pace F, Cillino G, Casuccio A. Biodegradable collagen matrix implant vs mitomycin-C as an adjuvant in trabeculectomy: a 24-month, randomized clinical trial. Eye (Lond). 2011;25:1598–606.
17. Walland MJ, Rose GE. Soft tissue infections after open lacrimal surgery. Ophthalmology. 1994;101:608–11.

21

Effect of dexamethasone intravitreal implant (Ozurdex®) on corneal endothelium in retinal vein occlusion patients

Corneal endothelium after dexamethasone implant injection

Hatice Ayhan Güler[1,3*], Nurgül Örnek[1], Kemal Örnek[2], Nesrin Büyüktortop Gökçınar[1], Tevfik Oğurel[1], Mehmet Erhan Yumuşak[1] and Zafer Onaran[1]

Abstract

Background: To assess corneal endothelial cell changes after intravitreal dexamethasone (DEX) implant (Ozurdex®) injection in patients with macular edema secondary to retinal vein occlusion (RVO).

Methods: Twenty-two eyes of 22 patients were assessed prospectively after intravitreal 0.7 mg DEX implant injection. Twenty-two eyes of 22 healthy volunteers served as control group. Corneal endothelial cell parameters including endothelial cell density (ECD), coefficient of variation of cell size (CV), percentage of hexagonality (Hex) and central corneal thickness (CCT) were analyzed before and 1 and 3 months after injection by specular microscopy. The results of the study were compared statistically.

Results: There were 17 (77.3%) patients with branch RVO and 5 (22.7%) patients with central RVO. Mean intraocular pressure (IOP) was 14.73 mmHg before injection, 17.05 mmHg at 1 month and 17.15 mmHg at 3 months after injection. Mean IOP at 1 and 3 months were significantly higher than pre-injection value ($p = 0.002$ and $p = 0.003$, respectively). There was a statistically significant reduction in mean ECD at 3 months after injection compared to pre-injection and 1 month ($p = 0.013$, $p = 0.009$, respectively) in the injected eyes. Mean ECD showed no significant difference in the uninjected fellow eyes during the follow up (p>0.05). Mean CV and Hex did not reveal a statistically significant difference in injected and uninjected fellow eyes ($p > 0.05$). No significant change was observed in mean CCT values during the follow up ($p = 0.8$).

Conclusion: Intravitreal dexamethasone implant may cause a transient reduction in corneal endothelial cell density in short term without changing cell morphology.

Keywords: Dexamethasone implant, Retinal vein occlusion, Corneal endothelium, Specular microscopy

Background

Corticosteroids are widely used in ophthalmology for their anti-inflammatory, antipermeability and antifibrotic properties. They modulate cellular proliferation, apoptosis, and development. Steroids suppress inflammation by immobilizing arachidonic acid, downregulating multiple cytokine pathways including vascular endothelial growth factor (VEGF) pathway, stabilizing cell membranes and mast cell granules, inhibiting leukocyte interaction and slowing diapedesis.

Dexamethasone is a type of synthetic corticosteroid. It is one of the most commonly used corticosteroid in ophthalmology with similar indications as other corticosteroid preparations. Anti-inflammatory activity of dexamethasone is about six times stronger than that of prednisone or prednisolone and 30 times that of cortisone.

Ozurdex® is an intravitreal implant containing 700 µg preservative-free dexamethasone (DEX) in a slow release drug delivery system. Because of its anti-inflammatory

* Correspondence: hatice_ayhanguler@hotmail.com
[1]Department of Ophthalmology, Faculty of Medicine, Kırıkkale University, Kırıkkale, Turkey
[3]Department of Ophthalmology, Bayburt State Hospital, Bayburt, Turkey
Full list of author information is available at the end of the article

and anti-angiogenic effect, DEX implant is indicated for various posterior segment diseases, like macular edema due to retinal vein occlusion (RVO), diabetic maculopathy and non-infectious posterior uveitis etc. [1–5].

Glucocorticoid receptors and messenger ribonucleic acids (mRNA) regulating glucocorticoid activity at these receptors were found in corneal endothelium [6, 7]. Effect of DEX implant on corneal endothelium has been studied in very few studies. Kwak et al. reported no toxic effect on cornea, retina and lens in a rabbit model following 400 mg intravitreal DEX injection [8]. İlhan et al. reported that 0.7 mg intravitreal DEX implant application probably have no side effect on corneal endothelium at six months in patients with macular edema caused by RVO [9].

The aim of the study was to evaluate effect of intravitreal dexamethasone implant (Ozurdex®) on corneal endothelium in patients with macular edema secondary to RVO.

Methods

This prospective clinical study was conducted between September 2015 and September 2016 at the Ophthalmology Department of Kırıkkale University Hospital. It was approved by local ethics committee and was in accordance with the Declaration of Helsinki. The patients were informed before the study and all signed the consent forms.

There were 22 eyes of 22 patients with RVO and macular edema in the study group. Twenty two eyes of 22 healthy volunteers served as controls. Participants who were under 18 years or over 80 years and those who had pregnancy, glaucoma, contact lens use, previous intravitreal injection, ocular trauma, uveitis, endothelial cell count less than 1500 cells/mm^2 and corneal opacity were excluded.

Complete ophthalmologic examination was performed at each visit including best-corrected visual acuity (BCVA), intraocular pressure (IOP) measurement, biomicroscopy, fundus examination and optical coherence tomography (OCT) imaging. IOP was measured by Goldman applanation tonometry (CSO®, Italy) before and at 1 and 3 months after intravitreal injection. OCT scans of macula were demonstrated using spectral domain OCT (Retinascan Advanced RS-3000, NIDEK, Gamagori, Japan). Fundus fluorescein angiography (Canon CF-1®, Japan) was performed before injection.

Endothelial cell density (ECD), coefficient of variation of cell size (CV), percentage of hexagonality (Hex) were measured from right eyes of volunteers and the injected and uninjected fellow eyes of patients before and at 1 and 3 months after injection using corneal specular microscopy (Konan Noncon Robo SP8000, Konan Medical, Hyogo, Japan). A single examiner evaluated corneal endothelial cell

parameters using central analysis method. In this method, at least 110 neighbouring cells were manually marked centrally for endothelial analysis and the imagenet software program displayed the results automatically. Central corneal thickness (CCT) was measured automatically by specular microscopy.

Dexamethasone implant was injected after topical anesthesia by proparacaine hydrochloride and surface disinfection with %5 povidone iodine. Dexamethasone implant was delivered through a 22-gauge needle, with a preloaded applicator and inserted into the vitreous cavity through pars plana. Topical moxifloxacine drop was used for 5 days after injection.

For assessing repeatability of corneal endothelial cell count measurements (ECD, CV, percentage of Hex) same baseline images of 22 injected eyes were analyzed twice on separate days by the same examiner using central analysis method. The difference between continuous variables was tested using one sample t test and repeatability of each pair of analysis was assessed using the 95% limit of agreement (LOA) calculated as mean difference ± 1.96 x SD of the difference according to Bland and Altman. Intraclass correlation coefficient (ICC) was measured to reveal reliability. ICC value should not be less than 0.9 in most clinical measurements.

Statistical analyses were performed using SPSS for Windows 22.0 (SPSS İnc., Chicago, IL). A p value below 0.05 was considered statistically significant.

Results

The study included 5 (22.7%) patients with central retinal vein occlusion (CRVO) and 17 (77.3%) patients with branch retinal vein occlussion (BRVO). Twenty-two eyes of 22 healthy volunteers served as control group. There were 14 females and 8 males. Mean age of the patients was 60.9 (range: 40–75) years. There were 14 phakic and 8 pseudophakic patients. There was no significant difference in terms of gender and age between control and study groups ($p = 0.678$, $p = 0.940$, respectively).

In comparison to control eyes, there was no statistically significant difference in mean ECD, CV, Hex and CCT measurements of injected and uninjected fellow eyes of the study group before injection (all $p > 0.05$) (Table 1).

Mean BCVA was 0.99 ± 0.75 logMAR (range: 0.20–2.20) and mean foveal thickness was 462.4 ± 96.1 μm (range: 306–600) before intravitreal dexamethasone implant injection. Argon laser treatment was applied to peripheral retina in 4 patients. Three months after intravitreal DEX implant, mean BCVA was increased to 0.46 ± 0.76 logMAR (range: 0–3.0) ($p = 0.033$) and mean foveal thickness was decreased to 316.41 ± 92.48 μm (range:186–552) ($p < 0.001$).

Table 1 ECD, CV, Hex and CCT values of control eyes and patient eyes before intravitreal injection

	Control Eyes	Injected Eyes	Uninjected Eyes	p value
ECD	2199.5 ± 325.1	2211.7 ± 370.6	2219.8 ± 263.2	0.608* 0.307**
CV	37.68 ± 5.7	37.86 ± 5.5	40.7 ± 8.5	0.883* 0.082**
Hex	54.5 ± 6.9	54.9 ± 6.8	53.7 ± 8.5	0.871* 0.241**
CCT	566.7 ± 42.4	567.5 ± 43.0	556.9 ± 35.2	0.830* 0.522**

ECD Endothelial cell density, *CV* Coefficient of variation of cell size, *Hex* Percentage of hexagonality and *CCT* Central corneal thickness by corneal specular microscopy. * shows statistical difference between control and injected eyes, ** shows statistical difference between control and uninjected fellow eyes

Mean CCT was measured 567.5 ± 43.0 μm before injection, 564.1 ± 43.9 μm at 1 month and 556.5 ± 44.3 μm at 3 months after intravitreal injection in injected eyes. There was no significant difference between mean CCT values before intravitreal injection and at 1 and 3 months after intravitreal injection ($p = 0.4$, $p = 0.5$, respectively) (Table 2).

Mean ECD at 3 months after intravitreal injection was statistically significantly lower compared to pre-injection and 1 month values in injected eyes ($p = 0.013$ and $p = 0.009$, respectively). There was no significant difference in ECD in uninjected fellow eyes of patients during follow up ($p > 0.05$). No significant difference was observed in mean CV, Hex and CCT values between injected and uninjected fellow eyes (all $p > 0.05$) (Table 2).

Mean difference (bias) was 3.77 cells/mm^2 for ECD, – 0.41 for CV and 0.27% for Hex. One sample t test showed no significant difference between 2 measurements ($p = 0.120$ for ECD, $p = 0.451$ for CV and $p = 0.718$ for Hex). Limit of agreement (LOA) (mean difference ± 1.96 x SD) values were 3.77 ± 21.39 cells/mm^2, – 0.41 ± 12.26 and 0.27 ± 6.85% for ECD, CV and percentage of Hex respectively. LOA values showed good agreement between two analyses. Intraclass correlation coefficient (ICC) value was measured as 0.99 for ECD, 0.93 for CV and 0.90 for Hex which suggested good reliability of measurements.

Mean IOP was 14.73 ± 3.58 mmHg before injection, 17.05 ± 4.40 mmHg at 1 month and 17.15 ± 6.65 mmHg at 3 months after intravitreal injection. Mean IOP at 1and 3 months after injection were statistically significantly higher than pre- injection value ($p = 0.002$, $p = 0.003$, respectively). Only 4 eyes (%18) had IOP higher than 21 mmHg. All were succesfully treated with anti-glaucomatous drops.

Two eyes (9%) had subconjunctival hemorrhage after intravitreal injection. According to the Lens Opasification Classification System (LOCS) 3 scale, mean cataract grade was increased significantly 3 months after intravitreal injection ($p = 0.001$). Mean LOCS 3 scale was 1.4 ± 0.5 (range:1–2) before intravitreal injection and was increased to 2.3 ± 1.1 (range:1–4) 3 months after intravitreal injection.

Discussion

Retinal vein occlusion is a common disease of retinal vasculature [10]. Macular edema is a frequent cause of visual loss in RVO patients. There are several methods available for treatment. Laser photocoagulation may decrease macular edema in BRVO patients but typically does not improve visual acuity [11].

Options for treatment of macular edema secondary to RVO have expanded in the past few years. Two types of drugs have emerged as an alternative treatment for macular edema in RVO; corticosteroids and anti-VEGF agents. Intravitreal steroid or anti-VEGF injections have been shown to effectively reduce macular edema and improve visual acuity in BRVO and CRVO patients [12, 13]. Good tolerance was observed for a 12-month period for 0.7 mgDEX implant with significantly lesser adverse effects compared to triamcinolone [14].

Sustained release DEX intravitreal implant is composed of a biodegradable copolymer of polylactic-co-glycolic acid containing micronized dexamethasone [3]. Ozurdex pharmocokinetics enable high concentrations of dexametasone release into retina and vitreous during first 3 months

Table 2 ECD, CV, Hex and CCT values of injected and uninjected eyes before intravitreal injection and follow-up visits

		Before injection	1st month	3rd month	p value*
CD	Injected eyes	2211.7 ± 370.6	2207.1 ± 351.9	2163.8 ± 357.7[ab]	0.018
	Uninjected eyes	2219.8 ± 263.2	2265.9 ± 254.2	2102.8 ± 551.9	0.179
CV	Injected eyes	37.86 ± 5.55	40.14 ± 6.47	40.05 ± 5.22	0.511
	Uninjected eyes	40.70 ± 8.46	41.35 ± 5.85	41.94 ± 9.22	0.842
Hex	Injected eyes	54.86 ± 6.84	55.81 ± 7.32	56.63 ± 8.25	0.481
	Uninjected eyes	53.70 ± 8.55	53.95 ± 7.52	53.72 ± 8.92	0.879
CCT	Injected eyes	567.5 ± 43.0	564.1 ± 43.9	556.5 ± 44.3	0.810
	Uninjected eyes	556.9 ± 35.2	558.8 ± 39.7	563.3 ± 41.2	0.104

*Friedman Test, aPost-hoc: Statistical difference detected before intravitreal injection and third month ($p = 0.013$), bPost-hoc: Statistical difference detected between first and third month ($p = 0.009$), *ECD* Endothelial cell density, *CV* Coefficient of variation of cell size, *HEX* Percentage of hexogonality and *CCT* Central corneal thickness by corneal specular microscopy

following injection and lower concentrations may still remain up to 6 months [15]. Ocular hypertension and cataract are two major long-term sequelae identified in large, randomized clinical trials. Case reports have shown implant migration, accidental injection into the lens, infection, posterior segment sequelae including vitreomacular traction et.. [16]. In the study, we observed elevated intraocular pressure and cataract formation as complications of intravitreal DEX implant.

Endothelial cell density was decreased at 3 months after intravitreal injection, but there was no statistically significant difference in pleomorphism and polymegatism. Despite increased IOP and decreased ECD at 3 month, there was no statistically significant change in CCT. Intraocular pressure may cause CCT variation by two possible mechanisms. First one is impairment of pump function of corneal endothelium when IOP reaches a critical level above 40 mmHg in human eyes. None of the patients had IOP above 40 mmHg after injection in the study. Another mechanism may be direct effect of elevated IOP on mechanical properties of cornea. Cornea is a nonlinear viscoelastic tissue that presents different mechanical properties under different IOP levels. Goldmann correlated IOP measured by ocular response analyser showed a positive correlation with CCT [17–19]. Endothelial cell function was compromised and corneal transparency was lost when cell density was decreased significantly from average of 3000 cells/mm^2 to nearly 1000 cells/mm^2 [20]. Decrease in ECD did not come to a critical level in the study, thus had no effect on CCT. Also increased pleomorphism and polymegatism might have reduced the ability of endothelial cells to hydrate the cornea [20]. Neither pleomorphism nor polymegatism showed statistically significant difference after intravitreal injection and had no effect on mean CCT.

Previous studies have reported different results about effect of intravitreal injections on corneal endothelium. Güzel et al. proposed that endothelial cell density and morphology did not change after intravitreal ranibizumab and bevacizumab injections [21]. Peraz Rico et al. showed that ranibizumab had no harmful effect on corneal endothelium [22]. Although previous immunohistochemistry studies detected mRNA encoding glucocorticoid receptor in corneal endothelium, [7], contraversies exist about effect of dexamethasone implant on corneal endothelium. In a study by İlhan et al., effect of intravitreal dexametasone implant on corneal endothelium has been studied and no statistical difference was found in ECD,CV and Hex during 6 month follow up [9]. Michalska-Małecka et al. reported no statistically significant difference in endothelial cell density of patients with macular edema secondary to BRVO and CRVO at 6 month [23]. Contrary to these studies, in an in vitro study in bovine eyes, corneal endothelial cells were cultured with different concentrations of dexamethasone and cellular apoptosis and necrosis were shown at high concentrations [6].

Unfavorable effect of corticosteroids on regeneration of corneal endothelial cells is well-known [24]. Although relatively rare, DEX implant may migrate to anterior chamber in aphakic eyes, pseudophakic eyes with capsular and zonular defects, vitrectomized eyes and eyes with long axial length. Kang et al. reported 4 patients out of 924 intravitreal DEX injections with 7 episode of anterior chamber migration. All 4 eyes had corneal edema and one eye required corneal transplantation. Corneal edema occured in all patients regardless of injection duration [25]. In a recent peer-reviewed literature, to date 51 cases of DEX implant migration to anterior chamber were reported by Rhimy et al. Corneal endothelial decompansation and edema were present in 74.5% of the patients (38 of 51 patients) and corneal edema was observed if migration occured within 3 weeks. Rhimy at el. hypothesized that mechanism of corneal edema may be secondary to chemical toxicity of implant or from mechanical trauma of the rigid device making direct contact with corneal endothelial surface [26]. In the study, there was no contact of DEX implant and corneal endothelium, therefore we may conclude that chemical toxicity of DEX implant seems to be more probable than mechanical trauma on corneal endothelium.

Small sample size and shorter follow-up time are the limitations of the current study. Also subgroup analysis such as pseudophakic or phakic patients could not be made because of small sample size.

Conclusions

In the study, dexamethasone implant caused a transient reduction in endothelial cell density but did not change cell morphology in injected eyes. Possible mechanism may be a kind of chemical toxicity from implant. Effect of DEX implant on corneal endothelium should be considered particularly in compromised corneas prior to decision making. Long-term studies with larger number of patients are still needed to clarify the effect of intravitreal dexamethasone implant on corneal endothelial cell layer.

Abbreviations

BRVO: Branch retinal vein occlussion; CCT: Central corneal thickness; CRVO: Central retinal vein occlusion; CV: Coefficient of variation of cell size; DEX: Dexamethasone; ECD: Endothelial cell density; Hex: Hexagonality; IOP: Intraocular pressure; LOCS: Lens opasification classification system; mRNA: Messenger ribonucleic acids; OCT: Optical coherence tomography; RVO: Retinal vein occlusion; VEGF: Vascular endothelial growth factor

Authors' contributions

Concept of design: NÖ, KÖ; Acquisition of data: HAG, NÖ, KÖ, NBG, TO; Analysis and interpretation of data: HAG, NÖ, MEY, ZO; Drafting the manuscript: NÖ, HAG, ZO; Critical revision of manuscript: NÖ, TO, NBG, MEY; Final approval: HAG, NÖ. All authors read and approved the final manuscript.

Competing interests
The authors declare that they have no competing interests.

Author details
[1]Department of Ophthalmology, Faculty of Medicine, Kırıkkale University, Kırıkkale, Turkey. [2]Department of Ophthalmology, Kudret Eye Hospital, Ankara, Turkey. [3]Department of Ophthalmology, Bayburt State Hospital, Bayburt, Turkey.

References
1. Kapoor KG, Wagner MG, Wagner AL. The sustained-release dexamethasone implant: expanding indications in vitreoretinal disease. Semin Ophthalmol. 2015;30(5–6):475–81.
2. London NJ, Chiang A, Haller JA. The dexamethasone drug delivery system: indications and evidence. Adv Ther. 2011;28(5):351–66.
3. Patil SD, Papadmitrakopoulos F, Burgess DJ. Concurrent delivery of dexamethasone and VEGF for localized inflammation control and angiogenesis. J Control Release. 2007;117(1):68–79.
4. Mutsaers HA, Tofighi R. Dexamethasone enhances oxidative stress-induced cell death in murine neural stem cells. Neurotox Res. 2012;22(2):127–3724.
5. Ruiz LM, Bedoya G, Salazar J, de García OD, Patiño PJ. Dexamethasone inhibits apoptosis of human neutrophils induced by reactive oxygen species. Inflammation. 2002;26(5):215–22.
6. Chen WL, Lin CT, Yao CC, Huang YH, Chou YB, Yin HS, Hu FR. In-vitro effects of dexamethasone on cellular proliferation, apoptosis, and Na+-K+-ATPase activity of bovine corneal endothelial cells. Ocul Immunol Inflamm. 2006; 14(4):215–23.
7. Stokes J, Noble J, Brett L, Phillips C, Seckl JR, O'Brien C, Andrew R. Distribution of glucocorticoid and mineralocorticoid receptors and 11beta-hydroxysteroid dehydrogenases in human and rat ocular tissues. Invest Ophthalmol Vis Sci. 2000;41(7):1629–38.
8. Kwak HW, D'Amico DJ. Evaluation of the retinal toxicity and pharmacokinetics of dexamethasone after intravitreal injection. Arch Ophthalmol. 1992;110(2):259–66.
9. Ilhan N, Coskun M, Ilhan O, Ayhan Tuzcu E, Daglioglu MC, Elbeyli A, Keskin U, Oksuz H. Effect of intravitreal injection of dexamethasone implant on corneal endothelium in macular edema due to retinal vein occlusion. Cutan Ocul Toxicol. 2015;34(4):294–7.
10. Rehak M, Wiedemann P. Retinal vein thrombosis: pathogenesis and managment. J Thromb Haemost. 2010;8(9):1886–94.
11. Hahn P, Fekrat S. Best practices for treatment of retinal vein occlusion. Curr Opin Ophthalmol. 2012;23(3):175–81.
12. Haller JA, Bandello F, Belfort R Jr, Blumenkranz MS, Gillies M, Heier J, Loewenstein A, Yoon YH, Jacques ML, Jiao J, Li XY, Whitcup SM, OZURDEX GENEVA Study Group. Randomized, sham-controlled trial of dexametasone intravitreal implant in patients with macular edema due to retinal vein occlusion. Ophthamology. 2010;117(6):1134–46.
13. Campochiaro PA. Anti-vascular endothelial growht factor treatment for retinal vein occlusions. Ophthalmologica. 2012;227(Suppl1):30–5.
14. Haller JA, Bandello F, Belfort R Jr, Blumenkranz MS, Gillies M, Heier J, Loewenstein A, Yoon YH, Jiao J, Li XY, Whitcup SM, for the OZURDEX GENEVA Study Group. Dexametasone intravitreal implant in patients with

maculer edema related to branch or central retinal vein occlusion twelve month study results. Ophtalmology. 2011;118(12):2453–60.
15. Chang Lin JE, Burke JA, Peng Q, Lin T, Orilla WC, Ghosn CR, Zhang KM, Kuppermann BD, Robinson MR, Whitcup SM, Welty DF. Pharmocokinetics and pharmocodynamics of a sustained release dexametasone intravitreal implant. Invest Opthalmol Vis Sci. 2011;52(7):80–6.
16. Fassbender Adeniran JM, Jusufbegovic D, Schaal S. Common and rare ocular side effects of the dexamethasone implant. Ocul Immunol Inflamm. 2016;5:1–7.
17. Park YW, Jeong MB, Lee ER, Lee Y, Ahn JS, Kim SH, Seo K. Acute changes in central corneal thickness according to experimental adjustment of intraocular pressure in normal canine eyes. J Vet Med Sci. 2013;75(11):1479–83.
18. Ytteborg J, Dohlman C. 1965. Corneal edema and intraocular pressure. II. Clinical results. Arch Ophthalmol. 1965;74(4):477–84.
19. Franco S, Lira M. Biomechanical properties of the cornea measured by the ocular response analyzer and their association with intraocular pressure and the central corneal curvature. Clin Exp Optom. 2009;92(6):469–75.
20. Zavala J, López Jaime GR, Rodríguez Barrientos CA, Valdez-Garcia J. Corneal endothelium: developmental strategies for regeneration. Eye (Lond). 2013; 27(5):579–88.
21. Guzel H, Bakbak B, Koylu MT, Gonul S, Ozturk B, Gedik S. The effect and safety of intravitreal injection of ranibizumab and bevacizumab on the corneal endothelium in the treatment of diabetic macular edema. Cutan Ocul Toxicol. 2017;36(1):5–8.
22. Pérez-Rico C, Benítez-Herreros J, Castro-Rebollo M, Gómez-Sangil Y, Germain F, Montes-Mollón MA, Teus MA. Effect of intravitreal ranibizumab on corneal endothelium in age-related macular degeneration. Cornea. 2010;29(8):849–52.
23. Michalska- Małecka K, Gaborek A, Nowak M, Halat T, Pawłowska M, Śpiewak D. Evaluation of the effectiveness and safety of glucocorticoids intravitreal implant therapy in macular edema due to retinal vein occlusion. Clin Interv Aging. 2016;23(11):699–705.
24. Solomon A, Solberg Y, Belkin M, Landshman N. Effect of corticosteroids on healing of the corneal endothelium in cats. Graefes Arch Clin Exp Ophthalmol. 1997;235(5):325–9.
25. Kang H, Lee MW, Byeon SH, Koh HJ, Lee SC, Kim M. The clinical outcomes of surgical management of anterior chamber migration of a dexamethasone implant (Ozurdex®). Graefes Arch Clin Exp Ophthalmol. 2017;255(9):1819–25.
26. Rahimy E N, Khurana RN. Anterior segment migration of dexamethasone implant: risk factors, complications, and management. Curr Opin Ophthalmol. 2017;28(3):246–51.

22

Assessment of the effect of age on macular layer thickness in a healthy Chinese cohort using spectral-domain optical coherence tomography

Qian Xu[1,2], Ying Li[1], Ying Cheng[1] and Yi Qu[1*]

Abstract

Background: To determine the effect of age on the thickness of individual retinal and choroidal vascular layers in the macula in an ophthalmologically healthy Chinese cohort by using spectral-domain optical coherence tomography (SD-OCT).

Methods: In all, 525 health eyes of 525 subjects were examined with SD-OCT. The instrument automatically obtained the regional retinal thickness of 8 layers. Subfoveal choroidal vascular layers' thickness was measured using enhanced depth imaging mode. The correlation of age with layer thickness measurements was determined.

Results: No age-associated variation was found on retinal thickness (RT) in the fovea; however, the foveal thickness of outer nuclear layer (ONL), retinal pigment epithelium (RPE) and vascular sublayers of the choroid decreased significantly with aging in this area ($P < 0.05$, respectively). Significant age-related reduction was seen in RT in the pericentral and peripheral rings ($P < 0.05$, respectively). The significant variation in thinning of the ganglion cell layer, inner plexiform layer, and ONL with aging is thought to be the main determinant of these results ($P < 0.05$, respectively). On the contrary, the RPE layout showed age-related thickening ($P < 0.05$, respectively) in the pericentral and peripheral regions.

Conclusions: The thickness of individual layers of the macula may be determinants of the age-related variations observed in the ophthalmologically healthy Chinese cohort, as assessed by SD-OCT examination.

Keywords: SD-OCT, Aging, Retina, Choroid, Layer thickness, Macula

Background

Detailed assessment of the macular area is critical in the diagnosis and management of a variety of ocular diseases. Traditional investigations such as fundus photography and fluorescein angiography can only provide qualitative and prospective information, therefore being subjective and relatively insensitive to small changes of the macula and unable to provide any cross-sectional or thickness-related data. The introduction of optical coherence tomography (OCT) has made it possible to noninvasively quantify macular structures in vivo with high resolution [1, 2]. In addition, because OCT is easy to use, ensures

patient comfort, and is economical, it has become an important diagnostic tool for fundus diseases.

Spectral domain-OCT (SD-OCT) is an advanced modification of time-domain OCT that provides better reproducibility for image acquisition, high-resolution three-dimensional images, and volumetric analyses [3, 4]. Techniques such as enhanced-depth imaging (EDI) permit improved analysis of the living choroid [5]. In addition, advances in layer segmentation algorithms have facilitated the automatic measurement of the thickness of individual retinal layers [6, 7].

Thickness measurement of the macula using SD-OCT has been shown to play an important role in understanding of the anatomy of individual macular layers, each of which has its own normal three-dimensional shape and may be affected in various ways by different diseases. Several studies

* Correspondence: yiqucn@sdu.edu.cn
[1]Department of Geriatrics, Qilu Hospital of Shandong University, No. 107, Wenhuaxi Road, Jinan 250012, Shandong, China
Full list of author information is available at the end of the article

have investigated morphological abnormalities of the macula in some ocular diseases by using SD-OCT. Macular thickening due to fluid accumulation is found in diabetic retinopathy and central serous chorioretinopathy (CSCR) [8–10]. The visual acuity of center-involved diabetic macular edema or CSCR eyes may be dependent on the disorganization of the retinal inner layers or the outer nuclear layer (ONL) in the fovea [8, 9]. Macular morphology is also an important parameter for monitoring and staging of glaucoma or age-related macular degeneration (AMD) [11, 12]. Moreover, clinically detected morphologic changes of different retinal layers were identified in many systemic diseases such as multiple sclerosis, [13] Parkinson's disease, [14] Alzheimer's disease, [15] and diabetes mellitus with preclinical retinopathy [16]. Therefore, measuring macular thickness by OCT is a powerful tool for physicians to evaluate progression of certain diseases, especially those that involve certain layers.

Recently, SD-OCT was used to study normal retinal and choroid thickness among subjects of different ethnicities, gender, and ages [17–20]. Age-related reduction in macular thickness was shown in a Caucasian and a Japanese population [18, 21]. However, the aforementioned reports were insufficient to facilitate the detailed analysis of the structure of specific retinal and choroidal layers. Moreover, to our best knowledge, there is no normative database available for the thickness of individual macular layers in the Chinese population.

Therefore, in this study, we used SD-OCT to measure the total retinal thickness (RT), the thickness of individual retinal layers of the macula that were divided into nine sectors, and the subfoveal choroidal thickness (SFCT) including vascular sublayers in 525 ophthalmologically healthy eyes in order to evaluate the effect of age on normal mean regional retinal and subfoveal choroidal layers on the macula.

Methods
Subjects
In this prospective observational study, self-reported, ophthalmologically healthy subjects of Chinese ethnicity aged ≥20 years were randomly recruited from May 2015 to December 2016. The study adhered to the tenets of the Declaration of Helsinki and was approved by the Ethics Committee of Qilu Hospital. Written consent was obtained from each subject.

All participants underwent a comprehensive ophthalmologic examination including best corrected visual acuity (BCVA), refraction, slit-lamp biomicroscopy, intraocular pressure (IOP) measurement by Goldmann applanation tonometry, and fundus photography obtained by two trained ophthalmologists. The inclusion criteria were as follows: BCVA≥20/25 Snellen (0.1 LogMAR), spherical equivalent refractive error not exceeding ±6.0 diopters, IOP < 21 mm

Hg, no history of any ocular abnormalities other than mild to moderate cataracts, no family history of glaucoma, and no systemic diseases such as hypertension, diabetes, or any other autoimmune or infectious diseases. One eye of each participant was randomly selected for OCT examination with the pupil dilated using 0.1% tropicamide.

Optical coherence tomography and layer segmentation
OCT measurements were performed with the Heidelberg Spectralis OCT (Heidelberg Engineering, Heidelberg, Germany). The instrument incorporates a real-time eye-tracking system that combines a confocal scanning laser ophthalmoscope and SD-OCT scanners to adjust for eye motion. The experienced operators performed all OCT scans under the same intensity of dim room lighting. If any scan was of insufficient quality, it was immediately repeated and reviewed until the image was satisfactory.

The macula was segmented into three concentric circles with diameters of 1 mm, 3 mm, and 6 mm, which were termed as the fovea, pericentral ring, and peripheral ring, respectively (Fig. 1a). Furthermore, the pericentral and peripheral rings were equally divided into four regions: superior, nasal, inferior, and temporal, according to the Early Treatment Diabetic Retinopathy Study (ETDRS). In all, 9 sectors were involved in the macular area (Fig. 1b and c). Each SD-OCT image was analyzed using an image segmentation algorithm, and thickness profiles of RT and eight individual retinal layers were automatically generated by the Spectralis OCT software (Fig. 2). The distance from the internal limiting membrane to the outer border of Bruch's membrane or external limiting membrane was taken as the RT or inner retinal thickness (IRT), and the individual retinal layers were identified as follows (from inner to outer surface): retinal nerve fiber layer (RNFL), ganglion cell layer (GCL), inner plexiform layer (IPL), inner nuclear layer (INL), outer plexiform layer (OPL), ONL, photoreceptor layer with retinal pigment epithelium (PRL + RPE), and the RPE alone.

SFCT was determined from images acquired by the Heidelberg Spectralis OCT device with enabled EDI mode and analyzed with the OCT-supplied software (Fig. 3). High-quality horizontal and vertical line scans centered on the fovea were obtained. In the fovea, the SFCT was manually measured from the hyperreflective line of the Bruch's membrane to the innermost surface of the choroido-scleral interface [5]. The thickness of Haller's layer was measured from the inner border of the choroido-scleral interface junction to the innermost point of the selected large choroidal vessel that was located close to the choroido-scleral border and within the closest proximity to the locations of the choroidal thickness measurement lines. The difference of these measurements was considered as the depth of the choriocapillaris/Sattler's layer [10]. Means were calculated as the average thicknesses measured from horizontal and vertical sections.

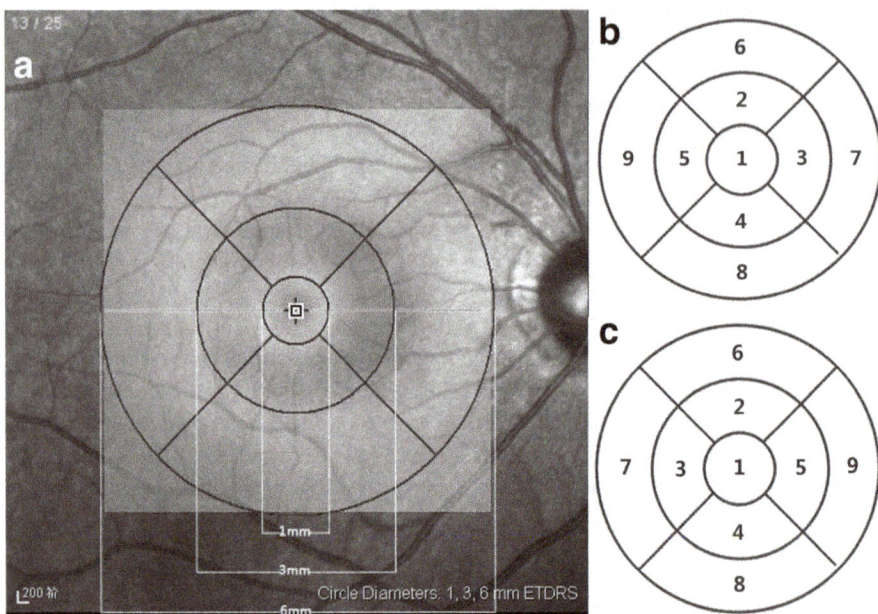

Fig. 1 Early Treatment Diabetic Retinopathy Study (ETDRS) grid. **a** Delineation of the nine macular sectors, according to the ETDRS, within which we measured macular layer thickness. **b** Nine ETDRS sectors in Right eye. **c** Nine ETDRS sectors in Left eye

Statistical analysis

All data were described as mean ± standard deviation (SD) where applicable. Statistical analyses were performed with commercial statistical software (IBM SPSS Statistics 21; SPSS Inc., Chicago, IL). The partial correlation test was used to determine the effect of age on individual layers' thicknesses with spherical equivalent and IOP as confounders that were known to influence OCT thickness measurements [17, 22]. Finally, simple linear regression analysis was performed for the layer whose thickness correlated significantly with age. P values < 0.05 were considered statistically significant.

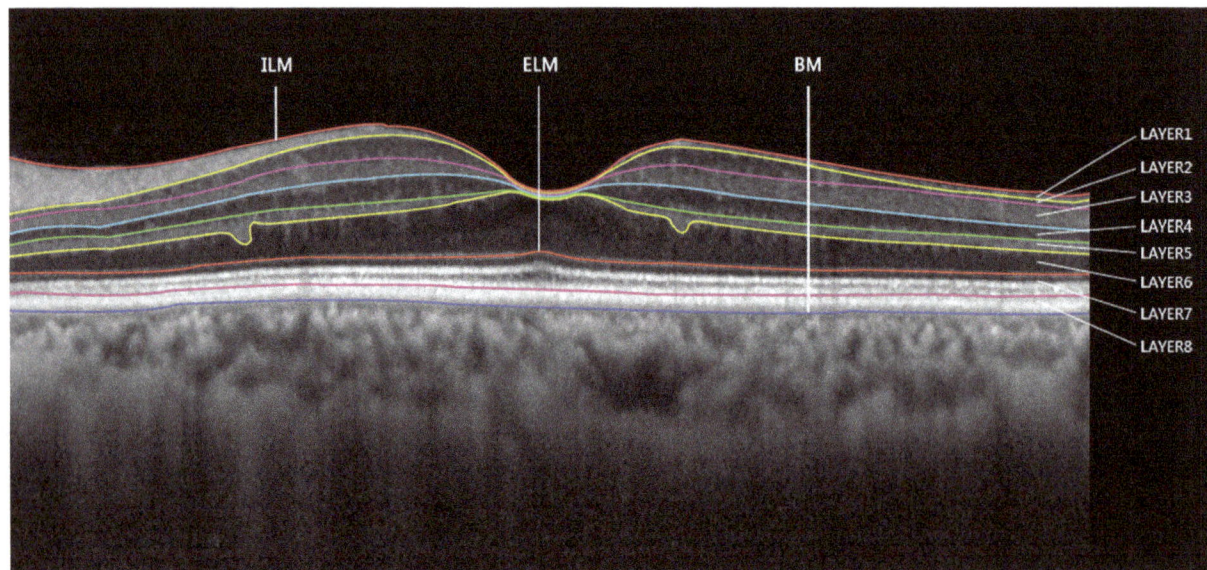

Fig. 2 An automated method (with manual correction) was used to segment retinal boundaries in each of the averaged B-scans in the spectral-domain optical coherence tomography examination. The individual retinal layers were identified as follows (from inner to outer surface): (Layer 1) Retinal nerve fiber layer (RNFL), (Layer 2) Ganglion cell layer (GCL), (Layer 3) Inner plexiform layer (IPL), (Layer 4) Inner nuclear layer (INL), (Layer 5) Outer plexiform layer (OPL), (Layer 6) Outer nuclear layer (ONL), (Layer 7) Photoreceptor layers (PRL), (Layer 8) Retinal pigment epithelium (RPE). Abbreviations: ILM: internal limiting membrane, BM: Bruch's membrane, ELM: external limiting membrane

Assessment of the effect of age on macular layer thickness in a healthy Chinese cohort...

143

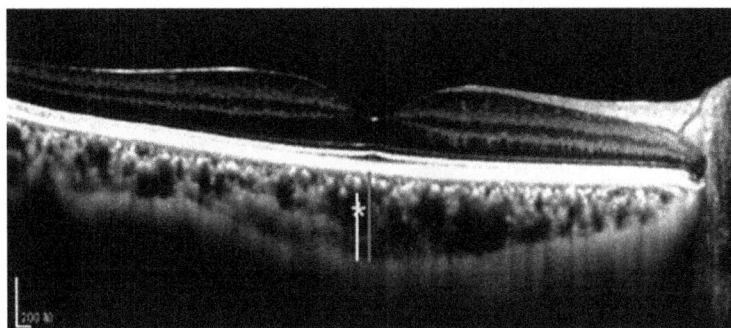

Fig. 3 Choroidal vasculature measurements. The vertical red bars delineate the subfoveal choroidal thickness from the retinal pigment epithelium to the choroido-scleral interface in the fovea. The yellow bars delineate the Haller's layer was measured from the inner border of the choroido-scleral interface to the innermost point of the selected large choroidal vessel. Asterisk is example of large choroidal vessel

Results

The study included 525 ophthalmologic healthy eyes of 525 subjects ranging in age from 20 to 87 years (mean age, 44.82 ± 17.74 years). Demographic and ocular features of the study population are presented in Table 1.

The mean thickness of RT and eight individual retinal layers in 9 macular EDTRS sectors of all participants are presented in Appendix: Table 6. IRT was excluded owing to similar results as that of RT (data not shown). After adjusting for spherical equivalence and IOP, no significant correlation was found on foveal RT ($P = 0.54$) (Table 2). In the fovea, the ONL and RPE correlated negatively with age (Correlation = -0.15, $P < 0.01$; Correlation = -0.09, $P = 0.03$, respectively) (Table 2); however, the RNFL, INL, and OPL correlated positively with age (Correlation = 0.13, 0.30, 0.10, respectively; all $P < 0.05$) (Table 2). Regression analysis indicated an increase for the RNFL boundary as well as the INL boundary and a loss for the RPE boundary with increasing age (Beta = 0.13, 0.10, -0.14, respectively; all $P < 0.05$) (Table 2).

As shown in Table 3, the total SFCT, thickness of the large choroidal vessel layer (Haller' s layer), choriocapillaris layer and Sattler' s layer (medium choroidal vessel layer) in the fovea showed significant negative correlation with age (Correlation = -0.55, -0.42, -0.46, respectively; all $P < 0.05$). In addition, our study found that SFCT and the thickness of

choroidal vascular sublayers decreased linearly with age (Beta = -0.61, -0.47, -0.52, respectively) (all $P < 0.05$).

Significant age-related reductions were seen for the RT, GCL, and IPL in the pericentral and peripheral rings (all $P < 0.05$; Tables 4 and 5). Moreover, the OPL of the temporal sector, ONL except the temporal sector in the pericentral ring (both $P < 0.05$; Table 4), RNFL of both superior and inferior sectors, INL except the superior sector, ONL of all sectors, and PRL + RPE of the inferior sector in the peripheral ring (all $P < 0.05$; Table 5) showed significant decreases with respect to age. However, significant age-related increase was demonstrated in the RNFL of the temporal sector, INL and OPL of the nasal sector, RPE of all sectors in the pericentral ring (all $P < 0.05$; Table 4), RNFL of the temporal sector, OPL of the nasal sector, and RPE of the superior and temporal sectors in the peripheral ring (all $P < 0.05$; Table 5).

Discussion

In this study, consistent with previous reports, [23–25] no significant correlation was found between age and foveal RT. However, the ONL, RPE and choroid vascular sublayers in this region showed significant age-related thinning, accompanied with age-related thickness of RNFL, INL, and OPL. To our best knowledge, we believe this is the first study to report the detailed age-related changes of foveal microstructure. On comparing with total thickness,

Table 1 Demographic and Ocular Features of Included Subjects

Age groups (y)	Number	Men/Women (ratio)	Mean Refractive Error (diopters)	Mean Intraocular Pressure (mm Hg)	Mean Age (y)
20–29	176	90/86(1.05)	-1.93 ± 1.71	14.1 ± 2.4	25.71 ± 1.52
30–39	50	27/23(1.17)	-0.74 ± 1.19	14.3 ± 2.1	35.38 ± 3.13
40–49	108	68/40(1.7)	-0.36 ± 1.29	13.8 ± 2.3	46.07 ± 2.33
50–59	79	41/38(1.08)	-0.54 ± 1.54	14.6 ± 2.1	53.90 ± 2.51
60–69	60	32/28(1.14)	0.08 ± 0.59	14.5 ± 2.6	64.53 ± 3.12
70+	52	27/25(1.08)	-0.04 ± 0.91	14.2 ± 2.0	79.40 ± 5.25
Total	525	285/240(1.19)	-0.87 ± 1.60	14.3 ± 2.3	44.82 ± 17.74

Mean refers to mean ± standard deviation

Table 2 Correlations of Age with Regional Retinal Thickness of Foveal Layers

Retinal Layer	RT	RNFL	GCL	IPL	INL	OPL	ONL	PRL + RPE	RPE
P Value[a]	0.54	< 0.01[c]	0.36	0.10	< 0.01[c]	0.02[c]	< 0.01[c]	0.77	0.03[c]
Correlation[a]	0.03	0.13	− 0.04	0.07	0.30	0.10	−0.15	− 0.01	− 0.09
P Value[b]	0.28	< 0.01[c]	0.15	0.25	< 0.01[c]	0.63	0.07	0.68	< 0.01[c]
Beta[b]	0.05	0.13	− 0.06	0.05	0.10	0.02	−0.08	−0.02	− 0.14

Abbreviations: RT Retinal thickness, RNFL Retinal nerve fiber layer, GCL Ganglion cell layer, IPL Inner plexiform layer, INL Inner nuclear layer, OPL Outer plexiform layer, ONL Outer nuclear layer, PRL Photoreceptor layer, RPE Retinal pigment epithelium, IOP Intraocular pressure
[a]Partial correlation coefficient after adjusting for spherical equivalent and IOP
[b]Simple linear regression analysis
[c]Statistically significant

assessment of macular layers provides a higher diagnostic power. The most significant observation herein was the age-related thinning of foveal ONL, RPE and choroid measurements even in ophthalmologically healthy subjects, which could be a potential anatomic predisposing factor for monitoring the age-related diseases in this eye region. The atrophy of RPE and choroid layer in the central retina is a feature of early/intermediate AMD, the incidence of which is increased with age. A 32% loss in the RPE/PRL thickness and a 22% loss in ONL thickness were found over the drusen as compared to the adjacent drusen-free regions in AMD patients [26]. The choriocapillaris degenerates in early stages of AMD, before loss of photoreceptor cells or RPE [12]. Although AMD is a complicated process that involves both age-related change and tissue damage caused by multiple stresses, age plays the most important role [27]. Functionally normal RPE and choroidal vasculature play a critical role in maintaining retinal health. Thinner RPE and choroid layer thickness may be anatomic features lead to increased risk in AMD. Our results showed that assessment of the foveal layer thickness with OCT in ophthalmologically healthy aged subjects' eyes may lead to early identification and treatment of AMD. Moreover, further investigations are needed on the mechanism of age-related variations of the ONL, RPE, RNFL, INL, and OPL in the fovea.

We have observed significant age-associated reductions of RT in the pericentral and peripheral rings that were distinct from the foveal results; these results were consistent with previous studies [19, 28, 29]. Notably, age-related changes of GCL, IPL, and ONL in the region likely contribute to this result. Parikh et al. [30] reported that age was related to the loss of neurons or glial cells in the inner retina, which may be responsible for the SD-OCT−examination outcome in this area.

Several studies have shown that assessment of GCL thickness could be a surrogate method to evaluate glaucomatous damage [31]. In this study, the observed age-related variation in GCL thickness in this ophthalmologically healthy cohort is a reminder that GCL thinning requires more accurate quantification before widespread adoption as a surrogate for glaucoma assessment.

The thickness of RPE in the pericentral and peripheral regions was significantly increased with aging. Many pathological changes led to the thickening of the RPE, which included the density of residual bodies and accumulation of lipofuscin, accumulation of basal deposits on or within the Bruch's membrane, formation of drusen, and thickening of the Bruch's membrane [32]. The age-related variation of RPE in the macular region requires future investigation.

This study has some limitations. The small sample size might have introduced some bias. Our data are limited to Chinese ethnicity and need to be tested in other ethnic groups in the future.

Conclusions

Using SD-OCT, we assessed age-related thinning of ONL, RPE, and choroidal layers accompanied with thickened RNFL, INL, and OPL of the fovea in an ophthalmologically healthy Chinese cohort. The variations of individual layers in the fovea may be related to age-independent RT. It is speculated that the age-related reductions of RT in the pericentral and peripheral rings were associated with age-related thinning of GCL, IPL and ONL in these regions. Regular monitoring of the macular architecture using SD-OCT in ophthalmologically healthy people, especially among the aged population, should be considered in future evaluations.

Table 3 Correlations of Age with Thickness of Suboveal Choroidal Layers

Suboveal Choroidal Layer	Thickness (mean ± SD, µm)	P Value[a]	Correlation[a]	P Value[c]	Beta[c]
Total Choroidal Thickness	225.02 ± 35.71	< 0.01[b]	− 0.55	< 0.01[b]	− 0.61
Haller's Layer Thickness	157.62 ± 26.57	< 0.01[b]	− 0.42	< 0.01[b]	− 0.47
Choriocapillaris /Sattler's layer Thickness	67.41 ± 17.83	< 0.01[b]	− 0.46	< 0.01[b]	− 0.52

[a]Partial correlation coefficient after adjusting for spherical equivalent and IOP
[b]Statistically significant
[c]Simple linear regression analysis

Table 4 Correlations of Age with Thickness of Macular Retinal Layers in Sectors of the Pericentral ring

Retinal Layer	Pericentral Superior				Pericentral Nasal				Pericentral Inferior				Pericentral Temporal			
	P Value[a]	Correlation[a]	P Value[b]	Beta[b]	P Value[a]	Correlation[a]	P Value[b]	Beta[b]	P Value[a]	Correlation[a]	P Value[b]	Beta[b]	P Value[a]	Correlation[a]	P Value[b]	Beta[b]
RT	< 0.01[c]	−0.27	< 0.01[c]	−0.24	<.01[c]	−.21	< 0.01[c]	−0.16	< 0.01[c]	−.26	<.01[c]	−.23	<.01[c]	−0.25	< 0.01[c]	−0.19
RNFL	0.72	−0.02	0.51	−0.03	0.74	0.01	0.66	0.02	0.17	−0.06	0.27	−0.05	< 0.01[c]	0.24	< 0.01[c]	0.31
GCL	< 0.01[c]	−0.31	< 0.01[c]	−0.32	< 0.01[c]	−0.24	< 0.01[c]	−0.24	< 0.01[c]	−0.32	< 0.01[c]	−0.34	< 0.01[c]	−0.35	< 0.01[c]	−0.37
IPL	< 0.01[c]	−0.37	< 0.01[c]	−0.39	< 0.01[c]	−0.33	< 0.01[c]	−0.33	< 0.01[c]	−0.36	< 0.01[c]	−0.37	< 0.01[c]	−0.28	< 0.01[c]	−0.29
INL	0.60	−0.02	0.20	0.06	< 0.01[c]	0.18	< 0.01[c]	0.27	0.29	−0.05	0.75	−0.01	0.08	−0.08	1.00	0.00
OPL	0.63	0.02	0.08	0.08	< 0.01[c]	0.18	< 0.01[c]	0.19	0.49	0.03	0.85	−0.01	< 0.01[c]	−0.13	< 0.01[c]	−0.19
ONL	< 0.01[c]	−0.13	< 0.01[c]	−0.14	< 0.01[c]	−0.28	< 0.01[c]	−0.26	0.01[c]	−0.11	0.36	−0.04	0.27	−0.05	0.39	0.04
PRL + RPE	0.16	0.06	0.31	0.01	0.91	−0.01	0.64	0.02	0.76	0.01	0.40	0.04	0.18	0.06	0.32	0.09
RPE	< 0.01[c]	0.19	< 0.01[c]	0.23	0.01[c]	0.12	0.01[c]	0.11	<.01[c]	.18	<.01[c]	0.23	< 0.01[c]	0.20	< 0.01[c]	0.21

Abbreviations: RT Retinal thickness, *RNFL* Retinal nerve fiber layer, *GCL* Ganglion cell layer, *IPL* Inner plexiform layer, *INL* Inner nuclear layer, *OPL* Outer plexiform layer, *ONL* Outer nuclear layer, *PRL* Photoreceptor layer, *RPE* Retinal pigment epithelium; IOP, Intraocular pressure

[a] Partial correlation coefficient after adjusting for spherical equivalent and IOP

[b] Simple linear regression analysis

[c] Statistically significant

Table 5 Correlations of Age with Thickness of Macular Retinal Layers in Sectors of the Peripheral ring

Retinal Layer	Pericentral Superior				Pericentral Nasal				Pericentral Inferior				Pericentral Temporal			
	P Value[a]	Correlation[a]	P Value[b]	Beta[b]	P Value[a]	Correlation[a]	P Value[b]	Beta[b]	P Value[a]	Correlation[a]	P Value[b]	Beta[b]	P Value[a]	Correlation[a]	P Value[b]	Beta[b]
RT	< 0.01[c]	− 0.37	< 0.01[c]	− 0.37	< 0.01[c]	− 0.23	< 0.01[c]	− 0.22	< 0.01[c]	− 0.31	< 0.01[c]	− 0.32	< 0.01[c]	− 0.28	< 0.01[c]	− 0.25
RNFL	0.01[c]	− 0.11	< 0.01[c]	− 0.18	0.19	− 0.06	< 0.01[c]	− 0.12	0.02[c]	− 0.10	< 0.01[c]	− 0.15	0.01[c]	0.11	< 0.01[c]	0.15
GCL	< 0.01[c]	− 0.39	< 0.01[c]	− 0.37	< 0.01[c]	− 0.31	< 0.01[c]	− 0.29	< 0.01[c]	− 0.32	< 0.01[c]	− 0.33	< 0.01[c]	− 0.36	< 0.01[c]	− 0.36
IPL	< 0.01[c]	− 0.40	< 0.01[c]	− 0.40	< 0.01[c]	− 0.35	< 0.01[c]	− 0.35	< 0.01[c]	− 0.26	< 0.01[c]	− 0.28	< 0.01[c]	− 0.28	< 0.01[c]	− 0.27
INL	0.08	− 0.16	0.01[c]	− 0.11	< 0.01[c]	− 0.18	< 0.01[c]	− 0.18	< 0.01[c]	− 0.17	< 0.01[c]	− 0.14	< 0.01[c]	− 0.33	< 0.01[c]	− 0.29
OPL	0.33	0.04	0.02[c]	0.11	< 0.01[c]	0.23	< 0.01[c]	0.30	0.36	0.04	0.29	0.05	0.41	− 0.04	0.77	0.01
ONL	< 0.01[c]	− 0.28	< 0.01[c]	− 0.29	< 0.01[c]	− 0.36	< 0.01[c]	− 0.39	< 0.01[c]	− 0.18	< 0.01[c]	− 0.16	< 0.01[c]	− 0.25	< 0.01[c]	− 0.24
PRL + RPE	0.87	− 0.01	0.59	0.02	0.10	− 0.07	0.25	− 0.05	0.04[c]	− 0.09	0.05	− 0.09	0.34	0.04	0.03	0.10
RPE	0.04[c]	0.09	< 0.01[c]	0.16	0.45	0.03	0.10	0.07	0.80	0.01	0.22	0.05	< 0.01c	0.20	< 0.01[c]	0.24

Abbreviations: RT Retinal thickness, *RNFL* Retinal nerve fiber layer, *GCL* Ganglion cell layer, *IPL* Inner plexiform layer, *INL* Inner nuclear layer, *OPL* Outer plexiform layer, *ONL* Outer nuclear layer, *PRL* Photoreceptor layer, *RPE* Retinal pigment epithelium, *IOP* Intraocular pressure

[a]Partial correlation coefficient after adjusting for spherical equivalent and IOP

[b]Simple linear regression analysis

[c]Statistically significant

Appendix

Table 6 Mean Thickness of Retina and eight individual retinal layers in nine Macular Sectors

Retinal Layer	fovea	Pericentral Superior	Pericentral Nasal	Pericentral Inferior	Pericentral Temporal	Peripheral Superior	Peripheral Nasal	Peripheral Inferior	Peripheral Temporal
RT	257.04±18.85	339.37±17.56	339.58±17.22	335.10±16.97	324.92±15.82	300.39±15.80	317.43±21.96	287.16±15.33	283.77±15.41
RNFL	10.78±2.24	23.44±3.68	20.11±2.32	24.50±3.10	16.82±1.33	37.52±5.14	46.12±6.85	38.93±5.70	19.21±8.37
GCL	12.31±3.20	52.03±5.76	50.12 ±6.04	51.33±5.33	46.66±5.51	36.58±3.88	40.48±4.26	34.03±3.69	36.92±4.74
IPL	18.28±2.85	41.18±3.82	42.34±3.84	40.90±3.67	41.01±3.64	29.67±2.96	31.20±3.19	27.81±3.06	32.61±3.00
INL	15.27±4.63	39.75±4.47	38.48±4.09	40.46±4.23	36.48±3.84	32.33±3.19	35.07±3.03	32.09±3.34	33.90±2.63
OPL	23.48±6.08	32.86±8.44	31.87±8.27	36.17±9.90	31.14±6.02	26.15±2.91	28.20±3.47	27.02±3.12	26.37±2.58
ONL	88.44±11.40	67.48±12.72	72.52±11.54	60.45±12.68	70.02±9.31	58.15±7.73	55.87±7.57	49.58±7.16	55.80±6.33
PRL+RPE	90.19±4.40	82.74±3.15	83.94±3.27	81.32±3.26	82.60±3.12	79.80±3.22	79.84±2.69	77.81±2.84	79.84±2.69
RPE	17.5±2.20	16.16±1.89	16.30±1.99	15.36±1.76	15.10±1.60	14.29±1.37	14.18±1.47	13.70±1.76	13.50±1.38

Values are mean ± SD (μm). RT, retinal thickness; RNFL, retinal nerve fiber layer; GCL, ganglion cell layer; IPL, inner plexiform layer; INL, inner nuclear layer; OPL, outer plexiform layer; ONL, outer nuclear layer; PRL, photoreceptor layer; RPE, retinal pigment epithelium.

Abbreviations
AMD: Age-related macular degeneration; BCVA: Best corrected visual acuity; BM: Bruch's membrane; CSCR: Central serous chorioretinopathy; EDI: Enhanced-depth imaging; ELM: External limiting membrane; ETDRS: Early Treatment Diabetic Retinopathy Study; GCL: Ganglion cell layer; ILM: internal limiting membrane; INL: Inner nuclear layer; IOP: Intraocular pressure; IPL: Inner plexiform layer; IRT: Inner retinal thickness; OCT: Optical coherence tomography; ONL: Outer nuclear layer; OPL: Outer plexiform layer; PRL: Photoreceptor layer; RNFL: Retinal nerve fiber layer; RPE: Retinal pigment epithelium; RT: Retinal thickness; SD-OCT: Spectral-domain optical coherence tomography; SFCT: Subfoveal choroidal thickness

Acknowledgements
The authors thank the subjects who participated in the study. We gratefully acknowledge those help us to prepare this research.

Funding
This study was partly supported by National Natural Science foundation of China (31570789), Fundamental Research Funds of Shandong University (2014JC015), Scientific & Technologic Project of Shandong Province (2014GSF118128). Natural Science foundation of Shandong Province (ZR2013HZ003).

Authors' contributions
YQ, QX, YL and YC conceived of and designed the experimental protocol. QX and YL collected the data. QX, YL and YC were involved in the analysis. QX wrote the first draft of the manuscript. YQ and QX reviewed and revised the manuscript and produced the final version. YQ, QX, YL and YC read and approved the final manuscript.

Competing interests
The authors declare that they have no competing interests.

Author details
[1]Department of Geriatrics, Qilu Hospital of Shandong University, No. 107, Wenhuaxi Road, Jinan 250012, Shandong, China. [2]Department of Ophthalmology, The Central Hospital of Taian, Tai'an 271000, Shandong, China.

References
1. Swanson EA, Izatt JA, Hee MR, Huang D, Lin CP, Schuman JS, Puliafito CA, Fujimoto JG. In vivo retinal imaging by optical coherence tomography. Opt Lett. 1993;18:1864–6.
2. Wang J, Gao X, Huang W, Wang W, Chen S, Du S, Li X, Zhang X. Swept-source optical coherence tomography imaging of macular retinal and choroidal structures in healthy eyes. BMC Ophthalmol. 2015;15:122.
3. Grover S, Murthy RK, Brar VS, Chalam KV. Comparison of retinal thickness in normal eyes using stratus and Spectralis optical coherence tomography. Invest Ophthalmol Vis Sci. 2010;51:2644–7.
4. Hirasawa H, Tomidokoro A, Araie M, Konno S, Saito H, Iwase A, Shirakashi M, Abe H, Ohkubo S, Sugiyama K, et al. Peripapillary retinal nerve fiber layer thickness determined by spectral-domain optical coherence tomography in ophthalmologically normal eyes. Arch Ophthalmol. 2010;128:1420–6.
5. Huang W, Wang W, Zhou M, Chen S, Gao X, Fan Q, Ding X, Zhang X. Peripapillary choroidal thickness in healthy Chinese subjects. BMC Ophthalmol. 2013;13:23.
6. Spaide RF, Koizumi H, Pozzoni MC. Enhanced depth imaging spectral-domain optical coherence tomography. Am J Ophthalmol. 2008;146:496–500.
7. Lang A, Carass A, Hauser M, Sotirchos ES, Calabresi PA, Ying HS, Prince JL. Retinal layer segmentation of macular OCT images using boundary classification. Biomed Opt Express. 2013;4:1133–52.
8. Matsumoto H, Sato T, Kishi S. Outer nuclear layer thickness at the fovea determines visual outcomes in resolved central serous chorioretinopathy. Am J Ophthalmol. 2009;148:105–10. e101
9. Sun JK, Lin MM, Lammer J, Prager S, Sarangi R, Silva PS, Aiello LP. Disorganization of the retinal inner layers as a predictor of visual acuity in eyes with center-involved diabetic macular edema. JAMA Ophthalmol. 2014; 132:1309–16.
10. Chung YR, Kim JW, Choi SY, Park SW, Kim JH, Lee K. Subfoveal Choroidal Thickness And Vascular Diameter In Active And Resolved Central Serous Chorioretinopathy. Retina. 2018;38:102–107.
11. Zucchiatti I, Parodi MB, Pierro L, Cicinelli MV, Gagliardi M, Castellino N, Bandello F. Macular ganglion cell complex and retinal nerve Fiber layer comparison in different stages of age-related macular degeneration. Am J Ophthalmol. 2015;160:602–607 e601.
12. Chirco KR, Sohn EH, Stone EM, Tucker BA, Mullins RF. Structural and molecular changes in the aging choroid: implications for age-related macular degeneration. Eye (Lond). 2017;31:10–25.
13. Garcia-Martin E, Polo V, Larrosa JM, Marques ML, Herrero R, Martin J, Ara JR, Fernandez J, Pablo LE. Retinal layer segmentation in patients with multiple sclerosis using spectral domain optical coherence tomography. Ophthalmology. 2014;121:573–9.
14. Sari ES, Koc R, Yazici A, Sahin G, Ermis SS. Ganglion cell-inner plexiform layer thickness in patients with Parkinson disease and association with disease severity and duration. J Neuroophthalmol. 2015;35:117–21.
15. Liu D, Zhang L, Li Z, Zhang X, Wu Y, Yang H, Min B, Zhang X, Ma D, Lu Y. Thinner changes of the retinal nerve fiber layer in patients with mild cognitive impairment and Alzheimer's disease. BMC Neurol. 2015;15:14.

16. Peng PH, Lin HS, Lin S. Nerve fibre layer thinning in patients with preclinical retinopathy. Can J Ophthalmol. 2009;44:417–22.

17. Song WK, Lee SC, Lee ES, Kim CY, Kim SS. Macular thickness variations with sex, age, and axial length in healthy subjects: a spectral domain-optical coherence tomography study. Invest Ophthalmol Vis Sci. 2010;51:3913–8.

18. Ooto S, Hangai M, Yoshimura N. Effects of sex and age on the normal retinal and choroidal structures on optical coherence tomography. Curr Eye Res. 2015;40:213–25.

19. Eriksson U, Alm A. Macular thickness decreases with age in normal eyes: a study on the macular thickness map protocol in the stratus OCT. Br J Ophthalmol. 2009;93:1448–52.

20. Alasil T, Wang K, Keane PA, Lee H, Baniasadi N, de Boer JF, Chen TC. Analysis of normal retinal nerve fiber layer thickness by age, sex, and race using spectral domain optical coherence tomography. J Glaucoma. 2013;22:532–41.

21. Ikuno Y, Kawaguchi K, Nouchi T, Yasuno Y. Choroidal thickness in healthy Japanese subjects. Invest Ophthalmol Vis Sci. 2010;51:2173–6.

22. Lim MC, Hoh ST, Foster PJ, Lim TH, Chew SJ, Seah SK, Aung T. Use of optical coherence tomography to assess variations in macular retinal thickness in myopia. Invest Ophthalmol Vis Sci. 2005;46:974–8.

23. Demirkaya N, van Dijk HW, van Schuppen SM, Abramoff MD, Garvin MK, Sonka M, Schlingemann RO, Verbraak FD. Effect of age on individual retinal layer thickness in normal eyes as measured with spectral-domain optical coherence tomography. Invest Ophthalmol Vis Sci. 2013;54:4934–40.

24. Grover S, Murthy RK, Brar VS, Chalam KV. Normative data for macular thickness by high-definition spectral-domain optical coherence tomography (spectralis). Am J Ophthalmol. 2009;148:266–71.

25. Huang D, Swanson EA, Lin CP, Schuman JS, Stinson WG, Chang W, Hee MR, Flotte T, Gregory K, Puliafito CA, et al. Optical coherence tomography. Science. 1991;254:1178–81.

26. Rogala J, Zangerl B, Assaad N, Fletcher EL, Kalloniatis M, Nivison-Smith L. In vivo quantification of retinal changes associated with drusen in age-related macular degeneration. Invest Ophthalmol Vis Sci. 2015;56:1689–700.

27. La Torre G, Pacella E, Saulle R, Giraldi G, Pacella F, Lenzi T, Mastrangelo O, Mirra F, Aloe G, Turchetti P, et al. The synergistic effect of exposure to alcohol, tobacco smoke and other risk factors for age-related macular degeneration. Eur J Epidemiol. 2013;28:445–6.

28. Ooto S, Hangai M, Tomidokoro A, Saito H, Araie M, Otani T, Kishi S, Matsushita K, Maeda N, Shirakashi M, et al. Effects of age, sex, and axial length on the three-dimensional profile of normal macular layer structures. Invest Ophthalmol Vis Sci. 2011;52:8769–79.

29. Sung KR, Wollstein G, Bilonick RA, Townsend KA, Ishikawa H, Kagemann L, Noecker RJ, Fujimoto JG, Schuman JS. Effects of age on optical coherence tomography measurements of healthy retinal nerve fiber layer, macula, and optic nerve head. Ophthalmology. 2009;116:1119–24.

30. Parikh RS, Parikh SR, Sekhar GC, Prabakaran S, Babu JG, Thomas R. Normal age-related decay of retinal nerve fiber layer thickness. Ophthalmology. 2007;114:921–6.

31. Distante P, Lombardo S, Verticchio Vercellin AC, Raimondi M, Rolando M, Tinelli C, Milano G. Structure/function relationship and retinal ganglion cells counts to discriminate glaucomatous damages. BMC Ophthalmol. 2015;15:185.

32. Bonilha VL. Age and disease-related structural changes in the retinal pigment epithelium. Clin Ophthalmol. 2008;2:413–24.

23

Outcomes of complex Descemet Stripping Endothelial Keratoplasty performed by cornea fellows

Jacquelyn Daubert[1], Terrence P. O'Brien[1], Eldad Adler[1] and Oriel Spierer[1,2]*

Abstract

Background: A major obstacle that academic institutions face is the steep learning curve for cornea fellows initially learning to perform Descemet Stripping Endothelial Keratoplasty (DSEK). The purpose of this study is to evaluate the outcomes of complex DSEK performed by cornea fellow supervised by an attending surgeon at an academic institution.

Methods: Patients who underwent a complex DSEK procedure performed by a cornea fellow during the years 2009-2013 were included. All the surgeries were supervised by the same cornea attending. All patients had a minimum follow-up of 6 months. Charts were reviewed for demographic data, intraoperative and postoperative complications and clinical outcomes. Corneal graft survival was calculated using the Kaplan-Meier analysis.

Results: Fifty-seven eyes of 55 patients (mean age 77.5 ± 8.5 years) were included in the study with a mean follow-up time of 16.4 ± 15.6 months. Previous graft failure, presence of a tube and history of trabeculectomy were the leading diagnoses to define the surgery as complex. No intraoperative complications occurred. In 21.1% of cases a corneal graft detachment was documented in the first postoperative day. Mean visual acuity improved from 1.06 LogMAR (20/230) preoperatively to 0.39 LogMAR (20/50, $p < 0.001$) by the sixth postoperative month and to 0.52 LogMAR (20/65, $p < 0.001$) at the last follow-up visit. Graft failure rate was 29.8%. Kaplan-Meier analysis found a 67.2% graft survival rate at 20 months.

Conclusions: Complex DSEK can be performed successfully with an acceptable postoperative complication rate by cornea fellows during their training period when supervised by an experienced attending.

Keywords: Cornea fellows, Descemet Stripping Endothelial Keratoplasty, DSEK, Ophthalmology fellowship training

Background

Descemet Stripping Endothelial Keratoplasty (DSEK) has been adopted worldwide as an alternative to penetrating keratoplasty in corneal pathologies restricted to the endothelium such as Fuchs endothelial dystrophy and pseudophakic bullous keratopathy. In these cases, DSEK has shown overall better results than penetrating keratoplasty [1] including a faster visual recovery, decreased astigmatic change, and reduced risk of suture related complications [2, 3].

DSEK has its limitations in complex cases such as in the presence of previous tube shunt procedures, trabeculectomies and previously failed DSEK or penetrating keratoplasty grafts [4–8]. For patients with tube shunts, the tube placement in the anterior chamber may interfere with the surgical placement of the corneal graft and allow air to escape causing possible graft detachment in the first postoperative day [4]. In DSEK performed on patients with tube shunts, the tube needs to be revised to provide enough room for the donor graft in the anterior chamber and to prevent future trauma to the endothelium [4]. Early graft detachment is also a concern in trabeculectomies, as the air can leak through the sclerotomy [5]. Patients with trabeculectomies and tube shunts usually have advanced optic nerve glaucomatous

* Correspondence: oriels1@yahoo.com
[1]Bascom Palmer Eye Institute, University of Miami Miller School of Medicine, Palm Beach Gardens, FL 33418, USA
[2]Department of Ophthalmology, Wolfson Medical Center, Sackler Faculty of Medicine, Tel Aviv University, Tel Aviv, Israel

damage. An elevation in intraocular pressure after DSEK surgery or during the procedure with the air bubble injection could cause loss of vision in these susceptible patients [5]. DSEK performed after a failed penetrating keratoplasty or failed DSEK is a technically challenging procedure and tends to have higher rates of postoperative complications [4, 6, 7].

There have been several studies evaluating resident and fellow outcomes during various ophthalmology surgical procedures [9]. When it comes to cataract surgery, fellows and residents have a higher complication rate as compared to the attending surgeons [10–12]. The major obstacle that academic institutions face is the steep learning curve for cornea fellows initially learning to perform DSEK [13]. Hashemi et al. concluded that DSEK can be performed successfully by cornea fellows in their training period with acceptable outcomes [14]. In the United States only one study, done by Chen et al., evaluated DSEK outcomes when performed by fellows as compared to an attending surgeon. The authors found no difference in visual outcome or endothelial cell loss between DSEK done by an experienced cornea surgeon and cornea fellow under the supervision of an attending surgeon [1]. They raised the question, however, of could these results be partially due to the attending surgeons choosing less complex cases for the fellows [1].

The purpose of this study is to report the outcomes of complex DSEK performed by cornea fellows supervised by an attending surgeon at an academic institution.

Methods

A retrospective chart review was performed of patients who underwent a complex DSEK procedure from January 2009 to November 2013 and was performed by a cornea fellow under the supervision of one cornea attending (T.P.O.) at the Bascom Palmer Eye Institute. The DSEK procedure was defined as complex if the patient had a functioning tube shunt or filtering bleb, presence of silicone oil in the anterior chamber, presence of vitreous in the anterior chamber, presence of peripheral anterior synechiae or iridocorneal adhesions, history of failed penetrating keratoplasty or failed DSEK, a history of angle closure glaucoma with the presence of a shallow anterior chamber or poor visualization necessitating the use of trypan blue during the DSEK procedure. Patients with less than 6 months of follow up were excluded. In this case series, patients in whom graft failure occurred in the first 6 months following surgery remained included in the study and were continued to be followed up. The medical charts were reviewed for demographic data, indication for DSEK, concurrent procedures, intraoperative and postoperative complications and clinical outcomes. Pre- and postoperative measurements included Snellen best-corrected visual acuity and

intraocular pressure measured by TONO-PEN (Medtronic, Doral, Florida, USA). When reporting visual acuity results, patients were divided into those with no other significant ocular pathology and to those with other ocular pathology limiting vision including previous retinal detachment involving the macula, chronic cystoid macular edema, proliferative diabetic retinopathy, advanced glaucoma and non-arteritic ischemic optic neuropathy. Postoperative data at 6 months and at final visit was included. Graft failure was defined as an edematous cornea with failure to maintain deturgescence lasting beyond a period of 1 month of intense corticosteroid therapy or vascularization and scarring resulting in irreversible loss of central graft clarity.

Surgical procedure

Prior to the surgery patients received a peribulbar block with intravenous sedation. The cornea was marked with an 8.25 mm manual trephine. Two 1 mm paracenteses tracts were made at the limbus and viscoelastic was injected into the anterior chamber. A 2.2 mm temporal beveled corneal incision was fashioned at the limbus. Using a reverse Sinskey hook (Bausch & Lomb, San Dimas, CA) the Descemet's membrane and endothelium were scored in a circular fashion and then stripped off with an endothelial stripper (Katena, Denville, NJ). Trypan blue was not used routinely to stain the endothelium. The Viscoelastic was removed from the anterior chamber using the irrigation/aspiration unit. The temporal incision was enlarged to 4.2 mm. The donor corneal tissue was trephined to 8.25-mm, separated from the donor stroma and placed into the anterior chamber. The graft was unfolded and balanced salt solution was used to form the anterior. The temporal wound was sutured with two 10-0 nylon sutures. The anterior chamber was completely filled with air to force the apposition of the graft to the recipient stromal bed and the patient was left face up for 10 min. A fluid-air exchange was then performed and using a 32-gauge needle air was injected to fill about 80% of the anterior chamber. At the end of the surgery, a topical cycloplegic drop was applied. The patient was then instructed to lie in the face-up position until the following day. Antibiotic and corticosteroid drops were applied after surgery and were tapered accordingly. Patients were examined 1 day, 1 week and 1 month after surgery and after that as needed.

Statistical analysis

Data was recorded on Microsoft Excel Software version 14.1 (Microsoft Corp., Redmond, WA, USA). Snellen best-corrected visual acuities were converted to logarithm of the minimal angle of resolution units (LogMAR) to allow for averaging and statistical analysis. BCVA and IOP before and after the surgery were compared using a t-test. Time to graft failure was determined using the Kaplan-Meier analysis log rank test (XLSTAT software, Addinsoft Inc., Brooklyn, NY, USA). A p-value < 0.05 was considered statistically significant. Data is presented as means ($\pm$ standard deviation).

Results

Fifty-seven eyes of 55 patients (56.4% female, 52.6% right eye) were included in this study. The mean age of the patients was 77.5 ± 8.5 years (range: 49-91 years). Mean follow-up time was 16.4 ± 15.6 months (range: 6-60 months). The main indication for DSEK was a history of failed DSEK or penetrating keratoplasty graft. Indications for DSEK are presented in Table 1. All eyes had a posterior chamber intraocular lens, with 6 eyes (10.5%) having scleral fixated intraocular lens. Table 2 summarizes the criteria for designating the DSEK as complex for the 57 eyes in this study. Fifteen eyes (26.3%) had more than one of these criteria: 11 eyes (19.3%) had two criteria and four eyes (7.0%) had 3 criteria. Concurrent surgical procedures during the DSEK are summarized in Table 3. No intraoperative complications were documented in any of the cases.

Visual acuity and intraocular pressure

Mean preoperative best-corrected visual acuity in all eyes was 1.06 LogMAR (20/230, range: 20/50 to hand motions). Mean best-corrected visual acuity improved to 0.39 LogMAR (20/50, range: 20/20 to 20/800, $p < 0.001$) by the sixth postoperative month and to 0.52 LogMAR (20/65, range: 20/25 to hand motions, $p < 0.001$) at the last follow-up visit. Twenty-two eyes (38.6%) had ocular pathology limiting vision beside the corneal pathology, including 8 cases (14%) of advanced glaucoma, 8 cases (14%) with chronic cystoid macular edema, 4 cases (7%) of previous retinal detachment, 1 case (1.8%) with proliferative diabetic retinopathy and 1 case (1.8%) of non-arteritic ischemic optic neuropathy. After excluding these patients, mean preoperative best-corrected visual acuity was 1.12 LogMAR (20/263, range: 20/70 to hand motions), which improved to 0.36 LogMAR (20/46, range: 20/20 to 20/800, $p < 0.001$) by the sixth postoperative month and to 0.48

Table 1 Indications for Descemet Stripping Endothelial Keratopalsty ($n = 57$ eyes)

Indication	N (%)
Previously failed graft	33 (57.9)
Pseudophakic bullous keratopathy	22 (38.7)
Fuchs endothelial dystrophy	1 (1.8)
Silicone oil keratopathy	1 (1.8)

Table 2 Criteria for designating Descemet Stripping Endothelial Keratoplasty as Complex ($n = 57$ eyes)

Cause	N (%)
Previous corneal graft failure	33 (57.9)
Presence of tube shunt	16 (28.1)
Previous trabeculectomy	13 (22.8)
Vitreous prolapse	4 (7.0)
peripheral anterior synechiae/iridocorneal adhesions	4 (7.0)
Shallow anterior chamber or angle closure glaucoma	3 (5.3)
Poor visualization necessitated trypan blue	2 (3.5)
Silicone oil in the anterior chamber	1 (1.8)

The total percent adds up to more than 100 because some patients had two or three criteria defining the Descemet Stripping Endothelial Keratoplasty as complex

LogMAR (20/60, range: 20/25 to hand motions, $p < 0.001$) at the last follow-up visit.

When compared to preoperative measures, mean intraocular pressure did not change 6 months and at last follow up: 14.1 ± 6.6 mmHg (range: 3 to 36 mmHg), 13.2 ± 6 mmHg (range: 3 to 31 mmHg, $p = 0.55$) and 13.3 ± 5 mmHg (range: 2 to 25 mmHg, $p = 0.38$), respectively.

Postoperative complications and graft failure

Postoperative complications were observed in 19 eyes (33.3%). Graft detachment occurred in 12 eyes (21.1%). Nine eyes (15.8%) were managed by one rebubbling, 2 (3.5%) required 2 rebubblings and 1 (1.8%) required 3 rebubblings. The lenticule reattached successfully in 9 cases. In the other 3 patients, the cornea never cleared after the surgery and 2 patients underwent another corneal transplantation. One patient refused additional intervention. IOP higher than 30 mmHg was seen in 6 patients (10.5%, range: 32 to 53 mmHg) on the first day after the surgery. Three had pupillary block and were treated with anterior chamber paracentesis. Suture abscess occurred in 1 patient (1.8%) 20 days after the surgery. Although prompt treatment with topical antimicrobials,

Table 3 Concurrent Surgical Procedures performed during the Descemet Stripping Endothelial Keratoplasty ($n = 57$ eyes)

Concurrent surgical procedure	N (%)
Tube revision/trimming	4 (7.0)
Anterior vitrectomy	4 (7.0)
Synechiolysis	2 (3.5)
Silicon oil removal from anterior chamber	1 (1.8)
Epithelial debridement	1 (1.8)
Tube revision/trimming + anterior vitrectomy + pupilloplasty	1 (1.8)
Anterior vitrectomy + synechiolysis	1 (1.8)

the DSEK graft eventually failed. There were no cases of endophthalmitis.

Secondary graft failure was observed in 17 cases (29.8%) and on average occurred 5.71 ± 4.54 months after surgery (range: 2 to 17 months). All of these patients had a previously failed corneal graft, a previous glaucoma surgery, or both. Five of these cases had a graft detachment on the first postoperative day necessitating rebubbling. Kaplan-Meier analysis found a 67.2% graft survival rate at 20 months (Fig. 1). No graft rejection episodes were documented.

Discussion

To our knowledge this is the first study to report the outcomes of complex DSEK performed by cornea fellows under the supervision of one experienced surgeon. In this study, mean best-corrected visual acuity improved significantly after the surgery. Postoperative complications were observed in 33.3% of cases and mainly included early graft detachments and spikes in intraocular pressure. Secondary graft failure was observed in 29.8% of the cases.

DSEK is more challenging and with higher rates of postoperative complications in complex eyes [4]. Previous glaucoma surgery is one of the significant risk factors for graft failure [8, 15–17]. It is associated with at least a 4-fold increase in the risk of failure when accounting for other factors [15, 18, 19]. Ward et al. assessed the association of glaucoma treatment with graft survival after penetrating keratoplasty and DSEK. Out of 156 DSEK-operated eyes, the 5-year Kaplan-Meier graft survival was higher than 90% in eyes without

any glaucoma surgery or with only medical glaucoma treatment, and as low as 50% in eyes with surgical intervention for glaucoma [17]. Iverson et al. reported that 76.9% of the grafts in eyes with prior trabeculectomy failed by 36 months [8], while Price et al. found that 60% failed by 5 years [16]. In our study, half of the patients had a history of a tube shunt or trabeculectomy. The Kaplan-Meier analysis showed a 67.2% graft survival rate at 20 months, which is in line with previous studies.

DSEK performed after a failed penetrating keratoplasty or failed DSEK can be technically more difficult, and tends to have higher rates of postoperative complications [4, 6, 7]. There is a risk that remnants of the friable Descemet membrane will be left behind leading to poor attachment of the new lenticule [7]. In DSEK performed after a failed penetrating keratoplasty with a glaucoma drainage device, the graft dislocation rate was reported by Clements et al. to be 67% [6]. This may be attributed to the compounded complexity of the glaucoma drainage device with the failed penetrating keratoplasty [6]. When looking at outcomes of DSEK after a failed penetrating keratoplasty, graft dislocations rates of 14- 43% have been reported [6, 7, 20]. In the present study, the majority of the cases were complex due to previous graft failure or the presence of a glaucoma drainage device. The graft dislocation rate was 21.1%, which is comparable to the published rate in the literature. Secondary graft failure rate was 29.8% (17 out of 57 eyes), which is on the low side compared to the range of 15.9% to 76.9% found in the literature for complex eyes [8, 15–17, 21].

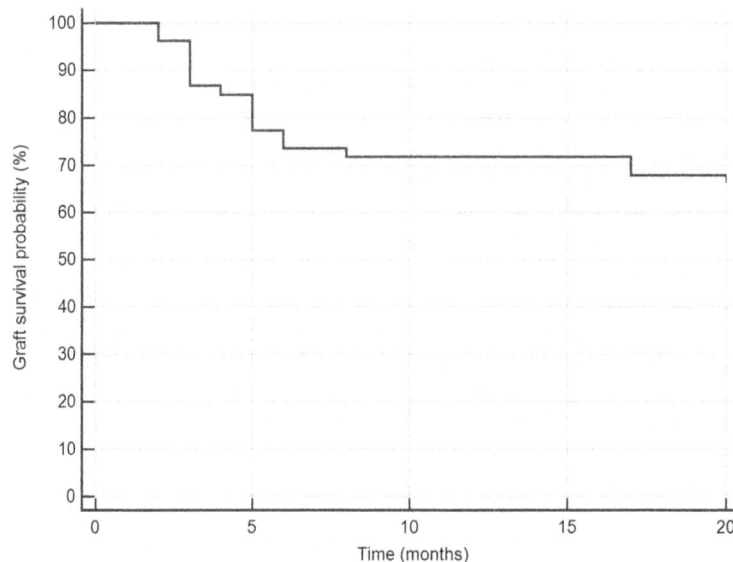

Fig. 1 Kaplan-Meier analysis showing the time to graft failure. At 2 months, 2 grafts failed. At 3 months, 5 grafts failed. At 4 months, 1 graft failed. At 5 months, 4 grafts failed. At 6 months, 2 grafts failed. At 8 months, 1 graft failed. At 17 months, 2 grafts failed

Attention in the literature has been directed towards the steep learning curve of endothelial keratoplasty procedures among experienced cornea surgeons [13]. Several authors reported relatively high donor dislocation rates in the early stages of their endothelial keratoplasty learning curve ranging from 25 to 27% [13, 22]. They also reported primary graft failure rates ranging from 7 to 11% in these cases [22, 23]. Excessive tissue handling by an inexperienced DSEK surgeon increases the endothelial trauma leading to an increased rate of postoperative complications [24, 25]. One study looked at the first 50 cases of novel DSEK surgeons compared with their second set of 50 cases and found that rates of primary failure, secondary graft failure and lenticule dislocation decreased as the surgeon gained experience with the procedure. Graft dislocation rates decreased from 20 to 10% between the early and late groups [24]. Terry claimed that the most important step for a successful DSEK is a strict surgical technique, regardless of a surgeon's experience [26]. In the present study, graft detachment occurred in 21.1% of cases. This rate is in agreement with the above studies. The graft dislocation rate was expected to be higher since all of our cases were complex and all were performed by inexperienced surgeons. The supervision of an experienced cornea attending and adherence to a strict surgical technique played a major role in our study's good results.

One of the biggest challenges academic institutions face is balancing the training of fellows with the risk of higher postoperative complications for their patients and possible poorer outcomes [1]. Only two studies have reported the outcomes of fellows performing non-complex DSEK. One, executed by Chen et al., was conducted in the United States and compared the outcomes of supervised fellows and attending surgeons. They found no significant difference between cornea fellows and attending surgeons in terms of visual acuity and postoperative complications [1]. Mean postoperative best-corrected visual acuity was 20/36 in the fellow cases. They also reported a very low graft dislocation rate (1%) which is much lower than the 21.1% dislocation rate we had. Nevertheless, their study population included mainly simple (non-complex) cases [1], as opposed to our study population consisting solely of complex cases. The second study done by Hashemi et al. at Tehran evaluated the performance of fellows mainly in non-complex DSEK cases without a control group. They reported a lenticule detachment rate of 21.8%, and a graft failure rate of 10.2% [14], results that are comparable to ours. They reported a mean postoperative best-corrected visual acuity of 20/118 at the 6-month follow-up visit [14]. Our 6 month mean postoperative best-corrected visual acuity was 20/50 which is slightly lower than the 20/36

reported by Chen et al. but better than the 20/118 in Hashemi et al. study [1, 14].

Limitations of this study include its retrospective nature and the reletedly small number of patients. In addition, consistent data regarding the patient's endothelial cell count throughout follow up was not available, so comparison to the preoperative endothelial cell count was not done.

Conclusions

For cornea pathology involving the endothelium, there has been an increasing trend over the last years from penetrating keratoplasty towards DSEK, offering a faster visual recovery with small refractive change [8]. Nevertheless, graft survival rates have not changed dramatically [8] and a substantial number of patients still require recurrent corneal grafting. It is estimated that 80 million people will have glaucoma by 2020 [27]. Academic institutions, as tertiary referral centers, are facing an enlarging number of patients with failed DSEK or penetrating ketaoplasty and patients with a history of glaucoma surgery who are now candidates for DSEK. These institutions face the challenge of training upcoming cornea surgeons while being a referral center for a large number of complex cases, causing their fellows to perform a rising number of complex cases. According to this study, complex DSEK can be performed successfully with an acceptable postoperative complication rate and outcomes by cornea fellows during their training period when supervised by an experienced attending.

Abbreviation
DSEK: Descemet Stripping Endothelial Keratoplasty

Funding
Not applicable.

Authors' contributions
JD, TPO, EA and OS have designed the study. JD and OS have collected the data. JD, TPO, EA and OS have analyzed the data. TPO and EA had administrative, technical, or logistical support. JD and OS wrote the manuscript. JD, TPO, EA and OS had critical revision and approval of the article.

Competing interests
The authors declare that they have no competing interests.

References

1. Chen ES, Terry MA, Shamie N, Hoar KL, Phillips PM, Friend DJ. Endothelial keratoplasty: vision, endothelial survival, and complications in a comparative case series of fellows vs attending surgeons. Am J Ophthalmol. 2009;148(1):26–31.

2. Wu EI, Ritterband DC, Yu G, Shields RA, Seedor JA. Graft rejection following descemet stripping automated endothelial keratoplasty: features, risk factors, and outcomes. Am J Ophthalmol. 2012;153(5):949–57.

3. Khor WB, Teo KY, Mehta JS, Tan DT. Descemet stripping automated endothelial keratoplasty in complex eyes: results with a donor insertion device. Cornea. 2013;32(8):1063–8.

4. Riaz KM, Sugar J, Tu EY, et al. Early results of Descemet-stripping and automated endothelial keratoplasty (DSAEK) in patients with glaucoma drainage devices. Cornea. 2009;28(9):959–62.

5. Banitt MR, Chopra V. Descemet's stripping with automated endothelial keratoplasty and glaucoma. Curr Opin Ophthalmol. 2010;21(2):144–9.

6. Clements JL, Bouchard CS, Lee WB, et al. Retrospective review of graft dislocation rate associated with descemet stripping automated endothelial keratoplasty after primary failed penetrating keratoplasty. Cornea. 2011;30(4):414–8.

7. Covert DJ, Koenig SB. Descemet stripping and automated endothelial keratoplasty (DSAEK) in eyes with failed penetrating keratoplasty. Cornea. 2007;26(6):692–6.

8. Iverson SM, Spierer O, Papachristou GC, et al. Comparison of primary graft survival following penetrating keratoplasty and Descemet's stripping endothelial keratoplasty in eyes with prior trabeculectomy. Br J Ophthalmol. 2015;99(11):1477–82.

9. Meeks LA, Blomquist PH, Sullivan BR. Outcomes of maual extracapsular versus phacoemulsification cataract extraction by beginner resident surgeons. J Cataract Refract Surg. 2013;39(11):1698–701.

10. Haripriya A, Chang DF, Reena M, Shekhar M. Complication rates of phacoemulsification and manual small-incision cataract surgery at Aravind eye hospital. J Cataract Refract Surg. 2012;28(8):1360–9.

11. Bhagat N, Nissirios N, Potdevin L, et al. Complications in resident-performed phacoemulsification cataract surgery at New Jersey medical school. Br J Ophthalmol. 2007;91:1315–7.

12. De Niro J, Biebesheimer J, Porco TC, Naseri A. Early resident performed cataract surgery. Ophthalmology 2011;118(6):1215.

13. Koenig SB, Covert DJ, Dupps WJ Jr, Meisler DM. Visual acuity, refractive error, and endothelial cell density six months after Descemet stripping and automated endothelial keratoplasty (DSAEK). Cornea. 2007;26(6):670–4.

14. Hashemi H, Asghari H, Amanzadeh K, Behrooz MJ, Beheshtnejad A, Mohammadpour M. Descemet stripping automated endothelial Keratoplasty performed by cornea fellows. Cornea. 2012;31(9):974–7.

15. Anshu A, Price MO, Price FW. Descemet's stripping endothelial keratoplasty: long-term graft survival and risk factors for failure in eyes with preexisting glaucoma. Ophthalmology. 2012;119(10):1982–7.

16. Price MO, Fairchild KM, Price DA, Price FW Jr. Descemet's stripping endothelial Keratopalsty five-year graft survival and endothelial cell loss. Ophthalmology. 2011;118(4):725–9.

17. Ward MS, Goins KM, Greiner MA, Kitzmann AS, Sutphin JE, Alward WL, Greenlee EC, Kwon YH, Zimmerman MB, Wagoner MD. Graft survival versus glaucoma treatment after penetrating or Descemet stripping automated endothelial keratoplasty. Cornea. 2014;33(8):785–9.

18. Anshu A, Price MO, Price FW Jr. Descemet's stripping endothelial keratoplasty under failed penetrating keratoplasty: visual rehabilitation and graft survival rate. Ophthalmology. 2011;118(11):2155–60.

19. Ritterband DC, Shapiro D, Trubnik V, Marmor M, Meskin S, Seedor J, Liebmann JM, Tello C, Koplin R, Harizman N, Shabto U, Ritch R. Penetrating keratoplasty with pars plana glaucoma drainage devices. Cornea. 2007;26(9):1060–6.

20. Price FW, Price MO. Endothelial keratoplasty to restore clarity to a failed penetrating graft. Cornea. 2006;25(8):895–9.

21. Aldave AJ, Chen JL, Zaman AS, Deng SX, Yu F. Outcomes after DSEK in 101 eyes with previous trabeculectomy and tube shunt implantation. Cornea. 2014;33(3):223–9.

22. Gorovoy MS. Descemet-stripping automated endothelial keratoplasty. Cornea. 2006;25(8):886–9.

23. Price FW Jr, Price MO. Descemet's stripping with endothelial keratoplasty in 200 eyes: early challenges and techniques to enhance donor adherence. J Cataract Refract Surg. 2006;32(3):411–8.

24. Pillar S, Tessler G, Dreznik A, Bor E, Kaiserman I, Bahar I. First 100: learning curve for Descemet stripping automated endothelial keratoplasty. Eur J Ophthalmol. 2013;23(6):865–9.

25. Lee JA, Djalilian AR, Riaz KM, Sugar J, Tu EY, Wadia H, Edward DP. Clinical and histopathologic features of failed Descemet-stripping automated endothelial keratoplasty (DSAEK) grafts. Cornea. 2009;28(5):530–5.

26. Terry MA. Precut tissue for Descemet stripping automated endothelial keratoplasty: complications are from technique not tissue. Cornea. 2008;27(6):627–9.

27. Cook C, Foster P. Epidemiology of glaucoma: what's new? Can J Ophthalmol. 2012;47(3):223–6.

24

A prospective case-control study comparing optical coherence tomography characteristics in neuromyelitis optica spectrum disorder- optic neuritis and idiopathic optic neuritis

Xiujuan Zhao[1], Wei Qiu[2], Yuxin Zhang[1], Yan Luo[1], Xiulan Zhang[1], Lin Lu[1*] and Hui Yang[1*]

Abstract

Background: Neuromyelitis optica spectrum disorder-optic neuritis (NMOSD-ON) can now be distinguished from other types of ON as a specific disease by the Aquaporin-4 antibody (AQP4-Ab) test. NMOSD-ON can cause severe retinal nerve fiber layer (RNFL) damage. The optical coherence tomography (OCT) characteristics between NMOSD- ON and idiopathic optic neuritis (IDON) were seldom studied in Asians.

Methods: This prospective case-control study involved 152 eyes from 143 optic neuritis (ON) patients. All the patients were divided into either the NMOSD-ON group or the IDON group based on the AQP4-Ab test. The retinal nerve fiber layer thickness (RNFLT), retinal thickness (RT), and choroidal thickness (CT) were measured by spectral-domain OCT and compared to the 60 age- and gender-matched healthy controls. The association between RNFLT and best corrected visual acuity (BCVA) was examined.

Results: The RNFLT was significantly thinner in all ON patients than in healthy controls, while NMOSD-ON eyes were significantly more affected than IDON eyes in all quadrants ($p < 0.01$). NMOSD-ON patients had stronger visual function impairment than IDON patients ($p < 0.01$). RNFLT was related to BCVA in both the NMOSD-ON and IDON groups. Microcystic macular edema (MME) was identified in 28 patients (19.58%) and in 29 of 152 eyes (19.08%), including 20 of 40 eyes (50%) previously affected by ON. MME was more common in patients with NMOSD-ON (32.2%) than in those with IDON (10.75%) ($p = 0.001$).

Conclusions: The NMOSD-ON group had more pronounced RNFLT thinning and visual function impairment than the IDON group. MME prevalence was higher in NMOSD-ON and was associated with higher frequency of clinical relapses.

Keywords: Optical coherence tomography, Optic neuritis, Retinal nerve fiber layer, Neuromyelitis optica

Background

Optic neuritis (ON) is an inflammatory demyelinating disease that involves the optic nerve and causes acute or subacute onset of vision loss [1]. ON is commonly involved in multiple sclerosis (MS), neuromyelitis optica (NMO), and other autoimmune diseases [2]. NMO spectrum disorder-optic neuritis (NMOSD-ON) is one of the common types of ON in Asian. With the finding of aquaporin-4 antibody (AQP4-Ab) [3], NMOSD-ON can now be distinguished from other types of ON as a specific disease [4], as it is present in most patients with NMOSD [5, 6]. What's more, in 2015, the International Panel for NMO Diagnosis (IPND) achieved consensus that ON with AQP4-Ab seropositivity can be diagnosed as NMOSD [7] and, therefore, ON related to NMOSD was named NMOSD-ON.

Since the definition of NMOSD, NMOSD-ON has been found to differ from other types of ON in many

---
* Correspondence: lulin888@126.com; 13710584767@163.com
[1]State Key Laboratory of Ophthalmology, Zhongshan Ophthalmic Center, Sun Yat-Sen University, No. 54 Xianlie South Road, Guangzhou 510060, People's Republic of China
Full list of author information is available at the end of the article

ways. In terms of pathogenesis, NMOSD is characterized by astrocytopathy with demyelination as a secondary involvement, while MS is primarily a demyelinating disease [5]. In laboratory exams, NMOSD differs from MS in serum and cerebrospinal fluid (CSF) examination [8]. For example, NMOSD had more coexisting autoimmunity [9]. Clinically, just as we have reported before [10] and as in many other reports [11, 12] NMOSD-ON has more female preponderance, more bilateral involvement, higher relapse rate, and worse visual prognosis than IDON [6].

Spectral-domain optical coherence tomography (SD-OCT) has been used extensively in ON for quantifying axon damage [13]. Although there have been many reports about OCT results in MS and NMO non-ON eyes [14], the OCT characteristics of ON eyes in Asians are rare. After an acute ON attack in NMOSD-ON and IDON, the OCT features are not so clear. This is especially true for NMOSD-ON, because the concept of NMOSD was only defined recently. As OCT improves in data acquisition speed, resolution and reproducibility [15], different layers in the retina as well as some subtle abnormalities, such as microcystic macular edema (MME), can be more clearly recognized. With the development of enhanced depth imaging (EDI) mode scan in OCT, choroidal thickness (CT) can be accurately measured. All of these advancements broaden the characteristics that can be compared between NMOSD-ON and IDON and improve our understanding about the differences between them. Ethnicity is significant for different types of ON. In Asian populations, the incidence of NMOSD-ON is much higher than reports from Caucasian populations [10]. Although there have been numerous studies about thinner retinal nerve fiber layer thickness (RNFLT), there was a higher incidence of MME in NMO than in MS [16, 17]. Due to the restricted availability of the AQP4-Ab test, research about the OCT characteristics of NMOSD-ON in Asian populations was rare.

To understand the influence of an acute ON attack on the retina and choroid, we analyzed the OCT characteristics six months after acute attacks in a Chinese cohort with NMOSD-ON or IDON, along with healthy controls. The OCT changes of the optic nerve and retinal and CT were then analyzed.

Methods

Patients with ON were recruited from the neuro-ophthalmology department of Zhongshan Ophthalmic Center. Recruitment took place from November 2013 to July 2015, and patients meeting the inclusion criteria in accordance with the optic neuritis treatment trial (ONTT) [18] with first or relapsing ON were offered participation in this study. Exclusion criteria included any of the following: any evidence of toxic, vascular, infiltrative, compressive,

metabolic, hereditary optic neuropathy, causative ocular diseases or retinal lesions [18], fulfilled the diagnostic criteria of MS McDonald's criteria [19].

Exclusion criteria also comprised an intraocular pressure higher than 21 mmHg, prior ocular trauma, systemic conditions that could affect the visual function, a significant refractive error more than 3D of spherical equivalent refraction or 2D of astigmatism, a history of glaucoma, retinal disease, laser therapy or media opacification. The data were analyzed after the patients had an episode of ON more than six months when the visual functional and structural changes were stabilized. Exclusion criteria also applied to the controls as for ON patients.

The patients were divided into three groups: NMOSD-ON, IDON, and healthy controls. NMOSD-ON included patients who met the established diagnostic criteria for NMO or NMOSD published by Wingerchuk et al. [7]. IDON group patients included those with typical acute demyelinating ON and AQP4-Ab seronegative, none of patients with AQP4-ab negative fullfiled NMOSD criteria or McDonald MS criteria [19].

This study complied with informed consent regulations and the Declaration of Helsinki. A verbal informed consent was needed before subject enrollment in the study.

Laboratory and radiological results were recorded. Serum was drawn for extractable nuclear antigen antibodies (SSA/SSB), antinuclear antibody (ANA), rheumatoid factor (RF), anti-double standard deoxyribonucleic acid (anti-ds DNA), anti-cardiolipin antibodies (ACLs), and AQP4-Ab at the Third Affiliated Hospital of Sun Yat-sen University. All serum samples were analyzed for the presence of AQP4-Ab by indirect immunofluorescence using human AQP4-transfected cells from a commercial BIOCHIP kit (Euroimmun, Germany) as described previously [20]. Clinical data was recorded along with the AQP4-Ab. Patients were sub-divided into the NMOSD-ON group or the IDON group according to the results of the AQP4-Ab test. All patients were treated with corticosteroids.

RNFLT was obtained on a high-definition spectral-domain optical coherence tomography (HD-OCT) with EDI mode (Heidelberg Engineering, Heidelberg, Germany). Measurements were taken using the Spectralis 3.5 mm standard circle scan protocol with version 5.3 software, with signal strength greater than 21. The RNFLT around the optic nerve head in a circle with a minimum of 50 automatic real time (ART) and yields a temporal, superior, nasal, inferior and mean overall graph. Nasal-to-temporal RNFL ratio (N/T ratio) were performed in all patients. A macular scan consisting of 25 horizontal scans centered on the fovea was performed. The central foveal thickness values were automatically generated by the imaging software. CT was defined as the distance between the retinal pigment epithelium (RPE) and the outer border of choroid

A prospective case-control study comparing optical coherence tomography characteristics...

157

at the subfoveal location. All OCT measurements were manually performed by one observer who was blinded with the clinical diagnosis and was not involved in the data analysis. MME [21–23] was defined as cystic, honeycombed, lacunar area of hyporeflectivity with clear boundaries in two or more consecutive SD-OCT macular raster scan images [24] (Fig. 1). The BCVA was converted to the logarithm of the minimum angle of resolution (logMAR) for statistical analysis.

Statistics

All of the data was analyzed using SPSS 19.0 (SPSS Inc., Chicago, IL, USA). First, we determined the mean value (presented as mean ± standard deviation) of RNFLT,

central foveal thickness, and CT before we used the one-way ANOVA test and Bonferroni adjustment to compare multiple variables between the different groups. Associations between BCVA and RNFLT were evaluated using the univariate linear regression. All p values were two-sided and statistical significance was established at $p < 0.05$.

Outcome measures

The primary outcome measures were RNFLT compared in NMOSD-ON, IDON patients, and healthy controls. Secondary outcome measures included MME, central foveal thickness, CT, correlations between RNFLT and BCVA.

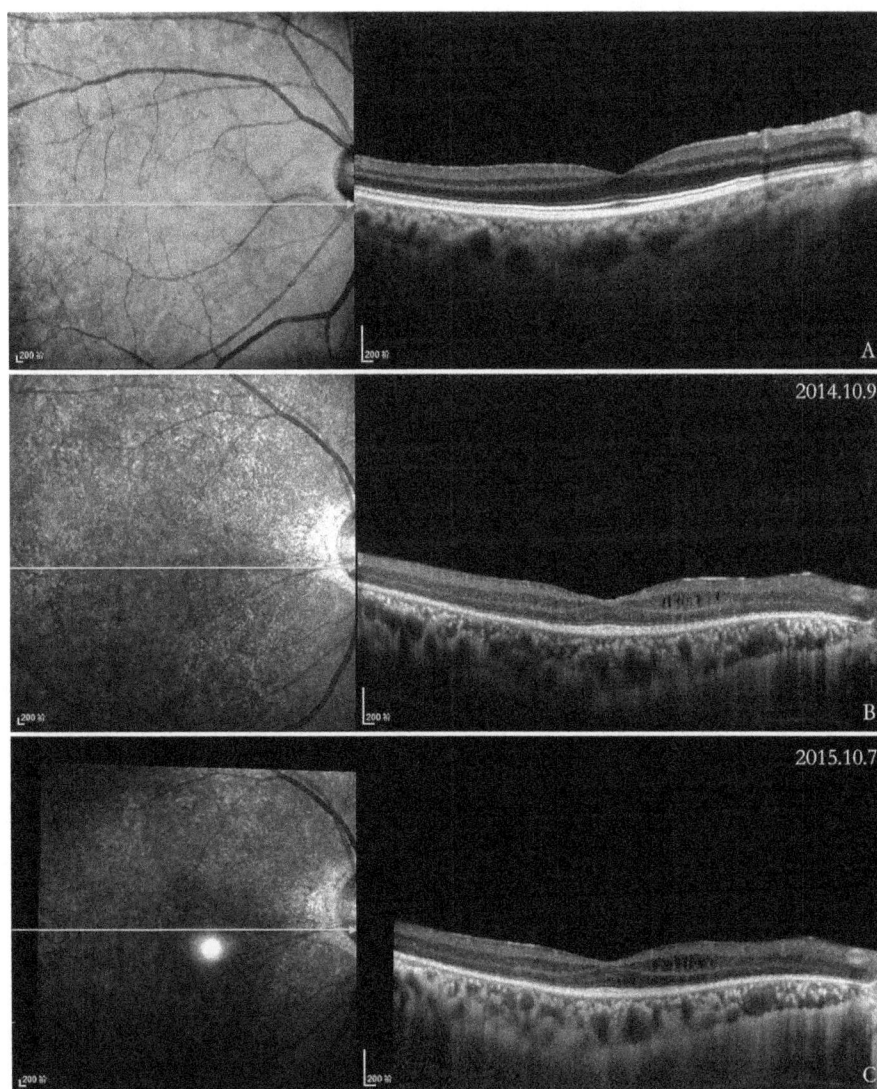

Fig. 1 Scans of a NMOSD-ON eyes with and without microcystic macular edema (MME). On the left, it is the infrared fundus image and the green line marks the position of the corresponding OCT image on the right. **a**, Macular scan of NMOSD-ON eye. **b**, MME of the inner nuclear layer on OCT in NMOSD-ON eye. **c**. At one year follow-up, the MME was increased (white arrow)

Results

A total of 143 patients were evaluated; among them, 59 eyes (52 patients) were in the NMOSD-ON group and 93 eyes (91 patients) were in the IDON group. All NMOSD-ON patients were AQP4-Ab positive. The demographic data of the study cohort is summarized in Table 1.

OCT measures in ON patients

Overall RNFLT and four quadrants RNFLT were significantly thinner in both NMOSD-ON and IDON eyes compared to healthy eyes, with NMOSD-ON eyes being more affected than IDON eyes significantly ($p < 0.01$) (Fig. 2). Central foveal thickness trended higher in ON eyes than healthy eyes, and NMOSD-ON eyes higher than IDON eyes ($p < 0.05$). The subfoveal CT in ON eyes was not different from the healthy controls ($p > 0.05$) (Fig. 3). In clinic work, a temporal preponderance was often seen in optic atrophy with ON and OCT showed particular damage to temporal axons [25, 26]. While peripapillary RNFLT (pRNFLT) was primarily thinned in the temporal quadrant

in both NMOSD-ON and IDON eyes, pRNFLT of other quadrants in NMOSD-ON eyes was much more reduced than IDON eyes. In order to identify whether a predilection of the temporal quadrant of pRNFL existed, we used the N/T ratio to compare quadrant thinning in the groups of NMOSD-ON and IDON patients [27], but the difference was not statistically significant (0.96 ± 0.43 vs. 1.01 ± 0.46; F = 0.298, $p = 0.586$). NMOSD-ON eyes with a history of one ON event were different from IDON eyes with one ON event ($p < 0.01$). NMOSD-ON eyes with more than one ON event were not different from MS-ON eyes with more than one ON event and NMOSD-ON eyes with one ON event ($p > 0.05$) (Table 2). Both in NMOSD-ON and IDON eyes, BCVA is strongly correlated with overall and four quadrants RNFLT ($p < 0.05$) (Table 3).

Role of microcystic macular edema (MME)

MME was identified on OCT in 28 patients (19.58%), and in 29 of 152 eyes (19.08%), including 20 of 40 eyes

Table 1 Demographic data of NMOSD-ON and IDON patients

Baseline characteristics	NMOSD-ON ($n = 52$)	IDON ($n = 91$)	P
Age at first clinical attack, y, median (IQR)	35.00 (20.75–47.00)	37.00 (27.00–49.00)	0.427[a]
Age at serum sampling, y, median (IQR)	36.50 (21.00–47.00)	37.00 (28.00–50.00)	0.196[a]
Sex, F:M	23:3	50:41	0.000[b]
No. of patients with recurrent ON	26	14	0.000[b]
No. of patients with ION	26	77	0.000[b]
No. of ON episodes, mean ± SD	1.58 ± 1.54	1.04 ± 0.19	0.007[a]
Interval relapsing time, m, median (IQR)	12.00 (6.00–48.00)	36.00 (20.25–63.00)	0.237[a]
Interval from onset of last ON attack to OCT test, m, mean ± SD	6.72 ± 1.32	6.31 ± 1.43	0.531[a]
Visual acuity at baseline (logMAR), mean ± SD	2.17 ± 1.38	1.49 ± 1.23	0.044[a]
ON event with visual acuity worse than 1.0 logMAR (n, %)	43, 82.69%	49, 53.85%	0.001[b]
At least one episode with no light perception (n, %)	13, 25.00%	8, 8.79%	0.008[b]
Abnormal brain MRI (n, %)	9, 17.31%	5, 5.49%	0.027[b]
Blood test	37	53	0.50[c]
SSA (n, %)	3, 8.11%	3, 5.66%	
Anti-ds DNA (n, %)	3, 8.11%	1, 1.89%	
ACL (n, %)	1, 2.70%	1, 1.89%	
Accelerated ESR (n, %)	3, 8.11%	1, 1.89%	
Increased CRP (n, %)	2, 5.41%	7, 13.21%	
ANCA positive (n, %)	2, 5.41%	2, 3.77%	
ANA (≥1:320, %)	9, 24.32%	6, 11.32%	
Follow-up outcomes			
No. of cases	48	85	
Visual acuity at last follow-up (logMAR), mean ± SD	1.35 ± 1.30	0.77 ± 0.97	0.001[a]
Cases with myelitis episodes (n, %)	12, 23.08%	1, 1.10%	0.000[b]

NMOSD-ON neuromyelitis optica spectrum disorder- optic neuritis, *IDON* idiopathic optic neuritis, *IQR* interquartile range, *ION* isolated optic neuritis, *SSA* anti-Ro/SSA antibody, *anti-ds DNA* anti-double standard deoxyribonucleic acid, *ACL* anti-cardiolipin antibody, *ESR* erythrocyte sedimentation rate, *CRP* C-reactive protein, *ANCA* antineutrophil cytoplasmic antibody, *ANA* antinuclear antibody, [a]Mann-Whitney U test, [b]Chi-squared test, [c]Fisher's exact test

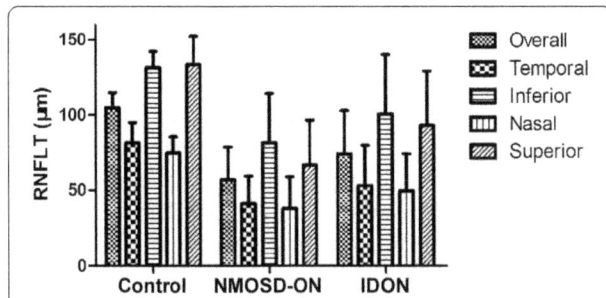

Fig. 2 Comparisons of Overall and quadrants RNFLT among control, NMOSD-ON and IDON. Overall and four quadrants RNFLT were significantly thinner in both NMOSD-ON and IDON eyes compared to healthy eyes, with NMOSD-ON eyes being more thinner than IDON eyes significantly ($p < 0.01$). RNFLT: retinal nerve fiber layer thickness; NMOSD-ON: neuromyelitis optica spectrum disorder- optic neuritis; IDON: idiopathic optic neuritis

(50%) with more than one episode of ON. MME was more common in patients with NMOSD-ON (32.20%, 19 of 59 eyes) than in those with IDON (10.75%, 10 of 93 eyes) ($p = 0.001$). A total of 69.0% of eyes with MME had prior ON. There were no appreciable differences in age or sex between patients with and without MME. Eyes with MME had lower vision, but the difference did not reach statistical significance. The overall RNFLT was 19.23 μm thinner in eyes with MME compared to all ON eyes without MME ($p = 0.03$). The overall RNFLT was 5.39 μm lower in eyes with MME compared to ON eyes with prior ON without MME ($p = 0.36$). Central foveal thickness was 10.42 μm higher in eyes with MME compared with eyes without MME ($p = 0.18$).

Discussion

In this study, a prospective case-control study was made to compare the OCT characteristics between NMOSD-ON and IDON. The study had a large NMOSD-ON sample size and the comparison was not limited to RNFLT, but also included macular and choroidal thicknesses.

As for the clinical features of these patients, there was a strong female predominance, higher recurrent ON

frequency, and more severe visual function damage in the NMOSD-ON group.

RNFLT was significantly thinner in NMOSD-ON and IDON patients six months after an ON attack compared to normal controls. It was reported that NMOSD-ON had no preponderant RNFLT thinning pattern [28]. In this study, no significant N/T ratio difference was found in NMOSD-ON versus IDON eyes, which means all quadrants were evenly affected in both types of ON. This was consistent with previous studies from the Asian cohort, which also failed to demonstrate the similar pattern [29]. On the other hand, the severity of the ON studied might also influence the RNFLT pattern. The temporal RNFLT contains the papillomacular bundle, which is more vulnerable to pathologic damage. When the ON attack was not as severe, quadrants other than the temporal might be relatively damaged. Further investigation is needed to identify whether there were indeed pattern differences or ethnic differences in the pathologic involvement of the optic nerve and severity of the ON attack.

Damage of the optic nerve from a single ON attack was more severe in NMOSD patients. RNFLT became much thinner in the NMOSD-ON group than IDON group, which was in line with previous OCT studies [30]. What's more, this study also demonstrated that RNFLT thinning in first-ever ON was significantly more severe in NMOSD-ON eyes than in IDON eyes. Ratchford et al. [31] suggested that RNFLT differences of more than 15 μm between eyes after a first episode of unilateral ON should prompt consideration of an NMOSD-ON. No significant difference in RNFLT thinning could be found between NMOSD-ON eyes with first-ever ON and those with recurrent ON (RON), which indicated that a single NMOSD-ON attack might be severe enough to destroy most of the RNFLT. This also implied that a functional index, such as visual field or visual evoked potentials, would be more suitable for evaluating the severity of visual damage in RON than RNFLT.

BCVA is strongly correlated with RNFLT, not only with average RNFLT, but also with all quadrants of

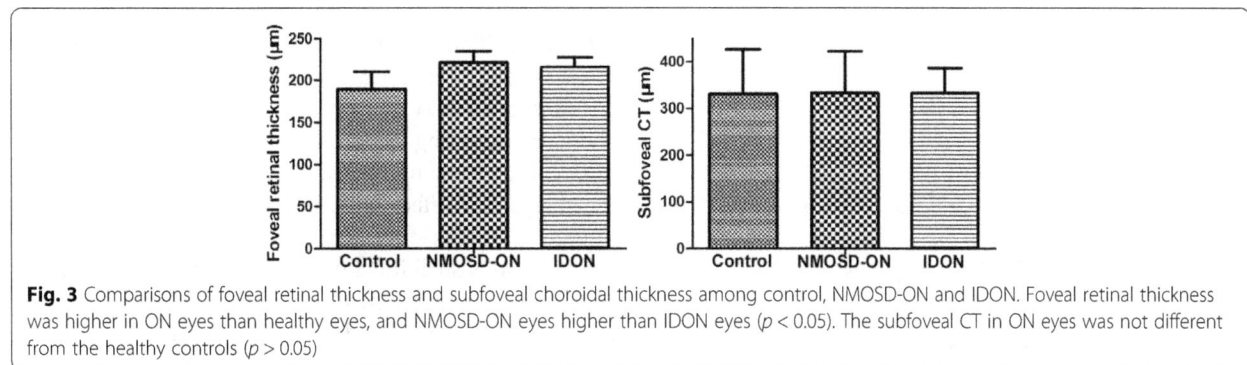

Fig. 3 Comparisons of foveal retinal thickness and subfoveal choroidal thickness among control, NMOSD-ON and IDON. Foveal retinal thickness was higher in ON eyes than healthy eyes, and NMOSD-ON eyes higher than IDON eyes ($p < 0.05$). The subfoveal CT in ON eyes was not different from the healthy controls ($p > 0.05$)

Table 2 Statistical analysis of overall RNFLT for optic neuritis patients and controls

Overall RNFLT		P values
NMOSD-ON with 1 ON (n = 32)	Healthy controls (n = 60)	0.000
59.67 ± 22.19	105.81 ± 10.60	
IDON with 1 ON (n = 79)	Healthy controls (n = 60)	0.000
75.48 ± 28.15	105.81 ± 10.60	
NMOSD-ON with 1 ON (n = 32)	IDON with 1 ON (n = 79)	0.001
59.67 ± 22.19	75.48 ± 28.15	
NMOSD-ON with > 1 ON (n = 27)	IDON with > 1 ON (n = 14)	0.644
45.44 ± 16.03	51.80 ± 32.51	
NMOSD-ON with 1 ON (n = 32)	NMOSD-ON with > 1 ON (n = 27)	0.120
59.67 ± 22.19	45.44 ± 16.03	
IDON with 1 ON (n = 79)	IDON with > 1 ON (n = 14)	0.038
75.48 ± 28.15	51.80 ± 32.51	

RNFLT retinal nerve fiber layer thickness, *ON* optic neuritis, *NMOSD-ON* neuromyelitis optica spectrum disorder- optic neuritis, *IDON* idiopathic optic neuritis. Wilcoxon Rank Sum Tests with Holm Correction

RNFLT in both NMOSD-ON and IDON eyes. This is in accordance with values reported by earlier studies [29, 32]. Schneider, E., et al. [27] reported that NMOSD-ON eyes showed more apparent association of structural retinal damage and impairment of visual function than in MS-ON eyes. The possible reason may be that half of the NMOSD-ON eyes had pRNFLT below 46.6 μm versus none of the IDON eyes in their study. In our study, there were 19 NMOSD-ON eyes and 17 IDON eyes with pRNFLT below 47 μm. The thinner the RNFLT becomes, the stronger the association between morphology and BCVA becomes. We suggest this might be due to the fact that visual function is no longer able to be maintained after RNFLT decreases to a certain threshold [29, 31].

As for retinal structures, the central foveal thicknesses of both groups were thicker than healthy controls, and

Table 3 Correlation between BCVA and RNFLT using univariate linear regression

RNFLT	NMOSD-ON BCVA		IDON BCVA	
	ß	P	ß	P
Global	−4.824	0.031	−2.425	0.042
Superior	−7.769	0.026	−1.465	0.028
Nasal	−5.173	0.034	−1.376	0.036
Inferior	−8.435	0.031	−1.168	0.033
Temporal	−4.907	0.044	−2.084	0.047

NMOSD-ON neuromyelitis optica spectrum disorder- optic neuritis, *IDON* idiopathic optic neuritis, *BCVA* best corrected visual acuity, *RNFLT* retinal nerve fiber layer thickness

NMOSD-ON eyes were thicker than IDON eyes. The differences were primarily driven by MME, which caused a thickening of the inner nuclear layer and outer retinal layers [27]. MME could be a manifestation of inner nuclear layer (INL) pathology. Both Sotirchos et al. [17] and Gelfand et al. [24] reported MME existed in NMO eyes affected by ON. Also, it can be seen in 5–6% of MS patients [6]. MME was associated with more severe MS and poorer VA [33]. In this study, MME was found in 32.2% of NMOSD-ON patients and 10.75% of IDON patients, but not in the healthy control. We also found that MME was associated with more severe RNFLT thinning and more profoundly impaired BCVA. MME occurred in various neuroinflammatory disorders associated with ON [34]. MME might be linked to Müller cell pathology [35], which is caused by AQP4-Ab via a leaky blood-retina barrier. Also, there might be a pathophysiological correlation between the extent of damage to the optic nerve and MME. The findings in this study showed that eyes with more severe ON had a higher incidence of MME.

CT is an index of eye circulation. The concentration of AQP4-Ab in serum was much higher than that in CSF [36–38] and there were reports of retina blood vessel abnormality in NMO [39]. All of these indicating mechanisms of retina blood barrier (RBB) and blood brain barrier (BBB) damage might be involved in the pathogenesis of NMO. Whether different types of ON have an effect on choroidal vessel structure has not yet been studied. Ebru Esen et al. [40] reported that the mean subfoveal CT was reduced significantly in MS patients versus the healthy controls. However, in this study, there was no significant difference between IDON and the normal controls, or between NMOSD-ON and IDON. Diurnal variations of CT [41] could have an effect on the results, because the data was not obtained at the same time of the day. In our study, the number of subfoveal CTs in the normal controls was in accordance with other reports [42, 43] while CT of the healthy control in Ebru Esen et al.'s study was much thicker [40]. Determining whether choroidal vessels are involved in the pathology of the disease requires a larger cohort and more detailed measurements.

Using OCT for differentiation of IDON from NMOSD-ON has long been desirable. However, so far, OCT alone has not been enough for differentiation, though OCT shows a promising effect in investigating the pathologic difference, managing the severity of ON, and evaluating the therapeutic effect on ON [44]. Still, there were some limitations to this study. The relationship between RNFLT change and visual function remains to be investigated. Multilayer segmentation of greater detail should be analyzed. Anti-myelin oligodendrocyte glycoprotein (MOG) antibodies are frequently associated with the recurrent

ON/chronic relapsing inflammatory ON phenotype, which is highly sensitive to even low doses of oral corticosteroids [45]. There is still a debate about whether MOG-Ab positive patients will be considered part of the NMOSD, or rather a distinct disease entity [46]. We did not test the anti-MOG antibody in AQP4-Ab negative patients in our study, which may somewhat skew the results. However, this could provide a direction for future research.

Conclusion

In summary, patients with NMOSD-ON had more pronounced RNFLT thinning than patients with IDON and was closely associated with visual function impairment.

Abbreviations

ACLs: Anti-cardiolipin antibodies; ANA: Antinuclear antibody; anti-ds DNA: anti-double standard deoxyribonucleic acid; AQP4-Ab: Aquaporin-4 antibody; BCVA: Best corrected visual acuity; CIS: Clinically isolated syndrome; CSF: Cerebrospinal fluid; CT: Choroidal thickness; EDI: Enhanced depth imaging; IDON: Idiopathic optic neuritis; MME: Microcystic macular edema; MS: Multiple sclerosis; MS-ON: MS-related optic neuritis; NMOSD: Neuromyelitis optica spectrum disorder; NMOSD-ON: NMOSD-related optic neuritis; OCT: Optical coherence tomography; ONTT: Optic neuritis treatment trial; RF: Rheumatoid factor; RNFT: Retinal nerve fiber layer thickness; RPE: Retinal pigment epithelium

Funding

National Basic Research Development Program of China (973 program: 2013CB967000), the National Natural Science Foundation of China to LIN LU (81570862), YAN LUO (81371020), the Natural Science Foundation of Guangdong Province of China to HUI YANG (S2012010008439).

Authors' contributions

HY and LL conceived the study, coordinated its design and drafted the manuscript. WQ and YL had significant input into study protocol. XJZ and XLZ were involved in critical appraisal and revision of the manuscript. YXZ provided statistical expertise. All authors read and approved the final manuscript.

Competing interests

The authors declare that they have no competing interest.

Author details

[1]State Key Laboratory of Ophthalmology, Zhongshan Ophthalmic Center, Sun Yat-Sen University, No. 54 Xianlie South Road, Guangzhou 510060, People's Republic of China. [2]Department of Neurology, The Third Affiliated Hospital of Sun Yat-Sen University, Guangzhou, China.

References

1. Beck RW, Cleary PA, Anderson MM Jr, et al. A randomized, controlled trial of corticosteroids in the treatment of acute optic neuritis. The optic neuritis study group. N Engl J Med. 1992;326(9):581–8.

2. Petzold A, Wattjes MP, Costello F, et al. The investigation of acute optic neuritis: a review and proposed protocol. Nat Rev Neurol. 2014;10(8):447–58.

3. Zekeridou A, Lennon VA. Aquaporin-4 autoimmunity. Neurol Neuroimmunol Neuroinflamm. 2015;2(4):e110.

4. Metz I, Beissbarth T, Ellenberger D, et al. Serum peptide reactivities may distinguish neuromyelitis optica subgroups and multiple sclerosis. Neurol Neuroimmunol Neuroinflamm. 2016;3(2):e204.

5. Lennon VA, Wingerchuk DM, Kryzer TJ, et al. A serum autoantibody marker of neuromyelitis optica: distinction from multiple sclerosis. Lancet. 2004; 364(9451):2106–12.

6. Bennett JL, de Seze J, Lana-Peixoto M, et al. Neuromyelitis optica and multiple sclerosis: seeing differences through optical coherence tomography. Mult Scler. 2015;21(6):678–88.

7. Wingerchuk DM, Banwell B, Bennett JL, et al. International consensus diagnostic criteria for neuromyelitis optica spectrum disorders. Neurology. 2015;85(2):177–89.

8. Jarius S, Paul F, Franciotta D, et al. Cerebrospinal fluid findings in aquaporin-4 antibody positive neuromyelitis optica: results from 211 lumbar punctures. J Neurol Sci. 2011;306(1–2):82–90.

9. Jarius S, Ruprecht K, Wildemann B, et al. Contrasting disease patterns in seropositive and seronegative neuromyelitis optica: a multicentre study of 175 patients. J Neuroinflammation. 2012;9:14.

10. Yang H, Qiu W, Zhao X, et al. The correlation between Aquaporin-4 antibody and the visual function of patients with demyelinating optic neuritis at onset. J Ophthalmol. 2015;2015:672931.

11. Kitley J, Leite MI, Nakashima I, et al. Prognostic factors and disease course in aquaporin-4 antibody-positive patients with neuromyelitis optica spectrum disorder from the United Kingdom and Japan. Brain. 2012;135(Pt 6):1834–49.

12. Merle H, Olindo S, Bonnan M, et al. Natural history of the visual impairment of relapsing neuromyelitis optica. Ophthalmology. 2007;114(4):810–5.

13. Pulicken M, Gordon-Lipkin E, Balcer LJ, et al. Optical coherence tomography and disease subtype in multiple sclerosis. Neurology. 2007;69(22):2085–92.

14. Outteryck O, Majed B, Defoort-Dhellemmes S, et al. A comparative optical coherence tomography study in neuromyelitis optica spectrum disorder and multiple sclerosis. Mult Scler. 2015;21(14):1781–93.

15. Bock M, Brandt AU, Dorr J, et al. Time domain and spectral domain optical coherence tomography in multiple sclerosis: a comparative cross-sectional study. Mult Scler. 2010;16(7):893–6.

16. Kaufhold F, Zimmermann H, Schneider E, et al. Optic neuritis is associated with inner nuclear layer thickening and microcystic macular edema independently of multiple sclerosis. PLoS One. 2013;8(8):e71145.

17. Sotirchos ES, Saidha S, Byraiah G, et al. In vivo identification of morphologic retinal abnormalities in neuromyelitis optica. Neurology. 2013;80(15):1406–14.

18. The clinical profile of optic neuritis. Experience of the Optic Neuritis Treatment Trial. Optic neuritis study group. Arch Ophthalmol. 1991;109(12):1673–8.

19. Polman CH, Reingold SC, Banwell B, et al. Diagnostic criteria for multiple sclerosis: 2010 revisions to the McDonald criteria. Ann Neurol. 2011;69(2):292–302.

20. Long Y, Qiu W, Lu Z, et al. Aquaporin 4 antibodies in the cerebrospinal fluid are helpful in diagnosing Chinese patients with neuromyelitis optica. Neuroimmunomodulation. 2012;19(2):96–102.

21. Cruz-Herranz A, Balk LJ, Oberwahrenbrock T, et al. The APOSTEL recommendations for reporting quantitative optical coherence tomography studies. Neurology. 2016;86(24):2303–9.

22. Schippling S, Balk LJ, Costello F, et al. Quality control for retinal OCT in multiple sclerosis: validation of the OSCAR-IB criteria. Mult Scler. 2015;21(2):163–70.

23. Tewarie P, Balk L, Costello F, et al. The OSCAR-IB consensus criteria for retinal OCT quality assessment. PLoS One. 2012;7(4):e34823.

24. Gelfand JM, Cree BA, Nolan R, et al. Microcystic inner nuclear layer abnormalities and neuromyelitis optica. JAMA Neurol. 2013;70(5):629–33.

25. Bock M, Brandt AU, Dorr J, et al. Patterns of retinal nerve fiber layer loss in multiple sclerosis patients with or without optic neuritis and glaucoma patients. Clin Neurol Neurosurg. 2010;112(8):647–52.

26. Kerrison JB, Flynn T, Green WR. Retinal pathologic changes in multiple sclerosis. Retina. 1994;14(5):445–51.

27. Schneider E, Zimmermann H, Oberwahrenbrock T, et al. Optical coherence tomography reveals distinct patterns of retinal damage in Neuromyelitis Optica and multiple sclerosis. PLoS One. 2013;8(6):e66151.

28. Mateo J, Esteban O, Martinez M, et al. The contribution of optical coherence tomography in Neuromyelitis Optica Spectrum disorders. Front Neurol. 2017;8:493.

29. Trip SA, Schlottmann PG, Jones SJ, et al. Retinal nerve fiber layer axonal loss and visual dysfunction in optic neuritis. Ann Neurol. 2005;58(3):383–91.

30. Nakamura M, Nakazawa T, Doi H, et al. Early high-dose intravenous methylprednisolone is effective in preserving retinal nerve fiber layer thickness in patients with neuromyelitis optica. Graefes Arch Clin Exp Ophthalmol. 2010;248(12):1777–85.

31. Ratchford JN, Quigg ME, Conger A, et al. Optical coherence tomography helps differentiate neuromyelitis optica and MS optic neuropathies. Neurology. 2009;73(4):302–8.

32. Fisher JB, Jacobs DA, Markowitz CE, et al. Relation of visual function to retinal nerve fiber layer thickness in multiple sclerosis. Ophthalmology. 2006;113(2):324–32.

33. Gelfand JM, Nolan R, Schwartz DM, et al. Microcystic macular oedema in multiple sclerosis is associated with disease severity. Brain. 2012;135(Pt 6):1786–93.

34. Brandt AU, Oberwahrenbrock T, Kadas EM, et al. Dynamic formation of macular microcysts independent of vitreous traction changes. Neurology. 2014;83(1):73–7.

35. Balk LJ, Killestein J, Polman CH, et al. Microcystic macular oedema confirmed, but not specific for multiple sclerosis. Brain. 2012;135(Pt 12):e226. author reply e7

36. Jarius S, Franciotta D, Paul F, et al. Cerebrospinal fluid antibodies to aquaporin-4 in neuromyelitis optica and related disorders: frequency, origin, and diagnostic relevance. J Neuroinflammation. 2010;7:52.

37. Majed M, Fryer JP, McKeon A, et al. Clinical utility of testing AQP4-IgG in CSF: guidance for physicians. Neurol Neuroimmunol Neuroinflamm. 2016;3(3):e231.

38. Wingerchuk DM, Lucchinetti CF. Comparative immunopathogenesis of acute disseminated encephalomyelitis, neuromyelitis optica, and multiple sclerosis. Curr Opin Neurol. 2007;20(3):343–50.

39. Vincent T, Saikali P, Cayrol R, et al. Functional consequences of neuromyelitis optica-IgG astrocyte interactions on blood-brain barrier permeability and granulocyte recruitment. J Immunol. 2008;181(8):5730–7.

40. Esen E, Sizmaz S, Demir T, et al. Evaluation of Choroidal vascular changes in patients with multiple sclerosis using enhanced depth imaging optical coherence tomography. Ophthalmologica. 2016;235(2):65–71.

41. Lee SW, Yu SY, Seo KH, et al. Diurnal variation in choroidal thickness in relation to sex, axial length, and baseline choroidal thickness in healthy Korean subjects. Retina. 2014;34(2):385–93.

42. Agawa T, Miura M, Ikuno Y, et al. Choroidal thickness measurement in healthy Japanese subjects by three-dimensional high-penetration optical coherence tomography. Graefes Arch Clin Exp Ophthalmol. 2011;249(10):1485–92.

43. Margolis R, Spaide RF. A pilot study of enhanced depth imaging optical coherence tomography of the choroid in normal eyes. Am J Ophthalmol. 2009;147(5):811–5.

44. Jacob A, Hutchinson M, Elsone L, et al. Does natalizumab therapy worsen neuromyelitis optica? Neurology. 2012;79(10):1065–6.

45. Chalmoukou K, Alexopoulos H, Akrivou S, et al. Anti-MOG antibodies are frequently associated with steroid-sensitive recurrent optic neuritis. Neurol Neuroimmunol Neuroinflamm. 2015;2(4):e131.

46. Zamvil SS, Slavin AJ. Does MOG Ig-positive AQP4-seronegative opticospinal inflammatory disease justify a diagnosis of NMO spectrum disorder? Neurol Neuroimmunol Neuroinflamm. 2015;2(1):e62.

25

Comparison of clinical outcomes of toric intraocular lens, Precizon vs Tecnis: a single center randomized controlled trial

Na Yeon Jung[1†], Dong Hui Lim[1,2†], Sung Soon Hwang[1], Joo Hyun[1,3] and Tae-Young Chung[1*]

Abstract

Background: To compare the clinical outcome of Precizon toric intraocular lens (IOL) (Ophtec Inc.) to that of Tecnis toric IOL (Abbott Medical Optics Inc.).

Methods: This randomized comparative study included 40 eyes (Precizon, 20 eyes; Tecnis, 20 eyes) of 40 patients with visually significant cataract and corneal astigmatism who underwent cataract surgery. Changes in uncorrected distant visual acuity (UCDVA), best corrected distant visual acuity (BCDVA), uncorrected intermediate visual acuity (UCIVA), refraction, residual astigmatism, rotation of the IOL axis, and higher order aberrations at 3 months postoperatively were evaluated. Vector analysis was performed using the Alpins method.

Results: Both groups showed significant reduction in refractive astigmatism after the surgery (Precizon: − 1.06 ± 0.94 Diopter (D) to − 0.31 ± 0.29 D, $p = 0.042$; Tecnis: − 1.83 ± 1.29 D to − 0.41 ± 0.33 D, $p = 0.015$). There was no significant ($p > 0.05$) difference in postoperative UCDVA, BCDVA, or residual astigmatism between the two groups, although a tendency of better UCIVA was observed in the Precizon group. Vector analysis parameters showed no statistically significant difference beween groups($P > 0.05$). Significant difference in rotation of toric IOL axis was found between the two groups (Precizon: 1.50° ± 0.84, Tecnis: 2.56° ± 0.68, $p = 0.010$). Spherical aberration in the Precizon group was significantly ($p = 0.005$) lower than that in the Tecnis group.

Conclusions: The Precizon toric IOL group had better rotational stability at 3-month postoperatively. Both Precizon toric IOL and Tecnis toric IOL could be effectively used by cataract surgeons to correct preexisting corneal astigmatism through cataract surgery.

Keywords: Precizon, Tecnis, Astigmatism, Toric, Intraocular Lens

Background

Approximately 40 to 45% of patients who have undergone cataract surgery have more than 1 diopter (D) of corneal astigmatism [1, 2]. Toric intraocular lenses (IOLs) are becoming more commonly available, allowing more improvement in clinical outcomes than other treatment options to correct corneal astigmatism during or after cataract surgery [3]. However, if unintended rotation of one degree from the target axis of toric IOL

occurs, it can result in a loss of approximately 3.3% of cylindrical power [4].

With growing interests in reducing undesirable residual astigmatism, several ideas have been suggested for the design of toric IOLs. Precizon toric IOL (Ophtec Inc., Netherlands), one of the relatively recently introduced toric IOL, is expected to have greater resistance in postoperative rotation due to its unique optic design (Fig. 1). However, only a few clinical results have been published on this aberration free toric IOL [5–7]. Therefore the aim of this study was to evaluate the clinical outcomes of Precizon toric IOL compared to commonly used Tecnis toric IOL (Abbott Medical Optics Inc., Santa Ana, CA, USA) which has

---
* Correspondence: tychung@skku.edu
†Na Yeon Jung and Dong Hui Lim contributed equally to this work.
[1]Department of Ophthalmology, Samsung Medical Center, Sungkyunkwan University School of Medicine, #81 Irwon-ro, Gangnam-gu, Seoul 06351, Korea
Full list of author information is available at the end of the article

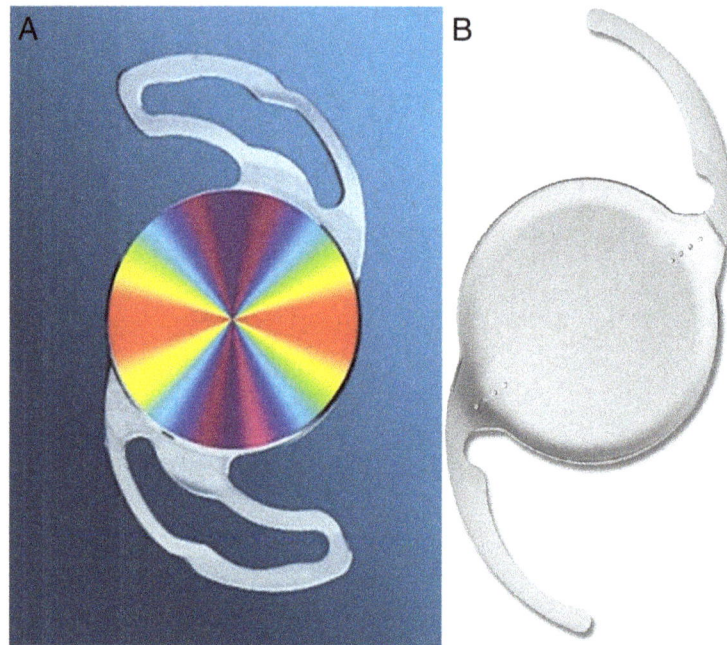

Fig. 1 Schematic images of the toric intraocualr lens. **a**: Precizon toric intraocular lens. **b**: Tecnis toric intraocular lens (**b**)

different characteristics in IOL after cataract surgery in patients with corneal astigmatism.

Methods
Patients selection
This prospective randomized comparative study included 40 eyes of 40 patients who were scheduled for cataract surgery with implantation of toric IOL from April 2016 at Samsung Medical Center, Seoul, Korea. Written informed consents were obtained from 40 consecutive patients before performing the study. These patients were randomly allocated into two groups to receive either Precizon toric IOL or Tecnis toric IOL during the cataract surgery. Inclusion criteria were visually significant cataract and regular corneal astigmatism measured with Scheimpflug imaging (Pentacam HR, Oculus, Wetzlar, Germany) between 0.50 diopter (D) and 2.50 D considering both anterior and posterior corneal surface. The surgically induced astigmatism (SIA) of the operating surgeon was found as 0.50 D for temporal clear corneal incision, so patients were included if their requiring corneal astigmatism correction considering surgically induced astigmatism was more than 1 D considering their steep axis. Each patients had a complete ophthalmological examination. Exclusion criteria were amblyopia, irregular astigmatism, corneal opacity, glaucoma, retinal disease, history of ocular inflammation, history of ocular trauma, and previous other intraocular surgery. Also patients were excluded if they take medications such as a-blocker. This study was approved by Institutional

Review Board of Samsung Medical Center(Permission number: SMC 2016–04-147). It was carried out in accordance with the Declaration of Helsinki. The manuscript reporting adheres to the CONSORT guidelines for the reporting of randomized trials. In South Korea, clinical trial registration is not mandatorily required for these randomized comparative study. However we registered the trial in 2017 when we submit the paper to meet the international guidelines. The authors confirm that all ongoing and related trials for this drug/intervention are registered. The enrolled eyes were randomized into two groups using a computer generated random number table with a 1:1 ratio at screening visit. One investigator (N.Y.J.) generated and implemented the randomization allocation process.

Preoperative evaluation
Preoperatively, all patients underwent complete ophthalmic evaluation including uncorrected distant visual acuity (UCDVA), best corrected distant visual acuity (BCDVA), refractive errors, and corneal topography using Scheimpflug imaging (Pentacam HR, Oculus, Wetzlar, Germany).

Biometry measurements (axial length and anterior chamber depth) used for IOL power calculation were obtained with optical coherence biometry (IOLMaster, software version 5.02, Carl Zeiss Meditec AG, Jena, Germany). The spherical power of the IOL was calculated using SRK-T formula. Emmetropia was target postoperative spherical equivalent (SE). Surgeon used his typical surgical induced astigmatism magnitude, and all main wound incision was planned to be at temporal side of the cornea. Total corneal astigmatism was calculated considering both anterior and posterior corneal surface measured with Pentacam HR using vector summation according to Alpins' method [8]. From these data, calculations of the cylindrical power and axis placement were performed using each IOL manufacturer's online calculator. For Precizon toric IOL, PRECIZON Online Calculator (available from: http://calculator.ophtec.com/) was used with A-constant of 118.5. For Tecnis toric IOL, Tecnis toric express calculator (available from: http://www.amoeasy.com/calc/) was used with A-constant of 119.3. Surgically induced astigmatism of 0.50 D was assumed for all cases.

Intraocular lenses
Characteristics of both IOLs are shown in Additional file 1: Table S1. The Precizon toric IOL Model 565 (Ophtec BV) is a piece of hydrophilic acrylic, monofocal, and aspheric IOL with a transitional conic toric surface (patent pending). It has consistent power from the center to the periphery, yielding a broader toric meridian. It is more resistant of IOL misalignment [9]. It has a closed-loop haptic design. This lens is also aberration free. Tecnis toric IOL has anterior toric surface with a proprietary wavefront-designed toric aspheric optic, resulting in negative spherical aberration [10]. It has open-loop C-haptics. Both toric IOL have two reference marks on the axis of the cylinder of their surface.

Surgical technique
Before surgery, 0° - 180° axis was marked with all patient seating upright at slit-lamp using a horizontal slit beam. Intraopertively, intended implantation axis was marked on the limbus after correctly aligning a Mendez ring to the primary marks to ascertain the intended angle of placement according to preoperative plan. One experienced surgeon (T.Y.C.) performed all surgeries under topical anesthesia (proparacaine hydrochloride 0.5%, Alcaine; Alcon Laboratories, Fort Worth, TX, USA). Phacoemulsification was performed through a 2.75 mm temporal clear corneal incision. After performing continuous curvilinear capsulorrhexis with an intended diameter 5.0 mm and hydrodissection, phacoemulsification of the nucleus and bimanual aspiration of the residual cortex were conducted using Centurion Vision System (Alcon, Laboratories, Fort Worth, TX, USA). Toric IOL was implanted in the capsular bag using injector and disposable cartridge system before removing ophthalmic viscosurgical device (OVD). After removing the OVD, the IOL was rotated to its final targeted position by exactly aligning the toric reference marks on the IOL surface with limbal axis marks. Finally, a balanced salt solution was injected into the incision site to close the corneal incision, causing edema. Before finishing the

surgery, intraoperative photographs were taken for all cases. After the surgery, postoperative eye drops of antibiotics (gatifloxacin 0.3%, Gatiflo; Handok, Seoul, Korea) and corticosteroid (lotepredrol etabonate, lotemax; Bausch + Lomb, Tampa, FL, USA) were used 4 times a day. They were tapered over a month. For all patients, non-steroidal anti-inflammatory drugs (NSAIDs) (ketorolac tromethamine 0.45%, Ocuveil; Allergan, Inc., Irvine, CA, USA) were used for 2 weeks.

Postoperative evaluation
Postoperative examinations were performed at 1 day, 1 week, 1 month, and 3 months after the surgery. All patients underwent measurement of UCDVA, BCDVA, uncorrected intermediate (80 cm) visual acuity (UCIVA), manifest refraction, and slit-lamp examination with IOP measurement. At 1-month and 3-month postoperatively, ocular wavefront aberrometry was performed using WASCA (Carl Zeiss Meditec AG, Jena, Germany). Parameters analyzed for a 5.0 mm pupil included vertical and horizontal coma, vertical and horizontal trefoil, spherical aberration, and root mean square (RMS) values of total aberrations and high order aberrations. The WASCA abberometer provided Zernike coefficients in Malacara notation. However, results are presented in standard notation of Optical Society of America(OSA).

Vector analysis
Vector analysis was performed using the Alpins method, facilitated by the ASSORT program version 5.04 (Assort Pty., Ltd., Victoria, Australia). Target induced astigmatism (TIA) was defined as the astigmatic change in the magnitude and axis the surgery was intended to correct. Therefore, actual measured preoperative corneal topographic astigmatism was used. Surgically induced astigmatism (SIA) was defined as the amount and axis of the astigmatism the surgery actually induced. Difference vector was defined as the induced astigmatic change by the magnitude and axis that would enable the initial surgery to achieve its intended astigmatic target. That means the difference vector is the actual measured postoperative refraction remaining after the surgery. Correction index calculated by determining ratio of SIA to TIA (correction index is preferably 1.0; if correction index > 1.0 overcorrection occurred and if correction index < 1.0 undercorrection occurred). Magnitude of error is the arithmetic difference between magnitudes of SIA and TIA (magnitude of error > 0 indicates overcorrection and magnitude of error < 0 undercorrection). Angle of error is the angle described by the vectors of SIA versus TIA (angle of error > 0: achieved correction index is counterclockwise to where it was intended; angle of error < 0: achieved correction is clockwise to its intended axis). Index of success is calculated by dividing the

difference vector by TIA, representing a relative measure of success (index of success is preferably 0).

Rotational stability analysis

Rotations of the IOL were assessed by analyzing digital photographs in retro-illumination of the IOL with full mydriasis. Conjunctival vessels, iris patterns, or conjunctival pigmented lesions were selected as a reference point to compare the axis between photographs. Postoperative rotation was defined as the difference between intraoperative axis and the achieved axis at 3 months postoperatively. The absolute rotation amount was analyzed by calculating differences between the angle of the IOL reference marks of intraoperative photographs and 3 months postoperative photographs using ImageJ program. One independent investigator performed the measurement.

Sample size

The study population was calculated according to previous conducted studies, Vale et al. [5] and Sheppard AL et al. [10] assuming 1:1 randomization with a significance level of 5% and a power of 80%. Based on previous data, the sample size was calculated to be 40 eyes were required, corresponding to 20 eyes in each group.

Statistical analysis

All data were inputted into Excel database (Microsoft Corporation, Redmond, WA, USA). Statistical analyses were performed using SPSS software system for Windows, Version 20 (SPSS Inc., Chicago, IL). Visual acuities were converted into logMAR for mathematical and statistical calculations. Paired t test was used to compare visual acuity and refractive parameters between preoperative and postoperative examinations. Independent t test was used for between-group comparisons. Results are expressed as means ± standard deviation of the means. Statistically significance was considered when P value was less than 0.05.

Results

Based on our study protocol, 40 eyes from 40 patients aged between 22 and 87 years were included in this study. Patient recruitment was from April 2016 to July 2016. The study was finished after 3 months postoperative follow up visit was completed for all patients in October 2016. The Precizon group included 20 eyes from 20 patients. The Tecnis group included 20 eyes from 20 patients. All patients received regular follow-up examinations for at least 3 months. Patients' demographics and IOL models used in the two groups are summarized in Table 1. Preoperatively, there was no significant ($P > 0.05$) difference between the two groups.

Visual acuity and refraction

After cataract surgery, UCDVA, BCDVA, and cylindrical errors were significantly ($P < 0.05$) improved in both groups (Table 2). In the Precizon group, UCDVA was significantly ($P < 0.05$) increased from 0.50 ± 0.17 (range, 0.30 to 0.82) logMAR preoperatively to 0.09 ± 0.09 (range, 0 to 0.30) logMAR after 3 months postoperatively. In the Tecnis group, UCDVA was also significantly ($P < 0.05$) improved from 0.38 ± 0.13 (range, 0.22 to 0.52) logMAR preoperatively to 0.08 ± 0.12 (range, 0 to 0.30) logMAR at

Table 1 Demographics and clinical information of patients included in this study

	Precizon	Tecnis	p value
Eyes (n)	20	20	
Patients (n)	20	20	
Age (y)	64.64 ± 19.55 (22.5 to 87.1)	64.51 ± 8.40 (46.6 to 87.8)	0.980
Male sex, n (%)	8 (40)	11 (55)	0.527
Right eyes, n (%)	8 (40)	10 (50)	0.751
UCDVA (logMAR)	0.50 ± 0.17 (0.30 to 0.82)	0.37 ± 0.13 (0.22 to 0.52)	0.123
BCDVA (logMAR)	0.30 ± 0.18 (0 to 0.7)	0.21 ± 0.13 (0 to 0.4)	0.266
Manifest Refraction			
Sphere (D)	−0.12 ± 1.32 (−1.75 to 2.75)	0.64 ± 2.82 (− 6.00 to 3.75)	0.418
Cylinder (D)	− 1.06 ± 0.94 (− 2.50 to − 0.50)	− 1.83 ± 1.29 (− 4.00 to − 0.50)	0.129
SE (D)	−0.66 ± 1.47 (− 2.50 to 2.75)	−0.28 ± 2.64 (− 6.50 to 1.88)	0.680
Corneal astigmatism (D)	1.32 ± 0.45 (0.53 to 2.15)	1.47 ± 0.47 (0.72 to 2.09)	0.465
IOL power (D)	19.56 ± 2.35 (15.75 to 23.75)	20.11 ± 3.52 (16.00 to 25.50)	0.629
IOL Cylinder power (D)	1.96 ± 0.84 (1.00 to 3.50)	2.36 ± 0.76 (1.50 to 4.00)	0.266
Axial length (mm)	23.86 ± 1.04 (22.01 to 25.57)	24.22 ± 0.83 (23.15 to 25.22)	0.387

Mean ± SD (range)
Y years, LogMAR Logarithm of the minimum angle of resolution, D diopter, UCDVA uncorrected distance visual acuity, BCDVA best corrected distance visual acuity, IOL intraocular lens, SE spherical equivalent refraction

Table 2 Preoperative and postoperative clinical data in the Precizon toric intraocular lens group and Tecnis toric intraocular lens group at 3-month postoperatively

Parameters	Precizon			Tecnis			P^{*} value
	Preop	Postop	p value	Preop	Postop	p value	
UCDVA (logMAR)	0.50 ± 0.17 (0.30 to 0.82)	0.09 ± 0.09 (0 to 0.30)	0.005	0.38 ± 0.13 (0.22 to 0.52)	0.08 ± 0.12 (0 to 0.30)	0.020	0.904
BCDVA (logMAR)	0.30 ± 0.18 (0 to 0.7)	0.02 ± 0.02 (0 to 0.05)	0.008	0.21 ± 0.13 (0 to 0.50)	0.01 ± 0.02 (0 to 0.05)	0.042	0.582
UCIVA (logMAR)	No data	0.26 ± 0.13 (0.09 to 0.49)		No data	0.40 ± 0.16 (0.20 to 0.60)		0.114
Manifest Refraction							
Sphere (D)	−0.12 ± 1.32 (− 1.75 to 2.75)	0.25 ± 0.35 (− 0.25 to 1.00)	0.324	0.64 ± 2.82 (− 6.00 to 3.75)	0.19 ± 0.48 (− 0.25 to 1.25)	0.260	0.753
Cylinder (D)	−1.06 ± 0.94 (− 2.50 to − 0.50)	−0.31 ± 0.29 (− 0.75 to 0)	0.042	−1.83 ± 1.29 (− 4.00 to − 0.50)	−0.41 ± 0.33 (− 0.75 to 0)	0.015	0.491
SE (D)	− 0.65 ± 1.47 (− 2.50 to 2.75)	0.06 ± 0.38 (− 0.50 to 0.75)	0.184	−0.28 ± 2.64 (− 6.50 to 1.88)	−0.04 ± 0.50 (− 0.63 to 1.00)	0.726	0.600
Rotation (°)	No data	1.50 ± 0.84 (0.18 to 3.02)		No data	2.56 ± 0.68 (1.50 to 3.50)		0.012

Mean ± SD (range)

SD standard deviation, *UCDVA* uncorrected distance visual acuity, *LogMAR* Logarithm of the minimum angle of resolution, *BCDVA* best corrected distance visual acuity, *UCIVA* uncorrected intermediate visual acuity, *D* diopter, *SE* spherical equivalent refraction

*P values between the two groups, $P < 0.05$

3 months postoperatively. The percentage of UCDVA that was 0.1 logMAR or better (Snellen chart 20/25 or better) was 91% in the Precizon group and 83% in the Tecnis group.

In the Precizon group, BCDVA was significantly ($P < 0.05$) increased from 0.30 ± 0.18 (range, 0 to 0.70) logMAR preoperatively to 0.02 ± 0.02 (range, 0 to 0.05) logMAR at 3 months postoperatively. In the Tecnis group, BCDVA was also significantly ($P < 0.05$) improved from 0.21 ± 0.13 (range: 0 to 0.50) logMAR preoperatively to 0.01 ± 0.02 (range, 0 to 0.05) logMAR at 3 months postoperatively (Table 2). The final BCDVA of all eyes in both groups achieved 0.05 logMAR (Snellen chart 20/25 or better).

The refractive cylinder was decreased from − 1.06 ± 0.94 D preoperatively to − 0.31 ± 0.29 D (70% decrease) at 3 months postoperatively in the Precizon group. It was decreased from − 1.83 ± 1.29 D preoperatively to − 0.41 ± 0.33 D (77% decrease) at 3 months postoperatively in the Tecnis group (Table 2). At the last follow-up, residual refractive cylinder which was less than 0.50 D occurred in 16 (80%) eyes in the Precizon group and in 14 (70%) eyes in the Tecnis group.

Results of postoperative visual acuity and refraction in both groups are shown in Table 2. No statistically significant difference in UCDVA or BCDVA ($P = 0.562$, $P = 0.368$, respectively) was found between the two groups. UCIVA in the Precizon group tended to be better compared to that of the Tecnis group. However, the difference was not statistically significant ($P = 0.147$). No significant difference in refractive outcomes (sphere,

cylinder, and spherical equivalent, $P = 0.423$, $P = 0.604$, and $P = 0.400$, respectively) was found between the two groups.

Vector analysis

Vector anlysis was perfeormed at 3 months postoperatively (Table 3). The TIA vector means were 1.41 ± 0.49 D in the Precizon group and 1.41 ± 0.43 D in the Tecnis group.

No statistically significant difference in average TIA vector nor average SIA vector ($P = 0.982$, $P = 0.468$, respectively) was found between the two groups. The average DV for the Precizon and Tecnis groups were 0.31 ± 0.23 versus 0.42 ± 0.24, respectively, and these were not significantly different ($P = 0.343$). The mean correction index (ratio SIA to TIA; preferably 1), were 0.97 ± 0.25 versus 1.08 ± 0.27, respectively, reflecting slight undercorrection in the Precizon group and slight overcorrection in the Tecnis group($P = 0.377$). Other vector analysis parameters show no statistically significant difference beween groups($P > 0.05$).

Rotational stability

The mean amount of toric IOL axis rotation was 1.50° ± 0.84° (range, 0.18° to 3.02°) in the Precizon group, which was significantly ($P = 0.01$) lower than that (2.56° ± 0.68°; range, 1.50° to 3.50°) in the Tecnis group (Table 2). No eye had IOL rotation for more than 4°. No eye required a second surgery to correct the IOL axis during the 3 months of follow-up period.

Table 3 Vector Analysis of astigmatism at 3-Month Postoperatively

Parameters	Mean ± SD (range)		p value
	Precizon	Tecnis	
TIA (D)	1.41 ± 0.49 (0.54 to 2.30)	1.41 ± 0.43 (0.75 to 2.18)	0.982
SIA (D)	1.35 ± 0.52 (0.53 to 2.15)	1.57 ± 0.79 (0.70 to 2.84)	0.468
DV (D)	0.31 ± 0.23 (0.01 to 0.76)	0.42 ± 0.26 (0.01 to 0.82)	0.343
Correction index (SIA/TIA)	0.97 ± 0.25 (0.62 to 1.45)	1.08 ± 0.27 (0.67 to 1.49)	0.377
Magnitude of error (arithematic SIA/TIA)	−0.06 ± 0.34 (− 0.58 to 0.46)	0.16 ± 0.45 (− 0.45 to 0.81)	0.233
Angle of error (degree)	0.19 ± 4.80 (− 6.7 to 14.4)	−2.78 ± 6.71 (− 20.4 to 1.6)	0.274
Absolute angle of error (degree)	2.42 ± 4.10 (0.00 to 14.4)	3.18 ± 6.52 (0.10 to 20.40)	0.761
Index of success (DV/TIA)	0.23 ± 0.20 (0.02 to 0.75)	0.30 ± 0.20 (0.01 to 0.68)	0.470

SD standard deviation, *TIA* target induced astigmatism, *SIA* Surgically induced astigmatism, *DV* difference vector

Ocular wavefront aberration

Ocular wavefront aberrometry values at 3 months postoperatively are shown in Table 4. Spherical aberration was significantly ($P = 0.004$) lower in the Tecnis group compared to that in the Precizon group. Other ocular wavefront aberrametry parameters showed no statistically significant ($P > 0.05$) difference between the two groups.

Discussion

Using toric IOLs to correct corneal astigmatism at the time of cataract surgery has greatly improved both postoperative visual performance and satisfaction of the patient [3, 11]. Many IOLs are available with different characteristics. They are designed to improve the clinical outcomes including visual acuity, correction of astigmatism, and rotational stability.

Although several studies have reported the clinical outcomes of different toric IOLs, to the best of our knowledge, Precizon toric IOL compared to other toric IOL has not been reported yet. Precizon toric IOL is a relatively recently introduced toric IOL. It has been reported that Precizon toric IOL is more resistant to reduction of astigmatic correcting effects because of its unique toric surface of conic design when unexpected IOL rotation occurs [9]. Due to its transitional conic toric surface, Precizon toric IOL has consistent toric power from the center to the periphery, yielding a broader toric meridian (Fig. 1a). Therefore, Precizon toric IOL is expected to more tolerable to postoperative rotation [9]. In an optical bench analsysis, precizon's transitional conic toric surface demonstrated maximal rotational resistance compared with other toric IOL models (AT Torbi 709, SN6AT4, ZCT 225) [12]. Together with AT Torbi Precizon also showed superior image quality despite the pupil size changes in the presence of decenteration [12]. Our aim was to determine the clinical outcomes of Precizon toric IOL in comparison with Tecnis toric IOL, a commonly used IOL. Precizon toric IOL has a closed-loop haptic design. This lens is also aberration free. Tecnis toric IOL has open-loop C haptics (Fig. 1b). It has anterior toric surface with a proprietary wavefront-designed toric aspheric optic, resulting in negative spherical aberration [10]. Both toric IOL have two reference marks on the axis of the cylinder of their surface (Fig 2). Because of their definite differences in IOL characteristics, we hypothesized that different clinical results would be obtained for the two groups. However, their postoperative clinical results for many parameters were similar to each other, except postoperative IOL rotation.

UCDVA is one of the most important parameters used to determine the success in patients who undergo the

Table 4 Ocular Aberrometry Analysis at 3-Month Postoperatively

Parameters	Mean ± SD (range)		p value
	Precizon	Tecnis	
Total Aberrations RMS (μm)	1.39 ± 0.86 (0.50 to 3.08)	0.78 ± 0.53 (0.24 to 1.67)	0.138
HOA RMS(μm)	0.37 ± 0.15(0.20 to 0.76)	0.22 ± 0.11 (0.10 to 0.38)	0.200
Vertical coma (μm)	0.07 ± 0.23 (− 0.22 to 0.47)	−0.05 ± 0.18 (− 0.30 to 0.23)	0.290
Horizontal coma (μm)	0.01 ± 0.73 (− 1.94 to 0.60)	−0.10 ± 0.73 (− 1.40 to 0.59)	0.757
Vertical trefoil (μm)	−0.01 ± 0.33 (− 0.47 to 0.50)	0.10 ± 0.24 (− 0.16 to 0.49)	0.495
Horizontal trefoil (μm)	0.37 ± 0.54 (− 0.63 to 1.02)	0.10 ± 0.67 (− 0.99 to 0.79)	0.412
Spherical aberration (μm)	0.33 ± 0.16 (0.18 to 0.68)	0.06 ± 0.16 (− 0.19 to 0.30)	*0.004*

SD standard deviation, *RMS* root mean square, *HOA* higher order aberrations Malacara notation was converted to Optical Society of America standard notation, $P < 0.05$

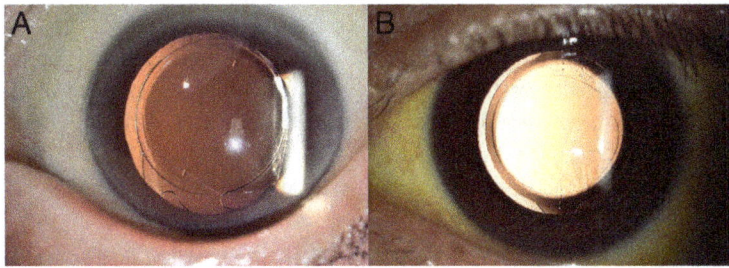

Fig. 2 Slit lamp images of the toric intraocular lens at 3 months postoperatively. **a**: Precizon toric intraocular lens. **b**: Tecnis toric intraocular lens. The axis markings can be clearly seen

surgery. In our study, the average UCDVA was 0.09 ± 0.09 logMAR in the Precizon group and 0.08 ± 0.12 log-MAR in the Tecnis group. The percentage of patients who achieved 0.1 logMAR (Snellen chart 20/25 or better) was 91% in the Precizon group and 83% in the Tecnis group. BCDVA of all eyes achieved 0.05 logMAR (Snellen acuity 20/22 or better) in both groups. Vale et al. [5] have reported that 100% of eyes have achieved a UCDVA of 0.20 logMAR (Snellen chart 20/30 or better) and Ferreira et al. [6] have reported that 82% of eyes have achieved a UCDVA of 0.10 logMAR (Snellen chart 20/25 or better) when Precizon toric IOL is used. Lubinski et al. [13] have also reported that all eyes have achieved 0.30 logMAR (Snellen chart 20/40 or better) when Tecnis toric IOL is used, similar to the outcome of the Tecnis toric IOL group in this study.

Rocha et al. [14] have shown that near and intermediate visual acuities are better in eyes with spherical IOLs compared to those with aspheric IOLs. They have concluded that residual spherical aberration can improve the depth of focus. Johansson et al. [15] have also found the depth of focus in aberration free IOLs is increased compared to negative spherical aberration IOLs. In our study, different toric IOLs (spherical aberration free and negative spherical aberration) were implanted to determine the difference in visual acuity between the groups. We planned to measure the visual acuity at 80 cm intermediate distance in postoperative evaluation because spherical aberration could increase the depth of focus [15, 16]. Although all parameters of visual acuity showed no significant difference between the two groups in this present study, UCIVA in the Precizon group did show a tendency to be better than that in the Tecnis group. The result of no significant difference in intermediate visual acuity between the two groups after the surgery might be due to the fact that the proportion of patients with large preoperative corneal astigmatism was relatively small in our sample size compared to previous studies.

The residual refractive cylinder at 3 months postoperatively was − 0.31 ± 0.29 D in the Precizon group, similar to the result of previous studies, Vale et al. [5] (0.27 ±

0.28 D at 6 months postoperatively), Ferreira et al. [6] (− 0.51 ± 0.29 D at 4 months postoperatively) and Thomas et al. [7] (− 0.25 D at 3 months postoperatively). The residual refractive cylinder in the Tecnis group was − 0.41 ± 0.33 D at 3 months postoperatively, which was smaller than − 0.56 ± 0.35 D at 8 weeks postoperatively or − 1.42 ± 0.88 D at 6 months postoperatively reported in previous studies [10, 13]. Because we considered both anterior and posterior corneal astigmatism, whereas other previous studies only considered anterior corneal astigmatism, we expected to have much smaller residual cylinder in both IOLs. However, the residual refractive cylinder in the Precizon group in our study was similar to that of a previous studies [5–7]. This might be due to the fact that preoperative corneal astigmatism in our study (1.32 ± 0.48 D) was much smaller than that in the previous studies, Vale et al. [5] (2.34 ± 0.95 D), Ferreira et al. [6] (2.38 ± 1.17 D) and Thomas et al. [7] (1.50 D). Subject component of the refraction and the effect of corneal incision might have also contributed to such result. Also the differences in postoperatve evaluation time between the studies might be the factor.

In the current study we analyzed the astigmatic change using Alpins method. No statistically significant difference in average TIA vector nor average SIA vector ($P = 0.982$, $P = 0.468$, respectively) was found between the two groups. The average DV for the Precizon and Tecnis groups were 0.31 ± 0.23 versus 0.42 ± 0.24, respectively, and these were not significantly different ($P = 0.343$). The mean correction index (ratio SIA to TIA; preferably 1), were 0.97 ± 0.25 versus 1.08 ± 0.27, respectively, reflecting slight undercorrection in the Precizon group and slight overcorrection in the Tecnis group, but there was no statistcally significant difference between two groups ($P = 0.377$). Also the Magnitude of error (arithmetic ration SIA to TIA: magnitude of error > 0 indicates overcorrection and magnitude of error < 0 undercorrection), were − 0.06 ± 0.34 versus 0.16 ± 0.45, respectively, which showed tendency of slight undercorrection in the Precizon group and slight overcorrection in the Tecnis group with no significant differences. In the previous study, Vale et al. [5] have also reported the mean difference vector as 0.24 ± 0.27, mean correction index as 0.95 ± 0.29, Absolute angle of error as 1.90 ± 0.60 (degree), and mean index of success as 0.12 ± 0.14, respectively. Kirwan C et al. [17] reported difference vector as 0.93 and correction index ratio as 1.17. There were few datas which conducted vector analysis using alpins method of the Precizon toric IOL and Tecnis toric IOL. Although the comparing with few previous data has some limitation, vector analysis of astigmatic change showed both two toric IOLs showed effective astigmatic correction.

Total aberration RMS, HOA RMS, coma, trefoil showed no significant difference between Precizon and Tecnis IOL in this current study. Spherical aberration was significantly higher in the Precizon IOL group($P = 0.004$). The Tecnis IOL has $- 0.27$ um spherical aberration and the Precizon IOL is aberration free IOL. Our results means both IOLs realized its aspheric feature. Residual spherical aberration could improve the depth of focus, and it can help the near and intermediated vision in certain part.

The main postoperative complication after implantation of toric IOLs might be rotation. It has been estimated that a rotation of 1 degree off axis can result in a loss of up to 3.3% of IOL cylinder power [4]. When misalignment is greater than 30 degrees, there might be no correction effect on the astigmatism and a shift in resultant astigmatic axis might occur. The rotational stability of the Precizon toric IOL in our study was significantly better than that in the Tecnis toric IOL group. Vale et al. [5], Ferreira et al. [6] and Thomas et al. [7] have reported that the rotation of the Precizon toric IOL was about $2.43° \pm 1.55°$, $1.98° \pm 1.78°$ and $3°$, respectively. Wasltz KL et al. [18] have found that the postoperative IOL rotation is $2.70° \pm 5.51°$ when Tecnis toric IOL is used, while Ferreira TB et al. [19] and Yang et al. [20] have reported postoperative IOL rotation of $3.15° \pm 2.62°$ and $3.2° \pm 2.2°$, respectively. In the present study, the absolute amount of postoperative rotation was $1.50° \pm 0.84°$ (range, $0.18°$ to $3.02°$) in the Precizon group and $2.56° \pm 0.68°$ (range, $1.50°$ to $3.50°$) in the Tecnis group, which were smaller than those reported previously for the two toric IOLs. Although there was a definite difference in the IOL design of the two toric IOLs (we also found significant less IOL rotation in the Precizon group compared to that in the Tecnis group), no significantly difference in clinical outcomes in terms of astigmatism correction of visual acuities at 3 months postoperatively was found between the two groups. Therefore, we conclude that such difference in rotational stability between the two groups might have minor clinical importance due to their small numerical amounts in both groups. Future studies with more participants of greater corneal astigmatism and longer postoperative follow up period are needed to determine whether the two will show different outcomes. In addition, if greater amount of rotation of IOL

occurs, clinical result might show significant difference in further studies.

There are some limitations of this study. Every study patient had undergone compelete ophthalmic examination before the surgery. If the patient showed asymmetry of capsular bag or absence of the zonules, they were excluded for study. No ocular adverse event occurred during the study. However, differences of capsular bag diameter between two groups might affect the differences in the rotational stability of the toric IOL in some part. Future study regarding size of the capsular bag can strengthen the clinical significancy.

Conclusions

In summary, our results showed that Precizon toric IOL was better than Tecnis toric IOL in rotational stability with follow up period of 3 months. Both Precizon toric IOL and Tecnis toric IOL appear to be effective alternatives for cataract surgeons to correct preexisting corneal astigmatism through cataract surgery.

Abbreviations
BCDVA: Best corrected distant visual acuity; D: Diopter; IOL: Intraocular lens; LogMAR: Logarithm of the minimum angle of resolution; RMS: Root mean square; SE: Spherical equivalent; SIA: Surgically induced astigmatism; UCDVA: Uncorrected distant visual acuity; UCIVA: Uncorrected intermediate visual acuity

Acknowledgements
None.

Funding
None.

Authors' contributions
TYC conceived and designed the study. NYJ, DHL, SSH and JH performed the study. NYJ, DHL, SSH, JH and TYC analyzed the data. NYJ, DHL and SSH contributed reagents/materials/analysis tools. NYJ and DHL wrote the manuscript. NYJ and DHL equally contributed to the manuscript as the first authors. TYC contributed to the manuscript as the corresponding authors. All authors read and approved the final manuscript.

Competing interests
The authors declare that they have no competing interests.

Author details
¹Department of Ophthalmology, Samsung Medical Center, Sungkyunkwan University School of Medicine, #81 Irwon-ro, Gangnam-gu, Seoul 06351, Korea. ²Department of Preventive Medicine, Graduate School, The Catholic University of Korea, Seoul, Korea. ³Department of Ophthalmology, Saevit Eye Hospital, Goyang, Korea.

Comparison of clinical outcomes of toric intraocular lens, Precizon vs Tecnis: a single center...

171

References

1. Khan MI, Muhtaseb M. Prevalence of corneal astigmatism in patients having routine cataract surgery at a teaching hospital in the United Kingdom. J Cataract Refract Surg. 2011;37:1751–5.
2. Guan Z, Yuan F, Yuan YZ, Niu WR. Analysis of corneal astigmatism in cataract surgery candidates at a teaching hospital in Shanghai, China. J Cataract Refract Surg. 2012;38:1970–7.
3. Kessel L, Andresen J, Tendal B, Erngaard D, Flesner P, Hjortdal J. Toric intraocular lenses in the correction of astigmatism during cataract surgery: a systematic review and meta-analysis. Ophthalmology. 2016;123:275–86.
4. Novis C. Astigmatism and toric intraocular lenses. Curr Opin Ophthalmol. 2000;11:47–50.
5. Vale C, Menezes C, Firmino-Machado J, Rodrigues P, Lume M, Tenedorio P, Meneres P, Brochado Mdo C. Astigmatism management in cataract surgery with Precizon((R)) toric intraocular lens: a prospective study. Clin Ophthalmol. 2016;10:151–9.
6. Ferreira TB, Berendschot TT, Ribeiro FJ. Clinical outcomes after cataract surgery with a new transitional toric intraocular lens. J Refract Surg. 2016;32:452–9.
7. Thomas BC, Khoramnia R, Auffarth GU, Holzer MP. Clinical outcomes after implantation of a toric intraocular lens with a transitional conic toric surface. Br J Ophthalmol 2017; pii: bjophthalmol-2017-310386. doi: https://doi.org/10.1136/bjophthalmol-2017-310386.
8. Alpins NA. A new method of analyzing vectors for changes in astigmatism. J Cataract Refract Surg. 1993;19:524–33.
9. Menezes C, Rodrigues P, J. Lemos, Gonçalves R, Coelho P, Vieira B, Serino J, Efficacy, "Rotational Stability and Tolerance for Misalignment of Precizon Toric IOL," presented at the XXXII Congress of the European Society of Cataract and Refractive Surgeons London, United Kingdom, September 2014. Abstract available at: http://www.escrs.org/london2014/programme/free-papers-details.asp?id=21889. Accessed 28 Aug 2015.
10. Sheppard AL, Wolffsohn JS, Bhatt U, Hoffmann PC, Scheider A, Hutz WW, Shah S. Clinical outcomes after implantation of a new hydrophobic acrylic toric IOL during routine cataract surgery. J Cataract Refract Surg. 2013;39:41–7.
11. Visser N, Bauer NJ, Nuijts RM. Toric intraocular lenses: historical overview, patient selection, IOL calculation, surgical techniques, clinical outcomes, and complications. J Cataract Refract Surg. 2013;39:624–37.
12. Kim MJ, Yoo YS, Joo CK, et al. Evaluation of optical performance of 4 aspheric toric intraocular lenses using an optical bench system: influence of pupil size, decentration, and rotation. J Cataract Refract Surg. 2015;41(10):2274–82.
13. Lubinski W, Kazmierczak B, Gronkowska-Serafin J, Podboraczynska-Jodko K. Clinical outcomes after uncomplicated cataract surgery with implantation of the Tecnis Toric intraocular Lens. J Ophthalmol. 2016;2016:3257217.
14. Rocha KM, Soriano ES, Chamon W, Chalita MR, Nose W. Spherical aberration and depth of focus in eyes implanted with aspheric and spherical intraocular lenses: a prospective randomized study. Ophthalmology. 2007;114:2050–4.
15. Johansson B, Sundelin S, Wikberg-Matsson A, Unsbo P, Behndig A. Visual and optical performance of the Akreos adapt advanced optics and Tecnis Z9000 intraocular lenses: Swedish multicenter study. J Cataract Refract Surg. 2007;33:1565–72.
16. Denoyer A, Denoyer L, Halfon J, Majzoub S, Pisella PJ. Comparative study of aspheric intraocular lenses with negative spherical aberration or no aberration. J Cataract Refract Surg. 2009;35:496–503.
17. Kirwan C, Nolan JM, Stack J, Dooley I, Moore J, Moore TC, Beatty S. Introduction of a Toric intraocular Lens to a non-refractive cataract practice: challenges and outcomes. Int J Ophthalmol Clin Res. 2016;25, 3(2):056.
18. Waltz KL, Featherstone K, Tsai L, Trentacost D. Clinical outcomes of TECNIS toric intraocular lens implantation after cataract removal in patients with corneal astigmatism. Ophthalmology. 2015;122:39–47.
19. Ferreira TB, Almeida A. Comparison of the visual outcomes and OPD-scan results 1of AMO Tecnis toric and Alcon Acrysof IQ toric intraocular lenses. J Refract Surg. 2012;28:551–5.
20. Yang SW, Lee JH, Lim SA, Chung SH. Comparison of the clinical outcomes of two types of Toric intraocular Lens. J Korean Ophthalmol Soc. 2016; 57:200.

26

Comparison of pars plana with anterior chamber glaucoma drainage device implantation for glaucoma: a meta-analysis

Bin Wang and Wenwei Li*

Abstract

Background: The purpose of this study was to compare the efficacy and safety of pars plana glaucoma drainage device (PP GDD) with anterior chamber glaucoma drainage device (AC GDD) for the treatment of glaucoma.

Methods: We comprehensively searched three databases, including PubMed, EMBASE, and the Cochrane Library databases, selecting the relevant studies. The continuous variables, namely, intraocular pressure (IOP) and glaucoma medications, were pooled by the weighted mean differences (WMDs), and the dichotomous outcomes, including corneal failure incidence and overall complications incidence, were pooled by the odds ratio (ORs).

Results: Four retrospective studies involving 275 eyes were evaluated, with 135 in the PP GDD group and 140 in the AC GDD group. The WMDs of the IOP reduction between the PP GDD group and the AC GDD group were -1.01 mmHg (95% CI -4.05 to 2.03, $p = 0.52$). The WMDs of the glaucoma medications reduction between the PP GDD group and the AC GDD group were 0.23 (95% CI -0.11 to 0.56, $p = 0.19$). The pooled ORs comparing PP GDD group with AC GDD group were 1.01 (95% CI 0.03 to 40.76, $p = 0.99$) for corneal failure incidence and 1.19 (95% CI 0.68 to 2.09, $p = 0.54$) for overall complication incidence. There were no significant differences between PP GDD group and AC GDD group on these aspects.

Conclusions: Both PP GDD and AC GDD procedures had similar efficacy of reduction in the IOP and number of medications. They are also both comparable on the safety with similar incidence of corneal failure and overall complications.

Keywords: Glaucoma drainage device, Pars plana, Anterior chamber, Meta analysis

Background

Glaucoma drainage device (GDD) was invented by Molteno in 1969 [1]. Since then, it has been widely used in the management of refractory glaucoma for more than 4 decades. A high success rate with an excellent intraocular pressure (IOP) control is achieved. In the last few years, some surgeons even recommended it as a first-line surgery for glaucoma.

In a standard procedure, the GDD is applied in the anterior chamber (AC) and serves as a shunter to draw aqueous humor through a tube to a subconjunctival end plate. However, it has been reported that many serious complications occurred during the follow up, especially in the anterior segment, such as corneal failure, flat anterior chamber, hyphema etc. [2–7]. Lots of attempts have been made to address these problems. This, in turn, usually aggravates the burden of patients both physically and mentally. Besides, for patients with inadequate anatomical space in the AC or those with previously compromised corneas, it is not feasible.

As an alternative surgery, pars plana (PP) insertion of a GDD into the vitreous cavity was first described in 1991 [8]. Nevertheless, it has its own operative risks as well, including vitreous incarceration of the tube, vitreous hemorrhage, and retinal detachment [9].

Until recently, only a few comparative studies have compared these two kinds of surgeries in the treatment of glaucoma [10–16]. To the best of our knowledge, comparisons of the efficiency and safety between these two methods

* Correspondence: wenwei60306@163.com
Department of Ophthalmology, Tongde Hospital of Zhejiang Province, 234 Gucui Road, Hangzhou 310012, China

have not been systematically reviewed and published. Therefore, we systematically analyzed the available literature to evaluate the efficiency and safety of PP GDD implantation versus AC GDD implantation for glaucoma.

Methods

Literature search

A comprehensive literature search of PubMed, EMBASE, and Cochrane library was performed to identify the relevant studies by two independent reviewers. The search methodology and search keywords are presented in Additional file 1. The search strategy used both keywords and Medical Subject Headings (MeSH) terms. No language or date restrictions were applied. The computerized searches covered the period from inception to April 2018.The full-text articles were retrieved for the manuscripts that potentially matched the inclusion criteria.

Inclusion and exclusion criteria

The inclusion criteria for eligibility were as follows: (1) comparisons of the efficacy and/or safety between PP GDD implantation and AC GDD implantation for glaucoma were reported; (2) prospective and retrospective comparative controlled clinical studies were included, because of the paucity of randomized controlled trials (RCTs) on PP GDD implantation and AC GDD implantation; and (3) the inclusion of at least one of the outcomes of interest. Exclusion criteria were as follows: (1) abstracts from conferences and full texts without raw data available for retrieval; (2) duplicate publications, letters, and reviews. For publications reporting on the same study, the most informative and recent article was included in this analysis. Slight disagreements between the reviewers were resolved by consensus.

Data extraction

Data were extracted from each included study by 2 independent reviewers. Slight discrepancies between the 2 independent data extractions were resolved by the discussion. For the eligible studies, the following data were extracted: (1) study characteristics, including the first author, year of publication, country, study design, number of eyes involved, patient demographics and follow-up time; (2) efficacy outcomes, including preoperative and postoperative IOP, preoperative and postoperative glaucoma medications; (3) safety outcomes, including the incidence of corneal failure and overall complications, such as tube obstruction, tube/plate exposure, device removal, retinal detachment, vitreous hemorrhage, hyphema, choroidal effusion, flat anterior chamber, corneal failure, cystoid macular edema, strabismus, diplopia, hypotony, loss of light perception, etc. Since other outcomes including visual field progression were not specifically recorded in the studies, we did not analyze these aspects.

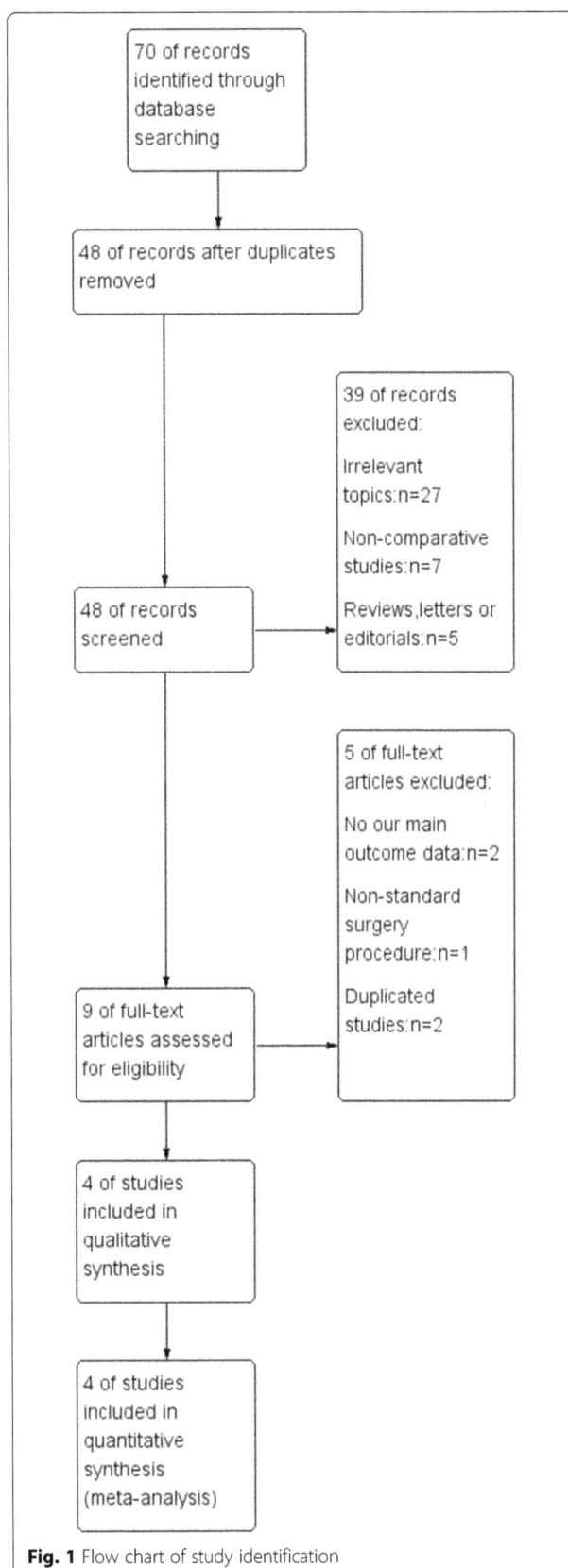

Fig. 1 Flow chart of study identification

Table 1 Study characteristics of eligible clinical studies

Study	Year	Country	Study Design	Gender(Female:Male)		Ethnicity(Black:White:Asian:other)		Assignments		No. of eyes		Mean Age(years)		Follow-up time(months)	
				Pars Plana	Anterior Chamber	Pars Plana	Anterior Chamber	Pars Plana	Anterior Chamber	Pars Plana	Anterior Chamber	Pars Plana	Anterior Chamber	Pars Plana	Anterior Chamber
Maris	2013	USA	R	19:12	18:13	2:17:1:11	3:10:3:15	PK,PAS,AACA	NA	31	31	67.3	65.7	20.9 ± 12.4	20.5 ± 13.1
Qin	2018	USA	R	30:27	36:21	20:35:2:0	23:32:1:1	LCEC,FD,CT	NA	57	57	63.1 ± 19.6	64.1 ± 20.5	43.5 ± 24.8	35.3 ± 16.7
Rososinski	2015	Australia	R	11:17	17:16	NA	NA	CP,CG,PV	NA	29	34	59	52	28	18
Seo	2015	Korea	R	9:9	10:8	NA	NA	NA	NA	18	18	52.9 ± 15.7	53.4 ± 17.8	18.0 (15~20)	18.0 (16~20)

PK penetrating keratoplasty, *PAS* peripheral anterior synechiae, *AACA* abnormal anterior chamber angle, *LCEC* low corneal endothelial count, *FD* Fuchs' dystrophy, *CT* corneal transplant, *CP* corneal pathology, *CG* corneal graft, *PV* previous vitrectom, *NA* not applicable

Table 2 Newcastle-Ottawa Scale table

Study	Selection	Comparability	Measurement	Total
Case-control studies				
Maris 2013	3	2	2	7
Qin 2018	3	1	2	6
Rososinski 2015	2	0	2	4
Seo 2015	3	1	2	6

Quality assessment

The methodological quality of each study was assessed based on the Newcastle-Ottawa Scale for quality of case–control studies in meta-analysis; for this assessment, and we used the Newcastle-Ottawa Scale star system (range, 0 to 9 stars) [17]. Two reviewers subjectively reviewed all studies and assessed all the aspects that influence the quality of a study, including selection, comparability and exposure.

Outcome measures

The primary outcome was the IOP reduction from preoperative to the last follow-up. The secondary outcome measure was the difference in the reduction in glaucoma medications from preoperative to the last follow-up. The outcomes of safety were complication rates in either group, including corneal failure and overall complications described before during the operation and whole follow-up time.

Statistical analysis

Data analysis was performed using Review Manager 5 software (RevMan 5, The Cochrane Collaboration, Oxford, UK). For continuous outcomes, the mean and SD were used to calculate weighted mean differences (WMDs). For dichotomous outcomes, odds ratios (ORs) were calculated. Statistical heterogeneity among studies was evaluated with the x^2 and I^2 tests [18]. $p < 0.05$ was considered statistically significant on the test for overall effect.

Results

Literature search

The selection of studies is shown in Fig. 1. A total of 70 articles were initially identified. 48 studies were left for further analysis after duplications removed. The abstracts were reviewed, and the remaining 9 studies were retrieved for a full-text review. Finally, 4 studies [10–12, 14] that enrolled a total of 275 eyes (135 in the PP GDD group and 140 in the AC GDD group) were included in this analysis.

Study characteristics and quality assessment

The main characteristics of the four included studies is listed in Table 1. These studies were conducted in several countries, as was shown in Table 1. In total, 275 eyes were enrolled, with 135 in the PP GDD group and 140 in the AC GDD group. Their mean age ranged from 52 to 67.3 years. All of them were retrospective studies. The average follow-up period varied from 18.0 months to 43.5 months. The qualitative assessment of these studies is summarized in Table 2.

Efficacy analysis

Since the time of follow-up in all the included studies lasted 1.5 years or more, the outcomes were believed to stabilize and may not make a difference on the statistical analysis. Therefore, the outcomes were analyzed from pre-operation to the final follow-up.

Intraocular pressure reduction

All the included studies reported preoperative and postoperative IOP. They demonstrated that the mean IOP reduction was similar in both groups, and the meta-analysis of pooled data did not show any statistically significant differences between the two groups (mean difference = – 1.01 mmHg, 95% CI -4.05 to 2.03, $p = 0.52$) (Fig. 2).

Glaucoma medications reduction

There were 3 outcomes illustrated in the 3 studies as to the glaucoma medications reduction. Examination of the forest plot showed that the differences between the two groups were not significantly different (mean difference = 0.23, 95% CI -0.11 to 0.56, $p = 0.19$) (Fig. 3).

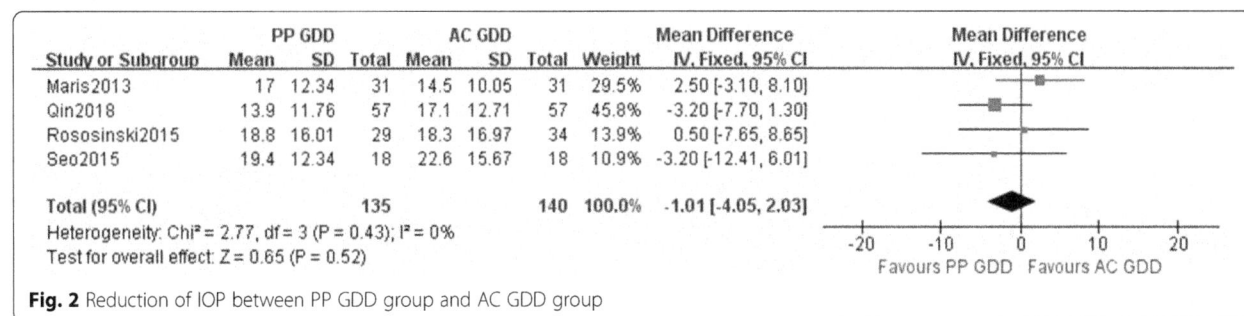

Study or Subgroup	PP GDD Mean	SD	Total	AC GDD Mean	SD	Total	Weight	Mean Difference IV, Fixed, 95% CI	Mean Difference IV, Fixed, 95% CI
Maris2013	17	12.34	31	14.5	10.05	31	29.5%	2.50 [-3.10, 8.10]	
Qin2018	13.9	11.76	57	17.1	12.71	57	45.8%	-3.20 [-7.70, 1.30]	
Rososinski2015	18.8	16.01	29	18.3	16.97	34	13.9%	0.50 [-7.65, 8.65]	
Seo2015	19.4	12.34	18	22.6	15.67	18	10.9%	-3.20 [-12.41, 6.01]	
Total (95% CI)			135			140	100.0%	-1.01 [-4.05, 2.03]	

Heterogeneity: Chi² = 2.77, df = 3 (P = 0.43); I² = 0%
Test for overall effect: Z = 0.65 (P = 0.52)

Favours PP GDD   Favours AC GDD

Fig. 2 Reduction of IOP between PP GDD group and AC GDD group

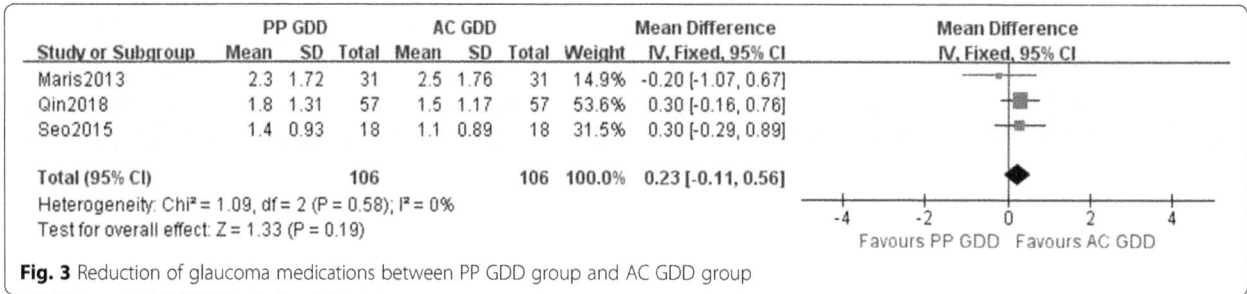

Fig. 3 Reduction of glaucoma medications between PP GDD group and AC GDD group

Safety analysis

Corneal failure

Three studies reported data for the corneal failure incidence. However, examination of the forest plots revealed that the differences were not statistically significant between the two groups (mean difference = 1.01, 95% CI 0.03 to 40.76, $p = 0.99$) (Fig. 4).

Overall complications

Overall complications comparing the two groups were described in all of the included studies. And these were displayed in Table 3. Pooled results showed similar overall complication incidence between the 2 groups (mean difference = 1.19, 95% CI 0.68 to 2.09, $p = 0.54$) (Fig. 5).

Discussion

In our present study, four retrospective clinical studies were reviewed. After pooling the results of these studies, we found that both procedures shared similar efficacy of reduction in the IOP and number of glaucoma medications. For safety, both procedures resulted in similar complications in terms of corneal failure and overall complications.

In a long time, glaucoma drainage devices have been reserved for patients diagnosed with refractory glaucoma. However, with its favorable advantages, it has been introduced to routine surgical management of glaucoma patients as well. In the traditional surgery, GDD is inserted into the anterior chamber. And it shunts aqueous outflow from the anterior chamber into the subconjunctival space, which could lower IOP to normal values. In spite of all these advantages, the routine placement of GDD has been

associated with serious anterior segment complications [19]. To avoid this, pars plana insertion of a GDD into the vitreous cavity was first described in 1991 [8]. Theoretically, the posterior location of GDD could reduce the risk of anterior segment complications. And in recent years, several clinical studies were designed to compare the therapeutic effects between the two methods [10–12, 14]. According to what we know, this is the first meta analysis to evaluate clinical effects and safety between PP GDD and AC GDD for glaucoma.

In our analysis, we found that the reductions of IOP and glaucoma medications in both groups were both remarkable. According to the four included studies, there was no statistically significant difference in efficiency between two procedures.

On the other hand, the incidence of corneal failure and overall complications were compared and analyzed respectively. Since PP GDD avoided the interference of anterior chamber, it was conjectured that it might come out with a lower corneal failure incidence. However, based on our analysis, we did not find any obviously difference. Of these, only in one study, Seo et al., 2015 compared the changes in corneal endothelial cells after PP GDD with those after AC GDD and its average follow-up was 18 months [12]. It showed significant difference between the 2 groups, which illustrated that endothelial cell damage in the PP GDD group appeared to be lower than that in the AC GDD group. Other clinical studies did not show specific details on endothelial cell number. Some further studies may be needed to confirm the effect on endothelial cell. So far, the two

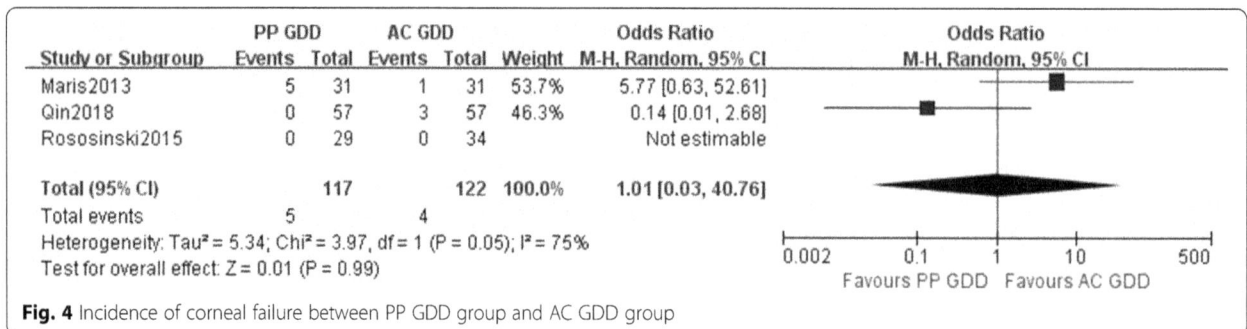

Fig. 4 Incidence of corneal failure between PP GDD group and AC GDD group

Table 3 All the complications included in the studies

Complications	Maris		Qin		Rososinski		Seo	
	PP(31)	AC(31)	PP(57)	AC(57)	PP(29)	AC(34)	PP(18)	AC(18)
Tube obstruction	4	2	NA	NA	NA	NA	NA	NA
Tube/plate exposure	2	0	NA	NA	NA	NA	NA	NA
Device removal	1	0	NA	NA	NA	NA	NA	NA
Retinal detachment	1	1	NA	NA	0	1	NA	NA
Vitreous hemorrhage	1	0	1	3	NA	NA	2	1
Hyphema	1	0	NA	NA	NA	NA	1	3
Choroidal effusion	3	4	NA	NA	NA	NA	NA	NA
Flat anterior chamber	0	6	NA	NA	NA	NA	NA	NA
Cystoid macular edema	1	1	NA	NA	NA	NA	NA	NA
Strabismus	1	0	NA	NA	NA	NA	NA	NA
Corneal failure	5	1	NA	NA	NA	NA	NA	NA
Loss of light perception	0	1	NA	NA	NA	NA	NA	NA
Diplopia	NA	NA	9	3	NA	NA		
Hypotony	NA	NA	5	5	NA	NA	1	0
Tube erosion	NA	NA	1	0	NA	NA		
Retinal hemorrhage	NA	NA	NA	NA	0	1	NA	NA
Tube replacement	NA	NA	NA	NA	0	1	NA	NA
Elevated IOP	NA	NA	NA	NA	NA	NA	2	1

NA not applicable

procedures had similar corneal failure incidence. This may be explained by the reason that the effect on corneal endothelial cells may not be so obviously different that the incidence of corneal failure was unable to detect this change in both groups. With regard to overall complications, the two groups did not show any significant advantages over the other one. This may be explained by the fact that clinicians have more effective means to intervene in case of anterior segment complications and the outcomes are better. However, when it comes to the posterior segment complications, the surgical intervention and treatment are limited with poor outcomes generally. Several studies analyzed this and our results were similar to theris [10–16].

However, several limitations should be taken into account when considering the results of this meta analysis. First, in reviewing the literature, the studies included are all retrospective studies because of the absence of randomized studies in the database, which may have potential sources of selection bias. There is still the possibility of underlying bias where there are different clinical indications for placing AC and PP GDD. As the PP is often reserved for cases where AC is not feasible or the cornea is at a high risk, we cannot exclude this bias. This needs to be confirmed with further RCTs, which are still rare in the publishing studies. Typically for meta-analysis research, publication bias cannot be excluded. Additionally, the pooled data were only from the mean follow up

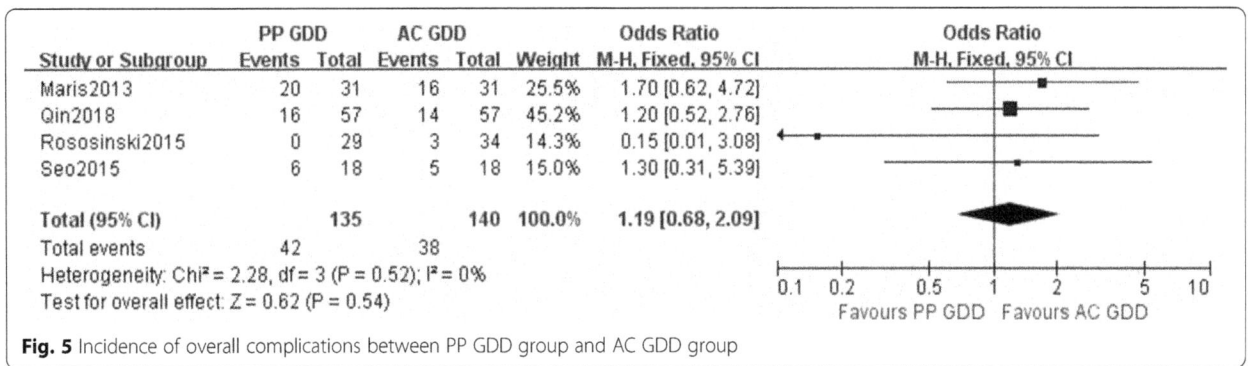

Fig. 5 Incidence of overall complications between PP GDD group and AC GDD group

of various studies of different durations, introducing a potential heterogeneity. And we speculated that outcomes were stabilized after 1.5 years. Later, the state of IOP, number of glaucoma medications and the incidence of corneal failure and overall complications became stable. The changes were subtle if the differences existed. On the other hand, different studies adopted different criteria for participants. It might be another source of heterogeneity in the results. Also, the antiglaucoma therapy difference among the studies served as another point of heterogeneity, which should not be neglected. Finally, because of the limited number of studies available in the analysis, we did not perform subgroup analysis.

Conclusions

Our results showed that both the PP GDD and AC GDD procedures had similar efficacy of reduction in the IOP and number of medications. They are also both comparable on the safety with similar incidence of corneal failure and overall complications. However, there is still an urgent need for pragmatic RCT with long duration and a large sample size to further determine the efficacy and safety (especially, the endothelial cell number change) of PP GDD in the treatment of glaucoma.

Abbreviations

AC: anterior chamber; CI: Confidence interval; GDD: Glaucoma drainage device; IOP: Intraocular pressure; OR: Odds ratio; PP: Pars plana; R: Retrospective; RCT: Randomized controlled clinical trial; WMD: Weighted mean difference

Authors' contributions

BW drafted the manuscript. BW and WL participated in the design of the study and performed the statistical analysis. Both authors read and approved the final manuscript.

Competing interests

The authors declare that they have no competing interests.

References

1. Molteno AC. New implant for drainage in glaucoma. Clinical trial. Br J Ophthalmol. 1969;53(9):606–15.
2. Sherwood MB, Joseph NH, Hitchings RA. Surgery for refractory glaucoma. Results and complications with a modified Schocket technique. Arch Ophthalmol. 1987;105(4):562–9.
3. Hill RA, Heuer DK, Baerveldt G, Minckler DS, Martone JF. Molteno implantation for glaucoma in young patients. Ophthalmology. 1991;98(7):1042–6.
4. Lloyd MA, Sedlak T, Heuer DK, Minckler DS, Baerveldt G, Lee MB, Martone JF. Clinical experience with the single-plate Molteno implant in complicated glaucomas. Update of a pilot study. Ophthalmol. 1992;99(5):679–87.
5. Netland PA, Walton DS. Glaucoma drainage implants in pediatric patients. Ophthalmic Surg. 1993;24(11):723–9.
6. Gandham SB, Costa VP, Katz LJ, Wilson RP, Sivalingam A, Belmont J, Smith M. Aqueous tube-shunt implantation and pars plana vitrectomy in eyes with refractory glaucoma. Am J Ophthalmol. 1993;116(2):189–95.
7. Siegner SW, Netland PA, Urban RC Jr, Williams AS, Richards DW, Latina MA, Brandt JD. Clinical experience with the Baerveldt glaucoma drainage implant. Ophthalmology. 1995;102(9):1298–307.
8. Varma R, Heuer DK, Lundy DC, Baerveldt G, Lee PP, Minckler DS. Pars plana Baerveldt tube insertion with vitrectomy in glaucomas associated with pseudophakia and aphakia. Am J Ophthalmol. 1995;119(4):401–7.
9. Lloyd MA, Heuer DK, Baerveldt G, Minckler DS, Martone JF, Lean JS, Liggett PE. Combined Molteno implantation and pars plana vitrectomy for neovascular glaucomas. Ophthalmology. 1991;98(9):1401–5.
10. Maris PJ Jr, Tsai JC, Khatib N, Bansal R, Al-Aswad LA. Clinical outcomes of Ahmed Glaucoma valve in posterior segment versus anterior chamber. J Glaucoma. 2013;22(3):183–9.
11. Rososinski A, Wechsler D, Grigg J. Retrospective review of pars plana versus anterior chamber placement of Baerveldt glaucoma drainage device. J Glaucoma. 2015;24(2):95–9.
12. Seo JW, Lee JY, Nam DH, Lee DY. Comparison of the changes in corneal endothelial cells after pars plana and anterior chamber ahmed valve implant. J Ophthalmol. 2015;2015:486832.
13. Parihar JK, Jain VK, Kaushik J, Mishra A. Pars Plana-modified versus conventional Ahmed Glaucoma valve in patients undergoing penetrating Keratoplasty: a prospective comparative randomized study. Curr Eye Res. 2017;42(3):436–42.
14. Qin VL, Kaleem M, Conti FF, Rockwood EJ, Singh A, Sood-Mendiratta S, Sears JE, Silva FQ, Eisengart J, Singh RP. Long-term clinical outcomes of pars Plana versus anterior chamber placement of Glaucoma implant tubes. J Glaucoma. 2018;27:1.
15. Wechsler D, Rososinski A, Grigg J. To compare outcomes of pars plana versus anterior chamber placement of baerveldt glaucoma drainage implant. Clin Exp Ophthalmol. 2011;39:61.
16. Qin V, Kaleem MA, Rockwood EJ, Singh A, Sood-Mendiratta S, Sears JE, Trace S, Silva FQDPA, Eisengart J, Singh RP. Long-term clinical outcomes of pars plana (PP) versus anterior chamber (AC) placement of glaucoma tube implants. Investig Ophthalmol Vis Sci. 2017;58(8).
17. Wells GA, Shea B, O'Connell D, Peterson J, Welch V, Losos M, Tugwell P.; The Newcastle-Ottawa Scale (NOS) for assessing the quality of nonrandomised studies in meta-analyses. http://www.ohri.ca/programs/clinical_epidemiology/oxford.htm. Accessed 29 Apr 2004.
18. Higgins JP, Thompson SG, Deeks JJ, Altman DG. Measuring inconsistency in meta-analyses. Bmj. 2003;327(7414):557–60.
19. Gedde SJ, Schiffman JC, Feuer WJ, Herndon LW, Brandt JD, Budenz DL. Tube versus trabeculectomy study G: treatment outcomes in the tube versus trabeculectomy (TVT) study after five years of follow-up. Am J Ophthalmol. 2012;153(5):789–803. e782

27

Comparative evaluation of refractive outcomes after implantation of two types of intraocular lenses with different diopter intervals (0.25 diopter versus 0.50 diopter)

Minjung Kim[1], Youngsub Eom[1,2]* ⓘ, Jong Suk Song[1] and Hyo Myung Kim[1]

Abstract

Background: Intraocular lenses (IOLs) with different diopter (D) intervals may have different tolerance, and may provide different accuracy of refractive outcome after cataract surgery. The aim of the study is to compare the accuracy of refractive outcome after implantation of IOLs with different D intervals after cataract surgery.

Methods: A total of 80 eyes from 40 patients who underwent phacoemulsification with implantation of a 0.50 D interval Akreos AO IOL in one eye and a 0.25 D interval Softec HD™ IOL in the other eye were enrolled. The percentages of eyes with refractive prediction error within ±0.50 D at one month after surgery were compared. To evaluate the effect of the dioptric errors of the IOL itself on refractive prediction error, the percentage of eyes with refractive prediction error within ±0.25 D of the IOL with a standard deviation (SD) of ±0.40 D was compared with that of the IOL with a SD of ±0.11 D through Monte Carlo simulations.

Results: In this clinical study, the percentage of eyes with refractive prediction error within ±0.50 D by the Haigis formula in the Softec HD™ group (85.0%) was significantly greater than that in the Akreos AO group (57.5%; $P = 0.027$). In Monte Carlo simulations, all percentages of eyes with refractive prediction error within ±0.25 D by the Haigis and SRK/T formulas in the Softec HD™ group were significantly greater than those in the Akreos AO group.

Conclusions: The IOL with a 0.25 D interval was more accurate than the IOL with a 0.50 D interval in predicting refractive outcome after cataract surgery.

Keywords: Intraocular lens power calculation, Refractive outcomes, Diopter intervals, Bilateral cataract extraction

Background

Intraocular lenses (IOLs) replace the human crystalline lens after cataract extraction by phacoemulsification. The advent of precise optical biometry and IOL power calculation formulas has greatly improved postoperative vision by decreasing refractive prediction error in cataract surgery. [1–3] However, it has always been a challenge for cataract surgeons to enhance refractive outcomes.

There are three main sources of error in IOL power calculation: preoperative estimation of effective lens position, measurement of axial length (AL), and corneal power (determined via keratometry [K]), which contribute to 42, 36, and 22% of errors, respectively. [1, 4] However, several factors such as surgical technique and dioptric power accuracy of the IOL can affect the refractive outcomes. [4] IOL power provided by the manufacturer has an allowed tolerance for power labelling, [5] although the IOL power error is known to contribute less than 1.0% to the total error in postoperative refractive prediction. [4, 6] Most of the IOLs used in cataract surgery are produced at 0.5 diopter (D) intervals. A previous study proposed that tolerance limits of ±0.40 D in the range of 15.5 D to 25.0 D

* Correspondence: hippotate@hanmail.net
[1]Department of Ophthalmology, Korea University College of Medicine, Seoul, South Korea
[2]Department of Ophthalmology, Ansan Hospital, Korea University College of Medicine, 123, Jeokgeum-ro, Danwon-gu, Ansan-si, Gyeonggi-do 15355, South Korea

is a suitable international standard for 0.5 D interval IOLs. [5, 7] However, 0.25 D interval IOLs have been developed and used in the IOL industry. Their manufacturer reported that these IOLs within the range of 15.5 D to 25.0 D have an error range of ±0.11 D. [8]

In this study, we hypothesized that implantation of IOLs with 0.25 D intervals, a value that is expected to have strict tolerance limits, would produce more accurate refractive outcomes than would IOLs with 0.50 D intervals after phacoemulsification. To test the hypothesis, this study compared refractive outcomes after implantation of 0.25 D interval IOL in one eye and 0.50 D interval IOL in the other eye in patients with bilateral cataract.

Methods
Study population

This prospective study was approved by the institutional review board (IRB) of Korea University Ansan Hospital (IRB number: 2016AS0020) and was registered as a clinical trial at https://cris.nih.go.kr (identification number: KCT0002192). All patients provided signed informed consent to participate in a clinical research study. All research and data collection practices adhered to the tenets of the Declaration of Helsinki and good clinical practices.

Eighty eyes from 40 patients with bilateral senile cataract who were scheduled to undergo consecutive phacoemulsification and IOL implantation within a period of one to four weeks at Korea University Ansan Hospital between November 1, 2016 and August 31, 2017 were enrolled in this study. The Softec HD™ (Lenstec Inc., St. Petersburg, FL, USA; 40 eyes) IOL with a 0.25 D interval was implanted in one eye of each subject, and the Akreos AO (Bausch & Lomb, Rochester, NY, USA; 40 eyes) IOL with a 0.50 D interval was implanted in the contralateral eye. The RANDBETWEEN(1,2) function in Microsoft Excel (Microsoft Inc., Redmond, WA, USA) was used to randomly decide which IOL would be used in the first eye. The Softec HD™ and Akreos AO IOLs employ similar material and optic design (hydrophilic acrylic bi-aspheric zero aberration with 1.46 refractive index), although their haptic design and overall length are different (Table 1 and Figure 1). We specifically included patients who were

scheduled to undergo implantation of IOL with a power range from 15.5 D to 25.0 D because the Softec HD™ IOL provides a 0.25 D interval in this range. Eyes with best corrected visual acuity (BCVA) of 20/40 or better postoperatively were included in this study. Patients with amblyopia, corneal disease such as keratoconus or corneal dystrophy, traumatic cataracts, or a history of previous ocular surgery (e.g., refractive surgery) were excluded. Also excluded from this study were those patients who had undergone complicated ocular surgery (e.g., anterior capsular tears); those who had had any postoperative complications; and those with noticeable postoperative IOL decentration or tilt.

Patient examination

Preoperative objective refraction measured with an autorefractor/keratometer (KR-8100; Topcon, Tokyo, Japan) was recorded at the screening visit. Subjective refraction was recorded when autorefraction was not available. Preoperative K, anterior chamber depth (ACD), and AL values were measured with optical biometry using an IOLMaster® 500 (Carl Zeiss Meditec, Jena, Germany). IOL power was calculated using the SRK/T and Haigis formulas of the device. The data-adjusted SRK/T A-constant was calculated using a spreadsheet (Microsoft Excel; Microsoft Inc.), and the data-adjusted a_0, a_1, and a_2 constants for the Haigis formula were calculated with linear regression analysis in order to obtain zero mean numerical error in IOL power prediction. [9–12] The data-adjusted SRK/T A-constant was 118.17 for the Softec HD™ IOL and 118.24 for the Akreos AO IOL. The optimized IOL constants for the Haigis formula (a_0, a_1, and a_2) were 0.565, 0.240, and 0.138, respectively, for the Softec HD™ IOL and 1.706, 0.279, and 0.087, respectively, for the Akreos AO IOL. Postoperative uncorrected distance visual acuity, BCVA, objective refraction measured with an autorefractor/keratometer, and subjective refraction were measured at one month after surgery. The refractionist was masked to type of IOL.

Surgical technique

All phacoemulsification and IOL implantations were performed by one experienced surgeon (Y.E.) under topical

Table 1 Characteristics of the IOLs used in this study

Parameter	Akreos AO	Softec HD™
Material	Hydrophilic acrylic (26% water content)	Hydrophilic acrylic (26% water content)
Refractive index	1.46	1.46
Overall length, mm	10.5–11.0	12.0
Optic size, mm	6.00	5.75
Optic design	Bi-aspheric zero aberration	Bi-aspheric zero aberration
Haptic design	Four loop	Modified C
Haptic angulation, degrees	0	0

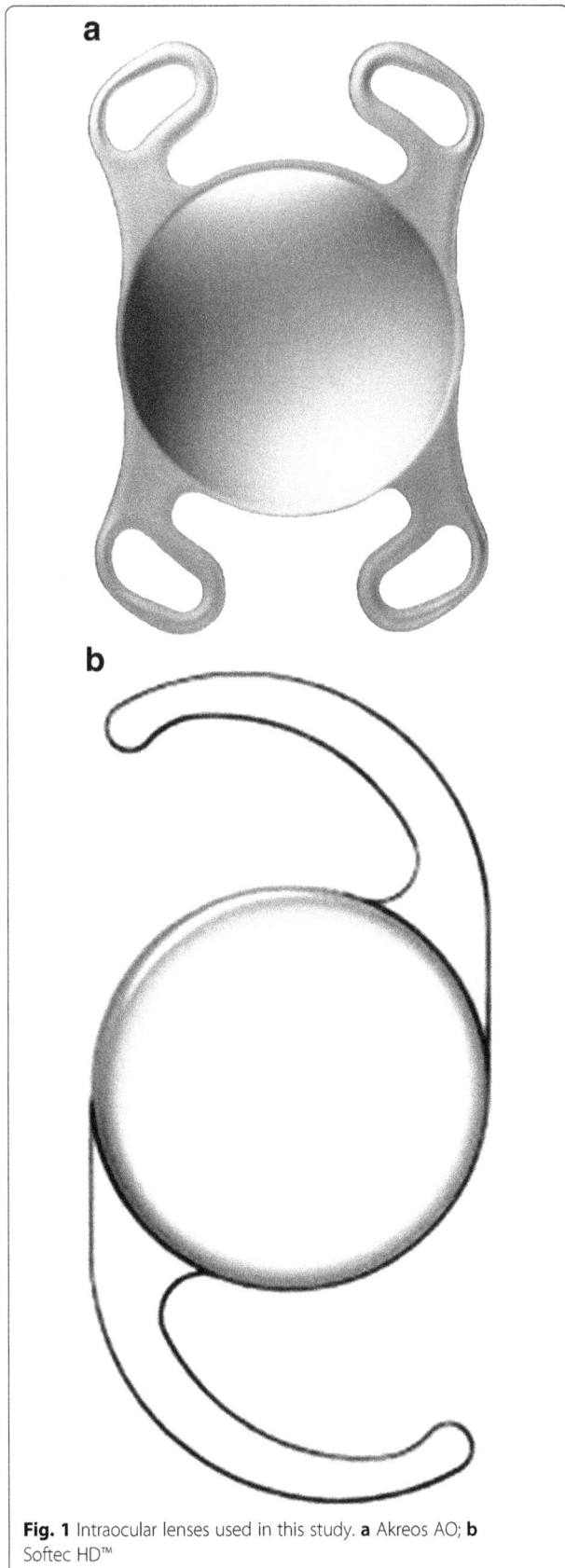

Fig. 1 Intraocular lenses used in this study. **a** Akreos AO; **b** Softec HD™

anesthesia with 0.5% proparacaine hydrochloride (Paracaine; Hanmi Pharm, Seoul, Korea). During surgery, a 2.75-mm clear corneal incision was made, and a continuous curvilinear capsulorrhexis slightly smaller in size than the IOL optic was created with a 26-gauge needle and capsulorrhexis forceps. After performing hydrodissection and hydrodelineation, superficial cortex and epinucleus were aspirated with a phaco probe. Then, the nucleus was held by the phaco probe, and the phaco chopper (Nagahara Chopper; ASICO, LLC, Westmont, IL) was placed on the opposite side of the equator of the nucleus. The phaco chopper was pulled and the phaco probe was pushed toward the phaco chopper to divide the nucleus into halves. Then the divided nucleus halves were rotated 90 degrees and divided into quadrants with the same technique. All pieces of segments of the divided nucleus were emulsified and aspirated. An irrigation/aspiration system was used to remove the epinucleus and cortex. The anterior chamber was filled with sodium hyaluronate 1.65% /chondroitin sodium sulfate 4.0% (DisCoVisc; Alcon Laboratories, Inc., Fort Worth, TX), and each IOL was implanted in a capsular bag using an injector system. After removing the ophthalmic viscosurgical device, the wound was sutured with 10–0 nylon, which was removed at postoperative 1 week.

Preoperative and postoperative medication
Preoperative medication 0.5% levofloxacin hydrate (Cravit®, Santen, Osaka, Japan) every 6 h and 0.1% bromfenac sodium hydrate (Bronuck®, Taejoon Pharm., Seoul, Korea) every 12 h were used for 3 days before surgery. At the day of surgery, 0.5% Moxifloxacin (Vigamox®, Alcon) every 2 h, 0.1% fluorometholone (Flucon®, Alcon) every 6 h, and 0.1% bromfenac sodium hydrate (Bronuck®) every 12 h were used. At the day after surgery, 0.5% Moxifloxacin was used every 6 h, along with the other eye drops used on 1 day for the next 1 month.

Monte Carlo simulation
To evaluate the effect of the dioptric error of the IOL produced during the manufacturing process on refractive outcome, only IOL power was used as a random variable in Monte Carlo simulation, and it was assumed that no error was caused by the preoperative estimation of effective lens position and/or the measurement of K, ACD, and AL in the IOL power calculation. In order to satisfy this assumption, IOL power, which has zero refractive prediction error, was calculated from preoperative biometry and postoperative spherical equivalent values in each patient. The mean and standard deviation (SD) values were used to generate random variables of IOL power for each patient with a normal distribution using the RAND() and NORMINV functions in Excel (Microsoft Inc.). The mean value of IOL power was defined as the IOL power that has

zero refractive prediction error in each patient, and SD was ±0.40 D in the Akreos AO group and ± 0.11 D in the Softec HD™ group. [7, 8] Generated IOL powers for each patient were used to calculate the refractive prediction error during Monte Carlo simulation. This study conducted 20 Monte Carlo simulations: 10 using the Haigis formula and 10 using the SRK/T formula.

Main outcome measures

The refractive prediction error was defined as the difference between postoperative spherical equivalent and preoperative predicted refraction as determined using two IOL calculation formulas (i.e., refractive prediction error = postoperative spherical equivalent – preoperative predicted refraction). The mean absolute error (MAE) was defined as the mean absolute value of the refractive prediction error, and the median absolute error (MedAE) was defined as the median absolute value of the refractive prediction error. The percentages of eyes that achieved a postoperative refractive prediction error within ±0.25 D, ± 0.50 D, and ± 0.75 D from the preoperative predicted refraction were estimated.

Statistical analysis

Descriptive statistics for all patient data were obtained using the Statistical Package for Social Sciences version 21.0 (IBM Corp., Armonk, NY, USA). Student's t-tests were used to compare K, ACD, AL, IOL power, and MAE, while Mann–Whitney U tests were used to compare MedAE between the two groups. Chi-square tests were conducted to compare the percentage of eyes that achieved a postoperative refractive prediction error within ±0.25 or ± 0.50 D from the preoperative predicted refraction by the SRK/T and Haigis formulas between the two groups. Results were considered statistically significant if the P-value was less than 0.05.

Results

The mean patient age was 70.2 ± 9.4 years (range: 43–88 years). Fourteen patients (35.0%) were male, and 26 patients were female. The Akreos AO group used 12 different IOLs (power range: 17.0–24.0 D), and the Softec HD™ group used 20 different IOLs (power range: 16.75–24.25 D). There was a significant correlation in the mean K ($R^2 = 0.926$, $P < 0.001$), ACD ($R^2 = 0.893$, $P < 0.001$), and AL ($R^2 = 0.934$, P < 0.001) values between the Akreos AO and Softec HD™ groups. In addition, there was a moderate to strong correlation in refractive prediction error between the two groups (Figure 2). The laterality, mean refractive error, K, ACD, AL, and calculated IOL power values are shown in Table 2.

Table 3 shows MedAE and mean refractive prediction error as determined by the Haigis and SRK/T formulas. The MedAE in the Softec HD™ group (0.30 D with the

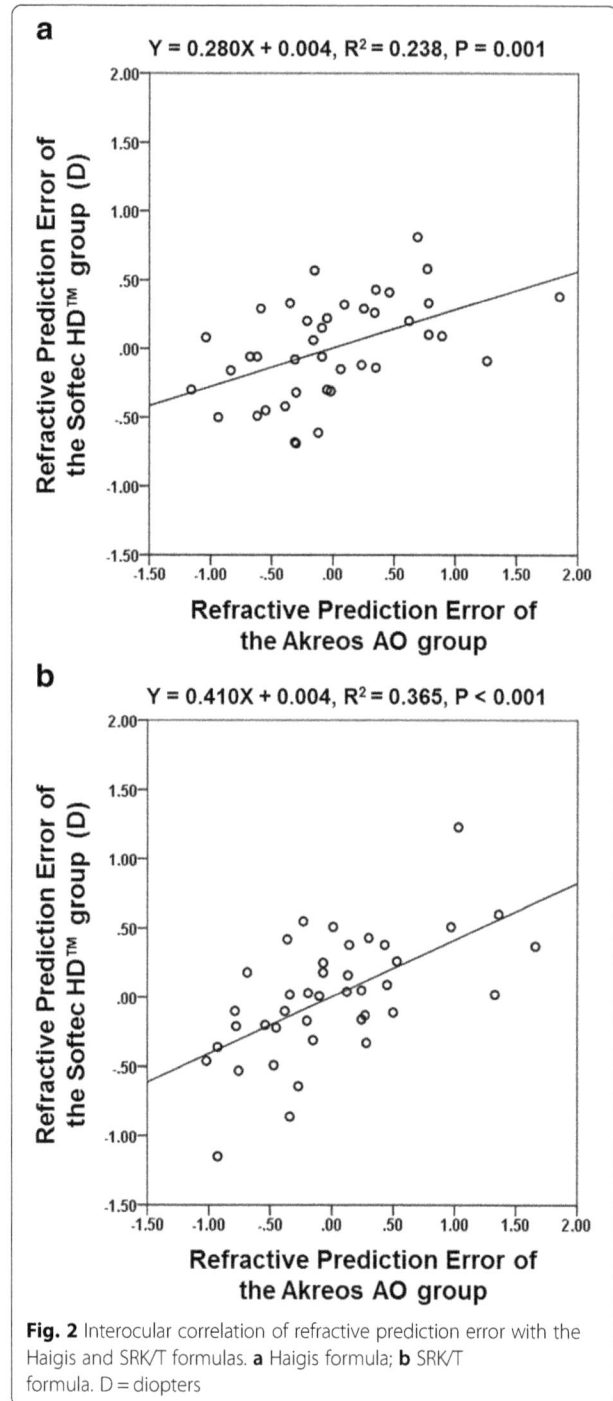

Fig. 2 Interocular correlation of refractive prediction error with the Haigis and SRK/T formulas. **a** Haigis formula; **b** SRK/T formula. D = diopters

Haigis formula and 0.26 D with the SRK/T formula) was significantly smaller than that in the Akreos AO group (0.35 D with the Haigis formula and 0.37 D with the SRK/T formula; $P = 0.037$ and $P = 0.049$, respectively). The percentage of eyes that achieved postoperative refractive prediction error within ±0.25 D, ± 0.50 D, and ± 0.75 D from the preoperative predicted refraction by the Haigis formula was 32.5, 57.5, and 75.0%, respectively, in the Akreos AO group and 42.5, 85.0, and 97.5%,

Table 2 Clinical characteristics of the cataract patients and their eyes

Parameter	Akreos AO (n = 40)	Softec HD™ (n = 40)	P-value[b]
Age, years	70.2 (9.4)		
Sex			
Male, n (%)	14 (35.0)		
Female, n (%)	26 (65.0)		
Laterality			> 0.999[c]
Right eye, n (%)	20 (50.0)	20 (50.0)	
Left eye, n (%)	20 (50.0)	20 (50.0)	
Refractive error, D[a]	− 0.92 (2.34)	−0.88 (2.44)	0.935
Keratometry, D[b]	44.41 (1.37)	44.36 (1.35)	0.880
Anterior chamber depth, mm[b]	3.14 (0.37)	3.17 (0.35)	0.769
Axial length, mm[b]	23.42 (0.70)	23.44 (0.69)	0.907
IOL power, D	20.50 (1.88)	20.37 (1.74)	0.747

Data are mean (SD) except for sex and laterality, which are n (%)

IOL Intraocular lens, *D* Diopters, *SD* Standard deviation

[a]Refractive error was measured by an autorefractor/keratometer (KR-8100). Subjective refraction was recorded when autorefraction was not available

[b]Keratometry, anterior chamber depth, and axial length were measured by the IOLMaster® 500

[b]Student's t-test

[c]Chi-square test

Table 3 Comparison of median absolute error and mean refractive prediction error between the Akreos AO and Softec HD™ groups in the Haigis and SRK/T formulas (n = 80)

	Akreos AO (n = 40)	Softec HD™ (n = 40)	P-value
Haigis formula			
MedAE, D[a]	0.35 (0.17: 0.75)	0.30 (0.13: 0.43)	0.037[c]
MAE, D[b]	0.49 (0.40)	0.30 (0.20)	0.009[d]
RE, D (range)	0.00 (−1.16–1.85)	0.00 (− 0.69–0.81)	
± 0.25 D, n (%)	13 (32.5)	17 (42.5)	
± 0.50 D, n (%)	23 (57.5)	34 (85.0)	0.027[e]
± 0.75 D, n (%)	130 (75.0)	39 (97.5)	
> ±1.00 D, n (%)	4 (10.0)	0 (0.0)	
SRK/T formula			
MedAE, D[a]	0.37 (0.21: 0.78)	0.26 (0.12: 0.48)	0.049[c]
MAE, D[b]	0.50 (0.40)	0.33 (0.26)	0.030[d]
RE, D (range)	0.00 (−1.02–1.66)	0.03 (−1.15–1.23)	
±0.25 D, n (%)	13 (32.5)	20 (50.0)	
±0.50 D, n (%)	26 (65.0)	31 (77.5)	0.323[e]
±0.75 D, n (%)	29 (72.5)	37 (92.5)	
> ±1.00 D, n (%)	4 (10.0)	2 (5.0)	

MedAE Median absolute error, *D* Diopters, *MAE* Mean absolute error, *RE* Mean refractive prediction error

[a]Values are presented as median (interquartile range)

[b]Values are presented as mean (SD)

[c]Mann–Whitney U test

[d]Student's t-test

[e]Chi-square test

respectively, in the Softec HD™ group. This percentage within ±0.50 D by the Haigis formula in the Softec HD™ group was significantly greater than that in the Akreos AO group (*P* = 0.027). On the other hand, there was no significant difference in the percentage of eyes that achieved a postoperative refractive prediction error within ±0.50 D from the preoperative predicted refraction by the SRK/T formula between the Akreos AO and Softec HD™ groups (Table 3).

In the Monte Carlo simulations, the MedAE as determined by the Haigis formula ranged from 0.14 D to 0.27 D, and that determined by the SRK/T formula ranged from 0.14 D to 0.24 D in the Akreos AO group. All MedAEs in the Akreos AO group were significantly greater than those in the Softec HD™ group (range: from 0.04 to 0.06 D in the Haigis formula and from 0.04 to 0.06 D in the SRK/T formula; Tables 4 and 5). Because the MedAE in the Monte Carlo simulations was about half or less than that in clinical study, the percentage of eyes that achieved a postoperative refractive prediction error within ±0.25 D from the preoperative predicted refraction was compared. The percentage of eyes that achieved a postoperative refractive prediction error within ±0.25 D as determined by the Haigis formula ranged from 45.0 to 72.5%, and that determined by the SRK/T formula ranged from 52.5 to 72.5% in the Akreos AO group. This percentage within ±0.25 D in the Akreos AO group was significantly smaller than that in the Softec HD™ group (range: 97.5 to 100.0% in the Haigis formula and 97.5% in the SRK/T formula; Tables 4 and 5).

Discussion

This study compared the accuracy of refractive outcomes of IOLs with different diopter intervals (0.50 D versus 0.25 D) in cataract surgery and showed that the IOL with a 0.25 D interval had a postoperative spherical equivalent closer to the target refraction predicted by the Haigis and SRK/T formulas than did the IOL with a 0.50 D interval. In addition, more eyes showed refractive prediction error within ±0.50 D with the IOLs with a 0.25 D interval than with the IOLs with a 0.50 D interval. The results of this study suggest that the implantation of IOLs with 0.25 D intervals, which are expected to have strict tolerance limits, would yield more accurate refractive outcomes than implantation of IOLs with 0.50 D intervals after phacoemulsification.

In this study, the percentages of eyes that achieved a refractive prediction error within ±0.50 D were 85.0 and 77.5% as determined by the Haigis and SRK/T formulas, respectively, in the Softec HD™ group. In line with this study, David et al. [13] performed a study involving 291 eyes that underwent cataract surgery with implantation of Softec HD™ IOLs and reported that 72.2% of these eyes achieved a refractive prediction error within ±0.50

Table 4 Comparison of median absolute error and percentage of eyes that achieved a postoperative refractive prediction error within ±0.25 D by the Haigis formula between the Akreos AO and Softec HD™ groups in Monte Carlo simulation

		Akreos AO (n = 40)	Softec HD™ (n = 40)	P-value
Simulation 1	MedAE, D[a]	0.21 (0.08: 0.27)	0.06 (0.02: 0.09)	< 0.001[b]
	RE < ± 0.25 D, n (%)	28 (70.0)	40 (100.0)	< 0.001[c]
Simulation 2	MedAE, D[a]	0.24 (0.09: 0.35)	0.06 (0.03: 0.10)	< 0.001[b]
	RE < ± 0.25 D, n (%)	22 (55.0)	40 (100.0)	< 0.001[c]
Simulation 3	MedAE, D[a]	0.14 (0.08: 0.29)	0.06 (0.04: 0.09)	< 0.001[b]
	RE < ± 0.25 D, n (%)	29 (72.5)	40 (100.0)	< 0.001[c]
Simulation 4	MedAE, D[a]	0.18 (0.11: 0.33)	0.05 (0.02: 0.07)	< 0.001[b]
	RE < ± 0.25 D, n (%)	26 (65.0)	40 (100.0)	< 0.001[c]
Simulation 5	MedAE, D[a]	0.23 (0.09: 0.33)	0.05 (0.03: 0.10)	< 0.001[b]
	RE < ± 0.25 D, n (%)	22 (55.0)	39 (97.5)	< 0.001[c]
Simulation 6	MedAE, D[a]	0.27 (0.13: 0.37)	0.05 (0.04: 0.08)	< 0.001[b]
	RE < ± 0.25 D, n (%)	18 (45.0)	40 (100.0)	< 0.001[c]
Simulation 7	MedAE, D[a]	0.22 (0.12: 0.39)	0.06 (0.04: 0.11)	< 0.001[b]
	RE < ± 0.25 D, n (%)	23 (57.5)	39 (97.5)	< 0.001[c]
Simulation 8	MedAE, D[a]	0.18 (0.06: 0.31)	0.06 (0.03: 0.10)	< 0.001[b]
	RE < ± 0.25 D, n (%)	24 (60.0)	40 (100.0)	< 0.001[c]
Simulation 9	MedAE, D[a]	0.24 (0.11: 0.34)	0.05 (0.02: 0.10)	< 0.001[b]
	RE < ± 0.25 D, n (%)	23 (57.5)	40 (100.0)	< 0.001[c]
Simulation 10	MedAE, D[a]	0.19 (0.11: 0.35)	0.04 (0.02: 0.09)	< 0.001[b]
	RE < ± 0.25 D, n (%)	23 (57.5)	40 (100.0)	< 0.001[c]

MedAE Median absolute error, *D* Diopters, *RE* Mean refractive prediction error
[a]Values are presented as median (interquartile range)
[b]Mann–Whitney U test
[c]Chi-square test

D of the target at one month postoperatively. On the other hand, a smaller proportion of eyes with IOLs with a 0.50 D interval (57.5 and 65.0%) achieved a refractive prediction error within ±0.50 D in this study. Similarly, in our previous study that investigated the refractive outcomes of 158 eyes that underwent cataract surgery with implantation of IOLs with 0.50 D intervals, 62.7 and 61.4% of them achieved a refractive prediction error within ±0.50 D according to the Haigis and SRK/T formulas, respectively. [14]

It is common knowledge that several factors affect achievement of accurate refractive outcomes after cataract surgery. These variables include surgical techniques, preoperative measures using biometry, IOL power calculation formulas, optimized IOL constants, and dioptric power accuracy of the implanted IOL. [2–4, 7] In this study, phacoemulsification was performed using the same surgical technique by a single surgeon using the same machine, and the biometry of both eyes was measured by a single examiner under the same environmental conditions. For comparison between the two groups, the Softec HD™ IOL was implanted in one eye of a patient, and the Akreos AO IOL in the contralateral eye.

Thus, there should be similar measurement error and effective lens position prediction error in both groups because there is a high degree of interocular symmetry of biometry and refractive prediction error between the two eyes of the same patient. [14, 15] Actually, there was a strong correlation in biometry and a moderate to strong correlation in refractive prediction error between the Akreos AO and Softec HD™ groups in this study. Thus, it seems reasonable to assume that there is only error in IOL power, and that there is no error caused by surgical techniques, preoperative biometry, or IOL power calculation formulas in the Monte Carlo simulations used to evaluate the effect of dioptric power accuracy of the implanted IOL.

In the Monte Carlo simulations of this study, the MedAE of IOLs with an SD of ±0.40 D ranged from 0.14 D to 0.27 D. On the other hand, the MedAE of IOLs with an SD of ±0.11 D ranged from 0.04 D to 0.06 D. According to the these results, if the dioptric power error of the implanted IOL has a normal distribution, the amount of the refractive error at the spectacle plane can be considered to be about half of the SD of the dioptric power error

Table 5 Comparison of median absolute error and percentage of eyes that achieved a postoperative refractive prediction error within ±0.25 D by the SRK/T formula between the Akreos AO and Softec HD™ groups in Monte Carlo simulation

		Akreos AO (n = 40)	Softec HD™ (n = 40)	P-value
Simulation 1	MedAE, D[a]	0.21 (0.11: 0.29)	0.05 (0.04: 0.10)	< 0.001[b]
	RE < ±0.25 D, n (%)	24 (60.0)	39 (97.5)	< 0.001[c]
Simulation 2	MedAE, D[a]	0.15 (0.06: 0.28)	0.06 (0.02: 0.10)	< 0.001[b]
	RE < ±0.25 D, n (%)	29 (72.5)	39 (97.5)	< 0.001[c]
Simulation 3	MedAE, D[a]	0.18 (0.11: 0.32)	0.05 (0.03: 0.07)	< 0.001[b]
	RE < ±0.25 D, n (%)	25 (62.5)	39 (97.5)	< 0.001[c]
Simulation 4	MedAE, D[a]	0.23 (0.13: 0.35)	0.06 (0.03: 0.10)	< 0.001[b]
	RE < ±0.25 D, n (%)	23 (57.5)	39 (97.5)	< 0.001[c]
Simulation 5	MedAE, D[a]	0.16 (0.07: 0.31)	0.05 (0.03: 0.07)	< 0.001[b]
	RE < ±0.25 D, n (%)	25 (62.5)	39 (97.5)	< 0.001[c]
Simulation 6	MedAE, D[a]	0.14 (0.08: 0.29)	0.06 (0.02: 0.09)	< 0.001[b]
	RE < ±0.25 D, n (%)	27 (67.5)	39 (97.5)	< 0.001[c]
Simulation 7	MedAE, D[a]	0.21 (0.11: 0.29)	0.04 (0.01: 0.09)	< 0.001[b]
	RE < ±0.25 D, n (%)	25 (62.5)	39 (97.5)	< 0.001[c]
Simulation 8	MedAE, D[a]	0.19 (0.13: 0.37)	0.06 (0.04: 0.11)	< 0.001[b]
	RE < ±0.25 D, n (%)	26 (65.0)	39 (97.5)	< 0.001[c]
Simulation 9	MedAE, D[a]	0.19 (0.10: 0.33)	0.06 (0.04: 0.09)	< 0.001[b]
	RE < ±0.25 D, n (%)	26 (65.0)	39 (97.5)	< 0.001[c]
Simulation 10	MedAE, D[a]	0.24 (0.07: 0.36)	0.06 (0.05: 0.10)	< 0.001[b]
	RE < ±0.25 D, n (%)	21 (52.5)	39 (97.5)	< 0.001[c]

MedAE median absolute error, *D* diopters, *RE* mean refractive prediction error
[a]Values are presented as median (interquartile range)
[b]Mann–Whitney U test
[c]Chi-square test

of the implanted IOL. The refractive error of 0.05 D at the spectacle plane may not be clinically meaningful, but an error of 0.20 D may have an effect on IOL power selection. However, it seems that the SD of the dioptric power error of the IOL that was actually produced and used is smaller than the reference value because of the IOL manufacturing technique. Although the dioptric power error of the IOL might be smaller than the international standard tolerance limits of ±0.40 D for 0.5 D interval IOLs, the surgeons performing these operations should know that refractive prediction errors could be caused by the IOL power error itself in the IOL power calculation.

To our knowledge, this is the first prospective, randomized, paired-eye study to consider the different manufacturing tolerances of IOLs to improve refractive outcomes. This study showed that tighter tolerance may contribute to refractions closer to the target value.

There are some limitations to this study. The designs of the haptics of the IOLs used in this study were not the same, although the material, optics design, and optic–haptic angulation were the same. A previous study showed that the nonangulated IOL has less postoperative axial movement than the angulated IOL. [16] The

Akreos AO IOL is a single-piece, four-haptic IOL with an overall length of 10.7 mm. In contrast, the Softec HD™ IOL is a single-piece, C loop IOL with an overall length of 12.0 mm. The relatively shorter IOL might not fully support the capsular bag during the early postoperative period and could affect postoperative IOL stability. [17, 18] However, we compared the refractive prediction error at one month postoperatively in order to exclude early postoperative IOL position change caused by capsular contraction. In addition, we additionally conducted Monte Carlo simulations and showed that the greater the dioptric errors of the IOL, the larger the number of refractive prediction errors that occurred.

Conclusions

In conclusion, the IOL with a 0.25 D interval considered in this study was more accurate than the IOL with a 0.50 D interval in predicting refractive outcome after cataract surgery. Surgeons should keep in mind that refractive errors may also occur due to the dioptric error of the implanted IOL itself when calculating IOL power in cataract surgery.

Abbreviations

ACD: Anterior chamber depth; AL: Axial length; BCVA: Best corrected visual acuity; D: Diopter; IOLs: Intraocular lenses; IRB: Institutional review board; K: Keratometry; MAE: Mean absolute error; MedAE: Median absolute error; SD: Standard deviation

Funding

This study was supported by Bumsuk Academic Research Fund in 2017. The funding source had no role in the design or conduct of this research.

Authors' contributions

MK participated in analysis and interpretation of data and drafting the manuscript. YE participated in conception and design of study, acquisition of data, analysis and interpretation of data, and drafting the manuscript. JSS and HMK participated in analysis and interpretation of data and the final design of the study. All authors have read and approved the final manuscript.

Competing interests

Youngsub Eom is a member of the editorial board of this journal.
The authors have no financial or proprietary interest in any product, method, or material described herein.

References

1. Olsen T. Calculation of intraocular lens power: a review. Acta Ophthalmol. 2007;85(5):472–85.
2. Olsen T. Improved accuracy of intraocular lens power calculation with the Zeiss IOLMaster. Acta Ophthalmol. 2007;85(1):84–7.
3. Mamalis N. Intraocular lens power accuracy: how are we doing? J Cataract Refract Surg. 2003;29(1):1–3.
4. Norrby S. Sources of error in intraocular lens power calculation. J Cataract Refract Surg. 2008;34(3):368–76.
5. International Organization for Standardization. Ophthalmic implants–intraocular lenses–part 2: Optical properties and test methods: (International Organization for Standardization). 2014. p. ISO 11979–2. https://www.iso.org/standard/55682.html.
6. Olsen T. Sources of error in intraocular lens power calculation. J Cataract Refract Surg. 1992;18(2):125–9.
7. Norrby NS, Grossman LW, Geraghty EP, Kreiner CF, Mihori M, Patel AS, Portney V, Silberman DM. Accuracy in determining intraocular lens dioptric power assessed by interlaboratory tests. J Cataract Refract Surg. 1996;22(7):983–93.
8. Lenstec. Products: Internationals: Softec series IOLs: Softec HD: Resources: Brochures: PKB07 Rev 10 Softec HD Flyer.pdf. Available at https://www.lenstec.com/resources2.html. Accessed 11 Dec 2017.
9. Eom Y, Kang SY, Song JS, Kim HM. Use of corneal power-specific constants to improve the accuracy of the SRK/T formula. Ophthalmology. 2013;120(3):477–81.
10. Eom Y, Song JS, Kim YY, Kim HM. Comparison of SRK/T and Haigis formulas for predicting corneal astigmatism correction with toric intraocular lenses. J Cataract Refract Surg. 2015;41(8):1650–7.
11. Eom Y, Kang SY, Song JS, Kim YY, Kim HM. Comparison of Hoffer Q and Haigis formulae for intraocular lens power calculation according to the anterior chamber depth in short eyes. Am J Ophthalmol. 2014; 157(4):818–24. e812.
12. East Valley Ophthalmology (doctor-hill.com) Physician Downloads: Haigis Formula Optimization – Haigis-300.xls. Available at https://doctor-hill.com/iol-power-calculations/resources-downloads. Accessed 11 July 2018.
13. Brown DC, Gills JP, Trattler WB, Newsom TH, Weinstock RJ, Sanders DR. Prospective multicenter trial assessing effectiveness, refractive predictability and safety of a new aberration free, bi-aspheric intraocular lens. Cont Lens Anterior Eye. 2011;34(4):188–92.
14. Choi Y, Eom Y, Song JS, Kim HM. Influence of corneal power on intraocular lens power of the second eye in the SRK/T formula in bilateral cataract surgery. BMC Ophthalmol. 2017;17(1):261.
15. Li Y, Bao FJ. Interocular symmetry analysis of bilateral eyes. J Med Eng Technol. 2014;38(4):179–87.
16. Petternel V, Menapace R, Findl O, Kiss B, Wirtitsch M, Rainer G, Drexler W. Effect of optic edge design and haptic angulation on postoperative intraocular lens position change. J Cataract Refract Surg. 2004;30(1):52–7.
17. Eom Y, Kang SY, Song JS, Kim HM. Comparison of the actual amount of axial movement of 3 aspheric intraocular lenses using anterior segment optical coherence tomography. J Cataract Refract Surg. 2013;39(10):1528–33.
18. Lim SJ, Kang SJ, Kim HB, Apple DJ. Ideal size of an intraocular lens for capsular bag fixation. J Cataract Refract Surg. 1998;24(3):397–402.

Retinal-image quality and contrast sensitivity function in eyes with epiretinal membrane: a cross-sectional observational clinical study

Limei Liu[1,2], Yi Wang[1], Ju Liu[1] and Wu Liu[1*]

Abstract

Background: To investigate the effect of idiopathic epiretinal membrane (ERM) on the retinal-image quality and psychophysical contrast sensitivity function (CSF).

Methods: Forty-four subjects with diagnosis of idiopathic unilateral ERM were enrolled in this cross-sectional observational clinical study. The fellow unaffected eyes were set as the control group. For retinal-image quality assessment, an Optical Quality Analysis System (OQAS) based on double-pass technique was used to evaluate objective scatter index (OSI) and Strehl ratio. For visual performance, the CSF under photopic condition was measured.

Results: For retinal-image quality, the result of double-pass device revealed a significant lower Strehl ratio and larger OSI in the ERM eyes compared to the fellow eyes (all $P < 0.05$). For visual performance, the CSF at all spatial frequencies under photopic condition were also significantly degraded in the ERM eyes compared to the fellow eyes (all $P < 0.05$). For the ERM eyes, the reduction of Strehl ratio and CSF was 29.41 and 54.39%, respectively, and the increase of OSI was 164.10% compared to the fellow eyes. Besides, BCVA significantly correlated to the total CSF (ERM eyes, $r = -0.53$, $P < 0.001$; the fellow eyes, $r = -0.467$, $P = 0.002$) and Strehl ratio (ERM eyes, $r = -0.485$, $P = 0.001$; the fellow eyes, $r = -0.311$, $P = 0.043$) in both of the ERM and the fellow eyes.

Conclusion: Eyes affected with ERM showed poorer retinal-image quality and visual performance than the normal eyes. Retinal-image quality measured by OQAS based on double-pass technique could be useful for assessing the retinal-image quality for ERM-affected eyes, in which retinal scattering was significantly increased.

Keywords: Epiretinal membrane, Retinal-image quality, Visual performance

Background

Epiretinal membrane (ERM) is a common retinal disease leading to significant visual impairment with an incidence of 2.2 and 28.9% [1–3]. In addition to the secondary ERM which can be caused by ocular pathology such as inflammation, trauma, tumors, or intraocular surgery, idiopathic ERM formation is a primary disease which can also often occur in the elderly [4]. It is characterized by a semi-translucent, glial and fibrocellular proliferative membrane at the vitreoretinal interface [5], which can exert tractional forces causing displacement of retina and retinal vessels [6, 7]. This pathology with characteristic morphological abnormalities, including curling and/or straightening of retinal vessels and deformation or displacement of the retinal tissues, may have a negative impact on the visual quality by changing the light reflected onto the altered retina.

For vision assessment, visual acuity (VA) is the most widely used parameter, but it cannot completely represent the whole visual performance at different degrees of contrast and spatial frequency in the real world. OQAS

* Correspondence: wuliubj@sina.com
[1]Beijing Tongren Eye Center, Beijing Tongren Hospital, Capital Medical University, Beijng Ophthalmology and Visual Sciences Key Laboratory, Beijing, China
Full list of author information is available at the end of the article

based on the double-pass technique has been used in the past to detect the retinal-image quality, such as optical aberration, diffraction and scattering, with good reliability [8–11]. The OQAS can provide parameters such as objective scatter index (OSI), Strehl ratio and modulation transfer function cut off requency (MTF cutoff), and it has been used extensively for visual asthenopia [8], eyes implanted with diffractive multifocal or monofocal intraocular lenses [9], endothelial keratoplasty [10] and healthy young population [11]. Contrast sensitivity function (CSF), providing the ability to detect difference in luminance and distinguishing details, is another good choice which can provide more information on visual function than VA [12]. It has been revealed that impaired CS may be found in cases of normal VA [13].

Although the superiority of retinal-image quality and CSF for assessing the visual function has been demonstrated and used in series of researches about many kinds of patients or healthy people, there is still a lack of information on the difference of retinal-image quality and psychophysical CSF between the ERM and healthy eyes. In this study, objective parameters of optical quality, including objective scatter index (OSI), Strehl ratio, and psychophysical CSF at five spatial frequencies (1.5, 3, 6, 12, and 18 cpd (cycles per degree)) were used to assess the effect of retinal structural change on the visual function in the ERM eyes.

Methods

This cross-sectional observational clinical study on patients with idiopathic unilateral ERM was conducted in the Beijing Tongren Hospital between October 2013 and July 2014. This study followed the tenets of the Declaration of Helsinki, and was approved by the ethical committee of the Beijing Tongren Hospital. Informed consent was obtained from each patient before the study.

The inclusion criterion was the presence of unilateral ERM. The exclusion criterion included: history of any intraocular surgery except for uncomplicated phacoemulsification, presence or history of age-related macular degeneration, diabetic retinopathy, retinal detachment, central or branch retinal vein occlusion, central or branch retinal artery occlusion, inflammatory eye disorders, different type and severity of cataract between the two eyes, ocular trauma, or any other potential cause of vision loss than ERM.

All the patients were assessed by two independent observers. Cycloplegic manifest refractions were conducted, and the best corrected VA (BCVA) was recorded as logMAR values for statistical analysis. LOCS III slitlamp grading was used to match the type and severity of cataract between the ERM and the fellow eyes.

A high-definition optical coherence tomography (Cirrus HD-OCT, Carl-Zeiss Meditec, Dublin, CA, USA) was conducted with a macular cube 512×128 combo across an area of 6×6 mm. The stages of ERM were identified with B-scan OCT images according the indication of Govetto et al. [14]:stage I: presence of mild ERM (the morphologic or anatomic disruption was negligible); stage II: the foveal depression was absent and the outer nuclear layer was characteristically stretched; stage III: the inner foveal layers anomalously crossed the central foveal area with a less pronounced widening of the outer nuclear layer, but all the retinal layers could be clearly identified on the OCT images; stage IV: the disruption of the macula was remarkable and the retinal layers could not be clearly identified on the OCT images.

Data of objective visual quality (retinal-image quality) were taken using an optical-quality device, OQAS (Optical Quality Analysis System, Visiometrics SL, Tarrasa, Spain), based on the double-pass technique. Spherical error was automatically corrected, and the cylindrical error was corrected with appropriate lens in order to optimize measurements on the double-pass system. In order to minimize the effect of tear film on the light scattering, all the measurements were taken after several eye blinks. The optical parameters including OSI and Strehl ratio were recorded for 4-mm pupil. The OSI parameter is often used to qualify the intraocular scattered light [15] that a small OSI value is usually correlated to eyes with low scattering. The Strehl ratio is often computed as the ratio between MTF area of the eye and the diffraction-limited MTF area. For normal people, it is about 30% [16], and a lower Strehl ratio value indicates a poor optical system aberration.

The Optec 6500 vision testing system (Stereo Optical Co. Inc., Chicago, IL, USA) was used to measure the functional acuity contrast testing (F.A.C.T). Tests were performed monocularly with best spectacle correction and natural pupil. The sinusoidal grating was set as the target chart and located at a fixed distance (2.5 m from the subjects) under a constant luminance of 85 cd/m^2. CS values were converted to numerical values at five spatial frequencies (1.5, 3, 6, 12, and 18 cpd) by using a conversion chart of F.A.C.T. All the measurements were conducted three times at all spatial frequencies to confirm an appropriate result.

For statistical analysis, SPSS Version 16.0 (SPSS 16.0, Inc., Chicago, IL) was used. Firstly, a Sample K-S test was used to test the data for normality. A paired-samples t test was used to compare the values of spherical equivalent refractive error (SER), BCVA, severity of cataract, parameters of retinal-image quality and CSF between the ERM and fellow eyes. Characteristics, optical performance and CSF in the 4 subgroups of the ERM eyes were compared using a one-way ANOVA. The CSF as a function of the Strehl ratio was analyzed to identify the correlation between visual performance and retinal-image quality using Pearson correlation analysis. The association between the BCVA with the total CSF and Strehl ratio was also tested using Pearson correlation analysis. For ERM eyes, association between the severity of ERM with BCVA, OSI, Strehl ratio and total CSF was assessed by excluding the effect of the grade of cataract using partial correlation analysis. P values lower than 0.05 at two tails were considered statistically significant.

Results

In all, 44 patients with unilateral ERM (15 males and 29 females) were enrolled in this study. The average age of patients was 63.70 ± 8.38 years (range from 38 to 74 years). The mean grade of LOCS III nuclear color (NC), nuclear opalescence (NO), cortical cataract (C) and posterior subcapsular cataract (P) was 2.80 ± 0.94, 2.56 ± 0.92, 0.61 ± 0.87 and 0.05 ± 0.21, respectively.

Table 1 summarizes the results of Paired-samples t test comparing the ERM eyes with the fellow eyes. The refraction error was best matched between the ERM and fellow eyes. Visual acuities accessed by logMAR of the ERM eyes were significantly worse than that of the fellow eyes (0.48 ± 0.28 vs. 0.02 ± 0.14, $P < 0.001$). Two subjects have accepted bilateral cataract surgery and intraocular lens implant, and the type and severity of cataract classified using LOCS III slitlamp grading system were similar between the two eyes of all the included patients (all $P > 0.05$). Retinal-image quality

Table 1 Difference between ERM eyes and the fellow eyes at presentation

Parameters	ERM eyes	Fellow eyes	P-value
SER (D)	0.08 ± 1.24	-0.09 ± 1.23	0.306
BCVA (logMAR)	0.48 ± 0.28	0.02 ± 0.14	< 0.001
LOCS III NC grade	2.80 ± 0.94	2.75 ± 0.87	0.486
LOCS III NO grade	2.56 ± 0.92	2.54 ± 0.89	0.781
LOCS III C grade	0.61 ± 0.87	0.65 ± 0.74	0.511
LOCS III P grade	0.05 ± 0.21	0.07 ± 0.25	0.323
OSI	3.09 ± 1.90	1.17 ± 1.11	< 0.001
Strehl ratio	0.12 ± 0.05	0.17 ± 0.05	< 0.001
Spatial frequency (cpd)			
1.5	31.55 ± 19.48	50.45 ± 22.38	< 0.001
3	33.52 ± 26.07	64.23 ± 36.89	< 0.001
6	28.73 ± 20.62	65.41 ± 26.44	< 0.001
12	4.61 ± 6.79	28.16 ± 18.72	< 0.001
18	0.86 ± 2.29	9.39 ± 6.90	< 0.001
Total	99.27 ± 64.84	217.64 ± 85.04	< 0.001

SER: spherical equivalent refractive error; D: diopter; BCVA: best corrected visual acuity; LOCS III: Lens Opacities Classification System III; NC: nuclear color; NO: nuclear opalescence; C: cortical cataract; P: posterior subcapsular cataract; OSI: objective scatter index; cpd: cycles per degree. P < 0.05 at two tails was considered to be statistically significant

accessed by OQAS of the ERM eyes was worse than that of the fellow eyes. For the ERM eyes, values of OSI was significantly larger, and values of the Strehl ratio were significantly less compared to the fellow eyes (all $P < 0.05$). In addition, for the ERM eyes, the reduction of Strehl ratio was 29.41%, and the increase of OSI was 164.10% compared to the fellow eyes. When compared to the fellow eyes, the CS values of the ERM eyes were significantly decreased at all spatial frequencies (1.5, 3, 6, 12, 18 cpd), under photopic condition (all $P < 0.05$, Fig. 1 & Table 2). Reduction of the total CS values was 54.39% for the ERM eyes.

The ERM eyes were identified to 4 stages according to the B-scan OCT images (stage II, $n = 11$; stage III, $n = 21$; stage IV, $n = 12$). Characteristics, optical performance and CSF in the 4 subgroups of the ERM eyes were summarized in Table 2. Statistically significant differences in BCVA, optical performance and CS values were found between the 4 subgroups (all $P<0.05$). BCVA was progressively deteriorated from stage II to stage IV ($P<0.001$). For optical performance, values of OSI steadily increased, and values of Strehl ratio significantly decreased from stage II to stage IV (all $P<0.05$). For CSF, values at all spatial frequency, except for at the spatial frequency of 18 cpd, were also progressively decreased as the stages increased (all $P<0.05$).

The CSF as a function of the Strehl ratio was analyzed to determine any correlation between visual performance and retinal-image quality. Significant correlation between the total CS value and the Strehl ratio were found for the ERM and the fellow eyes (both $P < 0.05$). The correlation coefficient of r for the ERM and the fellow eyes were 0.60 and 0.35, respectively. In addition, BCVA significantly correlated to the total CSF (ERM eyes, $r = -0.53$, $P < 0.001$; the fellow eyes, $r = -0.467$, $P = 0.002$) and Strehl ratio (ERM eyes, $r = -0.485$, $P =$

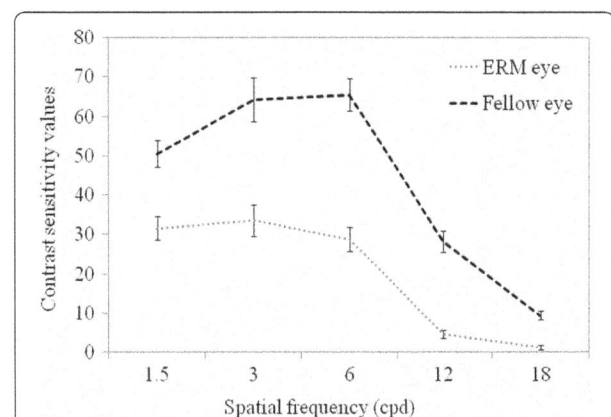

Fig. 1 Average CSF at five spatial frequencies for the ERM eyes and the fellow healthy Eyes. Data includes standard error

Table 2 Characteristics, optical performance and CSF of the ERM eyes

Parameters	Stage II ($n = 11$)	Stage III ($n = 21$)	Stage IV ($n = 12$)	P-value
Age (Years)	61.91 ± 9.29	64.00 ± 7.47	64.83 ± 9.49	0.698
SER (D)	−0.07 ± 1.46	0.22 ± 1.18	−0.04 ± 1.22	0.772
BCVA (logMAR)	0.37 ± 0.28	0.41 ± 0.25	0.73 ± 0.19	0.001
OSI	2.04 ± 1.43	2.89 ± 1.71	4.39 ± 1.99	0.007
Strehl ratio	0.15 ± 0.03	0.11 ± 0.05	0.10 ± 0.05	0.016
Spatial frequency (cpd)				
1.5	47.36 ± 15.76	32.05 ± 19.80	16.17 ± 5.97	< 0.001
3	56.36 ± 25.46	34.48 ± 22.85	10.92 ± 6.14	< 0.001
6	45.73 ± 17.33	30.14 ± 17.62	10.67 ± 13.25	< 0.001
12	10.82 ± 8.85	3.67 ± 5.08	0.58 ± 2.02	< 0.001
18	1.82 ± 3.28	0.52 ± 1.72	0.58 ± 2.02	0.285

SER: spherical equivalent refractive error; *D*: diopter; *cpd*: cycles per degree. P < 0.05 at two tails was considered to be statistically significant

0.001; the fellow eyes, $r = -0.311$, $P = 0.043$) in both of the ERM and the fellow eyes.

For the ERM eyes, the severity of the ERM was significantly correlated to the BCVA ($r = 0.41$, $P = 0.010$), OSI ($r = 0.35$, $P = 0.032$), Strehl ratio ($r = -0.35$, $P = 0.031$) and the total CS value ($r = -0.69$, $P < 0.001$) after adjusted for the grade of LOCS III NC, NO, C and P.

Discussion

Until today, the real effect of Idiopathic ERM on the visual function is not better understood, especially on the retinal-image quality and visual performance. In the current study, ERM eyes showed reductions in BCVA, CS values at five spatial frequencies and Strehl ratio, and increases in OSI compared to the fellow eyes. In addition, the total CS value was significantly correlated to the Strehl ratio for the ERM and the fellow eyes. Furthermore, in the ERM eyes, BCVA, CS and most of the optical parameters were progressively deteriorated as the stages increased with a significant deformation of retina. To our knowledge, this is the very few study demonstrating a strong effect of ERM on the visual function, including BCVA, retinal-image quality and CSF.

The precise pathophysiology of the ERM is not completely clear, but many studies indicated that the characteristic changes of the inner and outer retinal microstructure, such as increase in the inner retinal layer thickness [17, 18], disruption of the inner segment ellipsoid zone and photoreceptor outer segments [19–21], may have association with vision loss in eyes with ERM. Govetto et al. [14] established a new OCT-based classification system identifying novel morphologic features of retina and found that the presence of continuous ectopic inner foveal layers has a significant association with negative VA prognosis. Nevertheless, the relationship between this anatomic change in inner retina with the retinal-image quality and CSF remains unknown. In our

study, for the ERM eyes, the severity of the ERM was significantly correlated to the BCVA, OSI, Strehl ratio and the total CS value after adjusted for the grade of cataract, indicating that BCVA, CS and the optical parameters were progressively deteriorated as the severity of ERM increased with a significant deformation of retina.

OQAS can measure data on Strehl ratio and OSI which provides full information on optical performance, including aberrations, diffraction and scattering. The Strehl ratio, ranging from 0 to 1, is defined as the ratio between MTF area of the eye and the diffraction-limited MTF area. A lower value of Strehl ratio indicates poor optical quality with greater aberration and ocular scattering. In the current study, the results, that the Strehl ratio of the ERM eyes were lower compared to the fellow eyes, indicated a poor retinal-image quality for the ERM eyes. As demonstrated in previous studies [22, 23], interaction of light pass through the ocular media, reflected on the retina, all together influence the retinal-image quality. The OSI can quantitatively measure the intraocular scattering, which is correlated to the LOCS III system and macular thickness [15]. It indicated that OSI could be used as an index to reflect the abnormality in retina, if the crystalline lens was normal. In the current study, age-related cataract cannot be avoided because most of the patients included were elderly, but the type and severity of cataract were best matched using LOCS III slitlamp grading. Consequently, a higher OSI value found for the ERM eyes suggested that anatomic retinal change in ERM eyes would present more scattering than a relative healthy eye of a subject with the same age and refractive error. In addition, our result was consistent with previous studies [24, 25] that the Strehl ratio was lower and the OSI was higher as age increased. Also, the values of Strehl ratio and OSI for the fellow eyes in the current study were consistent with Ortiz et al.'s study [25] with similar age range (Strehl ratio, 0.17

± 0.05 vs. 0.17 ± 0.04, respectively; OSI, 1.17 ± 1.11 vs. 1.11 ± 0.50, respectively).

Both of VA and CSF are used as psychophysical testes which will be influenced by optical [26] and neural factors [27], but the CSF can evaluate the visual function more comprehensively than does VA. VA reflects the visual function under the same and high contrast, whereas the CSF measures the threshold contrast for seeing target under different spatial frequency. Nowadays, CSF has been widely accepted and used as a sensitive measure for evaluating visual function in many researches [28–30]. In the current study, significant differences were found at all spatial frequency between the ERM and fellow eyes. In addition, significant correlation between the CSF and the Strehl ratio were found for both the ERM and the fellow eyes, indicating a correlation between visual performance and retinal-image quality. Taking into account that the results for BCVA, retinal-image quality and visual performance, such as psychophysical CSF, showed a same trend for the ERM eyes, the objective devices, such as OQAS, and F.A.C.T charts could be used to assess the visual function in patients with ERM. These assessments may also be used as operational indications for the ERM or an index assessing the prognosis of surgery for the ERM, which warrants for further clinical researches.

It should be noted that we only measured the CSF under the photopic condition in this study, because the CSF test is time consuming and requires close cooperation of the patient which is difficult task especially for old patients. Therefore, further researches of ERM considered the CSF under both the photopic and mesopic conditions are warranted.

Conclusion

In conclusion, our result demonstrated that there is a higher ocular scattering in the ERM eyes than in the normal eyes, and this may degrade the retinal-image quality and CSF. The different level of retinal-image quality and CSF may be due to the fact that characteristic anatomic abnormality caused in the retina may change the light reflected onto the retina. Therefore, it is important to assess both of the retinal-image quality using objective device and CSF in patients with ERM. In addition, our results also indicated the feasibility of using a double-pass technique or F.A.C.T test in extensive clinical researches to assess the objective and psychophysical visual quality of ERM pathologies.

Abbreviations
BCVA: Best corrected visual acuity; C: Cortical cataract; CSF: Contrast sensitivity function; ERM: Epiretinal membrane; F.A.C.T: Functional acuity contrast testing; LOCS III: Lens opacities classification system III; NC: Nuclear color; NO: Nuclear opalescence; OQAS: Optical quality analysis system; OSI: Objective scatter index; P: Posterior subcapsular cataract

Acknowledgements
Not applicable

Funding
Not applicable.

Authors' contributions
Involved in the design of the study (LL, WL); conduct of the study (LL, YW, JL); collection, management, analysis of the data (LL, YW, JL, WL); preparation of the manuscript (LL, YW); and critical revision of the manuscript (WL, JL). All authors read and approved the final manuscript.

Competing interests
The authors declare that they have no competing interests.

Author details
[1]Beijing Tongren Eye Center, Beijing Tongren Hospital, Capital Medical University, Beijng Ophthalmology and Visual Sciences Key Laboratory, Beijing, China. [2]Department of Ophthalmology, Yantai Yuhuangding Hospital, Affiliated Hospital of Medical College, Qingdao University, Yantai, Shandong, China.

References
1. Ng CH, Cheung N, Wang JJ, et al. Prevalence and risk factors for epiretinal membranes in a multi-ethnic United States population. Ophthalmology. 2011;118(4):694–9.
2. Cheung N, Tan SP, Lee SY, et al. Prevalence and risk factors for epiretinal membrane: the Singapore epidemiology of eye disease study. Br J Ophthalmol. 2017;101(3):371–6.
3. You Q, Xu L, Jonas JB. Prevalence and associations of epiretinal membranes in adult Chinese: the Beijing eye study. Eye (Lond). 2008;22(7):874–9.
4. Fraser-Bell S, Guzowski M, Rochtchina E, Wang JJ, Mitchell P. Five-year cumulative incidence and progression of epiretinal membranes: the Blue Mountains eye study. Ophthalmology. 2003;110(1):34–40.
5. Michels RG. A clinical and histopathologic study of epiretinal membranes affecting the macula and removed by vitreous surgery. Trans Am Ophthalmol Soc. 1982;80:580–656.
6. Schmitz-Valckenberg S, Holz FG, Bird AC, Spaide RF. Fundus autofluorescence imaging: review and perspectives. Retina. 2008;28(3):385–409.
7. Dell'omo R, Cifariello F, Dell'omo E, et al. Influence of retinal vessel printings on metamorphopsia and retinal architectural abnormalities in eyes with idiopathic macular epiretinal membrane. Invest Ophthalmol Vis Sci. 2013; 54(12):7803–11.
8. Wee SW, Moon NJ. Clinical evaluation of accommodation and ocular surface stability relevant to visual asthenopia with 3D displays. BMC Ophthalmol. 2014;14:29.
9. Liao X, Lin J, Tian J, Wen B, Tan Q, Lan C. Evaluation of optical quality: ocular scattering and aberrations in eyes implanted with diffractive multifocal or Monofocal intraocular lenses. Curr Eye Res. 2018;43:1–6.
10. Kamiya K, Asato H, Shimizu K, Kobashi H, Igarashi A. Effect of intraocular forward scattering and corneal higher-order aberrations on visual acuity after Descemet's stripping automated endothelial Keratoplasty. PLoS One. 2015;10(6):e0131110.
11. Martínez-Roda JA, Vilaseca M, Ondategui JC, et al. Optical quality and intraocular scattering in a healthy young population. Clin Exp Optom. 2011; 94(2):223–9.
12. Arden GB. The importance of measuring contrast sensitivity in cases of visual disturbance. Br J Ophthalmol. 1978;62(4):198–209.
13. Plainis S, Anastasakis AG, Tsilimbaris MK. The value of contrast sensitivity in diagnosing central serous chorioretinopathy. Clin Exp Optom. 2007;90(4): 296–8.
14. Govetto A, Lalane RA, Sarraf D, Figueroa MS, Hubschman JP. Insights into Epiretinal membranes: presence of ectopic inner foveal layers and a new optical coherence tomography staging scheme. Am J Ophthalmol. 2017; 175:99–113.
15. Artal P, Benito A, Pérez GM, et al. An objective scatter index based on double-pass retinal images of a point source to classify cataracts. PLoS One. 2011;6(2):e16823.

16. Navarro R, Artal P, Williams DR. Modulation transfer of the human eye as a function of retinal eccentricity. J Opt Soc Am A. 1993;10(2):201–12.

17. Okamoto F, Sugiura Y, Okamoto Y, Hiraoka T, Oshika T. Associations between metamorphopsia and foveal microstructure in patients with epiretinal membrane. Invest Ophthalmol Vis Sci. 2012;53(11):6770–5.

18. Okamoto F, Sugiura Y, Okamoto Y, Hiraoka T, Oshika T. Inner nuclear layer thickness as a prognostic factor for METAMORPHOPSIA after EPIRETINAL membrane surgery. Retina. 2015;35(10):2107–14.

19. Kim JH, Kim YM, Chung EJ, Lee SY, Koh HJ. Structural and functional predictors of visual outcome of epiretinal membrane surgery. Am J Ophthalmol. 2012;153(1):103–10.

20. Itoh Y, Inoue M, Rii T, Hirota K, Hirakata A. Correlation between foveal cone outer segment tips line and visual recovery after epiretinal membrane surgery. Invest Ophthalmol Vis Sci. 2013;54(12):7302–8.

21. Watanabe K, Tsunoda K, Mizuno Y, Akiyama K, Noda T. Outer retinal morphology and visual function in patients with idiopathic epiretinal membrane. JAMA Ophthalmol. 2013;131(2):172–7.

22. Artal P, Ferro M, Miranda I, Navarro R. Effects of aging in retinal image quality. J Opt Soc Am A. 1993;10(7):1656–62.

23. Castro JJ, Jiménez JR, Hita E, Ortiz C. Influence of interocular differences in the Strehl ratio on binocular summation. Ophthalmic Physiol Opt. 2009; 29(3):370–4.

24. Wang YJ, Yang YN, Huang LY, Wang B, Han YC, Yan JB. Optical quality and related factors in ocular hypertension: preliminary study. J Ophthalmol. 2016;2016:3071036.

25. Ortiz C, Castro JJ, Alarcón A, Soler M, Anera RG. Quantifying age-related differences in visual-discrimination capacity: drivers with and without visual impairment. Appl Ergon. 2013;44(4):523–31.

26. Mutyala S, McDonald MB, Scheinblum KA, Ostrick MD, Brint SF, Thompson H. Contrast sensitivity evaluation after laser in situ keratomileusis. Ophthalmology. 2000;107(10):1864–7.

27. Elliott DB. Contrast sensitivity and glare testing. In: Benjamin WJ, editor. Borish's clinical refraction. Philadelphia: WB Saunders; 1998. p. 203–41.

28. Oshika T, Okamoto C, Samejima T, Tokunaga T, Miyata K. Contrast sensitivity function and ocular higher-order wavefront aberrations in normal human eyes. Ophthalmology. 2006;113(10):1807–12.

29. Preti RC, Ramirez LM, Monteiro ML, Carra MK, Pelayes DE, Takahashi WY. Contrast sensitivity evaluation in high risk proliferative diabetic retinopathy treated with panretinal photocoagulation associated or not with intravitreal bevacizumab injections: a randomised clinical trial. Br J Ophthalmol. 2013; 97(7):885–9.

30. Ortiz C, Jiménez JR, Pérez-Ocón F, Castro JJ, González-Anera R. Retinal-image quality and contrast-sensitivity function in age-related macular degeneration. Curr Eye Res. 2010;35(8):757–61.

29

Refractory macular hole repaired by autologous retinal graft and blood clot

An-Lun Wu[1,2], Lan-Hsin Chuang[2,3], Nan-Kai Wang[1,2,4], Kuan-Jen Chen[1,2], Laura Liu[1,2], Ling Yeung[2,3], Tun-Lu Chen[1,2], Yih-Shiou Hwang[1,2], Wei-Chi Wu[1,2] and Chi-Chun Lai[1,2]*

Abstract

Background: To evaluate the surgical technique using autologous retinal graft (ARG) and autologous blood clot (ABC) for the management of refractory macular holes (MHs).

Methods: This study was a retrospective, consecutive, interventional case series. Six eyes of 6 patients who underwent vitrectomy combined with ARG and ABC for the treatment of refractory MH were reviewed. Visual and anatomic outcomes were evaluated.

Results: The mean age was 59.0 ± 9.9 years. All cases had multiple vitreoretinal procedures including vitrectomy and gas fluid exchange before patient presentation. The average numbers of vitrectomies were 2.3 ± 0.5, and those of gas fluid exchange were 3 ± 1.7. Closure of the macular hole was achieved in four (66.7%) cases at last follow-up. The mean follow-up time was 25.2 ± 15.6 months. The averaged BCVA before and after 12 months of the surgery improved from 20/591 to 20/244.

Conclusions: This surgical technique using ARG and ABC provide an option for the treatment of refractory MHs.

Keywords: Refractory macular hole, Retinal graft, Autologous blood clot

Background

Pars plana vitrectomy combined with internal limiting membrane (ILM) peeling and gas tamponade is considered a standard approach for treating macular holes (MHs) [1]. The inverted ILM flap technique had been reported to improve the success rate in difficult cases [2]. The anatomic closure rate in a single operation could reach nearly 90% or higher [3, 4]. Repeat fluid-gas exchange closed most of the open holes after primary vitrectomy with ILM peeling [5]. However, surgical failure is still reported despite these high success rates.

Various surgical strategies have been introduced as adjunctive procedures to attempt closure of the refractory MH; these include enlargement of the previous ILM peel [6], use of heavy silicone oil for tamponade [7], pedicle ILM flap technique [8], lens capsular flap transplantation

[9], autologous free ILM flap [10–12], and autologous neurosensory retinal free flap [13].

Autologous neurosensory retinal free flap transplantation was first proposed by Grewal et al. [13], is a surgical technique used when no ILM was available to repair the MH. And another case report was presented to show the feasibility of using this method [14]. Although anatomical success and functional improvement could be reached, longer follow-up and larger sample sizes are needed for further study. Also, the risk of graft dislocation both intraoperatively and postoperatively remain an issue. Our group reported a surgical approach using the addition of autologous blood clot (ABC) appear to improve the limitation [15]. Therefore, we combined the autologous retinal graft (ARG) and ABC technique together as a macular plug to increase stability and keep the graft in place. The objective of this study was to present the efficacy of this technique in treating refractory MHs after failed surgeries with ILM removal or transplantation.

* Correspondence: chichun.lai@gmail.com
[1]Department of Ophthalmology, Chang Gung Memorial Hospital, No.5, Fu-Hsin Rd., Fuxing St., Guishan Dist, Taoyuan 33375, Taiwan
[2]College of Medicine, Chang Gung University, No.259, Wenhua 1st Rd., Guishan Dist, Taoyuan 333, Taiwan
Full list of author information is available at the end of the article

Methods

This study was a retrospective, consecutive, interventional case series. This ARG and ABC technique was conducted in six patients with refractory MH by 23-gauge vitrectomy. All surgeries were performed by one of the authors (C.-C.L.) at the Department of Ophthalmology, Chang Gung Memorial Hospital. This study adhered to the guidelines of the Declaration of Helsinki and was approved by the Institutional Review Board at Chung-Gang Memorial Hospital, Taiwan.

The inclusion criteria were as follows: (1) clinical presentation of an unclosed MH after previously receiving vitrectomy and ILM removal; (2) no remaining ILM within the vascular arcade in the posterior pole and treatment via combined pars plana vitrectomy with ARG and ABC; and (3) a follow-up period of more than 1 year after the vitrectomy with ARG and ABC. Patient records were reviewed, and the following data were collected: age, gender, past ocular history, preoperative best-corrected visual acuity (BCVA), and preoperative optical coherence tomography (OCT). Postoperative assessments were planned at 1 day, 1 week, 1 month, 3 months, 6 months, and 12 months after surgery; then, patients were followed up every 6 months. Extra visits may occur when there is a clinical need. BCVA and OCT were evaluated at each follow-up visit, except on the first postoperative day in which the fundus was prohibited from being viewed clearly. BCVA using a Snellen chart was converted to the logarithm of minimum angle of resolution (logMAR) for analysis purposes.

Diagrammatic representation of surgical procedure is outlined in Fig. 1. All cases underwent standard 23-gauge three-port, transconjunctival, sutureless microincision vitrectomy (Constellation; Alcon, Fort Worth, TX) with retrobulbar anesthesia. After the indocyanine green (ICG) staining procedure (concentration: 0.125 mg/ml in 5% glucose water) to make sure there was no remaining ILM within the vascular arcade in the posterior pole, excessive ICG was immediately removed via suction. The ARG harvest site was selected outside the vascular arcade and facilitated by laser photocoagulation in a circular manner. To achieve an effective laser burn, full thickness retinal burns were created at different power settings, from 200 mW to 300 mW and at different pulse durations, from 0.2 ms to 0.3 ms. The size of the graft was intended to be the same as the size of the MH and was harvested using scissors. Then, the retinal graft was gently moved to be inserted into the MH. Graft dislocation was prevented by lowering the intraocular pressure setting to reduce turbulence in the fluid stream. Further, the position of the graft proper was secured by trapping the edge of the graft under the edge of the hole. After the graft was manipulated into a proper position inside the hole, approximately 1 mL of fresh blood obtained from the patient's antecubital vein was collected into a syringe, with strict attention to aseptic precautions after disinfecting the entry site, and allowing it to dry completely as described before [15]. One to two drops of the fresh blood were then injected gently to cover the MH, using a back-flush needle mounted on a 1-mL syringe. The fresh blood soon became a clot on the surface of the macula, and the retina graft and blood clot sealed the hole in a few minutes as a macular plug. Afterwards, fluid–air exchange was performed. If the flap was disturbed during the gas-fluid exchange, more blood could be applied. At the end of the operation, the air was replaced with 20% sulfur hexafluoride gas. Patients were asked to remain face down for one week after surgery. The key steps of this technique are outlined in the Additional file 1.

Results

A total of six cases (six eyes in six patients: four female and two male) with refractory MH underwent surgery using the "ARG and ABC" technique. Characteristics of

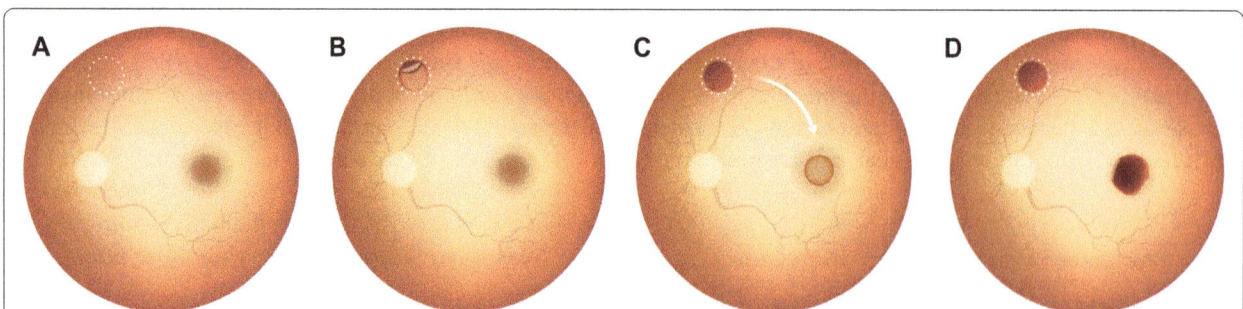

Fig. 1 Schematic drawings showing autologous retinal graft transposition with autologous blood clot surgical technique for repairing refractory macular holes. (**a**) Select the retinal graft harvest site outside the vascular arcade. White dotted circle indicates the area of an autologous retinal graft that is facilitated by laser photocoagulation. (**b**) The edge of the retinal graft was cut using vertical scissors. (**c**) Retinal graft was obtained and gently moved toward insertion within the macular hole. (**d**) Retinal graft was stabilized by placing autologous fresh blood over it. The fresh blood soon became a clot on the surface of the macula, and the retina graft and blood clots to seal the hole in a few minutes as a macular plug

the patients and surgical results are summarized in Tables 1 and 2 separately. Mean age at the time of the surgery was 59.0 ± 9.9 years. The mean basal MH size before autologous transposition of the graft was 978.5 ± 441.0 μm. The mean minimum opening of MH was 538.0 ± 184.9 μm. In failed cases, the mean basal MH size was 1047.5 ± 200.5 μm, and the mean minimum opening of MH was 697.0 ± 88.0 μm before surgery. Regarding the pathologies of MH in our study, 4 eyes (66.7%) were classified as idiopathic MH. And one MH occurred after successful rhegmatogenous retinal detachment surgery. The last case of MH had coexisting history of branch retinal vein occlusion with sectoral photocoagulation. All patients were pseudophakic at the beginning of the study. All cases had multiple vitreoretinal procedures including vitrectomy and gas fluid exchange before patient presentation. The average number of vitrectomies before ARG was 2.3 ± 0.5, and the average number of gas fluid exchanges was 3 ± 1.7. Closure of the MH was achieved in four out of the six (66.7%) patients after ARG in the study.

Intraoperatively, all eyes had successful transposition of the ARG and no intraoperative complications related to this technique were noted. The mean follow-up time was 25.2 ± 15.6 months. The averaged BCVA in logMAR before and after 12 months of the surgery were 20/591 (1.47 ± 0.31 logMAR) and 20/244 (1.09 ± 0.52 logMAR), respectively. Overall, 4/6 eyes with a closed hole after ARG gained visual acuity improvement, 2/6 eyes without a closed hole remained stable, and no eyes experienced a deterioration of the best corrected visual acuity after ARG surgery. The blood clot could be observed approximately one week after surgery. No postoperative complications developed during the follow up period. In the follow-up OCT, the graft appeared dislodged after the operation and no graft tissue was visible in the two eyes without closed holes. A reduced ellipsoid zone (EZ) line gap with partial restoration of the external limiting membrane and EZ was noted in one eye at last follow up regarding the recovery of the fovea microstructure post operatively 51 months later (Fig. 2).

Discussion

The treatment of an idiopathic macular hole could achieve a 90% closure rate or more with a modern vitrectomy [3, 4]. Some MH patients, such as those with a chronic large hole, high myopia, or trauma may require multiple surgeries. Treatment of refractory MH became a challenging issue for macular hole closure. Surgical management using ARG with ABC demonstrated the efficacy of a surgical option in refractory MHs.

The described technique may be used in patients with refractory MHs who underwent multiple surgeries and who had no remnant ILM. However, the closure rate of retinal graft transplantation for refractory MHs compares less favorably with those using ILM free flap transplantation [10–12]. This might be partly because anatomic success is more difficult to achieve in refractory MHs with repeated surgeries and when ILMs had been removed. Functional recovery after surgery is gradual and partial restoration of the external limiting membrane and EZ could continue suggesting that the retinal graft placed inside a macular hole may form a bridge to repair the fovea laminar structure from the graft edges. However, further studies are certainly needed to investigate if ARG could not only serve as a scaffold but also retain some function and further promote the reparation of the outer retinal layers.

Surgical approaches for refractory MH are limited. Improved outcomes have been reported with autologous ILM flaps [10–12]. However, harvesting a new suitable ILM free flap can be problematic in eyes with previous extensive ILM peeling. Lens capsular flap transplantation may be a solution for refractory MH when the ILM has already been removed [9]. However, the technique is not appropriate in phakic eyes if concomitant cataract surgery is not indicated and cannot be used in pseudophakic eyes with an open posterior capsule. Grewal and Mahmoud described an alternative approach involving the use of an autologous neurosensory retinal free flap for closure of refractory MH [13]. The differences between their

Table 1 Characteristics of patients undergoing autologous retinal graft and blood clot for refractory macular holes

Patient no.	Age (years)	Sex	Eye	Minimal diameter of MH (μm)	Basal MH size (μm)	MH status after ARG + ABC	Preoperative Lens status	Preoperative BCVA	Postoperative BCVA at 1 year	Follow-up
1	56	F	OS	219	576	Closed	Pseudophakic	20/1000	20/100	51
2	41	M	OS	657	832	Closed	Pseudophakic	20/400	20/200	36
3	61	M	OD	389	548	Closed	Pseudophakic	20/333	20/67	24
4	67	F	OS	569	1820	Closed	Pseudophakic	20/400	20/200	15
5	68	F	OS	785	1248	Open	Pseudophakic	20/400	20/400	13
6	61	F	OS	609	847	Open	Pseudophakic	20/2000	20/2000	12

ARG = autologous retinal graft, ABC = autologous blood clot, BCVA = best-corrected visual acuity, MH = macular hole

Table 2 Demographics and surgical results among all cases ($n = 6$)

Factor	
Male/Female (no.)	2/4
Age (yrs)	59.0 ± 9.9
Idiopathic MH, no. (%)	4 (66.7)
Axial length (mm)	25.63 ± 1.76
Follow-up (months)	25.2 ± 15.6
Basal MH size (μm)	978.5 ± 441.0
Minimum opening of MH (μm)	538.0 ± 184.9
Basal MH size in failed cases (μm)	1047.5 ± 200.5
Minimum opening of MH in failed cases (μm)	697.0 ± 88.0
Preoperative BCVA (logMAR)	20/591 (1.47 ± 0.31)
Postoperative BCVA (logMAR)	
1 mo	20/691 (1.54 ± 0.41)
3 mos	20/342 (1.23 ± 0.27)
6 mos	20/310 (1.19 ± 0.44)
12 mos	20/244 (1.09 ± 0.52)
BCVA at last visit, no. (%)	
Improved	4 (66.7)
No change	2 (33.3)
Worse	0 (0)
MH closed, no. (%)	4 (66.7)

BCVA = best-corrected visual acuity, logMAR = logarithm of the minimum angle of resolution, MH = macular hole

procedure and ours are in considering the size of the transplanted flap and its placement. In our surgical procedure, we placed a similarly sized retinal graft inside the macular hole instead of a free larger flap covering on it. We consider that persistent MHs close more efficiently and promptly when graft tissue becomes a filler, because the tissue may serve as a scaffold and a stronger bridge for glial cell proliferation. More importantly, we hypothesized to use ABC not only as a glue to keep the subsequently placed graft in place and reduce the risk of graft dislocation after the surgery, but also as a potential autologous adjuvant to augmenting the healing processes [15]. Additionally, the mixture of ARG and ABC formed a macular plug that sealed the MH shortly after application. This may maintain the dryness of the MH, prevent vitreous fluid from moving into the defect, and thereby ensure that the glial proliferation and migration closes the hole completely theoretically. However, further study is needed to arrive at a definitive conclusion of the mechanism.

The most difficult part of the transposition of the retinal graft technique is the transferring procedure from the harvest site to precisely insert the graft inside the macular hole. Grewal and Mahmoud developed the Perfluoro-n-octane heavy liquid (PFC) (Perfluoron; Alcon) assisted neurosensory retinal free flap transposition technique in their case [13]. The tamponade effect from the PFC could prevent the graft from floating away on intraocular currents during surgery before direct PFC–silicone oil exchange.

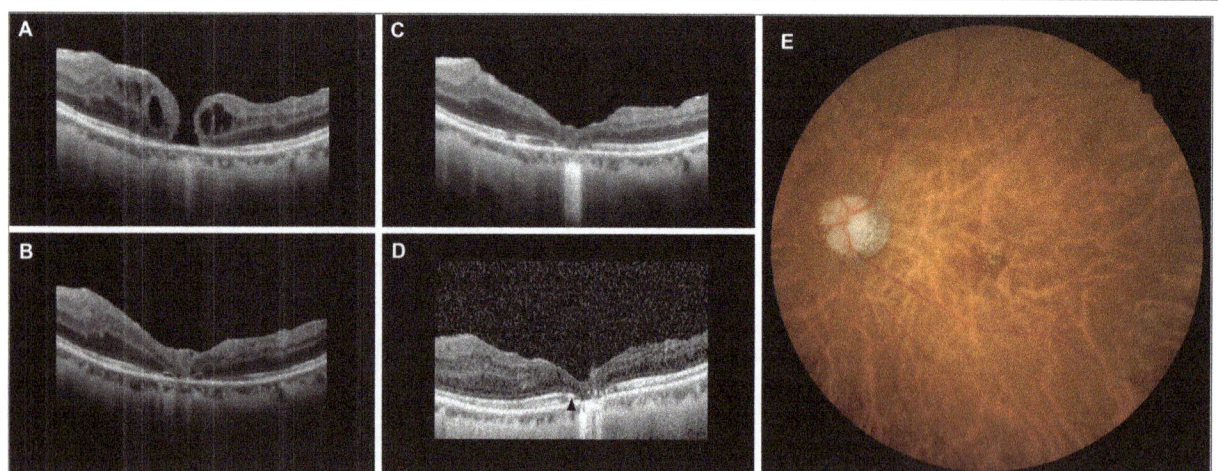

Fig. 2 Results of autologous retinal graft and blood clot in a 55-year-old refractory macular hole patient. Despite 4 pars plana vitrectomies with ILM peeling and additional 5 gas-fluid exchanges, spectral domain optical coherence tomography images (SD-OCT) showed the hole persisting (**a**). The base diameter of the MH before the retinal graft transplantation was 576 μm, and the minimum opening of the MH size was 219 μm. After the procedure, the macular hole was successfully closed at 3 months (**b**) and 12 months (**c**). The fovea remained stable and the patient's visual acuity improved from 20/1000 before the surgery to 20/100 at the final visit. SD-OCT imaging (**d**) and fundus photograph (**e**) obtained at 51 months postoperatively. SD-OCT showing partial restoration of external limiting membrane and gradually reconstructed ellipsoid zone (black arrowhead)

In contrast to their method, we found that the ARG tissue could be mechanically tucked and positioned inside the MH until completion of the autologous blood clot. However, the most important point during this procedure is to avoid potential iatrogenic trauma to the fovea tissue.

In this series, the aspiration of fluid was slowly performed via fluid-air exchange, and we did not perform further fluid aspiration after a 5 to 10-min wait after the initial fluid-air exchange to maximize vitreous cavity dehydration [16, 17]. Further, there is no need to aspirate the last drop of vitreous cavity fluid in avoidance of disturbing to the macular plug; this is because the hole is, theoretically, temporarily sealed after blood clot formation. And further gas tamponade is important to maintaining the dryness of the macula, which prevents the vitreous fluid from moving into the hole, and ensures that the retinal graft can be placed inside the MH as a bridge to help the repair process.

Graft dislocation was detected by OCT one month postoperatively in our two failure cases. The patients declined to receive any further treatment, however, the visual acuity revealed no deterioration after the surgery. We noted that these two cases were idiopathic MHs and the hole size was larger than the other four cases preoperatively. Given that hole and graft size cannot be accurately measured intraoperatively, the graft prepared may not have been large enough to fill the whole MH. Additionally, a shrinkage of the graft tissue may happen when cutting a graft, or contracture may occur during the healing process. In this situation, it was difficult to secure the graft tissue under the hole margin, causing graft dislodgement during the postoperative period. Regarding the toxicity issues due to blood products and fibrin degradation products used in this technique [18], although blood may leak into the subretinal space and cause damage to the photoreceptors, safety concerns are reduced because the graft tissue barrier serves as a filler at the hole. Although this study contains the postoperative visual acuity, further study measuring electroretinogram and microperimetry may provide more information regarding the functional outcomes.

Conclusion

Management of refractory MH presents a surgical challenge. ARG and ABC technique may be used in cases of refractory MH who have undergone multiple surgeries, and where no remnant ILM is present within the arcade vessels. Also, this surgical technique had a positive effect on visual function in all of the closure cases. Further study in a larger population that directly compares this technique with other techniques is warranted.

Abbreviations

ABC: Autologous blood clot; ARG: Autologous retinal graft; BCVA: Best-corrected visual acuity; EZ: Ellipsoid zone; ICG: Indocyanine green; ILM: Internal limiting membrane; logMAR: Logarithm of minimum angle of resolution; MH: Macular hole; OCT: Optical coherence tomography; PFC: Perfluoro-n-octane heavy liquid

Funding

This study was supported in part by the Chang Gung Memorial Hospital CMRPG3G0351. The funding sources had no role in the design and conduct of the study; the collection, management, analysis, and interpretation of the data; the preparation, review, or approval of the manuscript; or the decision to submit the manuscript for publication.

Authors' contributions

CL, AW, and LC conceived and designed the study protocol. NW, KC, LL and LY collected the data. TC, YH and WW were involved in the analysis. AW wrote the first draft of the manuscript. LL, LY, TC, YH, WW and CL reviewed and revised the manuscript and produced the final version. All authors have read and approved the final manuscript.

Competing interests

The authors declare that they have no competing interests.

Author details

[1]Department of Ophthalmology, Chang Gung Memorial Hospital, No.5, Fu-Hsin Rd., Fuxing St., Guishan Dist, Taoyuan 33375, Taiwan. [2]College of Medicine, Chang Gung University, No.259, Wenhua 1st Rd., Guishan Dist, Taoyuan 333, Taiwan. [3]Department of Ophthalmology, Chang Gung Memorial Hospital, No.222, Maijin Rd., Anle Dist, Keelung 204, Taiwan. [4]Edward S. Harkness Eye Institute, Department of Ophthalmology, Columbia University, 635 west, 165th street, New York, NY 10032, USA.

References

1. Kelly NE, Wendel RT. Vitreous surgery for idiopathic macular holes results of a pilot study. Arch Ophthalmol. 1991;109(5):654–9.
2. Michalewska Z, Michalewski J, Adelman RA, Nawrocki J. Inverted internal limiting membrane flap technique for large macular holes. Ophthalmology. 2010;117(10):2018–25.
3. Brooks HL Jr. Macular hole surgery with and without internal limiting membrane peeling. Ophthalmology. 2000;107(10):1939–48. discussion 1948-1939
4. Liu L, Enkh-Amgalan I, Wang NK, Chuang LH, Chen YP, Hwang YS, Chang CJ, Chen KJ, Wu WC, Chen TL, et al. RESULTS OF MACULAR HOLE SURGERY: evaluation based on the international Vitreomacular traction study classification. Retina. 2018;38(5):900–6.
5. Rao X, Wang NK, Chen YP, Hwang YS, Chuang LH, Liu IC, Chen KJ, Wu WC, Lai CC. Outcomes of outpatient fluid-gas exchange for open macular hole after vitrectomy. Am J Ophthalmol. 2013;156(2):326–33. e321
6. Che X, He F, Lu L, Zhu D, Xu X, Song X, Fan X, Wang Z. Evaluation of secondary surgery to enlarge the peeling of the internal limiting membrane following the failed surgery of idiopathic macular holes. Exp Ther Med. 2014;7(3):742–6.
7. Lappas A, Foerster AM, Kirchhof B. Use of heavy silicone oil (Densiron-68) in the treatment of persistent macular holes. Acta Ophthalmol. 2009;87(8):866–70.
8. Gekka T, Watanabe A, Ohkuma Y, Arai K, Watanabe T, Tsuzuki A, Tsuneoka H. Pedicle internal limiting membrane transposition flap technique for refractory macular hole. Ophthalmic Surg Lasers Imaging Retina. 2015;46(10):1045–6.
9. Chen SN, Yang CM. Lens capsular flap transplantation in the Management of Refractory Macular Hole from multiple etiologies. Retina. 2016;36(1):163–70.
10. Pires J, Nadal J, Gomes NL. Internal limiting membrane translocation for refractory macular holes. Br J Ophthalmol. 2017;101(3):377–82.
11. Dai Y, Dong F, Zhang X, Yang Z. Internal limiting membrane transplantation for unclosed and large macular holes. Graefes Arch Clin Exp Ophthalmol. 2016;254(11):2095 9.

12. Morizane Y, Shiraga F, Kimura S, Hosokawa M, Shiode Y, Kawata T, Hosogi M, Shirakata Y, Okanouchi T. Autologous transplantation of the internal limiting membrane for refractory macular holes. Am J Ophthalmol. 2014;157(4):861–9. e861

13. Grewal DS, Mahmoud TH. Autologous neurosensory retinal free flap for closure of refractory myopic macular holes. JAMA Ophthalmol. 2016;134(2):229–30.

14. De Giacinto C, D'Aloisio R, Cirigliano G, Pastore MR, Tognetto D. Autologous neurosensory retinal free patch transplantation for persistent full-thickness macular hole. Int Ophthalmol. 2018; https://doi.org/10.1007/s10792-018-0904-4.

15. Lai CC, Chen YP, Wang NK, Chuang LH, Liu L, Chen KJ, Hwang YS, Wu WC, Chen TL. Vitrectomy with internal limiting membrane repositioning and autologous blood for macular hole retinal detachment in highly myopic eyes. Ophthalmology. 2015;122(9):1889–98.

16. Iezzi R, Kapoor KG. No face-down positioning and broad internal limiting membrane peeling in the surgical repair of idiopathic macular holes. Ophthalmology. 2013;120(10):1998–2003.

17. Rubin JS, Thompson JT, Sjaarda RN, Pappas SS Jr, Glaser BM. Efficacy of fluid-air exchange during pars plana vitrectomy. Retina. 1995;15(4):291–4.

18. Glatt H, Machemer R. Experimental subretinal hemorrhage in rabbits. Am J Ophthalmol. 1982;94(6):762–73.

30

Behavior of hyperreflective foci in non-infectious uveitic macular edema, a 12-month follow-up prospective study

Barbara Berasategui[1]* , Alex Fonollosa[1], Joseba Artaraz[1], Ioana Ruiz-Arruza[2], Jose Ríos[3,4], Jessica Matas[5], Victor Llorenç[5], David Diaz-Valle[6], Marina Sastre-Ibañez[6], Pedro Arriola-Villalobos[6] and Alfredo Adan[5]

Abstract

Background: Hyperreflective foci have been described in OCT imaging of patients with retinal vascular diseases. It has been suggested that they may play a role as a prognostic factor of visual outcomes in these diseases. The purpose of this study is to describe the presence of hyperreflective foci in patients with non-infectious uveitic macular edema and evaluate their behavior after treatment.

Methods: We conducted a multicenter, prospective, observational, 12-month follow-up study. Inclusion criteria were age > 18 years and a diagnosis of non-infectious uveitic macular edema, defined as central macular thickness of > 300 μm as measured by OCT and fluid in the macula. Collected data included best corrected visual acuity, central macular thickness and the presence, number and distribution (inner or outer retinal layers) of hyperreflective foci. Evaluations were performed at baseline, and at 1, 3, 6, and 12 months after starting treatment.

Results: We included 24 eyes of 24 patients. The frequency of patients with ≥11 hyperreflective foci was 58.4% at baseline, falling to 20.8% at 12 months. Further, hyperreflective foci were observed in the outer retinal layers in 50% of patients at baseline and just 28.6% at 12 months. Mean LogMAR visual acuity improved from 0.55 (95% CI 0.4–0.71) at baseline to 0.22 (95% CI 0.08–0.35) at 12 months ($p < 0.001$). Mean central macular thickness decreased from 453.83 μm (95% CI 396.6–511) at baseline to 269.32 μm (95% CI 227.7–310.9) at 12 months ($P < 0.001$). Central macular thickness was associated with number ($p = 0.017$) and distribution ($p = 0.004$) of hyperreflective foci.

Conclusions: We have observed hyperreflective foci in most of our patients with non-infectious uveitic macular edema. During follow-up and after treatment, the number of foci diminished and they tended to be located in the inner layers of the retina.

Keywords: Hyperreflective foci, Intraocular inflammation, Microglia, Optical coherence tomography, Uveitic macular edema, Uveitis

Background

Macular edema is the main cause of vision loss in patients with uveitis [1]. Spectral domain optical coherence tomography (SD-OCT) is the gold standard for the diagnosis of this condition. Retinal thickness has come to be recognized as a remarkably valuable measure in the management of patients with uveitic macular edema (UME) and is almost universally used as a main outcome measure in clinical trials evaluating treatments in uveitis. Qualitative data provided by SD-OCT, i.e., the presence of subretinal fluid, distribution of cysts, and ellipsoid zone status, have also been considered in some papers where the analysis of these data has contributed to understanding the pathogenesis and prognosis of UME [2, 3].

In recent years, hyperreflective foci (HRF) have been described in SD-OCT imaging of patients with macular edema secondary to diabetic retinopathy [4], retinal vein occlusions [5], type 2 macular telangiectasia [6], and age-related macular degeneration [7]. Though their origin

* Correspondence: bberasateguif@gmail.com
[1]Department of Ophthalmology, BioCruces Health Research Institute, Cruces Hospital, University of the Basque Country, Cruces square s/n, CP 48903 Baracaldo, Vizcaya, Spain
Full list of author information is available at the end of the article

is not clear, it has been shown that the abundance of such foci may vary after treatment and has been suggested that there may be an association between a decrease in HRF and an improvement in visual function [8, 9]. The aim of this study was to evaluate the presence and behavior of HRF in UME. In addition, we assessed the potential association between these foci on macular thickness and visual acuity (VA).

Methods
Population
In this multicenter, prospective, observational, 12-month follow-up study, we included 24 eyes of 24 patients with UME. Patients were recruited from three referral centers for ocular inflammatory diseases in Spain (Hospital Clinic -Barcelona-, Hospital Universitario Cruces -Bilbao- and Hospital Clinico San Carlos –Madrid-) from january 2014 until september 2014. Local Ethics Committees approved the study (Comité ético de Investigación Clínica del Hospital Clínic de Barcelona 2013/8574; Comité de ética de la investigación con medicamentos de Euskadi, Hospital universitario Cruces PI201406; Comité ético de investigación clínica del hospital clínico San Carlos de Madrid 13/244-E). Informed consent was then obtained from each patient and the research was carried out in accordance with the Declaration of Helsinki.

Inclusion criteria were age > 18 years, and a diagnosis of macular edema (defined as central macular thickness [CMT] of > 300 µm as measured by OCT and fluid in the macula) secondary to non-infectious uveitis. Exclusion criteria were a diagnosis of infectious uveitis or any other retinal disease, a history of intraocular surgery in the last 4 months, and low quality OCT imaging that precluded adequate assessments.

Type of treatment for macular edema was left to the discretion of the treating physician.

The Standardization of Uveitis Nomenclature Working Group criteria were used to anatomically classify the uveitis [10].

Protocol-based assessments and other study procedures
For the purpose of this study, the following mandatory protocol-based assessments were performed and are reported in the present study: at baseline, and at 1, 3, 6 and 12 months after treatment. Other visits at different time-points (i.e., for monitoring pressure or any other reason) were allowed, at the discretion of the treating physician.

During each appointment, all patients underwent a full ophthalmic examination consisting of determination of best corrected visual acuity (BCVA), which was assessed with Snellen charts at a test distance of 6 m, anterior segment biomicroscopy, Goldmann applanation tonometry, 90-D lens biomicroscopy and SD-OCT. Other imaging methods, e.g., fluorescein angiography, were optional and were left to the discretion of the researcher. Inflammatory activity, that is the presence or absence of anterior chamber cells, vitritis or posterior segment inflammatory signs as judged by the investigator, was recorded at each protocol-based visit.

SD-OCT
A Cirrus OCT device (version 4.0, Carl Zeiss Meditec, Dublin, CA) was used in all patients. After pupillary dilatation, two scan protocols were performed: the Macular cube 512×128 A-scan, within a 6×6 mm^2 area centered on the fovea; and the Enhanced High Definition Single-Line Raster, which collected data along a 6 mm horizontal line consisting in 4096 A-scans, across the center of the fovea. This single line high definition scan was used to manually count the number of HRF, defined as discrete, punctiform hyperreflective white lesions (as hyperreflective as retinal pigment epithelium), and determine their distribution. As in previous publications [8], the abundance of HRF was assessed semi-quantitatively, each case being assigned to one of four groups: group A, 0 foci; group B, 1 to 10; group C, 11 to 20; and group D, more than 20 foci. Regarding the distribution of HRF, two locations were considered: the inner retina (IR), from the nerve fiber layer to the outer plexiform layer; and the outer retina (OR), from the outer nuclear layer to retinal pigment epithelium. When HRF were localized exclusively in the IR, the case was assigned to group 1, and if there were HRF in the OR (with or without foci in the IR) the case was assigned to group 2, while cases with no HRF were assigned to group 0.

All these assessments of the images were performed by two independent, experienced graders (AF and BB, from one of the participating centers) who were blind to clinical data of the corresponding patients. In the event of discrepancies, the two graders made the assessment together and reached a consensus.

Statistics
BCVA was converted to the logarithm of the minimum angle of resolution (logMAR) equivalents for statistical analyses. Qualitative variables have been described with percentages or frequencies. Results of logMAR VA and CMT are shown as estimated means and their 95% confidence intervals (95% CI). Other quantitative variables have been described using medians and ranges.

The evolution of LogMAR VA and CMT values has been estimated with a longitudinal lineal model using Generalized Estimated Equations methodology (GEE).

Estimations of LogMAR VA have been performed unadjusted (crude estimation) and adjusted for CMT, amount of HRF and distribution of HRF in order to assess a possible influence of these on VA. Estimations of CMT have been performed unadjusted (crude estimation) and adjusted for amount of HRF and distribution of HRF, in order to assess a possible influence of these on CMT.

GEE models use an unstructured matrix of correlations in order to account for intrasubject variability. All statistical analyses were performed using the Statistical Package for the Social Sciences (SPSS version 20.0 for Windows; SPSS Inc., Chicago, IL). $P < 0.05$ was considered statistically significant for all analyses.

Results

Baseline characteristics and clinical course

A total of 24 eyes from 24 patients (17 women) were included. The median age of the group was 49 years (21–67). Anatomic diagnosis classified five cases as anterior uveitis, five as intermediate, eight as posterior and six as panuveitis. Table 1 displays patients' demographic data, causes of uveitis and treatments for macular edema.

The overall logMAR VA improved from 0.55 (0.4–0.71) at baseline, to 0.42 (0.25–0.59) at 1 month ($p = 0.046$), 0.42 (0.18–0.66) at 3 months ($p = 0.255$), 0.31 (0.19–0.42) at 6 months ($p = 0.001$) and 0.22 (0.08–0.35) at 12 months ($p < 0.001$). In parallel, the CMT decreased,

from 453.83 μm (396.6–511) at diagnosis, to 358.34 μm (301.69–415) at 1 month ($p = 0.006$), 315.2 μm (258.4–372.1) at 3 months ($p < 0.001$), 328.87 μm (262.3–395.5) at 6 months ($p = 0.002$) and 269.32 μm (227.7–310.9) after 1 year ($p < 0.001$) Fig. 1 shows the evolution of logMAR VA and CMT during follow-up. Regarding the amount of HRF, we observed a progressive reduction in the percentage of eyes classified as group C or D, that is, with ≥11 HRF, from 58.4% at baseline, to 40.5% at 1 month, 45.8% at 3 months, 22.7% at 6 months and 21.7% at 12 months. Concerning the distribution of these foci at baseline, 50% of patients were classified as group 2 and 50% as group 1 or 0. During follow-up, at all time points, fewer than half of the patients were classified as group 2 (that is, patients with HRF in the outer retina) (month 1, 47.7% in group 2 vs 52.3%in group 0 + 1, month 3: 34.7% vs 65.3%, month 6: 28.6% vs 71.4%, and month 12: 28.6% vs 71.4%). Grader's assessments matched in 111 of 120 scans (92.5%).

Figure 2 shows the number of patients with inflammatory activity at each protocol-based visit.

Table 2 lists logMAR VA and SD-OCT parameters from all patients during follow-up.

Table 1 Patients' demographic data, causes of uveitis and treatments for macular edema

Patient	Gender	Age	SUN	Cause	Treatment
1	Male	34	Anterior	HLA-B27	Periocular Triamcinolone
2	Male	40	Anterior	HLA-B27	Intravitreal dexamethasone
3	Male	48	Anterior	HLA-B27	Oral steroids
4	Male	37	Anterior	Idiopathic	Oral steroids
5	Female	23	Anterior	Idiopathic	Oral steroids
6	Female	28	Intermediate	Idiopathic	Periocular Triamcinolone
7	Female	25	Intermediate	Idiopathic	Periocular Triamcinolone
8	Female	53	Intermediate	Idiopathic	Periocular Triamcinolone
9	Female	50	Intermediate	Idiopathic	Intravitreal dexamethasone
10	Female	35	Intermediate	Idiopathic	Intravitreal dexamethasone
11	Female	63	Posterior	Sarcoidosis	Oral steroids + Methotrexate
12	Female	54	Posterior	Sarcoidosis	Oral steroids + Methotrexate
13	Female	57	Posterior	Sarcoidosis	Oral steroids + Adalimumab
14	Female	61	Posterior	Sarcoidosis	Oral steroids + Adalimumab
15	Male	61	Posterior	Birdshot	Oral steroids + Tocilizumab
16	Male	34	Posterior	Birdshot	Oral steroids + Cyclosporine
17	Female	59	Posterior	Idiopathic	Oral steroids
18	Female	50	Posterior	Idiopathic	Oral steroids
19	Female	67	Panuveitis	Sarcoidosis	Oral steroids + Adalimumab
20	Female	21	Panuveitis	Sarcoidosis	Oral steroids + Adalimumab
21	Female	35	Panuveitis	Chronic VKH	Oral steroids + Azathioprine
22	Female	47	Panuveitis	Chronic VKH	Periocular triamcinolone+Azathioprine
23	Female	61	Panuveitis	Idiopathic	Oral steroids
24	Male	53	Panuveitis	Idiopathic	Oral steroids

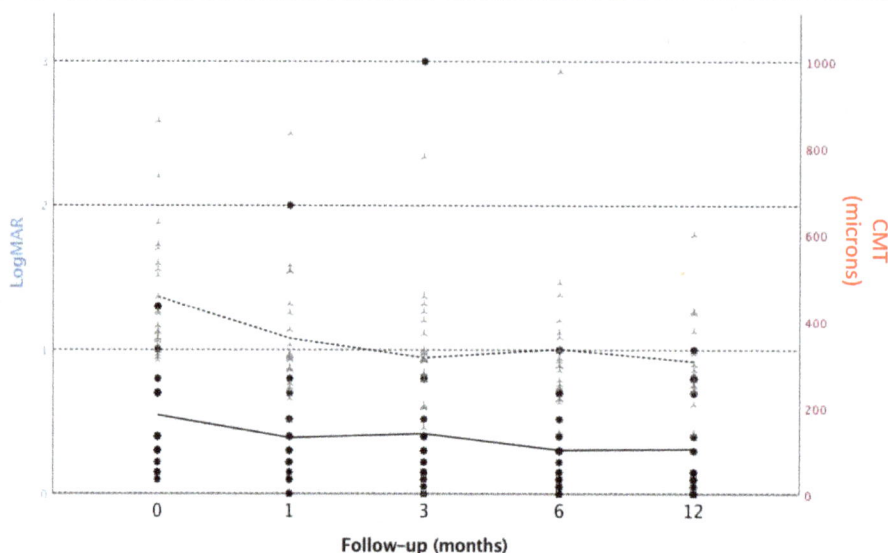

Fig. 1 Evolution of logMAR visual acuity (solid line) and central macular thickness (CMT, dashed line) during follow-up

Tables 3, 4, 5 and 6 show logMAR VA and HRF related data in patients with anterior, intermediate, posterior and panuveitis respectively.

Influence of OCT parameters on visual acuity

The adjusted model for the estimation of VA showed that the decrease in CMT was associated with the increase in VA ($p = 0.002$). However VA was not associated with either HRF number or distribution ($p = 0.513$ and $p = 0.324$ respectively). On the other hand, the adjusted model for the estimation of CMT showed that both HRF number ($p = 0.017$) and distribution ($p = 0.004$) had an influence on CMT values, that is, the decrease in CMT was associated with a decrease in the number of HRF and the distribution of the foci.

Discussion

In this prospective study we describe, to our knowledge for the first time, the behavior of HRF in patients with UME. At baseline, patients had larger numbers of foci and half of them had at least some foci in the outer retina. During follow-up, while macular edema resolved, OCT showed fewer foci and those that remained were more frequently located in the inner retina. Figure 3 illustrates this behavior. Moreover, macular thickness was found to be associated with both the number and the distribution of the foci.

Although HRF have been described in several diseases including diabetic macular edema, age-related macular degeneration, retinal vein occlusions and type 2 macular telangiectasia, the precise nature of these foci and their

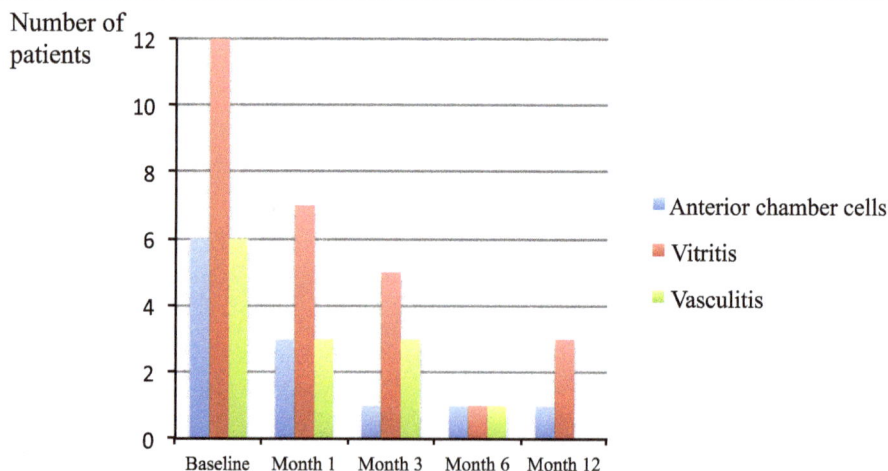

Fig. 2 Number of patients with inflammatory activity at each protocol-based visit

Table 2 Changes in SD-OCT parameters and visual acuity over follow-up (all patients)

	Baseline	Month 1	Month 3	Month 6	Month 12
Frequency of patients with ≥11 foci(groups C or D)	58.3%	40.5%	45.8%	22.7%	21.7%
Distribution (% patients in each group)					
Group 0 (no foci)	4.2%	4.8%	8.7%	14.3%	4.7%
Group 1 (inner retina)	45.8%	47.5%	56.6%	57.1%	66.7%
Group 2 (outer retina)	50%	47.7%	34.7%	28.6%	28.6%
logMAR VA[a]	0.55 (0.4–0.71)	0.42 (0.25–0.59)	0.42 (0.18–0.66)	0.31 (0.19–0.42)	0.22 (0.08–0.35)
CMT (µm)[b]	453.83 (396.6–511)	358.34 (301.69–415)	315.2 (258.4–372.1)	328.87 (262.3–395.5)	269.32 (227.7–310.9)

[a]logMAR VA: logarithm of the minimum angle of resolution visual acuity
[b]CMT: Central macular thickness

molecular constituents remain unclear. Three main theories have been put forward in publications concerning these foci. Some authors have hypothesized that HRF represent precursors of hard exudates [4, 11]. Others suggested that they are degenerated photoreceptors or macrophages engulfing such cells, since they have been observed close to disrupted external limiting membrane and ellipsoid zone and have been associated with decreased VA [12]. Finally, other authors have interpreted them as microglial cells activated during an inflammatory reaction [13, 14]. All these theories are plausible and it is possible that all three mechanisms may occur in the same disease but it is likely that each one of them plays a predominant role in a given disease.

Shape of foci is described as round or oval in previous publications regarding HRF in patients with retinal vascular diseases. Our cases showed also round or oval foci. Regarding the size, hyperreflective foci are defined as "small" in publications that evaluate this feature in patients with retinal vascular diseases, though precise size is not reported. In SD-OCT figures provided in these publications displaying foci, variable sizes may be observed. Though it is a subjective judgement, we believe that in our uveitic patients, foci are usually smaller than those observed in patients with diabetic macular edema or retinal vein occlusions. We speculate that this may be explained by a different origin of foci in different diseases. In retinal vascular diseases bigger foci may correspond to lipid exudation; on the other hand smaller foci

seen in our patients may correspond to inflammatory cells. A microglial and leukocytic origin of the HRF would seem the most plausible in the context of UME, given the clear inflammatory origin of this condition, and the absence of hard exudates in UME. This may support the view that HRF should not be considered an initial lipidic extravasation in these cases. In this regard, a study assessing SD-OCT imaging of the vitreous and retina of seven patients with posterior segment inflammatory disease described HRF of a size consistent with that expected for inflammatory cells [15]. Interestingly, data from studies performed in murine experimental autoimmune uveoretinitis assessing correlations of OCT imaging of inflammatory lesions and their histopathologic analysis have shown that HRF may represent cellular infiltration [16].

In our patients, HRF decreased over time after starting treatment, whilst macular thickness decreased and edema resolved. Similar findings have been described by other researchers in patients with retinal vasculopathies and age-related macular degeneration. In diabetic macular edema, Vujosevic et al. [9] assessed the presence of HRF and the effect of treatment with anti-vascular endothelial growth factor on their abundance. They observed that the number of foci decreased after treatment, but did not find a correlation between the number of HRF and retinal thickness. In patients with macular edema secondary to diabetic retinopathy or branch retinal vein occlusions treated with intravitreal implant of dexamethasone or

Table 3 Behavior of foci and evolution of visual acuity in patients with anterior uveitis

	Baseline	Month 1	Month 3	Month 6	Month 12
Frequency of patients with ≥11 foci(groups C or D)	40%	40%	40%	0%	0%
Distribution (% patients in each group)					
Group 0 (no foci)	20%	20%	40%	0%	0%
Group 1 (inner retina)	20%	40%	40%	100%	75%
Group 2 (outer retina)	60%	40%	20%	0%	25%
Mean logMAR VA[a]	0.56	0.32	0.32	0.2	0.125

[a]logMAR VA: logarithm of the minimum angle of resolution visual acuity

Table 4 Behavior of foci and evolution of visual acuity in patients with intermediate uveitis

	Baseline	Month 1	Month 3	Month 6	Month 12
Frequency of patients with ≥11 foci(groups C or D)	60%	20%	60%	20%	20%
Distribution (% patients in each group)					
Group 0 (no foci)	0%	0%	0%	0%	25%
Group 1 (inner retina)	40%	100%	80%	100%	50%
Group 2 (outer retina)	60%	0%	20%	0%	25%
Mean logMAR VA[a]	0.28	0.25	0.23	0.24	0.21

[a] logMAR VA: logarithm of the minimum angle of resolution visual acuity

ranibizumab, Chatziralli et al. observed a decrease in HRF in parallel with resolution of the macular edema [17]. Framme et al. described a reduction in the number of HRF in 54% of their patients with neovascular choroidal neovascularization after treatment with ranibizumab [7]. Moreover, this reduction correlated with a decrease in CMT. Abri Aghdam et al. assessed the behavior of HRF in patients with neovascular age related macular degeneration after treatment with intravitreal aflibercept [18]. They observed a decrease in the number of foci within radius of 500 and 1500 µm, as well as a correlation between the CMT and number of foci within a 500-µm radius. To explain this behavior, these researchers suggested that HRF were precursors of lipid exudates and hence a sign of hyperpermeability, which might explain the association found between number of foci and macular thickness.

In patients with UME, the inflammatory process induces the invasion of leukocytes into the retina and the activation of microglia. These undergo significant changes in shape and size, from ramified multidirectional extensions to polarized dendrites and then to larger rounded cells which aggregate [19]. Leukocytes and activated microglial cells produce cytokines that increase vascular and epithelial permeability. When the inflammation resolves, the level of retinal cellular infiltrates decreases. These phenomena may support our finding of an association between HRF number and macular thickness.

As mentioned above, almost half of our cases showed HRF in the outer retina at baseline. During follow-up, as the edema resolved, foci were more frequently located in the inner retina. Similar observations have been described

in diabetic macular edema. Vujosevic et al. [9], in their study assessing the effect of ranibizumab on HRF in diabetic macular edema, reported that the main decrease in foci occurred in the outer nuclear layer when edema resolved. Zheng et al. [19] showed that resting microglia are physiologically located in the inner retinal layers in human eyes. In the same study it was shown that activated microglia migrate towards the outer retinal layers in human eyes with diabetic macular edema and it is suggested that proinflammatory cytokines are responsible for the activation of microglia. Interestingly, in a rat model of experimental autoimmune uveoretinitis, Rao et al. showed that microglia had migrated from the nerve fiber layer and other inner retinal layers to the photoreceptor layer at day 9 after the induction of uveitis [20]. Moreover, Ding X et al. showed that rat microglial cells activated by lipopolysaccharides secreted proinflammatory cytokines (tumour necrosis factor and interleukin beta) which could promote vascular dysfunction and hence permeability [21]. These findings could explain the high frequency of patients with HRF in the outer retina at baseline, when macular edema was present and hence the inflammatory process was active. It has been shown that glucocorticoids inhibit microglial migration [22]. We speculate that the treatment given in our patients (mainly glucocorticoids) may explain the behavior of the HRF after treatment, that is, a more frequent location of foci in the inner retina.

We have not found the number or location of the HRF to have an independent influence on VA. Previous studies have evaluated possible associations between HRF and visual outcomes in diabetic macular edema, retinal vein occlusions and neovascular age-related

Table 5 Behavior of foci and evolution of visual acuity in patients with posterior uveitis

	Baseline	Month 1	Month 3	Month 6	Month 12
Frequency of patients with ≥11 foci(groups C or D)	62.5%	28.5%	25%	14.2%	12.5%
Distribution (% patients in each group)					
Group 0 (no foci)	0%	0%	0%	0%	0%
Group 1 (inner retina)	50%	28.5%	57%	62.5%	85.7%
Group 2 (outer retina)	50%	71.5%	43%	37.5%	14.3%
Mean logMAR VA[a]	0.5	0.3	0.41	0.25	0.18

[a] logMAR VA: logarithm of the minimum angle of resolution visual acuity

Table 6 Behavior of foci and evolution of visual acuity in patients with panuveitis uveitis

	Baseline	Month 1	Month 3	Month 6	Month 12
Frequency of patients with ≥11 foci(groups C or D)	66.7%	80%	66.7%	60%	60%
Distribution (% patients in each group)					
Group 0 (no foci)	0%	0%	0%	16.7%	0%
Group 1 (inner retina)	67%	40%	50%	33.3%	50%
Group 2 (outer retina)	33%	60%	50%	50%	50%
Mean logMAR VA[a]	0.85	0.8	0.69	0.55	0.40

[a] logMAR VA: logarithm of the minimum angle of resolution visual acuity

macular degeneration. In the study by Vujosevic et al., the number of foci was correlated inversely with retinal sensitivity and directly with non-stable fixation, as measured by microperimetry [9]. Uji et al. found an association between the presence of HRF in the outer retinal layers and poor VA in patients with diabetic macular edema [12]. Moreover, both HRF and VA were associated with disruptions in the external limiting membrane and in the junction between the inner and outer segment of the photoreceptors (nowadays known as the ellipsoid zone). In the study by Chatziralli et al. performed in patients with diabetic macular edema and retinal vein occlusions, a higher number of HRF was associated with poorer VA [17]. Kang et al. found that the number of HRF at baseline was inversely associated with final VA in patients with diabetic macular edema treated with

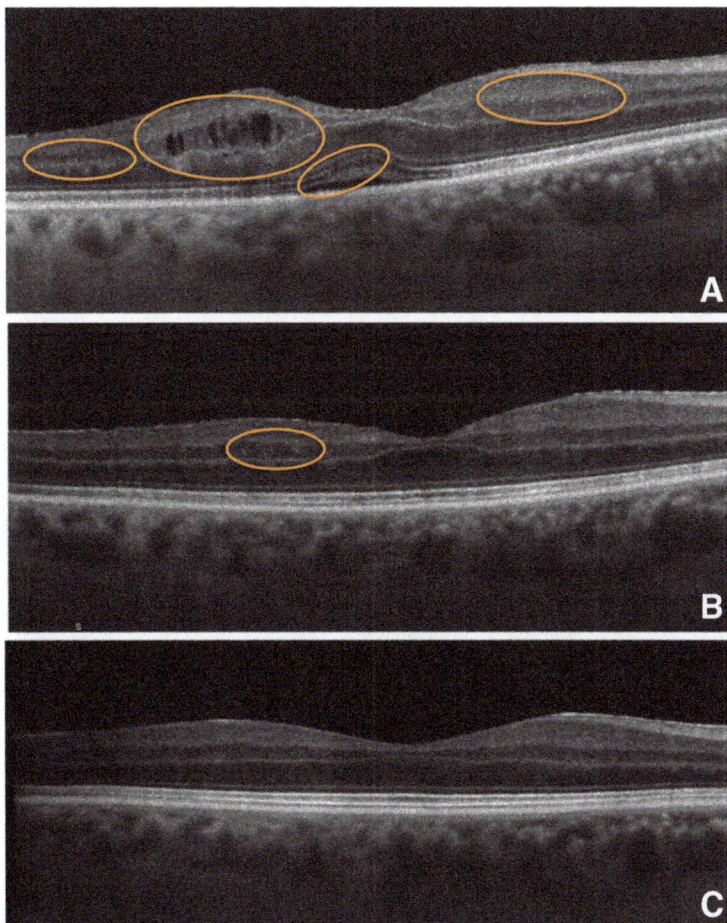

Fig. 3 Example of behavior of HRF number and distribution as detected by SD-OCT over the course of follow-up. Circles highlight foci. Left eye of a 61-year-old man with chronic idiopathic anterior uveitis. **a** At baseline, multiple HRF scattered across all retina layers and macular edema (assigned to groups D and 2. **b** At 6 months, HRF number reduced and outer retina not affected (assigned to groups B and 1). **c** At 12 months, no visible foci (assigned to groups A and 0)

intravitreal bevacizumab [23]. The same group reported similar findings in patients with branch retinal vein occlusion [8], neovascular age-related macular degeneration and polypoidal choroidal neovascular vasculopathy [24].

In most of the aforementioned studies, HRF are assumed to be extravasations of lipoproteins and precursors of lipid exudates and the researchers consistently suggest that the underlying pathogenesis of poorer visual outcomes may be related to a toxic effect of lipids on photoreceptors. Regarding UME, it has been shown in a rat model of experimental autoimmune uveoretinitis that activated microglia located at the photoreceptor layer secrete peroxynitrite, which is the most potent biological oxidant known and capable of oxidizing cellular components [20]. Assuming a microglial origin of the foci, one could expect some deleterious effect on photoreceptors and hence on VA, due to the presence of microglia in the outer retina. We failed, however, to demonstrate an association between BCVA and HRF number or distribution. A protective effect of the treatment administered, usually local or systemic steroids, on photoreceptors and/ or an insufficient capability of the BCVA test to highlight functional damage may explain this finding.

The main limitation of our study is the subjective assessment and counting of HRF. Nevertheless, agreement between graders of the scans was high. In the future, software able to automatically measure the amount of HRF may help us objectively define the behavior of such foci and clarify their meaning and relevance. Other limitations are the relatively small size of the sample and that the SD-OCT device used lacks software capable of performing consecutive scans in the same retinal section. Strengths of our study are its prospective nature and the long-term follow-up.

Conclusions

In conclusion, SD-OCT scans showed HRF in eyes with UME in our study. After treatment, the number of foci decreased and their distribution changed, remaining foci locating preferentially in the inner retina, and this was associated with a decrease in macular thickness. Further studies with larger numbers of patients are needed to confirm these results and shed light on their implications for clinical practice.

Abbreviations
BCVA: Best corrected visual acuity; CI: Confidence interval; CMT: Central macular thickness; GEE: Generalized estimated equations methodology; HRF: Hyperreflective foci; IR: Inner retina; logMAR: Logarithm of the minimum angle of resolution; OR: Outer retina; SD-OCT: Spectral domain Optical coherence tomography; SPSS: Statistical Package for the Social Sciences; UME: Uveitic macular edema; VA: Visual acuity

Acknowledgements
Presented at the 13th Meeting of the International Ocular Inflammation Society, September 25-27 2015, San Francisco, California, USA.

Funding
This work was supported by grants from: Spanish Ministry of Economy, Industry and Competitivity, Carlos III Health Institute: PI 13/02148, cofinanced by the European Regional Development Fund.

Authors' contributions
BB and AF were involved in the assesment of OCT images. AF, JA, IRA, VL, DDV, MS, PA and AA were involved in medical management of the patients and OCT performance. JM was involved in collection of data. AF and BB were involved in literature review, conception, design and preparation of manuscript draft. JR was involved in statistics analyses. All authors have read and approved the final manuscript.

Competing interests
The authors declare that they have no competing interests.

Author details
[1]Department of Ophthalmology, BioCruces Health Research Institute, Cruces Hospital, University of the Basque Country, Cruces square s/n, CP 48903 Baracaldo, Vizcaya, Spain. [2]Autoimmune Diseases Research Unit, Department of Internal Medicine, BioCruces Health Research Institute, Cruces Hospital, University of the Basque Country, Bilbao, Spain. [3]Medical Statistics Core Facility, Institut d'Investigacions Biomèdiques August Pi i Sunyer (IDIBAPS), and Hospital Clinic, Barcelona, Spain. [4]Biostatistics Unit, Faculty of Medicine, Universitat Autònoma de Barcelona, Barcelona, Spain. [5]Ophthalmology Institute, Hospital Clinic of Barcelona, Barcelona, Spain. [6]Ophthalmology Department and Health Research Institute (IdISSC), Hospital Clinico San Carlos, Madrid, Spain.

References
1.   Okhravi N, Lightman S. Cystoid macular edema in uveitis. Ocul Immunol Inflamm. 2003;11:29–38.
2.   Tortorella P, D'Ambrosio E, Iannetti L, et al. Correlation between visual acuity, inner segment/outer segment junction, and cone outer segment tips line integrity in uveitic macular edema. Biomed Res Int. 2015;2015:5. Article ID 853728. https://doi.org/10.1155/2015/853728.
3.   Munk MR, Bolz M, Huf W, et al. Morphologic and functional evaluations during development, resolution, and relapse of uveitis-associated cystoid macular edema. Retina. 2012;33:1673–83.
4.   Bolz M, Schmidt-Erfurth U, Deak G, et al. Diabetic Retinopathy Research Group Vienna. Optical coherence tomographic hyperreflective foci: a morphologic sign of lipid extravasation in diabetic macular edema. Ophthalmology. 2009;116:914–20.
5.   Ogino K, Murakami T, Tsujikawa A, et al. Characteristics of optical coherence tomographic hyperreflective foci in retinal vein occlusion. Retina. 2012;32: 77–8.
6.   Baumüller S, Charbellssa P, Schmitz-Valckenberg S, Holz FG. Outer retinal hyperreflective spots on spectral-domain optical coherence tomography in macular telangiectasia type 2. Ophthalmology. 2010;117:2162–8.
7.   Framme C, Wolf S, Wolf-Schnurrbusch U. Small dense particles in the retina observable by spectral-domain optical coherence tomography in age-related macular degeneration. Invest Ophthalmol Vis Sci. 2010;51:5965–9.
8.   Kang JW, Lee H, Chung H, Kim HC. Correlation between optical coherence tomographic hyperreflective foci and visual outcomes after intravitreal bevacizumab for macular edema in branch retinal vein occlusion. Graefes Arch Clin Exp Ophthalmol. 2014;252:1413–21.
9.   Vujosevic S, Berton M, Bini S, et al. Hyperreflective retinal spots and visual function after anti-vascular endothelial growth factor treatment in center-involving diabetic macular edema. Retina. 2016;36:1298–308.
10. Jabs DA, Nussenblatt RB, Rosenbaum JT. Standardization of uveitis nomenclature (SUN) working group. Standardization of uveitis nomenclature for reporting clinical data. Results of the first international workshop. Am J Ophthalmol. 2005;40:509–16.
11. Framme C, Schweizer P, Imesch M, Wolf S, Wolf-Schnurrbusch U. Behavior of SD-OCT-detected hyperreflective foci in the retina of anti-VEGF-treated patients with diabetic macular edema. Invest Ophthalmol Vis Sci. 2012;53: 5814–8.

12. Uji A, Murakami T, Nishijima K. Et al: association between hyperreflective foci in the outer retina, status of photoreceptor layer, and visual acuity in diabetic macular edema. Am J Ophthalmol. 2012;153:710–7.

13. Vujosevic S, Bini S, Midena G, et al. Hyperreflective intraretinal spots in diabetics with and without non proliferative diabetic retinopathy: an in vivo study using spectral domain optical coherence tomography. J Diabetes Res. 2103;2013:5. Article ID 491835. https://doi.org/10.1155/2013/491835

14. De Benedetto U, Sacconi R, Pierro L, Lattanzio R, Bandello F. Optical coherence tomographic hyperreflective foci in early stages of diabetic retinopathy. Retina. 2015;35:449–53.

15. Saito M, Barbazetto IA, Spaide RF. Intravitreal cellular infiltrate imaged as punctate spots by spectral-domain optical coherence tomography in eyes with posterior segment inflammatory disease. Retina. 2013;33:559–65.

16. Chu CJ, Herrmann P, Carvalho LS, et al. Assessment and in vivo scoring of murine experimental autoimmune uveoretinitis using optical coherence tomography. PLoS One. 2013;14(8):e63002.

17. Chatziralli IP, Sergentanis TN, Sivaprasad S. Hyperreflective foci as an independent visual outcome predictor in macular edema due to retinal vascular diseases treated with intravitreal dexamethasone or ranibizumab. Retina. 2016;36:2319–28.

18. AbriAghdam K, Pielen A, Framme C, Junker B. Correlation between hyperreflective foci and clinical outcomes in neovascular age-related macular degeneration after switching to aflibercept. Invest Ophthalmol Vis Sci. 2015;56:6448–64455.

19. Zeng HY, Green WR, Tso MO. Microglial activation in human diabetic retinopathy. Arch Ophthalmol. 2008;126:227–32.

20. Rao NA, Kimoto T, Zamir E, et al. Pathogenic role of retinal microglia in experimental uveoretinitis. Invest Ophthalmol Vis Sci. 2003;44:22–31.

21. Ding X, Zhang M, Ruiping G, Xu G, Wu H. Activated microglia induce the production of reactive oxygen species and promote apoptosis of co-cultured retinal microvascular pericytes. Graefes Arch Clin Exp Ophthalmol. 2017;255:777–88.

22. Zhou Y, Ling EA, Deen ST. Dexamethasone suppresses monocyte chemoattractant protein-1 production viamitogen activated protein kinase phosphatase-1 dependent inhibition of JunN-terminal kinase and p38 mitogen-activated protein kinase in activated rat microglia. J Neurochem. 2007;102:667–78.

23. Kang JW, Chung H, Chan Kim H. Correlation of optical coherence tomographic foci with visual outcomes in different patterns of diabetic macular edema. Retina. 2016;36:1630–09.

24. Lee H, Ji B, Chung H, Kim HC. Correlation between optical coherence tomographic hyperreflective foci and visual outcomes after anti-VEGF treatment in neovascular age-related macular degeneration and polypoidal choroidal vasculopathy. Retina. 2016;36:465–75.

31

Dry eye symptoms and impact on vision-related function across International Task Force guidelines severity levels in the United States

Laurie Barber[1*], Omid Khodai[2], Thomas Croley[3], Christopher Lievens[4], Stephen Montaquila[5], Jillian Ziemanski[6], Melissa McCart[7], Orsolya Lunacsek[7], Caroline Burk[8] and Vaishali Patel[9]

Abstract

Background: International Task Force (ITF) guidelines established a grading scheme to support treatment of dry eye disease based on clinical signs and symptoms. The purpose of this study was to assess the impact of dry eye on vision-related function across ITF severity levels using the Ocular Surface Disease Index (OSDI) questionnaire.

Methods: Non-interventional, cross-sectional study of prescription treatment-naïve dry eye patients seeking symptom relief at 10 ophthalmology and optometry practices. Clinicians assessed corneal and conjunctival staining, tear break-up time, Schirmer's test (type I with anesthesia), and best-corrected visual acuity. Patients completed the OSDI questionnaire and OSDI overall and domain (Symptoms, Visual Function, and Environmental Triggers) scores were compared across ITF guidelines severity levels (1–4).

Results: Of 158 patients (mean age, 55 years) enrolled, 52 (33%) were ITF level 1, 54 (34%) ITF level 2, and 52 (33%) ITF levels 3/4 combined. No significant differences were observed in most baseline characteristics. Overall OSDI scores (mean [standard deviation]) were 26.5 [20.0] for ITF level 1, 33.8 [17.5] for ITF level 2, and 44.9 [26.1] for ITF level 3/4 cohorts ($P < 0.0001$). Component OSDI Symptoms, Visual Function, and Environmental Triggers domain scores all worsened with increasing ITF severity level ($P \leq 0.01$).

Conclusions: Dry eye disease has significant deleterious impact on vision-related function across all ITF severity levels.

Keywords: Dry eye disease, Ocular Surface Disease Index, International Task Force guidelines, Vision-related function

Background

Dry eye is a multifactorial disease of the ocular surface resulting in discomfort, visual disturbance, and instability of the tear film [1]. In the early 2000s, it was estimated that dry eye affected over 7 million people over the age of 40 years in the United States [2, 3]. Prevalence has likely increased significantly over the past 10 years with the escalation of risk factors such as an aging population, a greater number of refractive laser surgeries, and more frequent use of contact lenses, computers, smartphones, and tablets [2–5]. Additionally, women are known to experience dry eye more frequently than men, potentially owing to hormone fluctuations during the menstrual cycle or menopause, and from use of oral contraceptives or hormone replacement therapy [6].

The symptoms that commonly compel patients with dry eye to seek treatment from ophthalmologists and optometrists include ocular discomfort and irritation, burning, itching, and blurred vision [7, 8]. In addition to blurring of vision, other changes in visual function noted in dry eye patients include reductions in functional visual acuity [9] and contrast sensitivity [10], optical

* Correspondence: barberlauried@gmail.com
[1]Little Rock Eye Clinic, 203 Executive Court, Suite A, Little Rock, AK 72205, USA
Full list of author information is available at the end of the article

aberration due to tear film irregularity [11], and degradation of retinal image quality [12]. Dry eye disease significantly affects patients' visual function and greatly impacts social and physical functioning, workplace productivity, and quality of life [13, 14]. For example, ocular discomfort and dryness are often reported as the primary reason for discontinuation of contact lens wear [15–18], negatively affecting patients' quality of life. In one study conducted in the United Kingdom using utility assessment (Time Trade-Off and Standard Gamble methods) to quantify and understand the impact of a given health condition relative to other diseases, severe dry eye utilities were similar to those associated with dialysis or severe angina [19].

Symptomatic dry eye disease can present without evidence of ocular surface damage or changes in tear flow [13, 14, 20]. Poor correlation has been found between symptoms and clinical measures of dry eye disease [21–24], and patient-reported dry eye symptoms have been demonstrated to be more reproducible from visit to visit than many of the clinical signs used to diagnose and monitor dry eye [25]. Consequently, quality of life or patient-reported outcomes (PRO) evaluations have been used to provide clinicians with valuable information on the impact of dry eye disease and the effectiveness of treatment [26, 27]. The Ocular Surface Disease Index (OSDI) is a validated PRO instrument that provides a measure of the ocular symptoms and disability associated with dry eye [20, 28]. The OSDI was developed as a brief, self-administered questionnaire to provide rapid evaluation of the range and frequency of ocular symptoms associated with dry eye disease, and their impact on patients' visual functioning. The questionnaire includes 3 subscales, which cover ocular discomfort, limitations in performance of daily activities affected by dry eye, and the susceptibility of dry eye symptoms to environmental factors. As an instrument, OSDI shows internal consistency, with good to excellent test-retest reliability and excellent discriminant validity for measuring dry eye symptoms [28].

The International Task Force (ITF) guidelines for diagnosis and treatment of dry eye were established by an expert panel that considered dry eye disease severity to be the most important factor in making treatment decisions [29]. The ITF panel established a 4-level dry eye severity grading scheme based on signs and symptoms [29]. A study evaluating the implementation of this scheme by clinicians found these guidelines to be simple and efficient for assessing dry eye severity and for supporting treatment decisions [30]. Notably, use of the ITF guidelines led clinicians to focus on patient symptoms and initiating early treatment rather than relying on dry eye diagnostic tests [30].

As standard clinical measures of dry eye provide only a partial picture of the disease experience, it is difficult to appreciate how dry eye is perceived by the patient. The current study was conducted to quantify the frequency of dry eye symptoms and their impact on vision-dependent functioning across different ITF levels, using the OSDI questionnaire. Patients were prescription treatment-naïve (received no prescription therapy for dry eye disease) presenting to their clinicians with complaints of dry eye. Although studies have assessed symptoms in patients with dry eye [7, 13, 14, 20], to date no real-world, clinic-based studies assessing dry eye symptoms and the impact of disease based on ITF severity categories have been reported in the published literature.

Methods

Study design and patient selection

This was a non-interventional, cross-sectional study conducted from July 2014 to October 2014. To ensure real-world representation of dry eye patients' access to care, 5 ophthalmology and 5 optometry clinical practices across the United States were recruited to enroll patients. Prescription treatment-naïve dry eye patients at least 18 years of age, seeking routine consultation for relief of dry eye symptoms, were enrolled consecutively. For study eligibility, patients were required to show clinical signs of dry eye, as assessed from conjunctival (lissamine green) and corneal (fluorescein staining and Schirmer's test (type I with anesthesia), during screening. The study excluded patients with prior use of prescription dry eye medication or punctal plugs; ocular surgery within the previous 6 months; use of antibiotics, corticosteroids, immunosuppressant medications, topical nonsteroidal anti-inflammatory drugs or antivirals within 30 days of the start of the study; a diagnosis of active ocular allergies; infection of the anterior segment or uveitis; and a systemic or ocular disorder or condition deemed by the investigator to potentially affect interpretation of study results. The study protocol was reviewed and approved by the following independent review boards: Liberty Institutional Review Board (DeLand, FL), Southern College of Optometry Institutional Review Board (Memphis, TN), and Western Institutional Review Board (Puyallup, WA). Patients provided written informed consent prior to study participation.

Data collection and study measurements

During the enrollment visit, patient demographics as well as medical and medication histories were recorded for ocular and nonocular conditions. Clinicians conducted an examination of the worse eye (as reported by the patient) or the right eye if both eyes were reported to be equally affected. Clinicians were selected on the basis of their expertise in ocular surface disease and were instructed to use clinical standard of care in their grading of ocular surface staining. For corneal punctate staining with fluorescein, the entire cornea was examined using slit-lamp evaluation with a yellow barrier filter and cobalt blue illumination, and staining was graded as "none", "mild", "marked", "severe", as well as "central" or "non-central". For conjunctival staining with lissamine green, interpalpebral staining was measured between 30 s and 2 min after instillation of the dye and likewise graded according to the clinician's judgement as "none", "mild", "marked", or "severe". Tear break-up time (TBUT), the time (seconds) until random location tear break-up between blinks, and the amount of wetting (mm) on Schirmer's test (type I with anesthesia) performed for 5 min also were assessed. Since the study was performed within the setting of routine clinical practice, best-corrected visual acuity was evaluated (both eyes) using Snellen notation. No safety assessment was performed, as there was no intervention in this study.

Clinicians' assessments of dry eye severity were based on objective measures and patient-reported visual symptoms of disease. In accordance with ITF guidelines, disease severity in the study eye was graded on a 4-point scale ranging from level 1 (mild-to-moderate symptoms plus mild-to-moderate conjunctival signs), via level 2 (moderate-to-severe symptoms plus either tear film signs, conjunctival staining, mild corneal punctate staining, or visual signs) and level 3 (severe symptoms plus either marked corneal punctate staining, central corneal staining, or filamentary keratitis), to level 4 (severe symptoms plus either severe corneal staining, with erosions or conjunctival scarring) [29]. Dry eye symptoms identified by the ITF panel as being of particular relevance in determining disease severity are ocular discomfort (itchiness, burning, foreign body sensation, and sensitivity to light) and visual disturbance [29]. Stratification by ITF severity was not disclosed to patients to ensure unbiased completion of survey questionnaires following their clinical examination.

The OSDI questionnaire was used to quantify the symptomatic and functional impact of dry eye, as perceived by the patient. The questionnaire consists of 12 items (questions) included in 3 subscale domains measuring the frequency of (1) ocular symptoms (specifically sensitivity to light, grittiness, sore/painful eyes, blurred vision, and poor vision) (questions 1–5), (2) visual problems impacting daily activities (reading, television viewing, computer work, and night-time driving) (questions 6–9), and (3) ocular discomfort triggered by environmental factors (wind, low humidity, and air conditioning) (questions 10–12) over the previous week. The response to each question is graded on an analog scale of 0 (none of the time), 1 (some of the time), 2 (half of

the time), 3 (most of the time), and 4 (all the time). Overall OSDI and subscale domain scores range from 0 to 100, with higher scores representing greater ocular disability, and based on the overall score, patients can be classified as mild (13–22), moderate (23–32), or severe (≥33) [31].

Patient and Clinician Assessment Forms were used to record patient data and results of diagnostic and survey tests. Prior to study initiation, 2 clinicians took part in 60-min interviews and 3 patients participated in 30-min interviews to ensure that the survey's wording and directions were clear and easily understood. The final Clinician Assessment Form and Patient Assessment Form were slightly revised as a result.

Study endpoints and data analysis

Study endpoints were clinicians' assessments of dry eye signs (ocular surface staining intensity, TBUT, and Schirmer score) as well as OSDI overall and Symptoms, Visual Function, and Environmental Triggers domain scores, categorized by ITF severity level.

Data were summarized using descriptive statistics for continuous and categorical variables. Frequencies reported for individual OSDI questions were collapsed into 2 groups according to how often each item was reported to have occurred: less than half of the time versus at least half of the time. Comparisons between ITF severity levels for demographics, clinical characteristics, and diagnostic tests were performed using 1-way analysis of variance (means) and chi-square test (proportions). The mean overall and subscale domain OSDI scores were compared across ITF severity levels using general linear models adjusted for age, gender, and hypertension. The percent of patients responding to individual OSDI questions among ITF severity levels was compared using the chi-square test. Statistical significance was set at $P < 0.05$.

Sample size estimates for analysis of variance of OSDI scores across ITF severity levels were based on previous reports of a minimal clinically important difference in overall OSDI score of approximately 5 points for patients with mild-to-moderate dry eye and 10 points for those with severe dry eye, where the standard deviation (SD) for the minimal clinically important difference in OSDI score ranged from 2.5 to 23.1 points [28, 31]. A sample size of at least 150 patients was determined to have > 90% power to detect a minimal clinically important difference of at least 5 points when the SD was 13 or less, assuming $\alpha = 0.05$ for a 1-way analysis of variance. For analysis, patients were grouped into 3 cohorts based on ITF severity level, with an estimated 50 patients in ITF level 1, 50 patients in ITF level 2, and 50 patients in ITF level 3/4 combined. It was anticipated that there would be fewer treatment-naïve patients in the more severe ITF levels who would meet study eligibility criteria, making it difficult to enroll 50 patients in each of the ITF level 3 and 4 categories. The F test statistic threshold to reject the null hypothesis of no difference in OSDI scores between the 3 ITF severity levels was 2.662. Power calculations based on a planned sample size of 150 patients indicated that 1-way analysis of variance would have 80% power to detect an effect size of 0.26 at $\alpha = 0.05$.

Results

Patient demographics and clinical characteristics

A total of 158 patients were recruited for the study; 52 (33%) were categorized in ITF level 1, 54 (34%) in ITF level 2, and 52 (33%) in ITF level 3/4 combined (of which 39 [25%] were in ITF level 3 and 13 [8%] were in ITF level 4). The study population had a mean age of 55 years and was predominantly female (82%) and white (86%); 76% of patients had college education or higher, and 65% were employed at the time of the study (Table 1). There were no differences in patient demographics, including education, employment status, geographic location, household income, or health care coverage, between the 3 ITF severity level cohorts. Additionally, no significant differences in concomitant non-dry eye-related ocular and non-ocular comorbidities were observed across the 3 ITF cohorts, except for hypertension ($P < 0.01$). Individual comparisons between ITF severity levels revealed differences in hypertension, diabetes and hyperlipidemia, which were significantly more frequent ($P < 0.05$) in the ITF level 3/4 cohort compared with ITF level 1 or ITF level 2 (Table 1).

Clinical assessments

Table 2 summarizes the intensity of ocular surface staining and tear film signs for each ITF level. Central corneal staining, which is indicative of more severe dry eye [29], was present in 56% of patients in ITF level 3/4 but no more than 2% of patients in either ITF level 1 or ITF level 2 ($P < 0.0001$ across all ITF levels). In addition, the mean grade of both corneal and conjunctival staining rose as ITF level increased ($P < 0.0001$ across all ITF levels). TBUT decreased significantly as ITF severity increased from level 1 (mean [SD], 8.4 [3.6] s) to level 3/4 (3.7 [2.0] s; $P < 0.0001$ across all ITF levels). In addition, Schirmer's test scores were significantly lower in ITF level 3/4 (mean [SD], 7.2 [5.6] mm) compared with ITF level 1 (mean [SD], 13.6 [7.9] mm; $P < 0.0001$ across all ITF levels). The proportion of study eyes with visual acuity better than 20/40 declined numerically as ITF severity increased, while the proportion of eyes with visual acuity of 20/40 or worse rose numerically with increasing ITF severity (Table 2).

OSDI questionnaire scores by ITF severity level

Analysis of the OSDI questionnaire responses revealed that as ITF severity level increased, patients had worse OSDI overall and Symptoms, Visual Function, and Environmental Triggers domain scores (Table 3). Overall OSDI scores (mean [SD]) were 26.5 [20.0], 33.8 [17.5], and 44.9 [26.1] for ITF level 1, ITF level 2, and ITF level 3/4 cohorts, respectively ($P < 0.0001$ across all ITF levels). As expected, OSDI Symptoms domain score increased, indicating greater frequency of symptoms, as ITF severity level increased ($P < 0.0001$ across all ITF levels). However, OSDI Visual Function domain score and Environmental Triggers domain score also increased, suggesting more frequent disability, as ITF level increased ($P = 0.0013$ and $P = 0.0107$, respectively, across all ITF levels). Comparison of OSDI overall and subscale domain scores between individual ITF severity levels indicated that patients in ITF level 3/4 had significantly higher scores than those in ITF level 1 ($P \le 0.005$) and ITF level 2 ($P \le 0.03$, except for the Environmental Triggers domain). Patients in ITF level 2 also had significantly higher OSDI overall and Symptoms subscale domain scores compared with ITF level 1 ($P \le 0.04$) (Table 3).

Generally, a greater percentage of patients in ITF level 2 and ITF level 3/4 experienced frequent (at least half of the time) symptoms of light sensitivity, eye grittiness, painful/sore eyes, blurred vision and poor vision (Fig. 1a) and frequent dry-eye-related impairment of reading, night-time driving, computer work, and watching television (Fig. 1b) than patients in ITF level 1. The percentage of patients who reported frequent eye discomfort in windy and low humidity conditions was generally similar across ITF severity levels; however, the proportion of patients who reported frequent eye discomfort in air-conditioned areas was higher in ITF levels 2 and 3/4 compared with ITF level 1 (Fig. 1c).

Discussion

Variation in diagnostic criteria and clinical measures of dry eye disease and its severity have been reported [25], and poor correlation between clinical signs and patient-reported symptoms has been documented in previously published literature [21–23]. Discordance between ocular surface findings and symptoms of dry eye may occur in the early stages of disease where symptoms can exist without clinical signs of dry eye [32]. Some investigators have hypothesized that chronic dry eye symptoms occurring in the absence of clinical signs of dry eye might be of neuropathic origin, arising as a result of central sensitization and manifesting as neuropathic ocular pain [33, 34]. The ITF guidelines were developed from expert consensus to establish severity criteria and treatment recommendations for dry eye [29], and formed a

Table 1 Patients' demographic and clinical characteristics by ITF severity level

Baseline characteristic	Overall (N = 158)	Dry eye severity level		
		ITF 1 (n = 52)	ITF 2 (n = 54)	ITF 3/4 (n = 52)
Age, mean (SD), y	55 (16)	53 (13)	57 (17)	56 (17)
Female, n (%)	130 (82)	43 (83)	41 (76)	46 (88)
White, n (%)	136 (86)	41 (79)	47 (87)	48 (92)
Geographic region, n (%)				
Midwest	7 (4)	3 (6)	4 (7)	0
Northeast	37 (23)	12 (23)	12 (22)	13 (25)
South	80 (51)	28 (54)	28 (52)	24 (46)
West	34 (22)	9 (17)	0 (19)	15 (29)
Education level, n (%)				
High school or less	38 (24)	12 (23)	12 (22)	14 (27)
Some college or higher	120 (76)	40 (77)	42 (78)	38 (73)
Employment status, n (%)				
Employed	103 (65)	36 (69)	36 (67)	31 (60)
Retired/disabled	47 (30)	12 (23)	16 (30)	19 (37)
Nonemployed	8 (5)	4 (8)	2 (4)	2 (4)
Ocular comorbidity, n (%)				
Cataract	48 (30)	13 (25)	16 (30)	19 (37)
Primary open-angle glaucoma	8 (5)	3 (6)	2 (4)	3 (6)
Ocular hypertension	2 (1)	0	0	2 (4)
Sjögren's syndrome	4 (3)	1 (2)	1 (2)	2 (4)
Ocular allergy	2 (1)	2 (4)	0	0
Nonocular comorbidity, n (%)				
Hypertension	55 (35)	12 (23)*	16 (30)*	27 (52)
Hyperlipidemia	37 (23)	10 (19)	9 (17)*	18 (35)
Gastrointestinal disorders[a]	20 (13)	5 (12)	16 (11)	9 (17)
Diabetes	17 (11)	3 (6)*	4 (7)	10 (19)
Rheumatologic disease	14 (9)	3 (6)	3 (6)	8 (15)
Asthma	11 (7)	1 (2)	7 (13)	3 (6)
Peripheral vascular disease	2 (1)	1 (2)	1 (2)	0
Congestive heart failure	2 (1)	0	1 (2)	1 (2)
Angina	2 (1)	0	0	2 (4)
Other	26 (16)	7 (13)	13 (24)	6 (12)

*P < 0.05 versus ITF 3/4 by chi-square test
[a]Gastroesophageal reflux disease or peptic ulcer disease
ITF International Task Force, SD standard deviation

foundation for the 2007 International Dry Eye Workshop management and therapy of dry eye guidelines [35]. To date, there are no studies that have evaluated the impact of disease, in particular its functional impact, in prescription-naïve dry eye patients across ITF severity levels in a real-world, clinic-based setting.

In this observational study of patients with symptomatic dry eye, no significant overall differences were observed in patient demographics, concomitant non-dry eye-related ocular conditions, and comorbidities (other than hypertension) across the 3 dry eye patient cohorts based on ITF severity level (ITF level 1, ITF level 2, and ITF level 3/4 combined). Almost one-third of the patients enrolled in the study had cataracts and less than 10% had glaucoma. Very few (3%) patients enrolled in this study had Sjögren's syndrome, an autoimmune condition associated with severe dry eye. Of the 30 patients enrolled who presented with central corneal staining, 29 were in ITF severity level 3/4. This, together with the higher prevalence of cataract in ITF severity level 3/4, may have

Table 2 Clinical assessment of dry eye by ITF severity level

Dry eye assessment	Overall (N = 158)	Dry eye severity level		
		ITF 1 (n = 52)	ITF 2 (n = 54)	ITF 3/4 (n = 52)
Left eye visual acuity, n (%)				
< 20/20	11 (7)	4 (8)	5 (9)	2 (4)
20/20 to < 20/40	134 (85)	46 (88)	45 (83)	43 (83)
20/40 to 20/60+	13 (8)	2 (4)	4 (7)	7 (14)
Right eye visual acuity, n (%)				
< 20/20	12 (8)	3 (6)	6 (11)	3 (6)
20/20 to < 20/40	133 (84)	47 (90)	45 (83)	41 (79)
20/40 to 20/60+	13 (9)	2 (4)	3 (6)	8 (15)
Central corneal staining, n (%)	30 (19)	0[†]	1 (2)[†]	29 (56)
Corneal staining, mean (SD)	1.2 (0.8)	0.7 (0.5)[*,†]	1.2 (0.6)[†]	2.3 (0.5)
Conjunctival staining, mean (SD)	1.3 (0.8)	0.8 (0.5)[*,†]	1.2 (0.7)[†]	2.0 (0.8)
TBUT, mean (SD), s	6.2 (4.3)	8.4 (3.6)[*,†]	6.4 (5.3)[†]	3.7 (2.0)
Schirmer's test type I, mean (SD)	10.3 (7.0)	13.6 (7.9)[*,†]	10.3 (6.0)[†]	7.2 (5.6)

*$P \leq 0.01$ versus ITF 2; [†]$P \leq 0.01$ versus ITF 3/4 by 1-way analysis of variance (means) and chi-square test (proportions)

ITF International Task Force, *SD* standard deviation, *TBUT* tear break-up time

contributed to the greater proportion (≥2 times) of patients in the ITF level 3/4 cohort who reported poorer visual acuity (20/40 to 20/60+) in both eyes compared with the lower ITF severity level 1 and 2 cohorts.

The study demonstrated that all OSDI subscale scores, including those for Visual Function and Environmental Triggers, were significantly worse in higher ITF severity level cohorts. This would indicate that the observed deterioration in OSDI overall score with increasing ITF severity was not driven solely by worsening dry eye symptoms. Pairwise tests demonstrated that overall and subscale domain OSDI scores were significantly higher in the ITF level 3/4 cohort compared with ITF level 1 and ITF level 2 cohorts, except for the Environmental Triggers domain score, which was not significantly different between ITF level 3/4 and ITF level 2 cohorts. In addition, analysis of individual OSDI questions demonstrated that a higher percentage of ITF level 3/4 patients experienced not only more frequent symptoms of dry eye, but also more frequent disruption of daily tasks and more frequent symptoms from environmental triggers of dry eye. Assessed against the published OSDI guideline

categories of mild (13–22), moderate (23–32), and severe (≥33) ocular surface disease [31], patients in this study generally had frequent ocular disability, as reflected in overall mean OSDI scores of 26.5, 33.8, and 44.9 in ITF level 1, 2, and 3/4 cohorts, respectively, although intracohort variation in overall OSDI score was appreciable (based on standard deviation values in Table 3). Observed differences from the published guidelines may be associated with a different anchor (such as Global Clinician's Assessment versus ITF guidelines) that was used to establish disease severity [31].

Our study results, obtained from a sample of prescription treatment-naïve patients presenting with symptomatic dry eye in the real-world setting, are consistent with previously reported clinical study findings that OSDI overall scores increase as levels of dry eye severity worsen. In a study by Schiffman et al. [28], patients' severity of dry eye was categorized using 2 evaluations: physician assessment and a composite score that combined traditional clinical measures (Schirmer's test and lissamine green staining) and a symptoms-based measure (patients' perception of ocular symptoms, as

Table 3 OSDI questionnaire scores

OSDI score, mean (SD)	Overall (N = 158)	Dry eye severity level			P value[a]
		ITF 1 (n = 52)	ITF 2 (n = 54)	ITF 3/4 (n = 52)	
Overall	35.1 (22.6)	26.5 (20.0)[*,†]	33.8 (17.5)[‡]	44.9 (26.1)	< 0.0001
Symptoms domain	32.8 (22.2)	23.3 (18.1)[*,†]	32.3 (17.2)[‡]	42.7 (26.2)	< 0.0001
Visual-Related Function domain	32.8 (25.1)	26.8 (23.0)[†]	28.6 (21.0)[‡]	42.7 (28.2)	0.0013
Environmental Triggers domain	43.3 (30.1)	34.2 (27.7)[†]	43.2 (29.1)	52.2 (33.0)	0.0107

*$P < 0.05$ compared with ITF level 2; [†]$P \leq 0.005$ compared with ITF level 3/4; [‡]$P < 0.05$ compared with ITF level 3/4

[a]Comparison of scores across all ITF levels using general linear models adjusted for gender, ethnicity (overall, Symptoms domain), and hypertension

ITF International Task Force, *OSDI* Ocular Surface Disease Index, *SD* standard deviation

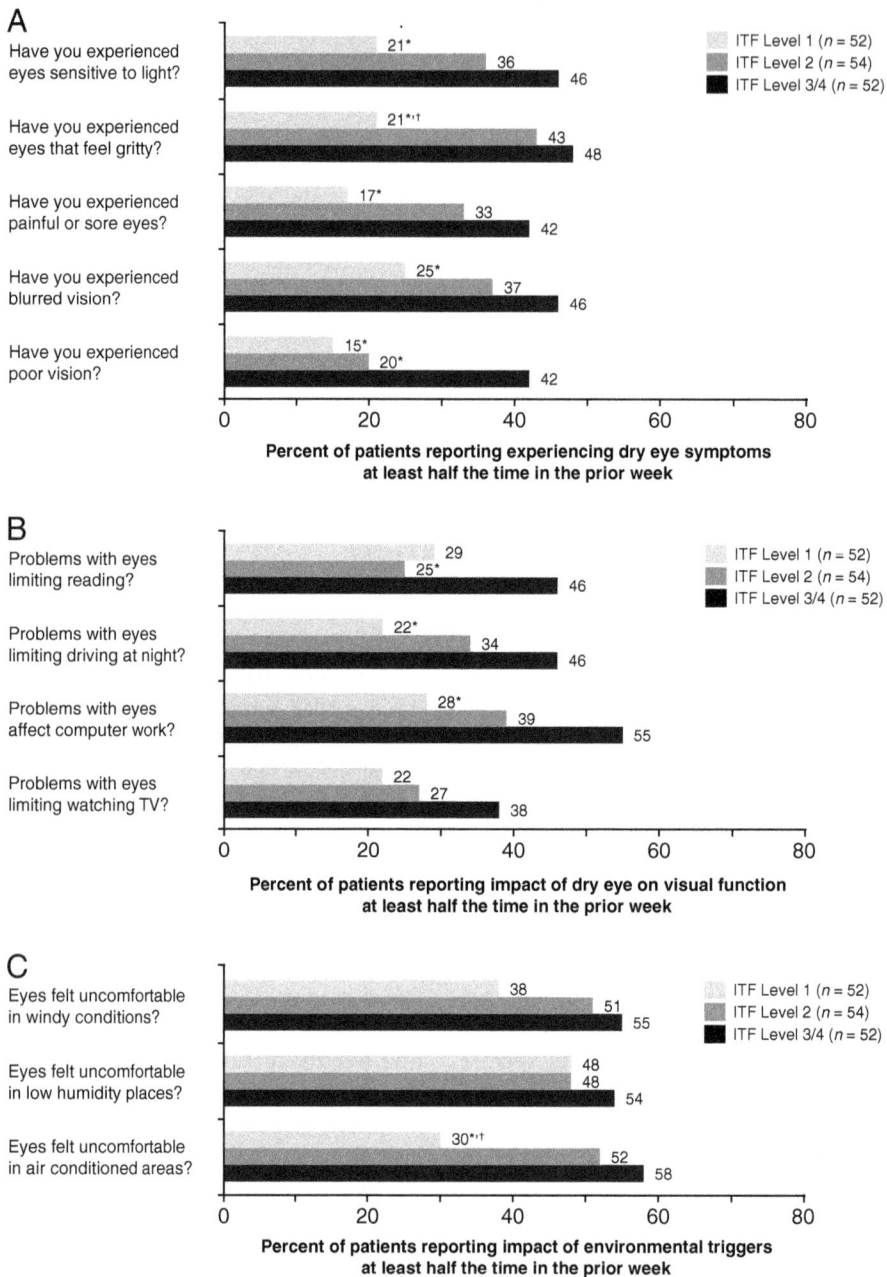

Fig. 1 Proportion of patients indicating on OSDI questionnaire components that at least half of the time in the past week: (**a**) experienced dry eye symptoms (questions 1–5); (**b**) had problems with their eyes limiting visual function (questions 6–9); and (**c**) had eyes that felt uncomfortable in certain environmental conditions (questions 10–12) by ITF dry eye severity level. *$P < 0.05$ compared with ITF level 3/4; †$P < 0.05$ compared with ITF level 2 by chi-square test; sample size varied for visual function and environmental triggers, as not all patients performed tasks over the previous week. *OSDI* Ocular Surface Disease Index, *ITF* International Task Force, *TV* television

assessed using the McMonnies Dry Eye Questionnaire [36] and the National Eye Institute Visual Functioning Questionnaire [NEI VFQ-25] [37]). Overall mean OSDI scores grouped into "normal", "mild/moderate", and "severe" categories were 9.6, 20.8, and 36.3 based on physician assessment, respectively, and 4.5, 18.1, and 36.3 based on patients' composite score, respectively [28]. In

another study by Sullivan et al. [38], a composite score of dry eye severity was established by converting clinical measures (tear osmolarity, Schirmer's test, TBUT, Meibomian score, corneal and conjunctival staining) and symptoms (from the OSDI) into a common unit system, whereby 0 represented least evidence of the disease and 1 represented most evidence of disease. Based on the composite score, overall mean OSDI scores in patient groups categorized as having "normal", "mild/moderate", or "severe" disease were 5.5, 21.0, and 41.2, respectively [38]. Compared with both the Schiffman [28] and Sullivan [38] studies, patients in our study categorized in ITF level 1 had higher overall OSDI scores, and patients in ITF level 2 had similar OSDI scores to patients categorized as having "severe disease" in the study by Schiffman et al. [28]. This suggests that mild-to-moderate dry eye as defined by the ITF guidelines may be associated with a relatively high level of ocular disability compared to other composite signs- and symptoms-based measures of dry eye severity.

Our study is limited by the cross-sectional survey design and lack of patient follow-up. Clinicians were not intentionally masked to patients' previous dry eye diagnoses and treatments, and hence their assessments of dry eye severity (ITF grading) were subject to possible bias. In addition, no specific method for assessment of conjunctival and corneal staining was stipulated for use at the various study sites, other than clinicians' standard of care. While the absence of formal grading definitions may have resulted in greater variability, the results are likely to be more reflective of a real-world, clinic-based setting. Despite the inherent variability based on this aspect of the study design, statistical significance was still obtained. On the other hand, as a result of restricting study participation to patients seeking medical consultation for their dry eye symptoms, demonstration of statistical significance may have been facilitated by a selection bias toward homogeneity of the patient sample. Accordingly, the generalizability of our study findings remains to be established using a randomly drawn sample from an unselected dry eye population. Prospective studies with follow-up after initiation of treatment will help further define patients' perceptions of the impact of dry eye on their overall quality of life.

Conclusions

Dry eye disease is frequently undertreated [32, 39, 40]. Barriers to appropriate treatment include the time required to adequately diagnose and determine appropriate treatment based on the patient's severity level, the perception by clinicians that the condition has minor impact on patient well-being, the perception by patients that the disease is normal or less important than other conditions that require treatment, lack of understanding of the disease process [41], and a perceived paucity of therapeutic options [42, 43]. Supplemental artificial tears and eyelid hygiene are common treatment modalities for dry eye disease, yet many patients continue to experience significant disruption to their daily lives. Our findings suggest that dry eye symptoms are frequently troublesome to the patient at all levels of disease severity, and require attention and adequate treatment. A complete and comprehensive medical and ocular history conducted by clinicians should help correctly identify patients who may have ambiguous symptoms without clinical signs or vice versa, and allow proper treatment and management of dry eye disease.

Abbreviations

ITF: International Task Force; OSDI: Ocular Surface Disease Index; PRO: Patient-reported outcomes; SD: Standard deviation; TBUT: Tear break-up time; VA: Visual acuity

Acknowledgements

Allergan plc, Irvine, CA, USA participated in the design of the study, data analysis, interpretation of the data, and preparation, review, and approval of the manuscript. We thank Kakuri Omari, PhD, of Evidence Scientific Solutions, Inc (Philadelphia, PA) who provided writing and editorial assistance. All authors met the ICMJE authorship criteria. Neither honoraria nor payments were made for authorship.
We thank the following participating investigators who provided and cared for the study patients: Jason Bacharach, Laurie Barber, Thomas Croley, Edward Holland, Omid Khodai, Thomas Kislan, Christopher Lievens, Jillian Ziemanski, Kelly Nichols, Stephen Montaquila, and Lee Shettle.

Funding

This study was sponsored by Allergan plc, Dublin, Ireland. Writing and editorial assistance in preparation of the manuscript was funded by Allergan plc, Irvine, CA, USA.

Authors' contributions

LB, MM, VP and CB participated in the design of the study. LB, OK, TC, CL, SM and JZ participated in data collection. All authors participated in data interpretation. OL performed the statistical analysis of the study data. All authors helped to draft the manuscript, and all authors read and approved the final manuscript.

Competing interests

LB and SM were consultants for the study. OK and TC declare that they have no conflicts of interest to disclose. JZ has served as a consultant to Allergan plc. CL has served as an advisor to Allergan plc. MM and OL are employees of Xcenda, which has received fees for data and statistical analysis from Allergan plc. CB is a consultant to Allergan plc. VP is an employee of Allergan plc.

Author details

[1]Little Rock Eye Clinic, 203 Executive Court, Suite A, Little Rock, AK 72205, USA. [2]Mobile Medical Solutions, Inc., Foothill Ranch, CA, USA. [3]Central Florida Eye Institute, Ocala, FL, USA. [4]Southern College of Optometry, Memphis, TN, USA. [5]West Bay Eye Associates, Warwick, RI, USA. [6]School of Optometry, University of Alabama at Birmingham, Birmingham, AL, USA. [7]Xcenda, Palm Harbor, FL, USA. [8]Health Outcomes Consultant, Laguna Beach, CA, USA. [9]Allergan plc, Irvine, CA, USA.

References

1. Craig JP, Nichols KK, Akpek EK, Caffrey B, Dua HS, Joo C-K, et al. TFOS DEWS II definition and classification report. Ocul Surf. 2017;15:276-3.
2. Moss SE, Klein R, Klein BE. Prevalence of and risk factors for dry eye syndrome. Arch Ophthalmol. 2000;118:1264–8.
3. Schaumberg DA, Sullivan DA, Buring JE, Dana MR. Prevalence of dry eye syndrome among US women. Am J Ophthalmol. 2003;136:318–26.
4. Stapleton F, Alves M, Bunya VY, Jalbert I, Lekhanont K, Malet F, et al. TFOS DEWS 2 Epidemiology Report. Ocular Surface. 2017;15:334-365.
5. Sweeney DF, Millar TJ, Raju SR. Tear film stability: a review. Exp Eye Res. 2013;117:28–38.
6. Schaumberg DA, Buring JE, Sullivan DA, Dana MR. Hormone replacement therapy and dry eye syndrome. JAMA. 2001;286:2114–9.
7. Begley CG, Caffery B, Nichols K, Mitchell GL, Chalmers R, DREI Study Group. Results of a dry eye questionnaire from optometric practices in North America. Adv Exp Med Biol. 2002;506:1009–16.
8. O'Brien PD, Collum LM. Dry eye: diagnosis and current treatment strategies. Curr Allergy Asthma Rep. 2004;4:314–9.
9. Goto E, Yagi Y, Matsumoto Y, Tsubota K. Impaired functional visual acuity of dry eye patients. Am J Ophthalmol. 2002;133:181–6.
10. Rolando M, Iester M, Macri A, Calabria G. Low spatial-contrast sensitivity in dry eyes. Cornea. 1998;17:376–9.
11. Montes-Mico R, Caliz A, Alio JL. Wavefront analysis of higher order aberrations in dry eye patients. J Refract Surg. 2004;20:243–7.
12. Tutt R, Bradley A, Begley C, Thibos LN. Optical and visual impact of tear break-up in human eyes. Invest Ophthalmol Vis Sci. 2000;41:4117–23.
13. Mertzanis P, Abetz L, Rajagopalan K, Espindle D, Chalmers R, Snyder C, et al. The relative burden of dry eye in patients' lives: comparisons to a U.S. normative sample. Invest Ophthalmol Vis Sci. 2005;46:46–50.
14. Miljanović B, Dana R, Sullivan DA, Schaumberg DA. Impact of dry eye syndrome on vision-related quality of life. Am J Ophthalmol. 2007;143:409–15.
15. Pritchard N, Fonn D, Brazeau D. Discontinuation of contact lens wear: a survey. Int Contact Lens Clin. 1999;26:157–62.
16. Young G, Veys J, Pritchard N, Coleman S. A multi-centre study of lapsed contact lens wearers. Ophthalmic Physiol Opt. 2002;22:516–27.
17. Richdale K, Sinnott LT, Skadahl E, Nichols JJ. Frequency of and factors associated with contact lens dissatisfaction and discontinuation. Cornea. 2007;26:168–74.
18. Dumbleton K, Woods CA, Jones LW, Fonn D. The impact of contemporary contact lenses on contact lens discontinuation. Eye Contact Lens. 2013;39:93–9.
19. Buchholz P, Steeds CS, Stern LS, Wiederkehr DP, Doyle JJ, Katz LM, et al. Utility assessment to measure the impact of dry eye disease. Ocul Surf. 2006;4:155–61.
20. Vitale S, Goodman LA, Reed GF, Smith JA. Comparison of the NEI-VFQ and OSDI questionnaires in patients with Sjögren's syndrome-related dry eye. Health Qual Life Outcomes. 2004;2:44.
21. Schein OD, Tielsch JM, Munõz B, Bandeen-Roche K, West S. Relation between signs and symptoms of dry eye in the elderly. A population-based perspective. Ophthalmology. 1997;104:1395–401.
22. Hay EM, Thomas E, Pal B, Hajeer A, Chambers H, Silman AJ. Weak association between subjective symptoms or and objective testing for dry eyes and dry mouth: results from a population based study. Ann Rheum Dis. 1998;57:20–4.
23. Nichols KK, Nichols JJ, Mitchell GL. The lack of association between signs and symptoms in patients with dry eye disease. Cornea. 2004;23:762–70.
24. Vehof J, Sillevis Smitt-Kamminga N, Nibourg SA, Hammond CJ. Predictors of discordance between symptoms and signs in dry eye disease. Ophthalmology. 2017;124:280–6.
25. Nichols KK, Mitchell GL, Zadnik K. The repeatability of clinical measurements of dry eye. Cornea. 2004;23:272–85.
26. Friedman NJ. Impact of dry eye disease and treatment on quality of life. Curr Opin Ophthalmol. 2010;21:310–6.
27. Abetz L, Rajagopalan K, Mertzanis P, Begley C, Barnes R, Chalmers R. Impact of dry eye on everyday life (IDEEL) study group. Development and validation of the impact of dry eye on everyday life (IDEEL) questionnaire, a patient-reported outcomes (PRO) measure for the assessment of the burden of dry eye on patients. Health Qual Life Outcomes. 2011;9:111.
28. Schiffman RM, Christianson MD, Jacobsen G, Hirsch JD, Reis BL. Reliability and validity of the Ocular Surface Disease Index. Arch Ophthalmol. 2000;118:615–21.
29. Behrens A, Doyle JJ, Stern L, Chuck RS, McDonnell PJ, Azar DT and Dysfunctional Tear Syndrome Study Group. Dysfunctional tear syndrome: a Delphi approach to treatment recommendations. Cornea. 2006;25:900–7.
30. Wilson SE, Stulting RD. Agreement of physician treatment practices with the international task force guidelines for diagnosis and treatment of dry eye disease. Cornea. 2007;26:284–9.
31. Miller KL, Walt JG, Mink DR, Satram-Hoang S, Wilson SE, Perry HD, et al. Minimal clinically important difference for the ocular surface disease index. Arch Ophthalmol. 2010;128:94–101.
32. Bron AJ, Tomlinson A, Foulks GN, Pepose JS, Baudouin C, Geerling G, et al. Rethinking dry eye disease: a perspective on clinical implications. Ocul Surf. 2014;12:S1–31.
33. Galor A, Levitt RC, Felix ER, Martin ER, Sarantopoulos CD. Neuropathic ocular pain: an important yet underevaluated feature of dry eye. Eye (Lond). 2015;29:301–12.
34. Shtein RM, Harper DE, Pallazola V, Harte SE, Hussain M, Sugar A, et al. Discordant dry eye disease (an American Ophthalmological Society thesis). Trans Am Ophthalmol Soc. 2016;114:T4.
35. Pflugfelder SC, Geerling G, Kinoshita S, Lemp MA, McCulley J, Nelson D, et al. Management and therapy of dry eye disease: report of the Management and Therapy Subcommittee of the International Dry Eye WorkShop (2007). Ocul Surf. 2007;5:163–78.
36. McMonnies CW, Ho A. Patient history in screening for dry eye conditions. J Am Optom Assoc. 1987;58:296–301.
37. Mangione CM, Lee PP, Gutierrez PR, Spritzer K, Berry S, Hays RD. Development of the 25-item National Eye Institute Visual Function Questionnaire. Arch Ophthalmol. 2001;119:1050–8.
38. Sullivan BD, Whitmer D, Nichols KK, Tomlinson A, Foulks GN, Geerling G, et al. An objective approach to dry eye disease severity. Invest Ophthalmol Vis Sci. 2010;51:6125–30.
39. Geerling G, Tauber J, Baudouin C, Goto E, Matsumoto Y, O'Brien T, et al. The international workshop on meibomian gland dysfunction: report of the subcommittee on management and treatment of Meibomian gland dysfunction. Invest Ophthalmol Vis Sci. 2011;52:2050–64.
40. Stonecipher KG, Chia J, Onyenwenyi A, Villanueva L, Hollander DA. Health claims database study of cyclosporine ophthalmic emulsion treatment patterns in dry eye patients. Ther Clin Risk Manag. 2013;9:409–15.
41. Foulks GN, Nichols KK, Bron AJ, Holland EJ, McDonald MB, Nelson JD. Improving awareness, identification, and management of meibomian gland dysfunction. Ophthalmology. 2012;119(10 Suppl):S1–12.
42. Colligris B, Crooke A, Huete-Toral F, Pintor J. An update on dry eye disease molecular treatment: advances in drug pipelines. Expert Opin Pharmacother. 2014;15:1371–90.
43. Sullivan DA, Hammitt KM, Schaumberg DA, Sullivan BD, Begley CG, Gjorstrup P, et al. Report of the TFOS/ARVO Symposium on global treatments for dry eye disease: an unmet need. Ocul Surf. 2012;10:108–16.

32

Microglia enhanced the angiogenesis, migration and proliferation of co-cultured RMECs

Xinyi Ding[1,2,3,4], Ruiping Gu[1,2,3,4], Meng Zhang[1,2,3,4], Hui Ren[1,2,3,4], Qinmeng Shu[1,2,3,4], Gezhi Xu[1,2,3,4] and Haixiang Wu[1,2,3,4]*

Abstract

Background: Attention is increasingly being given to microglia-related inflammation in neovascular diseases, such as diabetic retinopathy and age-related macular disease. Evidence shows that activated microglia contribute to disruption of the blood–retinal barrier, however, the mechanism is unclear. In this study, we aimed to clarify whether and how microglia affect the function of retinal microvascular endothelial cells (RMECs).

Methods: We activated microglia by Lipopolysaccharides (LPS) stimulation. After co-culturing static or activated microglia with RMECs using the Transwell system, we evaluated the function of RMECs. Vascular endothelial growth factor-A (VEGF-A) and platelet-derived growth factor-BB (PDGF-BB) levels in the supernatant from the lower chamber were evaluated by ELISA. Angiogenesis, migration, and proliferation of RMECs were assessed by tube formation, wound healing, and WST-1 assays. The expression levels of tight junction proteins (ZO-1 and occludin) and endothelial markers (CD31 and CD34) were examined by Western blot analysis.

Results: We successfully established an LPS-activated microglia model and co-culture system of static or activated microglia with RMECs. In the co-culture system, we showed that microglia, especially activated microglia stimulated VEGF-A and PDGF-BB expression, enhanced angiogenesis, migration, proliferation, and permeability, and altered the phenotype of co-cultured RMECs.

Conclusions: Microglia, especially activated microglia, play important roles in angiogenesis and maintenance of vascular function hemostasis in the retinal microvasculature. The mechanism needs further investigation and clarification.

Keywords: Microglia, Retinal microvascular endothelial cells, Angiogenesis, Inflammation, Retinopathy

Background

Microglia are important immune cell residents of the central nervous system, as well as the retina [1]. Microglial activation is involved in many important retinopathies, including light-induced photoreceptor degeneration, uveitis, age-related macular degeneration (AMD), and diabetic retinopathy [2–5].

Vascular endothelial cells are key components involved in the blood–retina barrier function and angiogenesis. Increased levels of blood glucose, advanced glycosylation end products (AGEs), and oxidative stress in diabetes drastically alter endothelial cell metabolism and induce endothelial cell dysfunction [6].

Increasing attention has recently been given to microglia-related inflammation in neovascular diseases, both in the central nervous system (CNS) and the retina. For example, it has been reported that diabetic retinopathy is closely related to retinal microvascular system damage, such as breakdown of the blood–retina barrier and angiogenesis and activation of hyperglycemia and/or hypoxia [7]. Recent studies have shown that retinal inflammation also contributes to the pathogenesis of

* Correspondence: whx577@163.com; drwhx577@163.com
Xinyi Ding and Ruiping Gu are co-first authors.
Xinyi Ding and Ruiping Gu contributed equally to this work.
[1]Department of Ophthalmology, Eye and ENT Hospital of Fudan University, 83 Fen Yang Road, Shanghai 200031, People's Republic of China
[2]Institute of Eye Research, Eye and ENT Hospital of Fudan University, Shanghai, China
Full list of author information is available at the end of the article

diabetic retinopathy, and that activated microglia are present during the early stages of diabetic retinopathy and cluster in the retinal microvasculature [8–13]. However, the mechanism by which microglia affect retinal microvascular pericytes and endothelial cells needs further clarification. In our previous study, we showed that activated microglia induce production of reactive oxygen species (ROS) and promote apoptosis in co-cultured retinal microvascular pericytes [14]. Thus, in this study, we aimed to clarify whether microglia affect the functions of RMECs such as angiogenesis, migration, and proliferation.

Methods

RMECs culture

Rat primary RMECs were purchased from the Cell Biologics Company (catalogue no. RA-6065; Chicago, IL, USA). The cell line was recovered and cultured in accordance with the supplier's instructions. Cells from passages 4–10 were used in this study.

Primary retinal microglia culture

Microglia were isolated from the retinas of newborn Sprague–Dawley rats. Newborn Sprague–Dawley rats (1–3 days old) were obtained from the Shanghai SLAC Laboratory Animal Company, and were sacrificed by decapitation. Treatment of animals was complied with the rules of the "Instruction and Administration of Experimental Animals", and was approved by the Eye and ENT Hospital of Fudan University. The dissected retinas were collected and digested with 0.25 mg/mL trypsin at 37 °C. After 5 min, the trypsin was deactivated with DMEM/F12 (Gibco, Carlsbad, CA, USA) containing 20% FBS (Gibco) and 1% penicillin/streptomycin (Sigma-Aldrich, Billerica, MA, USA). The digested tissues were mechanically dissociated into a single cell suspension and collected by centrifugation. The cells were then resuspended in a DMEM: F12 (1:1) solution containing 20% FBS and plated in T75 cell culture dishes at 10^6 cells/dish. After 12 days, the supernatant containing microglia was collected and centrifuged, and the cells were resuspended at the appropriate density, depending on the experiment. The microglia were identified by immunocytochemical staining using microglia-specific antibodies, OX42 (targeting CD11b/c) and ED1 (targeting CD68). The morphology of the isolated microglia was examined by phase-contrast microscopy (Nikon) and fluorescence microscopy (Leica Microsystems).

Flow cytometry

Isolated microglia were collected in DMEM/F12 containing 20% FBS and centrifuged for 10 min. After washing in PBS, the cell precipitate was resuspended in blocking solution (PBS containing 5% FBS and 1% BSA) and labelled with Alexa-Fluor-647-conjugated mouse anti-OX42 (1:100, Abcam, Cambridge, MA) for 15 min at 4 °C. The

OX42-positive cells were counted by flow cytometry (Coulter Epics XL, Beckman-Coulter, Fullerton, CA).

Immunofluorescence assay

For immunofluorescence assays, cell cultures were fixed with 4% paraformaldehyde in 0.01 M PBS for 10 min and then washed with PBS. After washing, the cultures were incubated in blocking buffer (5% normal goat serum) for 30 min at 37 °C. The cells were then incubated overnight at 4 °C with primary antibodies specific for markers of microglia (mouse OX42, 1:100, and mouse ED1, 1:100; Abcam, Cambridge, MA, USA) or RMECs (mouse anti-von Willebrand factor (vWF, 1:100; Abcam). After washing with PBS, the cells were incubated with the appropriate secondary antibodies for 30 min at 37 °C and counterstained with DAPI (1:1000; Molecular Probes/Thermo Fisher Scientific, Waltham, MA, USA). The labelled cells were examined by fluorescence microscopy (Leica Microsystems).

Activation of microglia by LPS

The harvested microglia were seeded at 10^6 cells/well in a six-well culture plate pre-coated with 20 μg/mL poly-d-lysine (Sigma-Aldrich). Twenty-four hours after seeding, each well was washed three times with 0.1 M PBS and incubated with culture medium containing 0, 0.1, 1, 10, 100, or 1000 ng/mL lipopolysaccharide (LPS) (*Escherichia coli* OB4:1111; Sigma-Aldrich) for 24 h.

Assessment of microglial viability

The effects of LPS on the viability of microglia were measured using the cell proliferation reagent water soluble tetrazolium-1 (WST-1; Roche, Basel, Switzerland). The WST-1 assay is based on the cellular reduction of WST-1 by viable cells. Microglia were seeded in a 96-well microplate at 4×10^3 cells/well in 100 μL culture medium containing 0, 0.1, 1, 10, 100, or 1000 ng/mL LPS. The cells were incubated for 48 h at 37 °C in 5% CO_2, and 10 μL WST-1 reagent was added to each well and incubated for 4 h at 37 °C in 5% CO_2. The plate was thoroughly shaken for 1 min on a shaker. To detect the production of formazan, the absorbance of each well at 420–480 nm was measured relative to the blank wells on a microplate reader.

Measurement of microglial cytokine concentrations

After exposure to LPS, the culture media was collected and centrifuged. Aliquots of the supernatant (50 μL) were collected to measure the concentrations of TNFα and IL-1β using enzyme-linked immunosorbent assay (ELISA) kits (R&D Systems, Minneapolis, MN, USA).

Transwell co-culture of microglia and RMECs

Freshly collected microglia were seeded onto 12-well Transwell collagen-coated membrane inserts (Corning Co.,

Corning, NY, USA). Separately, RMECs were grown to confluence in a collagen-coated 12-well plate. The microglia and RMECs were incubated in basal media for 24 h before co-culturing, and the Transwell inserts containing the retinal microglia (treated with or without LPS for 24 h) were placed into the wells containing RMECs. The 0.4 μm pore size of the Transwell prevents direct cell–cell interactions but allows the diffusion of soluble factors across the membrane (Fig. 1). After 24 h, the co-cultured cells were separated and cultured in fresh culture mediums for another 24 h, and then, the supernatant and cells were collected for further research. The experiment was divided into three groups: Con (RMECs without microglia), MG: (RMECs with static microglia), LPS-MG (RMECs with activated microglia).

Levels of angiogenesis-related growth factors in RMECs measured by ELISA

The supernatant of RMECs was collected and subjected to ELISA. The levels of vascular endothelial growth factor-A (VEGF-A) and platelet-derived growth factor-BB (PDGF-BB) were evaluated by sandwich ELISA (human VEGF-A and PDGF-BB ELISA kits, Abcam) according to the manufacturer's instructions. Colorimetric analysis was performed and the absorbance was measured using an ELISA plate reader.

Tube formation assays

Tube formation assays were conducted on Matrigel (BD Biosciences, Franklin Lakes, NJ, USA). A 96-well plate was coated with 50 μL/well Matrigel at 37 °C for 30 min. After co-culturing with microglia for 24 h, RMECs were seeded on the Matrigel at 1.5×10^4 cells/well in 100 μL medium. After 4 h, tube formation was observed and photographed with a microscope (Leica Microsystems). Images were analyzed using ImageJ (NIH public domain), and four parameters were measured for quantification of tube formation: total tube length, number of nodes, number of branches, and total branch length.

Wound healing assays

RMECs were plated at a density of 10^4 in 24-well plates and grown to 100% confluence. To investigate the migration capability of RMECs, a wound was created by scratching the confluent monolayer down the middle of each well using a 10 μL pipette tip. Scratched RMECs were washed with PBS, and then 500 μL of fresh DMEM without serum was added to each well. Cells were imaged immediately after stimulation (0 h) and then at 6, 12, and 18 h after wounding. ImageJ software was utilized to determine the percentage of wound closure.

Assessment of RMEC proliferation

RMECs were collected and seeded in 96-well plates at 1×10^4 cells/well and treated with WST-1 for 4 h. The absorbance of the wells was read at 450 nm using the Benchmark Plus microplate reader to evaluate RMEC proliferation.

Phenotype and tight junction of RMECs

ZO-1 and occludin are markers of tight junctions in RMECs.CD31 and CD34 are markers of endothelial cells. RMECs were harvested, and the protein expression levels of zonula occludens-1(ZO-1), occludin, CD31 and CD34, were determined by Western blotting. After the proteins were transferred onto a PVDF membrane, the blots were incubated with primary antibodies (mouse anti-ZO-1, 1:100; mouse anti-occludin, 1:100; mouse anti-CD31, 1:100; mouse anti-CD34, 1:100; all from Abcam) and probed with a horseradish-peroxidase-conjugated secondary antibody. Protein expression was detected using an enhanced chemiluminescence kit. The density of each band was quantified using ImageQuant software (ImageQuant TL v. 7.0, GE Healthcare, Piscataway, NJ, USA). All samples were assayed in triplicate.

Statistical analysis

All statistical analyses were performed using GraphPad Prism 5.0. Measurement data were presented as x ± s. Differences between groups were evaluated using

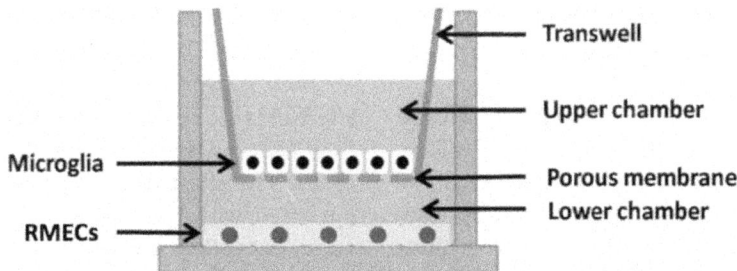

Fig. 1 Schematic diagram of the Transwell coculture system. The Transwell system consists of two chambers separated by a porous membrane. The RMECs were placed on the bottom of the lower chamber and the microglia were placed on the membrane of the upper chamber. (Page7, Paragraph 1)

unpaired one-way ANOVA and LSD post-hoc tests. Each experiment was repeated three times. $P < 0.05$ was considered statistically significant.

Results

Characterization of rat retinal microglia and RMECs

Microglia were harvested from 14-day-old primary mixed glial cultures using the "shaking-off" method. Twenty-four hours after purification and reseeding, the microglia had recovered from the isolation process and resumed their normal morphology of a short, single process and small cell soma (Fig. 2A). The purity of isolated microglia detected by low cytometry through its specific surface marker CD11b, was 93.6% (Fig. 2B). The cultured RMECs had round nuclei and a fusiform shape (Fig. 2C), and vWF was abundantly expressed throughout the RMECs (Fig. 2 D1). Immunofluorescence studies showed cell staining of CD11b/c (by OX42) (Fig. $2E_1$), and CD68 (by ED1) (Fig. $2E_2$).

Effects of LPS on microglial morphology

To complete our following experiment, we needed to establish a model of activated microglia using LPS. To confirm LPS activation of microglia, the morphology of the microglia was evaluated. The purified microglia presented a static morphology with a branching shape, and immunofluorescence staining confirmed expression of CD11b/c and CD68 in the resting microglia (Fig. $2E_1$–E_4). After treatment with 100 ng/mL LPS for 24 h, the microglia became rounder and larger, developing a characteristic amoeboid shape consistent with their activation (Fig. $2F_1$–F_4), as we reported previously [14].

Effects of LPS on microglial viability

To confirm that LPS had no cytotoxic effect on the activated microglia, cell viability was evaluated using WST-1 reagent. At concentrations of 0.1–100 ng/mL, LPS did not significantly reduce cell viability. However, at 1000 ng/mL, LPS significantly reduced the viability of the microglia, indicating that 1000 ng/mL LPS has a cytotoxic effect on the microglia (Fig. 3a), as we reported previously [14]. Thus, we chose 100 ng/mL LPS to activate microglia, avoiding its cytotoxic effect on cells.

Effects of LPS on TNFα and IL-1β secretion from microglia

To confirm LPS activation of microglia, the pro-inflammatory factors of the microglia were evaluated. As shown in Fig. 3, TNFα and IL-1β were significantly overexpressed after adding 100 ng/mL LPS to the microglial culture medium. The TNFα and IL-1β levels were 3.22 ± 0.14 and 2.35 ± 0.08 times higher, respectively, than the levels in unstimulated microglia after 24 h LPS activation (Fig. 3b). Activation of microglia by LPS was shown by microglia morphology change and increased TNFα and IL-1β secretion.

Effects of static or activated microglia on the expression of angiogenesis-related factors in RMECs

After successfully establishing activated model of microglia, we co-cultured pretreated microglia with RMECs in the Transwell system to see the effects of microglia on RMECs. Freshly collected microglia were seeded onto 12-well Transwell collagen-coated membrane inserts (Corning Co., Corning, NY, USA) (treated with or without LPS for 24 h). Separately, RMECs were grown to confluence in a collagen-coated 12-well plate for 24 h. After co-culture for 24 h, as shown in Fig. 1, the cells were separated and cultured in fresh culture mediums for another 24 h, then then, the supernatant and cells were collected for further research. The experiment is divided into three groups: Con (RMECs without microglia), MG: (RMECs with static microglia), LPS-MG (RMECs with activated microglia).

The effects of microglia on the expression of angiogenesis-related factors in RMECs were evaluated by ELISA using the supernatant collected from the lower chamber. In the co-culture system, microglia significantly increased the release of VEGF-A and PDGF-BB from RMECs, compared to the RMECs without microglia. Furthermore, LPS-activated microglia enhanced the effects of static microglia on RMECs (Fig. 4). We conclude that microglia, especially activated microglia induced VEGF-A and PDGF-BB secretion of RMECs.

Effect of static or activated microglia on RMECs tube formation

Preprocessing and grouping of cells were as mentioned above. The effect of microglia on the angiogenesis ability of RMECs was measured with the tube formation assay, an important in vitro model for angiogenesis. As shown in Fig. 5, both static and activated microglia stimulated tube formation in the RMECs. In addition, the effects on RMECs tube formation were enhanced by the activated microglia compared with the static microglia (Fig. 5). The tube formation assay suggested that microglia, especially activated microglia induced the angiogenic abilities of RMECs.

Effect of static or activated microglia on RMECs migration

Preprocessing and grouping of cells were as mentioned above. The effect of microglia on RMEC migration was measured with the wound healing assay. As shown in Fig. 6, both static and activated microglia induced RMEC migration. Static microglia significantly stimulated wound recovery at 18 h, while activated microglia significantly stimulated wound recovery at 6, 12, and 18 h (Fig. 6). The wound healing assay revealed that microglia,

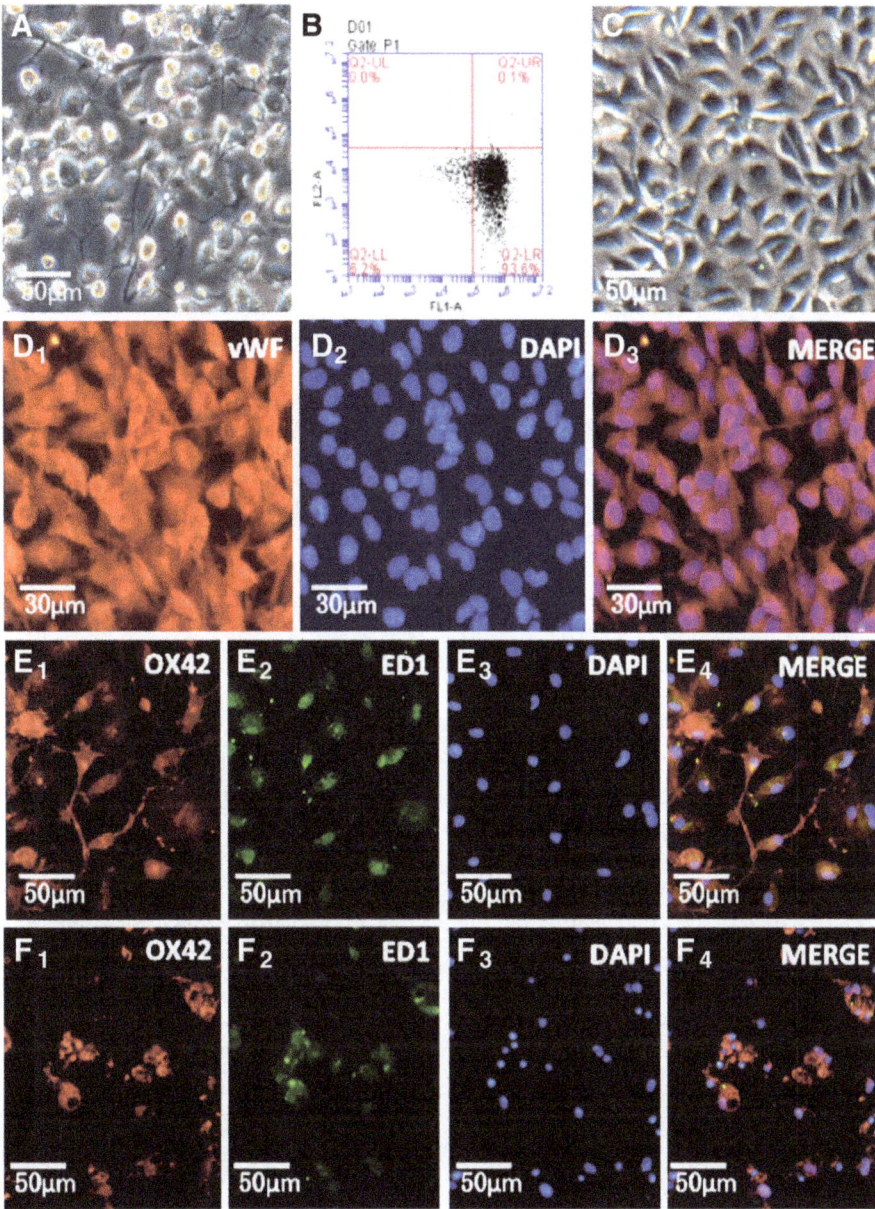

Fig. 2 Characterization of rat retinal microglia and RMECS. A: Cultures of primary isolated microglia. B: The purity of isolated microglia detected by low cytometry through its specific surface marker CD11b is 93.6%. C: Culture of RMECs. D1-D3: Immunofluorescent detection of RMECs marked by vWF, DAPI and both. E1-E4: Normal microglia are static. F1 – F4: Exposure to 100 ng/mL LPS for 24 h altered the morphology of the microglia from a ramified state with long processes to the activated state with an amoeboid appearance. E1-E4, F1-F4 has been published in our previous research. Abbreviations: vWF, von-Willebrand factor; LPS, lipopolysaccharide. (Page9–10)

especially activated microglia increased the migration of RMECs.

Effect of static or activated microglia on RMEC proliferation

Preprocessing and grouping of cells were as mentioned above. The effect of microglia on RMECs proliferation was measured with WST-1 reagent. We found that both static and activated microglia induced RMEC proliferation,

and LPS further enhanced the stimulatory effect of microglia on RMECs (Fig. 7a). The WST-1 assay showed that microglia, especially activated microglia promoted migration of RMECs.

Effects of static or activated microglia on tight junctions and the phenotype of RMECs

Preprocessing and grouping of cells were as mentioned above. For evaluation of the tight junction and phenotype

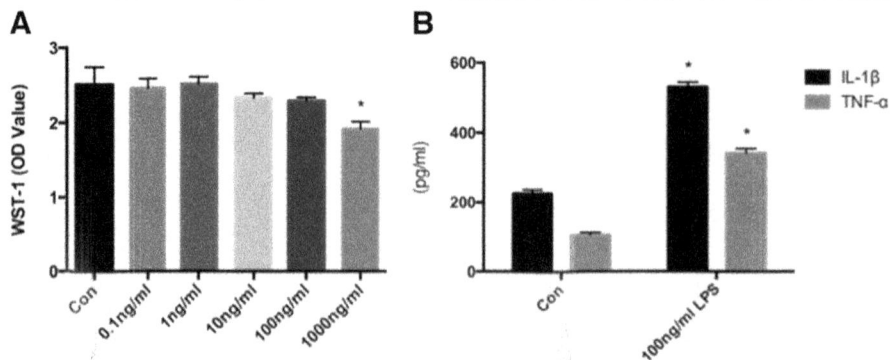

Fig. 3 a Concentration-dependent effects of LPS on the viability of microglia. Microglia were exposed to LPS (0, 0.1, 1, 10, 100, or 1000 ng/mL) for 24 h. Microglial viability was measured with WST-1 reagent. LPS at 1000 ng/mL significantly reduced the viability of microglia. This part has been published in our previous research. **b** Effects of LPS on TNF and IL-1beta secretion. Microglia were exposed to LPS (0 and 100 ng/mL) for 24 h. The TNFα and IL-1beta concentration in the supernatant was measured using an ELISA kit. LPS at concentrations of 100 ng/mL significantly increased the production of TNF and IL-1beta. Results are means ± SD (n = 3 per group). *P < 0.05 vs Con using one-way ANOVA. Abbreviations: Con, microglia without LPS; WST-1, water soluble tetrazolium-1; LPS, lipopolysaccharide; TNFα, tumor necrosis factor; IL-1β, interleukin 1β. (Page 10, paragraph3–4)

of RMECs, protein levels of occludin, ZO-1, CD-31, and CD-34 were measured with Western blotting. Both static and activated microglia significantly reduced the expression of tight junction occludin and ZO-1, markers of cell permeability, in RMECs compared with control cells. Regarding phenotype, both static and activated microglia significantly reduced CD31 and increased CD34 expression, which are endothelial markers, in RMECs (Fig. 7b). We concluded from these data that microglia, especially activated microglia, destroyed the tight junction of RMECs, which may contribute to the increased permeability of vasculature. In addition, microglia, especially activated microglia changed phenotype of RMECs, and the specific effect of these changes needs further investigation.

Discussion

The retinal microvasculature is composed of endothelial cells and pericytes. Diabetic retinopathy is first considered to be a simple microangiopathy. In the early stages of diabetic retinopathy, endothelial cell proliferation and pericytes apoptosis leads to damage of the blood-retinal barrier (BRB) [15].

Recently, new insights into retinal physiology have led to the emergence of the concept of the retinal neurovascular unit, [16–18] which is composed of retinal neurons (photoreceptors, horizontal, etc), their supporting cells (astrocytes and Müller glial cells), and the vascular beds (endothelial cells and pericytes). In diabetic retinopathy, metabolic alterations may first lead to glial dysfunction,

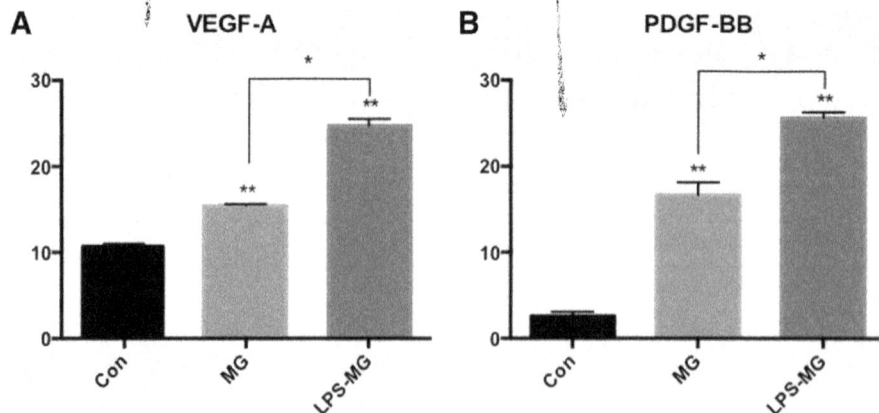

Fig. 4 Effects of static or activated microglia on angiogenesis relative factors expression of RMECs. **a** VEGF-A. **b** PDGF-BB. Compared with control RMECs, microglia significantly increased expression and release of VEGF-A and PDGF-BB in RMECs. LPS activated microglia enhanced the effects of static microglia to RMECs. Each bar graph indicates means ± SD of three independent experiments. *Significant difference in results between the two compared groups. *P < 0.05 using one-way ANOVA. **P < 0.01 using one-way ANOVA. Abbreviations: Con, control RMECs (i.e., cultured without microglia); MG, REMCs co-cultured with static microglia; LPS-MG, REMCs co-cultured with activated microglia; LPS, lipopolysaccharide; VEGF-A, Vascular endothelial growth factor-A; PDGF-BB, Platelet-derived growth factor-BB. (Page 11, paragraph 2)

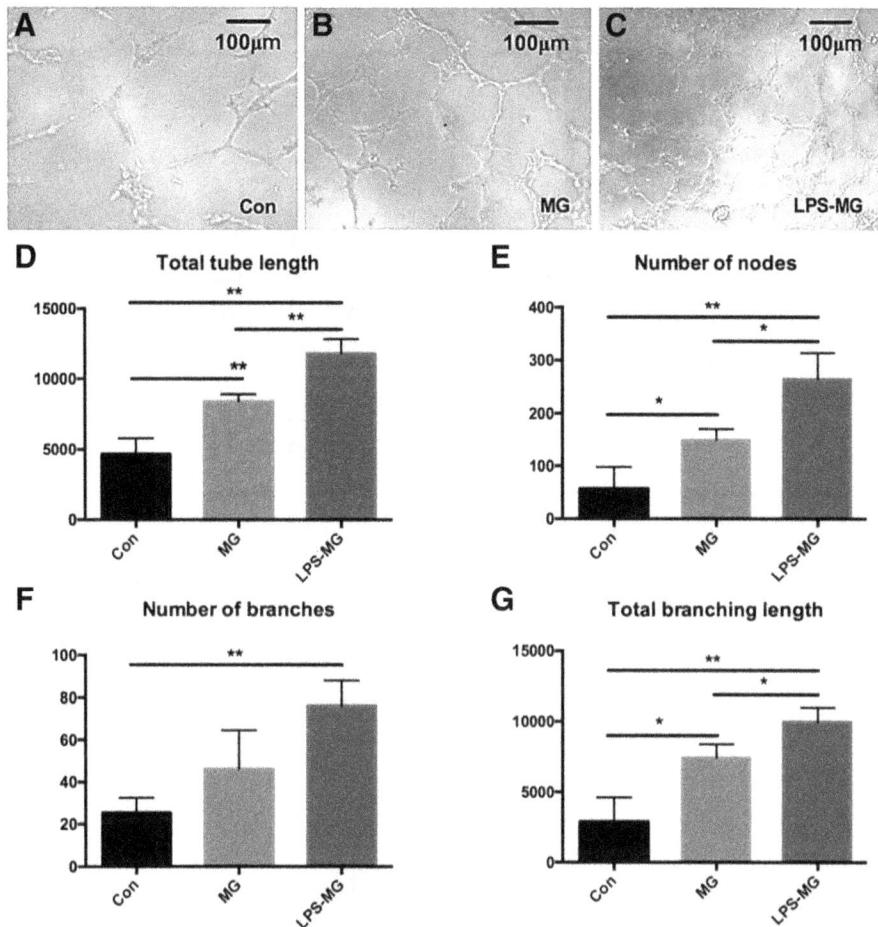

Fig. 5 Effects of static or activated microglia on tube formation of RMECs. **a-c** One representative experiment of tube formation of three different groups at 4 h. **d-g** Total tube length, number of nodes, number of branches, total branching length quantified by ImageJ. Both static and LPS-activated microglia stimulated tube formation in the RMECs. In addition, the effects on RMEC tube formation were enhanced by the activated microglia compared with the static microglia. Each bar graph indicates means ± SD of three independent experiments. Significant difference in results between the two compared groups. *$P < 0.05$ using one-way ANOVA. **$P < 0.01$ using one-way ANOVA. Abbreviations: Con, control RMECs (i.e., cultured without microglia); MG, REMCs co-cultured with static microglia; LPS-MG, REMCs co-cultured with activated microglia; LPS, lipopolysaccharide. (Page 11, paragraph 3)

then induces inflammation, and neuronal apoptosis. Neurodegeneration also contributes to the breakdown of the blood–retinal barrier (BRB) [16, 17].

In addition, the role of microglia in diabetic retinopathy is currently of particular interest. However, the mechanisms by which the microglia affect the retinal microvascular pericytes and endothelial cells in diabetic retinopathy needs further clarification.

Combining our previous study with the present study, we showed that activated microglia increased oxidative stress damage and promoted apoptosis in pericytes; [14] and induced VEGF production, angiogenesis, migration, and proliferation. Activated microglia also destroyed the tight junction of endothelial cells affecting the integrity of the microvasculature, leading to BRB breakdown and contributing to neovascularization.

As the most important immune monitoring cell in the retina, microglia may manifest as static or activated states. It has been documented that microglia cells are abnormally activated in a variety of retinal diseases,, including diabetic retinopathy [8, 19]. LPS stimulation is the most commonly used and effective method to activate microglia in vitro [20–22]. LPS could induce NF-κB activation and inflammatory cytokines release [23]. We initially used 100 ng/ml of LPS to successfully establish an activated model of microglia, which was proved by an increased expression of the pro-inflammatory cytokines TNFα and IL-1β and the typical morphological changes in the cells. In our study, we co-cultured static or activated microglia with RMECs using the Transwell co-culture system. After 24 h of co-culturing, we collected the RMECs to evaluate their functions. VEGF is a

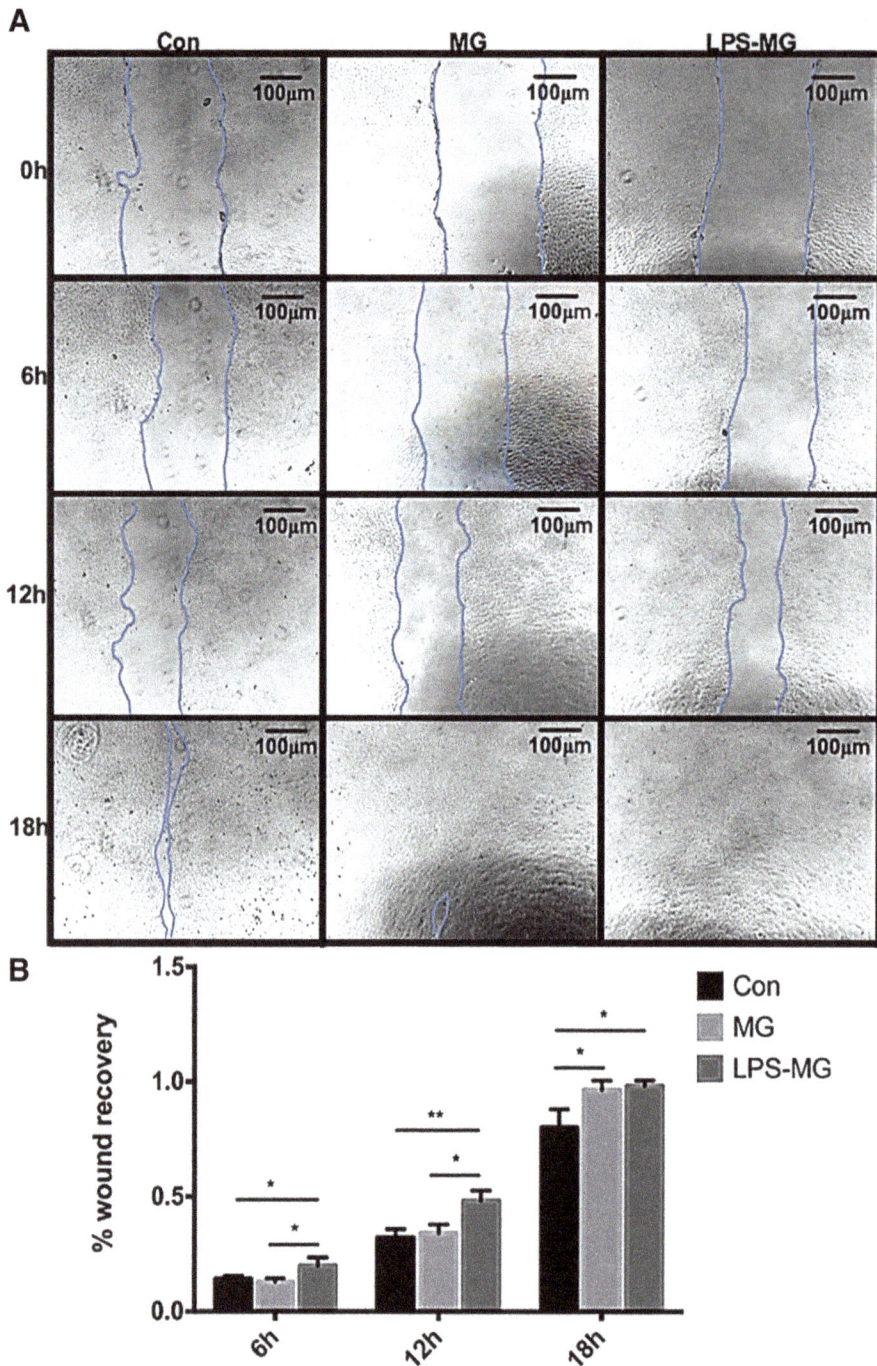

Fig. 6 Effects of static or activated microglia on migration of RMECs. **a** One representative experiment of three different groups at 0 h, 6 h, 12 h, 18 h. **b** Wound recovery percentage analyzed by ImageJ. We see static microglia significantly stimulated wound recovery at 18 h, at the same time, activated microglia significantly stimulated wound recovery at 6 h, 12 h and 18 h. Each bar graph indicates means ± SD of three independent experiments. *Significant difference in results between the two compared groups. *P < 0.05 using one-way ANOVA. **P < 0.01 using one-way ANOVA. Abbreviations: Con, control RMECs (i.e., cultured without microglia); MG, REMCs co-cultured with static microglia; LPS-MG, REMCs co-cultured with activated microglia; LPS, lipopolysaccharide. (Page 11, paragraph 4)

key regulator among growth factors involved in angiogenesis [24]. VEGF-A is the most prevalent member of the VEGF family [25]. In addition to VEGF, PDGF is another well-studied angiogenic growth factor [26, 27]. PDGF-BB is the predominant isoform of the PDGF family expressed in the eye [28]. VEGF and PDGF have a synergic effect on vascular homeostasis [29, 30]. In the second part of our study, we found that microglia stimulate VEGF-A and PDGF-BB

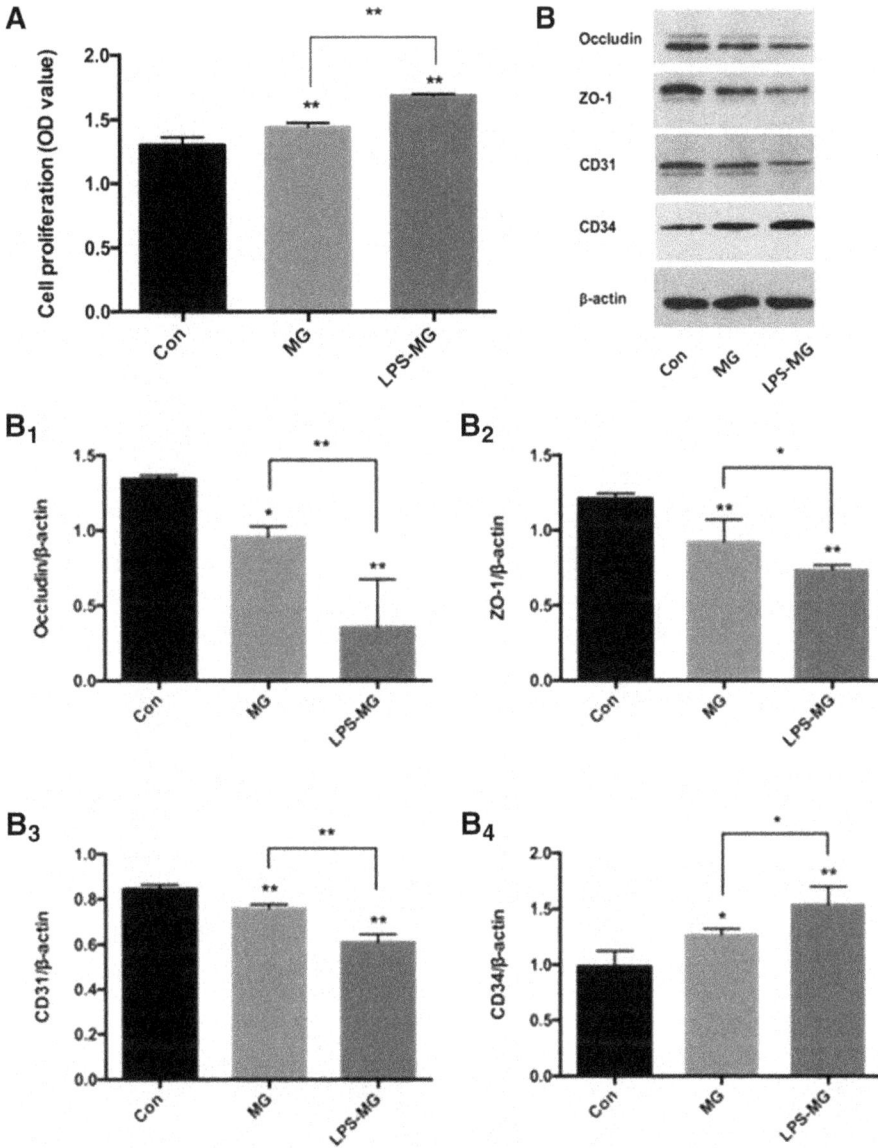

Fig. 7 A. Effects of static or activated microglia on proliferation of RMECs. RMECs were cocultured with microglia (with or without LPS) for 24 h, WST-1 reagent was used to evaluate RMECs proliferation ability. We found that both static and activated microglia induced RMECs proliferation, and LPS further enhanced the stimulatory effect of microglia on RMECs. B. Effects of static or activated microglia on permeability and phenotype of RMECs. For evaluation of permeability and phenotype of RMECs, after cocultured with microglia (with or without LPS) for 24 h, we collected RMECs and tested protein expression of occludin, ZO-1, CD-31, and CD-34. Both static and activated microglia significantly reduced the expression of occludin and ZO-1, markers of cell permeability, in RMECs compared with RMECs without microglia. Regarding phenotype, both static and activated microglia reduced CD31 and increased CD34 expression, which are endothelial markers, in RMECs (B). *$P < 0.05$ using one-way ANOVA. **$P < 0.01$ using one-way ANOVA. Abbreviations: Con, control RMECs (i.e., cultured without microglia); MG, REMCs co-cultured with static microglia; LPS-MG, REMCs co-cultured with activated microglia; LPS, lipopolysaccharide; ZO-1, zonula occludens-1. (Page 12, paragraph 2–3)

expression in, and secretion from, RMECs, with an even stronger effect induced by activated microglia. As shown in the first part of the study, static microglia secreted basal levels of TNFα and IL-1β, which were markedly increased after activation by LPS. Thus, we hypothesize that TNFα and IL-1β function to stimulate VEGF-A and PDGF-BB, as suggested by previous studies [31, 32]. TNFα is able to increase the expression of VEGF, [33] stimulate NF-κB, JNK

and p38 signaling pathways, [34, 35] all of which contribute to angiogenic activity [36]. IL-1β induced VEGF production through an src-dependent pathway and MAPK/ERK signal pathways, and both of VEGF and IL-1beta up-regulated vascular angiogenesis and permeability [37–39].

Angiogenesis, migration, and proliferation are the most representative indices of endothelial cell function. The angiogenic growth factors VEGF and PDGF can enhance endothelial angiogenesis, migration, and the proliferation [30, 39–41]. We showed that microglia promoted tube formation, wound healing, and proliferation of co-cultured RMECs, and activated microglia significantly enhanced these effects, in accordance with increased VEGF and PDGF levels.

Hyperpermeability is an important change associated with vascular dysfunction in neovascular diseases [42]. The paracellular permeability of the endothelium depends on the integrity of protein complexes involved in the inter-endothelial junctions [43]. ZO-1 and occludin are indispensable components of tight junctions regulated by pro-inflammatory cytokines and growth factors [44–49]. We showed that microglia downregulated ZO-1 and occludin expression, in agreement with previous studies [50–52]. The inhibitory effects of activated microglia on tight junction proteins were stronger than those of static microglia.

CD31 and CD34 are specific markers of endothelial cells. CD31 (also known as platelet/endothelial cell adhesion molecule-1) is a transmembrane protein that is strongly expressed at cell borders and plays a role in supporting the integrity of endothelial cell–cell junctions [53–55]. CD34, a marker of angiogenesis, is a single-chain transmembrane glycoprotein expressed on the surfaces of hematopoietic precursor cells and capillary endothelial cells [56–58]. In this study, we found that microglia downregulated the expression of CD31 but upregulated the expression of CD34 in co-cultured endothelial cells, and activation of the microglia enhanced these effects. This result is additional evidence illustrating the effects of microglia on tight junction proteins and angiogenesis of endothelial cells.

Vascular endothelial cells and microglia interact in direct or indirect ways. In this study, we used the Transwell system to study their indirect contact mainly through evaluating the release of soluble cytokines. Similar approaches have been evaluated in the CNS system. Endothelial angiogenesis and blood-brain barrier (BBB) dysfunction were caused by the soluble tumor necrosis factor α (TNF-α) released from microglial cells [59, 60]. Circulating micro-vesicles containing miR-27a obtained from LPS-stimulated microglia supernatant damaged the tight junction of RMECs under the OGD condition [61]. In addition, the literature shows that microglia and endothelial cells can also directly interact through the interaction of CD200/CD200R and CX3CL1/CX3CR1, by which endothelial cells are able to regulate the function of microglia [62, 63]. The mechanism and pathways need further investigation.

Conclusion

In this study, we demonstrated that co-culturing RMECs with microglia resulted in upregulation of VEGF-A and PDGF-BB expression, angiogenesis, migration, and proliferation and downregulated the expression of tight junction proteins in RMECs, and these effects were significantly enhanced by microglial activation. The mechanisms underlying the effects of microglia on the function of adjacent endothelial cells, including the cytokines/proteins and specific pathways involved, need further clarification.

Abbreviations

IL-1β: Interleukin 1β; LPS: Lipopolysaccharide; MG: Microglia; PDGF-BB: Platelet-derived growth factor-BB; RMECs: Retinal microvascular endothelial cells; TNFα: Tumor necrosis factor; VEGF-A: Vascular endothelial growth factor-A; vWF: von-Willebrand factor; WST-1: Water soluble tetrazolium-1; ZO-1: Zonula occludens-1

Acknowledgements

Thanks for the contributions of all the authors.

Funding

This work was supported by funding from the National Natural Science Foundation for Young Scholars of China (nos. 81300781,81400410,81300805,81700862), National Natural Science Foundation of China (nos. 81570854).

Authors' contributions

HW conceived and designed the experiments; XD and RG performed the experiments with the assistance of MZ, HR and QS. XD and RG analyzed the data and prepared the manuscript. GX aided the technical support. GX and QS helped revise the manuscript. All authors read and approved the final manuscript.

Competing interests

All authors certify that they have no affiliations with or involvement in any organization or entity with any financial interest (such as honoraria; educational grants; participation in speakers' bureaus; membership, employment, consultancies, stock ownership, or other equity interest; and expert testimony or patent-licensing arrangements) or non-financial interest (such as personal or professional relationships, affiliations, knowledge or beliefs) in the subject matter or materials discussed in this manuscript.

Author details

[1]Department of Ophthalmology, Eye and ENT Hospital of Fudan University, 83 Fen Yang Road, Shanghai 200031, People's Republic of China. [2]Institute of Eye Research, Eye and ENT Hospital of Fudan University, Shanghai, China. [3]Key Laboratory of Myopia of State Health Ministry (Fudan University), Shanghai, China. [4]Shanghai Key Laboratory of Visual Impairment and Restoration(Fudan University), Shanghai, China.

References

1. Li L, Eter N, Heiduschka P. The microglia in healthy and diseased retina. Exp Eye Res. 2015;136:116–30.
2. Zhu SH, et al. Paeoniflorin suppressed high glucose-induced retinal microglia MMP-9 expression and inflammatory response via inhibition of TLR4/NF-kappaB pathway through Upregulation of SOCS3 in diabetic retinopathy. Inflammation. 2017;40(5):1475–86.
3. Ma W, et al. Microglia in the mouse retina alter the structure and function of retinal pigmented epithelial cells: a potential cellular interaction relevant to AMD. PLoS One. 2009;4(11):e7945.
4. Rutar M, et al. Analysis of complement expression in light-induced retinal degeneration: synthesis and deposition of C3 by microglia/macrophages is associated with focal photoreceptor degeneration. Invest Ophthalmol Vis Sci. 2011;52(8):5347–58.
5. Gullapalli VK, et al. Hematopoietically derived retinal perivascular microglia initiate uveoretinitis in experimental autoimmune uveitis. Graefes Arch Clin Exp Ophthalmol. 2000;238(4):319–25.
6. Eelen G, et al. Endothelial cell metabolism in normal and diseased vasculature. Circ Res. 2015;116(7):1231–44.
7. Armulik A, Abramsson A, Betsholtz C. Endothelial/pericyte interactions. Circ Res. 2005;97(6):512–23.
8. Grigsby JG, et al. The role of microglia in diabetic retinopathy. J Ophthalmol. 2014;2014:705783.
9. Adamis AP, Berman AJ. Immunological mechanisms in the pathogenesis of diabetic retinopathy. Semin Immunopathol. 2008;30(2):65–84.
10. Rungger-Brandle E, Dosso AA, Leuenberger PM. Glial reactivity, an early feature of diabetic retinopathy. Invest Ophthalmol Vis Sci. 2000;41(7):1971–80.
11. Zeng XX, Ng YK, Ling EA. Neuronal and microglial response in the retina of streptozotocin-induced diabetic rats. Vis Neurosci. 2000;17(3):463–71.
12. Krady JK, et al. Minocycline reduces proinflammatory cytokine expression, microglial activation, and caspase-3 activation in a rodent model of diabetic retinopathy. Diabetes. 2005;54(5):1559–65.
13. Zeng HY, Green WR, Tso MO. Microglial activation in human diabetic retinopathy. Arch Ophthalmol. 2008;126(2):227–32.
14. Ding X, et al. Activated microglia induce the production of reactive oxygen species and promote apoptosis of co-cultured retinal microvascular pericytes. Graefes Arch Clin Exp Ophthalmol. 2017;255(4):777–88.
15. Wong JS, Aiello LP. Diabetic retinopathy. Ann Acad Med Singap. 2000;29(6):745–52.
16. van der Wijk AE, et al. Spatial and temporal recruitment of the neurovascular unit during development of the mouse blood-retinal barrier. Tissue Cell. 2018;52:42–50.
17. Busch S, et al. Systemic treatment with erythropoietin protects the neurovascular unit in a rat model of retinal neurodegeneration. PLoS One. 2014;9(7):e102013.
18. Feng Y, et al. Crosstalk in the retinal neurovascular unit - lessons for the diabetic retina. Exp Clin Endocrinol Diabetes. 2012;120(4):199–201.
19. Antonetti DA, Klein R, Gardner TW. Diabetic retinopathy. N Engl J Med. 2012;366(13):1227–39.
20. Yousif NM, et al. Activation of EP2 receptor suppresses poly(I: C) and LPS-mediated inflammation in primary microglia and organotypic hippocampal slice cultures: contributing role for MAPKs. Glia. 2018;66(4):708–24.
21. Zheng X, et al. Propofol attenuates inflammatory response in LPS-activated microglia by regulating the miR-155/SOCS1 pathway. Inflammation. 2018;41(1):11–19.
22. Wang YM, et al. Blocking the CD38/cADPR pathway plays a double-edged role in LPS stimulated microglia. Neuroscience. 2017;361:34–42.
23. Covert MW, et al. Achieving stability of lipopolysaccharide-induced NF-kappaB activation. Science. 2005;309(5742):1854–7.
24. Guo D, et al. VEGF stimulated the angiogenesis by promoting the mitochondrial functions. Oncotarget. 2017;8(44):77020–7.
25. Kaigler D, et al. VEGF scaffolds enhance angiogenesis and bone regeneration in irradiated osseous defects. J Bone Miner Res. 2006;21(5):735–44.
26. Carmeliet P. Angiogenesis in health and disease. Nat Med. 2003;9(6):653–60.
27. Yancopoulos GD, et al. Vascular-specific growth factors and blood vessel formation. Nature. 2000;407(6801):242–8.
28. Klinghoffer RA, et al. Platelet-derived growth factor-dependent activation of phosphatidylinositol 3-kinase is regulated by receptor binding of SH2-domain-containing proteins which influence Ras activity. Mol Cell Biol. 1996;16(10):5905 14.
29. Erber R, et al. Combined inhibition of VEGF and PDGF signaling enforces tumor vessel regression by interfering with pericyte-mediated endothelial cell survival mechanisms. FASEB J. 2004;18(2):338–40.
30. Siedlecki J, et al. Combined VEGF and PDGF inhibition for neovascular AMD: anti-angiogenic properties of axitinib on human endothelial cells and pericytes in vitro. Graefes Arch Clin Exp Ophthalmol. 2017;255(5):963–72.
31. Herrmann JL, et al. IL-6 and TGF-alpha costimulate mesenchymal stem cell vascular endothelial growth factor production by ERK-, JNK-, and PI3K-mediated mechanisms. Shock. 2011;35(5):512–6.
32. Vinores SA, et al. Upregulation of vascular endothelial growth factor (VEGF) in the retinas of transgenic mice overexpressing interleukin-1beta (IL-1beta) in the lens and mice undergoing retinal degeneration. Histol Histopathol. 2003;18(3):797–810.
33. Chen WH, Chen Y, Cui GH. Effects of TNF-alpha and curcumin on the expression of VEGF in Raji and U937 cells and on angiogenesis in ECV304 cells. Chin Med J. 2005;118(24):2052–7.
34. Zhou P, et al. Attenuation of TNF-alpha-induced inflammatory injury in endothelial cells by Ginsenoside Rb1 via inhibiting NF-kappaB, JNK and p38 signaling pathways. Front Pharmacol. 2017;8:464.
35. Ohba T, et al. TNF-alpha-induced NF-kappaB signaling reverses age-related declines in VEGF induction and angiogenic activity in intervertebral disc tissues. J Orthop Res. 2009;27(2):229–35.
36. Shin MR, et al. TNF-alpha and LPS activate angiogenesis via VEGF and SIRT1 signalling in human dental pulp cells. Int Endod J. 2015;48(7):705–16.
37. Tipton DA, Christian J, Blumer A. Effects of cranberry components on IL-1beta-stimulated production of IL-6, IL-8 and VEGF by human TMJ synovial fibroblasts. Arch Oral Biol. 2016;68:88–96.
38. Huang F, et al. MAPK/ERK signal pathway involved expression of COX-2 and VEGF by IL-1beta induced in human endometriosis stromal cells in vitro. Int J Clin Exp Pathol. 2013;6(10):2129–36.
39. Sheikpranbabu S, et al. Silver nanoparticles inhibit VEGF-and IL-1beta-induced vascular permeability via Src dependent pathway in porcine retinal endothelial cells. J Nanobiotechnol. 2009;7:8.
40. Sufen G, et al. bFGF and PDGF-BB have a synergistic effect on the proliferation, migration and VEGF release of endothelial progenitor cells. Cell Biol Int. 2011;35(5):545–51.
41. Vinals F, Pouyssegur J. Transforming growth factor beta1 (TGF-beta1) promotes endothelial cell survival during in vitro angiogenesis via an autocrine mechanism implicating TGF-alpha signaling. Mol Cell Biol. 2001;21(21):7218–30.
42. Mathews MK, et al. Vascular endothelial growth factor and vascular permeability changes in human diabetic retinopathy. Invest Ophthalmol Vis Sci. 1997;38(13):2729–41.
43. Matsunaga T, et al. Enhancement of endothelial barrier permeability by Mitragynine. Biol Pharm Bull. 2017;40(10):1779–83.
44. Ni Y, et al. TNFalpha alters occludin and cerebral endothelial permeability: role of p38MAPK. PLoS One. 2017;12(2):e0170346.
45. Zhang L, et al. Vascular endothelial growth factor increases GEnC permeability by affecting the distributions of occludin, ZO-1 and tight juction assembly. Eur Rev Med Pharmacol Sci. 2015;19(14):2621–7.
46. Li R, et al. Diesel exhaust particles modulate vascular endothelial cell permeability: implication of ZO-1 expression. Toxicol Lett. 2010;197(3):163–8.
47. Abbruscato TJ, et al. Nicotine and cotinine modulate cerebral microvascular permeability and protein expression of ZO-1 through nicotinic acetylcholine receptors expressed on brain endothelial cells. J Pharm Sci. 2002;91(12):2525–38.
48. Murakami T, Felinski EA, Antonetti DA. Occludin phosphorylation and ubiquitination regulate tight junction trafficking and vascular endothelial growth factor-induced permeability. J Biol Chem. 2009;284(31):21036–46.
49. Harhaj NS, et al. VEGF activation of protein kinase C stimulates occludin phosphorylation and contributes to endothelial permeability. Invest Ophthalmol Vis Sci. 2006;47(11):5106–15.
50. Denieffe S, et al. Classical activation of microglia in CD200-deficient mice is a consequence of blood brain barrier permeability and infiltration of peripheral cells. Brain Behav Immun. 2013;34:86–97.
51. Mehrabadi AR, et al. Poly(ADP-ribose) polymerase-1 regulates microglia mediated decrease of endothelial tight junction integrity. Neurochem Int. 2017;108:266–71.
52. Sumi N, et al. Lipopolysaccharide-activated microglia induce dysfunction of the blood-brain barrier in rat microvascular endothelial cells co-cultured with microglia. Cell Mol Neurobiol. 2010;30(2):247–53.

53. Privratsky JR, Newman PJ. PECAM-1: regulator of endothelial junctional integrity. Cell Tissue Res. 2014;355(3):607–19.

54. RayChaudhury A, et al. Regulation of PECAM-1 in endothelial cells during cell growth and migration. Exp Biol Med (Maywood). 2001;226(7):686–91.

55. Rothermel TA, Engelhardt B, Sheibani N. Polyoma virus middle-T-transformed PECAM-1 deficient mouse brain endothelial cells proliferate rapidly in culture and form hemangiomas in mice. J Cell Physiol. 2005;202(1):230–9.

56. Jackson DE, et al. Platelet endothelial cell adhesion molecule-1 (PECAM-1/CD31) is associated with a naive B-cell phenotype in human tonsils. Tissue Antigens. 2000;56(2):105–16.

57. Vasconcelos MG, et al. Expression of CD34 and CD105 as markers for angiogenesis in oral vascular malformations and pyogenic granulomas. Eur Arch Otorhinolaryngol. 2011;268(8):1213–7.

58. Yao Y, et al. Endoglin (CD105) expression in angiogenesis of primary hepatocellular carcinomas: analysis using tissue microarrays and comparisons with CD34 and VEGF. Ann Clin Lab Sci. 2007;37(1):39–48.

59. Li Y, et al. Ephrin-A3 and ephrin-A4 contribute to microglia-induced angiogenesis in brain endothelial cells. Anat Rec (Hoboken). 2014;297(10):1908–18.

60. Nishioku T, et al. Tumor necrosis factor-alpha mediates the blood-brain barrier dysfunction induced by activated microglia in mouse brain microvascular endothelial cells. J Pharmacol Sci. 2010;112(2):251–4.

61. Lyu Y, et al. Microvesicles derived from LPS-induced microglia aggravate the injury of tight junction in rat brain microvascular endothelial cells under oxygen-glucose deprivation. Xi Bao Yu Fen Zi Mian Yi Xue Za Zhi. 2018;34(3):211–7.

62. Liu Y, et al. Role of microglia-neuron interactions in diabetic encephalopathy. Ageing Res Rev. 2018;42:28–39.

63. Jerath MR, et al. Dual targeting of CCR2 and CX3CR1 in an arterial injury model of vascular inflammation. Thromb J. 2010;8:14.

33

Ectopic orbital meningioma: a retrospective case series

Xiaoming Huang[1], Dongrun Tang[2,3], Tong Wu[2,3], Tianming Jian[2,3] and Fengyuan Sun[1,2,3]*

Abstract

Background: To evaluate the ophthalmic manifestations and radiographic features of ectopic orbital meningioma to improve diagnostic accuracy.

Methods: Patient data from patients admitted to our institution during a 217-month period from August 1999 to September 2017 were included. Patient ophthalmic manifestations, radiographic features (CT and MRI), diagnosis, pathology, therapeutic regimens, and prognosis were retrospectively reviewed.

Results: Six patients with ectopic orbital meningioma were identified. The mean age at the first visit was 33.2 years (range, 7–56 years). All six patients displayed manifestations of exophthalmos, upper eyelid oedema, and motility impairment with a mean history of illness of 20.3 months (range 3–72 months). Optical lesions were located in the superonasal extraconal compartment (3/6, 50%), bitemporal extraconal compartment (1/6, 16.7%) and orbital intraconal compartment (2/6, 33%). Radiographic features were ill-defined, heterogeneous, enhancing soft tissue masses with extraocular muscular adhesion (6/6, 100%) and calcification (1/6, 16.7%), not adjacent to the optic nerve and not extending along the dura. Six cases were treated intraoperatively with complete surgical resection, indicating that all lesions were independent of the optic nerve and sphenoid ridge. The histopathologic classification was mostly of meningothelial cells (5/6, 83%). Immunohistochemistry revealed EMA and vimentin to have positive expression in all six cases, while two cases were calponin-positive and strongly expressed in the olfactory bulb. Postoperatively, lesions caused no visual impairment, and there were no cases of recurrence.

Conclusions: Ectopic orbital meningiomas are rare tumours that are not easily diagnosed without postoperative histopathology. This report highlights some of the distinguishing features of isolated orbital lesions, especially around the location of frontoethmoidal suture. Accompanying upper eyelid oedema and eye mobility restriction were observed to be dissimilar to other orbital tumours. In these cases, a diagnosis of ectopic orbital meningioma should be considered.

Keywords: Ectopic orbital meningioma, Ophthalmic manifestations, Radiographic features, Pathological diagnosis

Background

The meninges have three membranes, including the dura mater, the arachnoid mater, and the pia mater, that envelop the brain and spinal cord. Meningiomas are a variety of tumours caused by arachnoid "cap" cells of meningeal arachnoid villi [1]. Orbital meningiomas can be considered to be primary and secondary in origin [2]. Primary orbital meningioma accounted for 5–10% of all orbital tumours and 30% of all orbital meningiomas; they were also mainly observed in adults and rarely in children [3]. Primary

orbital meningiomas originate from the arachnoid layer of the optic nerve sheath. Approximately 70% of orbital meningiomas are secondary intracranial meningiomas, usually originating at the sphenoid ridge, with orbital, intracranial, and intraluminal intrusions [4].

A rare subset of orbital meningiomas that do not involve the optic nerve sheath or sphenoid ridge were initially considered to be "ectopic". Ectopic orbital meningiomas are occasionally reported as single or multiple case series in the literature. However, there exists a paucity of published clinical evidence regarding the distinguishing features of ectopic orbital meningioma. Preoperative diagnosis is often difficult, which is not

* Correspondence: eyesunfy@126.com
[1]The School of Medicine, Nankai University, Tianjin 300071, China
[2]Tianjin Medical University Eye Hospital, Tianjin 300384, China
Full list of author information is available at the end of the article

conducive to the establishment of surgical methods, surgical operation, and follow-up treatment success.

All cases reported in this report were admitted to the Tianjin Medical University Eye Hospital during a 217-month period. Clinical manifestations, radiographic features, and therapeutic regimens of these patients were retrospectively analysed in the following report.

Methods
Study population
The present study was approved by the Tianjin Medical University Eye Hospital Foundation Institutional Review Board (REC No.2017KY(L)L-56) and adhered to HIPAA regulations as well as the principles of the Declaration of Helsinki. The six patients included in this study were selected from 162 cases with a pathological diagnosis of orbital meningioma at Tianjin Medical University Eye Hospital during a 217-month period between August 1999 and September 2017. Patients with known optic nerve sheath meningiomas and intracranial meningiomas were excluded.

Data collection
Data were collected on patient symptoms, such as headache, nausea, vomiting, and other intracranial symptoms, and the results of regular eye examination, including (i) a visual acuity and best corrected visual acuity test using international visual chart; (ii) examination of the exophthalmos by a Hertel exophthalmometer (differences in the bilateral exophthalmos of more than 2 mm were regarded as abnormal); (iii) examination of eye movement and periorbital changes; and (iv) indirect ophthalmoscopy to check the fundus after mydriasis. All patients underwent radiographic examination, including computed tomography (CT) or magnetic resonance imaging (MRI), to identify the location of their tumour and relative location to the optic nerve, extraocular muscle, and other peripheral tissues.

Therapeutic regimen and pathological diagnosis
Surgery was the preferred therapeutic regimen. All patients underwent complete surgical resection, and surgical approaches were divided into lateral orbitotomy or anterior orbitotomy according to lesion location. All tumour specimens were sent for pathological examination. The two-step method for immunohistochemical staining was employed to detect the expression of EMA, vimentin, S-100, Ki-67 and calponin and was performed according to the manufacturer's instructions (Shanghai Bioleaf Biotech Co, Ltd., Shanghai, China). Phosphate buffered saline (PBS) was used as the negative antibody control, and the EMA antibody for clinical pathology diagnosis was used as the positive control. Diaminobenzidine (DAB)-staining, haematoxylin staining, dehydration,

transparentisation and sealing with neutral balsam were performed in that order. Positive staining presented as a tan colour in staining assessment.

Results
Characteristics of the study population and their medical conditions
All patients were diagnosed with monocular diseases. Among them, four were male, and two were female, with a male to female ratio of 2:1. The mean age at first visit and age range were 33.2 and 7 to 56 years, respectively; the mean disease history and range were 20.3 and 3 to 72 months, respectively. The main complaints recorded at the first visit were upper eyelid oedema (6/6, 100%), exophthalmos (5/6, 83%), ptosis (4/6, 66.7%), impaired vision (2/6, 33%), diplopia (2/6, 33%) and tumours detected by physical examination (2/6, 33%). Three patients developed intracranial symptoms; two of whom had symptoms of nausea and vomiting due to diplopia. One such patient had a headache in accordance with a history of migraines for many years. Two patients had a history of remote head trauma, but this was considered unrelated to their intracranial symptoms. Patients were misdiagnosed as having neurofibromatosis (one case), eosinophilic granuloma (one case), venous haemangioma (one case), and capillary haemangioma (two cases) (Table 1).

Ophthalmic manifestations
In most cases, the visual acuity of patients was better than 1.0 (4/6, 67%). All cases were observed to have different degrees of unilateral exophthalmos (Additional file 1: Figure. a and c). Other ophthalmic manifestations included upper eyelid oedema, mobility restriction, light diplopia, different levels of increased intraorbital pressure, and fundus abnormalities, including papilledema and optic nerve compression with an increased cup-disc ratio (Table 1).

Radiographic features
All cases underwent either CT or MRI examination. CT examination was indicative of ill-defined and heterogeneous lesions, with calcium spots present in one case. Most cases were recognised as having neither optic nerve nor sphenoid ridge involvement. Some cases were observed to have tumours in close proximity to the optic nerve. These were likely to be mistaken as originating from the optic nerve because the human eye is limited when identifying CT values. Indeed, completely preserved optic nerves were observed in all cases after surgery, and the periosteal nerve had no proliferation and no bone involvement. T1WI MRI was hypointense and T2WI MRI was hyperintense in all cases. CT and MRI images are shown in Fig. 1.

Table 1 Clinical manifestations in six patients with ectopic orbital meningioma

No.	Age/Sex	History (months)	Visual acuity	Head trauma	Exophthalmos (mm)	Ptosis	Upper eyelid edema	Mobility restriction/ diplopia	Fundus abnormality	Intraorbital pressure	Initial misdiagnosis	Treatment	prognosis
1	7/M	5	1.2	–	14 (95)11	–	+	+	–	–	capillary haemangioma	surgical resection	No recurrence
2	18/F	24	1.2	–	22.5 (105)14.5	+	+	+	–	–	capillary haemangioma	surgical resection	No recurrence
3	31/M	12	LP	+	14 (109)13	–	+	+	Papilledema and increased cup-disc ratio	+	venous haemangioma	surgical resection	No recurrence
4	35/M	72	1.0	+	21 (98)13	+	+	+	papilledema	–	eosinophilic granuloma	surgical resection	No recurrence
5	56/M	3	1.0	–	16.5 (93)13	+	+	+	–	+	undiagnosed	surgical resection	No recurrence
6	52/F	6	0.5	–	18 (105)13	+	+	+	–	+	neurofibromatosis	surgical resection	No recurrence

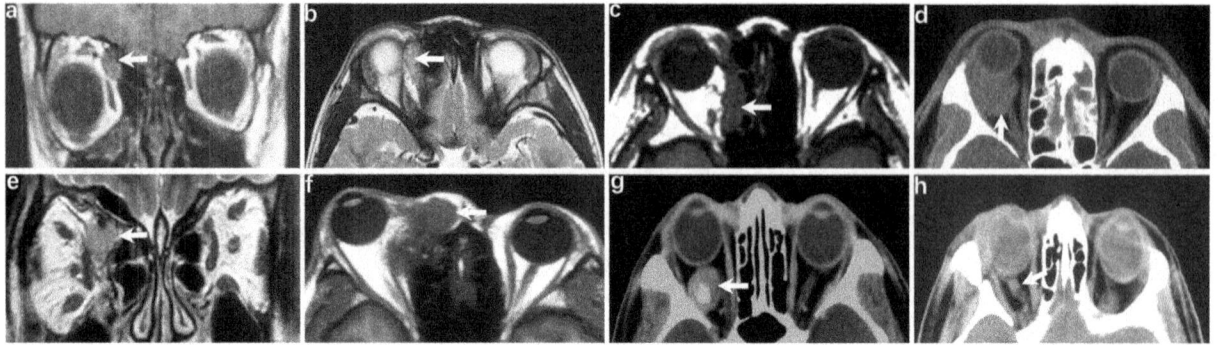

Fig. 1 a and **b** MRI of case 1. **a** coronal T1WI showing the superonasal mass (arrow). **b** Axial T2WI showing an ill-defined and heterogeneous mass and adjacent medial rectus (arrow). **c** MRI of case 2. Axial T1 showing an ill-defined and heterogeneous superonasal mass and adjacent medial rectus (arrow). **d** Axial CT of case 3. A well-defined intraconal mass adjacent to the anterior optic nerve (arrow). **e** and **f** MRI of case 4. **e** Coronal T1 W1 showing the superonasal mass and no adjacent medial rectus (arrow). **f** Axial T1 W1 showing the ill-defined and heterogeneous superonasal mass (arrow). **g** and **h**: CT of case 5. **g** Axial CT showing a well-defined intraconal lesion with a calcified mass (arrow). **h** Optic nerve was compressed and dislocated but integrated into the structure (arrow)

Therapeutic regimen and pathological diagnosis

All cases underwent complete surgical resection. The following surgical methods were used: four cases of lateral orbitotomy, one case of transconjunctival orbitotomy, and one case of supraorbital orbitotomy. During surgery, the optic nerves remained intact while tumour resection was performed, and no orbital bone involvement or periosteal proliferation was observed. However, most tumours were observed as having different degrees of adhesion with extraocular muscles, including the medial rectus (two cases), lateral rectus (two cases), both medial rectus and lateral rectus (two cases), and both medial rectus and superior oblique (one case).

The postoperative histopathologic classification of five cases revealed meningothelial cells, and one case revealed psammomatous meningioma (Fig. 2b). In the WHO grading system, the tumours of all six cases were considered to be grade I[5]. However, case NO.1 was considered to have low malignancy because of its invasion of surrounding adipose tissue (Fig. 2a). All cases underwent immunohistochemistry (IHC) (Table 2). IHC revealed EMA and vimentin to be positive (Fig. 2c and e); Ki-67 levels of all cases were less than 3% (Fig. 2d). S-100 was expressed in the two youngest cases, which showed low malignancy (Fig. 2f); Two patients had calponin expression (Fig. 2g). Calponin is an actin-binding protein, and there is clear evidence from previous reports that calponin is strongly expressed by meningeal cells from the lamina propria of the olfactory bulb (OB) [6]. Two patients in this report had calponin expression, and both of these tumours were located in the superonasal extraconal compartment. For this reason, we speculated that meningeal cells were supposed to pass through the frontoethmoidal suture to the orbit and grow into tumours.

After surgeries, all patients' exophthalmos was obviously relieved (Additional file 1: Figure. b and d). During the follow-up period (1–72 months), no postoperative diminution of vision was noted, and no recurrence was observed.

Discussion

The existence of ectopic orbital meningiomas is still debated in the field of ophthalmology. Some previous cases have likely been diagnosed as central nervous system or atypical optic nerve sheath meningiomas, so ectopic orbital meningiomas may be underreported.

There is no definitive evidence as to the origin of ectopic orbital meningiomas. One theory, advanced by Craig and Cogela [7], states that no meningeal tissue in normal orbits other than the arachnoid of the optic nerve should be observed after inspecting several autopsy specimens histologically. It was also suggested that ectopic orbital meningiomas originate from the optic nerve sheath and migrate to ectopic locations. Tan and Lim [8] suggested that ectopic orbital meningiomas could originate from the arachnoid sheath of the cranial nerves, as opposed to the optic nerve, in orbit. Furthermore, there is no evidence that arachnoid courses with the cranial nerves into the orbit, in which cases the involved arachnoid tissue must originate outside the orbit. Another theory suggested that ectopic orbital meningiomas may originate from a regressed orbital meningocele or from meningeal tissue trapped outside the centre [9]. Irwin Tendler et al. [10] reported a case involving the sinus and proposed sinus enlargement as a marker of a congenital event that displaced meningeal cells. This may have caused the formation of an ectopic lesion or mechanical stress induced by the presence of an ectopic orbital tumour, thereby causing sinus asymmetry.

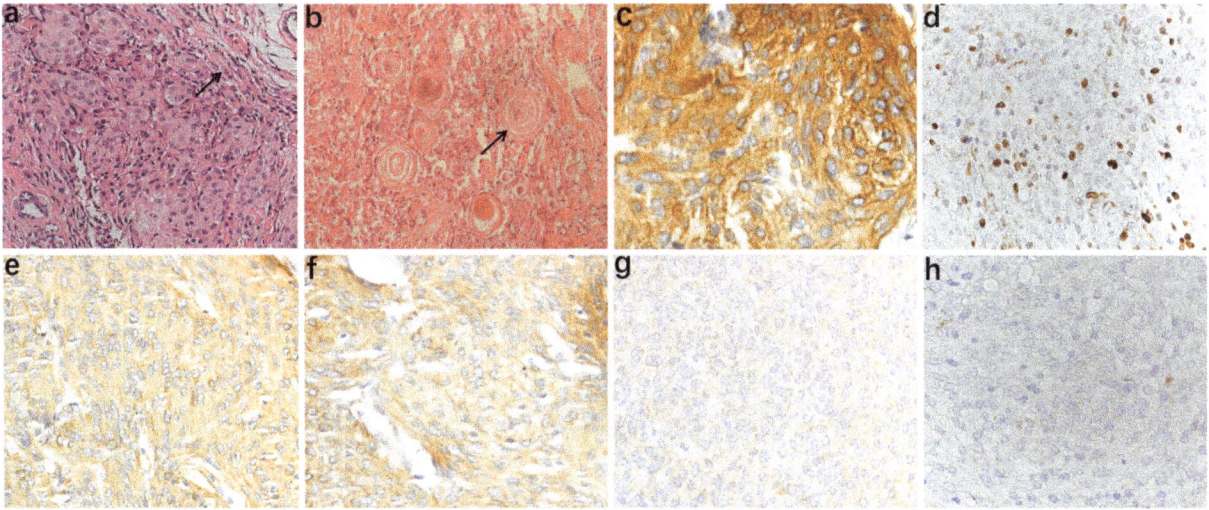

Fig. 2 a Epithelial-type meningioma with low malignancy. Tumours indicated an infiltrative growth pattern with invasion of surrounding adipose tissue (arrow), HE× 40. **b** Image of psammomatous meningioma, HE× 200. **c-g** immunohistochemistry revealed positive staining for EMA, Ki-67, Vimentin, S-100 and calponin respectively, IHC × 200. **h** PBS was used to replace the primary antibody as the negative control, IHC × 200

However, obvious sinus enlargement was not observed in the present study.

In our study, we hypothesised that some ectopic meningiomas originate from meningeal cells of the OB, in which case meningeal cells could pass through the frontoethmoidal suture to the orbit. EMA and vimentin are important markers of meningioma cells, and these proteins were strongly expressed by tumour cells in all cases in the present study. However, we also found only two cases positive for calponin in tumours which were just in the location of the lateral antorbital frontoethmoidal suture. Interestingly, calponin has been reported to be strongly expressed by connective tissue cells, mesenchymal-derived cells, fibroblasts and meningeal cells from the lamina propria of the olfactory mucosa (OM) and the OB [5, 11, 12].

To date, only 20 cases are described. Among them, 14 cases are from other studies in the literature, and the six cases presented here were treated at our hospital over the last 18 years. Among these cases, the male to female ratio and the mean age at presentation were 11:9 and 32.6 years (range 7–77 years), respectively. This is a marked difference from typical meningiomas, where females are more commonly affected, with detection occurring in the fourth or fifth decade of life. The tumour itself was observed to have little impact on vision, as most visual impairment was caused by excessive tumour growth leading to optic nerve compression (4/20, 20%). This finding differs from nerve sheath meningioma, which affects vision early in its development.

All cases presented here were identified during surgery. Remarkably, the tumours from 11 cases, including three cases in our study and eight cases in previous reports, were located in the superonasal extraconal compartment near the frontoethmoidal suture (11/20, 55%). Two cases reported in the previous literature were noted to have neither CT nor MRI data because they were diagnosed before these radiographic instruments came into use. Among the other 18 cases, radiographic features in most cases were ill-defined, heterogeneous orbital masses (15/18, 83%). MRI showed T1WI as hypointense and T2W as hyperintense fat suppression signal enhancement. Some cases of CT indicated calcium spots (4/18, 22%), and recurrence was rare with complete excision (2/20, 10%). Finally, some of the tumours were obviously separated from the optic nerve, and no evidence suggested bony hyperostosis (Table 3) [3, 4, 8–10, 13–17].

Although the cases outlined here did not have a definite diagnosis before pathological testing, our study may offer ophthalmologists cues to improve the diagnostic accuracy for future patients. We found that most

Table 2 Tumors with immunohischemistry in different locations

NO.	Location	EMA	Vimetin	S-100	Calponin	Ki-67
1	SEC	+	+	+	+	2%
2	SEC	+	+	+	–	0.5%
3	IC	+	+	–	–	0.2%
4	SEC	+	+	–	+	0.7%
5	IC	+	+	–	–	0.8%
6	BEC	+	+	–	–	1%

SEC superonasal extraconal compartment, *IC* intraconal compartment, *BEC* bitamporal extraconal compartment

Table 3 Results of our 6 cases and 14 cases from literature review of ectopic orbital meningioma

Clinical Characteristics	Literature Review (N = 14)	Our Data (N = 6)	Total Data (N = 20)
Sex			
Male	7	4	11 (55%)
Female	7	2	9 (45%)
Range of age(years)(mean)	7–77 (32.4)	7–56 (33.2)	7–77 (32.6)
History(months)	6–60 (22.4)	3–72 (20.3)	3–72 (20.8)
History of head trauma	2	2	4 (20%)
Symptoms or sign			
Exophthalmos	9	5	14 (70%)
Ptosis	2	4	6 (30%)
Upper eyelid edema	3	6	9 (45%)
Mobility restriction	4	6	10 (50%)
Fundus abnormality	2	2	4 (20%)
Tumor locations			
Superonasal extraconal compartment	8	3	11 (55%)
Bitamporal extraconal compartment	1	1	2 (10%)
Intraconal compartment	5	2	7 (35%)
CT and MRI			
Ill-defined	9	4	13 (65%)
Well-defined	3	2	5 (25%)
Calcification	3	1	4 (20%)
Therapeutic regimen			
Complete resection	12	6	18 (90%)
Radiotherapy	2	0	2 (10%)
Histopathology			
Meningothelial meningioma	12	5	17 (85%)
Fibrous meningioma	2	0	2 (10%)
Psammomatous meningioma	0	1	1 (5%)

patients with ectopic orbital meningioma had upper eyelid oedema and eye mobility restriction through this 18-year clinical retrospective analysis, even though most of the tumours did not involve the eyelids or cause increased intraorbital pressure resulting in obstruction of the returning fluid to the lower eyelid. Such findings are not particularly common in other orbital tumours and may be related to some unknown properties of meningioma cells.

Conclusions

In summary, orbital isolate lesions, especially around the location of the frontoethmoidal suture, had accompanying upper eyelid oedema and eye mobility restriction not observed in other orbital tumours. Therefore, ectopic orbital meningioma should be considered in such cases. Ideally, further research into the origin and pathogenesis of ectopic orbital meningiomas should be conducted.

Abbreviations

CT: Computed tomography; MRI: Magnetic resonance imaging; OB: Olfactory bulb; OM: Olfactory mucosa

Acknowledgement

We would like to thank Professor Guoxiang Song for his advice on this manuscript.

Funding

This study was supported by the Tianjin Medical University 13th Five-Year Discipline Construction Fund, award number: 2016XK030505. The funders had the opportunity to review the final version of the manuscript to address any factual inaccuracies or request the revision of information deemed to be proprietary or confidential and ensure that study support was disclosed.

Authors' contributions

XH designed the study, wrote the ethics proposal and received Tianjin Medical University Eye Hospital Foundation Institutional Review Board approval, collected patient materials, performed the analyses, prepared monitoring of the study and drafted the manuscript. DT gave advice on the study design and helped with the approvals from the Institutional Review Board. TW, TJ and FS critically reviewed and revised the manuscript. All authors read and approved the final manuscript.

Competing interests
The authors declare that they have no competing interest.

Author details
[1]The School of Medicine, Nankai University, Tianjin 300071, China. [2]Tianjin Medical University Eye Hospital, Tianjin 300384, China. [3]Tianjin Orbital Disease Institute, Tianjin 300384, China.

References
1. Eggers H, Jakobiec FA, Jones IS. Tumors of the optic nerve. Doc Ophthalmol. 1976;41(1):43–128.
2. Fortuna A, Nicole S, Palma L, Di Lorenzo N. Primary intraorbital meningiomas. Riv Neurol. 1978;48(3):251–70.
3. Johnson TE, Weatherhead RG, Nasr AM, Siqueira EB. Ectopic (extradural) meningioma of the orbit: a report of two cases in children. J Pediatr Ophthalmol Strabismus. 1993;30(1):43–7.
4. Pushker N, Shrey D, Kashyap S, Sen S, Khurana S, Sharma S. Ectopic meningioma of the orbit. Int Ophthalmol. 2013;33(6):707–10.
5. Louis DN, Ohgaki H, Wiestler OD, et al. World Health Organization classification of tumours of the central nervous system. 4th ed. Lyon, France: IARC; 2007.
6. Ibanez C, Ito D, Zawadzka M, Jeffery ND, Franklin RJ. Calponin is expressed by fibroblasts and meningeal cells but not olfactory ensheathing cells in the adult peripheral olfactory system. Glia. 2007;55(2):144–51.
7. Craig WM, Gogela LJ: Intraorbital meningiomas; a clinicopathologic study. Am J Ophthalmol 1949, 32(12):1663–1680, illust.
8. Tan KK, Lim AS. Primary extradural intra-orbital meningioma in a Chinese girl. Br J Ophthalmol. 1965;49(7):377–80.
9. Farah SE, Konrad H, Huang DT, Geist CE. Ectopic orbital meningioma: a case report and review. Ophthal Plast Reconstr Surg. 1999;15(6):463–6.
10. Tendler I, Belinsky I, Abramson DH, Marr BP. Primary Extradural Ectopic Orbital Meningioma. Ophthal Plast Reconstr Surg. 2017;33(3S):S99–S101.
11. Tome M, Siladzic E, Santos-Silva A, Barnett SC. Calponin is expressed by subpopulations of connective tissue cells but not olfactory ensheathing cells in the neonatal olfactory mucosa. BMC Neurosci. 2007;8:74.
12. Rizek PN, Kawaja MD. Cultures of rat olfactory ensheathing cells are contaminated with Schwann cells. Neuroreport. 2006;17(5):459–62.
13. Yokoyama T, Nishizawa S, Sugiyama K, et al. Primary intraorbital ectopic meningioma. Skull Base Surg. 1999;9(1):47–50.
14. Arai H, Sato K, Matsumoto T. Free-lying ectopic meningioma within the orbit. Br J Neurosurg. 1997;11(6):560–3.
15. Decock CE, Kataria S, Breusegem CM, Van Den Broecke CM, Claerhout IJ. Ectopic meningioma anterior to the lacrimal gland fossa. Ophthal Plast Reconstr Surg. 2009;25(1):57–9.
16. Gunduz K, Kurt RA, Erden E. Ectopic orbital meningioma: report of two cases and literature review. Surv Ophthalmol. 2014;59(6):643–8.
17. Wolter JR, Benz SC. Ectopic meningioma of the superior orbital rim. Arch Ophthalmol. 1976;94(11):1920–2.

34

Association between diabetic retinopathy in type 2 diabetes and the *ICAM-1* rs5498 polymorphism: a meta-analysis of case-control studies

Zikang Xie and Hao Liang[*] ⓘ

Abstract

Background: Genetic studies have reported contradictory results on the association between the intercellular adhesion molecule-1 (*ICAM-1*) rs5498 polymorphism and diabetic retinopathy (DR) risk in type 2 diabetic patients. We aimed to perform a systematic literature search and conduct random-effects meta-analysis to provide a quantitative evaluation.

Methods: We searched Pubmed, Embase, Scopus, Web of Science and Wanfang databases from inception up to January 2018. Allelic and genotype frequencies of rs5498 was compared between DR cases and controls. Odds ratios (OR) and 95% confidence intervals (CI) were calculated using a random effects model.

Results: Nine studies involving a total of 1792 cases and 1400 controls met our inclusion criteria. We did not find any significant association between rs5498 and DR risk at the dominant model (GG + GA versus AA, OR = 1.00, 95% CI: 0.66–1.50, $P = 0.987$), the recessive model (GG versus GA + AA, OR = 1.24, 95% CI: 0.86–1.77, $P = 0.245$), the GG versus AA contrast (OR = 1.14, 95% CI: 0.68–1.92, $P = 0.611$), and the G allele versus A allele contrast (OR = 1.08, 95% CI: 0.81–1.45, $P = 0.592$). Subgroup analysis by ethnicity showed no association in Asian populations (G allele versus A allele: OR = 1.05, 95% CI: 0.76–1.44, $P = 0.790$). Subgroup analysis by DR subtype also did not reveal any association of rs5498 with proliferative DR (G allele versus A allele: OR = 1.34, 95% CI: 0.71–2.52, $P = 0.364$) and non-proliferative DR (G allele versus A allele: OR = 0.71, 95% CI: 0.43–1.17, $P = 0.180$).

Conclusion: Our meta-analyses provide no evidence of the association of rs5498 with DR in type 2 diabetic patients.

Keywords: ICAM-1, rs5498, Meta-analysis, Diabetic retinopathy

Background

Diabetic retinopathy (DR) is the single most common complication of diabetes mellitus and the leading cause of blindness in working-aged adults worldwide [1]. Despite numerous breakthroughs in the development of novel pharmacological agents for DR in the last decade, the incidence of DR remains high and 90% of type 1 and 60% of type 2 diabetes patients suffer from the disease. Body mass index (BMI), increased duration of diabetes, ineffective blood glucose control, and ineffective blood pressure control are the major risk factors for DR [1, 2].

However, they do not adequately predict disease progression in individual patients, suggesting the presence of a genetic component. Identification of the specific genetic risk factors for DR susceptibility is an area of substantial research and could unravel druggable targets for the purpose of treatment or even prevention.

In recent years, emerging evidence has highlighted the potential role of intercellular adhesion molecule-1 (ICAM-1) in the development of DR. ICAM-1 is a immunoglobulin-(Ig)-like transmembrane glycoprotein expressed on the surface of leukocytes, endothelial cells, and epithelial cells [3]. It influences the adhesion of circulating immune cells to the endothelium and contributes to immune cell migration and perivascular infiltration. Increased levels

* Correspondence: liangh@gxmu.edu.cn
Department of Ophthalmology, First Affiliated Hospital, Guangxi Medical University, Nanning, China

of ICAM-1 and its ligands have been observed in patients with DR and retina of animal models [4–7]. ICAM-1 blockade with monoclonal antibodies effectively prevents diabetic retinal leukostasis, vascular leakage, and capillary nonperfusion in experimental DR [4]. Similarly, when the bioactivity of the ICAM-1 counter receptor CD18 is inhibited, diabetic retinal leukocyte adhesion is potently suppressed [5].

Because ICAM-1 has been implicated in DR development, multiple studies have investigated how genetic variation at *ICAM-1* is related to DR risk. More than 100 single-nucleotide polymorphisms (SNPs) were identified in the *ICAM-1* gene. The best studied SNP is a G/A polymorphism in exon6 at codon 469 (rs5498), resulting in a lysine (Lys) to glutamine (Glu) substitution in Ig-like domain 5 that is essential for dimerisation, surface presentation and solubilisation of the protein [8]. This polymorphism has been shown to influence the interaction of ICAM-1 with leukocyte function-associated antigen-1 (LFA-1) and the macrophage-1 antigen during leukocyte adhesion [8]. In the present study, we aimed to provide a quantitative evaluation of the association between DR in type 2 diabetes and the *ICAM-1* rs5498 polymorphism.

Methods

Literature search

The search strategy for this meta-analysis was comprehensive, aiming to retrieve the largest possible number of relevant studies. We systematically screened 5 electronic databases including Pubmed (Additional file 1), Embase, Scopus, Web of Science and Wanfang for articles published between January 1990 and January 2018. The following keywords were used: intercellular adhesion molecule-1, K469E, rs5498, diabetic retinopathy, type 2 diabetes, and polymorphism. In addition, the reference lists of all the retrieved papers and relevant reviews were manually searched for eligible papers. We only included published studies with full-text articles available. In case of overlap between articles reporting on the same cohort, we included the study with the largest cohort. Our meta-analysis adhered to the Preferred Reporting Items for Systematic Reviews and Meta-Analyses (PRISMA) Statement (Additional file 2) [9].

Inclusion and exclusion criteria

One reviewer performed the initial screen of all papers identified by the electronic searches. Studies were excluded when the title clearly indicated that it did not meet the inclusion criteria. Where a title/abstract could not be rejected with certainty, the full text of the publications was obtained for assessment. Studies were considered eligible if they met the following criteria: 1) evaluated the frequency of the *ICAM-1* rs5498 polymorphism in relation to the number of retinopathy cases

and controls; 2) published in English or Chinese; and 3) published prior to January 2018 unless an online version of the study had been released prior to this date; and 4) reported odds ratios (ORs) and 95% confidence intervals (95% CIs) or data to calculate them. Case-only and case series studies with no control population were excluded, as well as studies based only on phenotypic tests, reviews, meta-analysis. We also excluded unpublished studies or gray literature because we expected them to contain insufficient reporting for our analysis.

Data extraction and quality assessment

Data extraction was performed by the first author and entered into predesigned electronic tables. The second author checked the extracted data. Disagreements were resolved by discussion between the two authors. The following items were considered: first author, year of publication, location of the study, ethnicity, number of cases and controls, diagnostic criteria, allele or genotype frequency, Hardy-Weinberg equilibrium (HWE) status, and genotyping method. The methodological quality of each study was assessed by the Newcastle-Ottawa Scale, which was used for its simplicity in comparing observational studies. Studies were evaluated based on cohort selection, comparability and ascertainment of exposure using nine multiple-choice questions. Studies were deemed of low quality if the total score was 5 or lower [10].

Statistical analyses

Statistical analysis was performed using STATA 11 (StataCorp, College Station, TX). To assess HWE status, we used a publicly available program (http://ihg.gsf.de/cgi-bin/hw/hwa1.pl). For our main analysis, we compared allele frequencies (the -encoding allele G versus the -encoding allele A) between cases and controls. We also evaluated a dominant model (GG + AG versus AA) and a recessive model (GG versus AG + AA) for the G allele. All associations were presented as ORs with their corresponding 95% CIs. Heterogeneity was evaluated by Cochran's Q and the I^2 statistic. When heterogeneity was high ($I^2 > 50\%$, $P < 0.10$), a pooled analysis was conducted using DerSimonian and Laird random effects models [11]. The significance of the summary OR was determined using an asymptotic Z-test. We evaluated publication bias or selective reporting by using funnel plots as well as Egger's regression intercept test.

Results

Study characteristics

Our search yielded 476 records, with 14 articles being possibly eligible after review on abstract level. After full-text review, we excluded 5 studies. Overall, 9 studies involving 1792 cases and 1400 controls met the selection criteria and could be used for meta-analysis [12–20].

Figure 1 showed the process of identifying eligible studies. The mean (range) year of publication was 2010 (2002–2016). The mean (range) sample size was 355 (70–792). Studies had been performed in 4 countries, including China ($n = 5$), India ($n = 2$), Japan ($n = 1$), and Slovenia ($n = 1$). Study characteristics and methodological quality of included studies are shown in Table 1.

Data synthesis

The minor allele frequency (MAF) for the *ICAM-1* rs5498 polymorphism varied from 16.7 to 54.8%. The pooled effect estimates among all studies did not find statistically significant associations between the *ICAM-1* rs5498 polymorphism and retinopathy in type 2 diabetes at the dominant model (GG + GA versus AA, OR = 1.00, 95% CI: 0.66–1.50, $P = 0.987$), the recessive model (GG versus GA + AA, OR = 1.24, 95% CI: 0.86–1.77, $P = 0.245$), the GG versus AA contrast (OR = 1.14, 95% CI: 0.68–1.92, $P = 0.611$), and the G allele versus A allele contrast (OR = 1.08, 95% CI: 0.81–1.45, $P = 0.592$) (Table 2 and Figs. 2 and 3). Among the included studies, 8 studies with 1597 cases and 1257 controls were performed on Asian populations. We conducted subgroup analyses by ethnicity using Asian studies, but we did not find any significant associations of the *ICAM-1* rs5498 polymorphism with retinopathy in Asians (dominant model: OR = 0.96, 95% CI: 0.61–1.50, $P = 0.843$; recessive model: OR = 1.15, 95% CI: 0.79–1.68, $P = 0.469$; GG versus AA contrast: OR = 1.04, 95% CI: 0.60–1.81, $P =$

0.887; G allele versus A allele: OR = 1.05, 95% CI: 0.76–1.44, $P = 0.790$) (Table 2 and Figs. 2 and 3). The single Caucasian study showed a statistically significant association between rs5498 and retinopathy at the recessive model (OR = 2.00, 95% CI: 1.15–3.48, $P = 0.014$), the GG versus AA contrast (OR = 2.21, 95% CI: 1.16–4.22, $P = 0.016$) and the G allele versus A allele contrast (OR = 1.44, 95% CI: 1.06–1.95, $P = 0.021$) (Table 2) [14]. When DR was subdivided into non-proliferative DR and proliferative DR, subgroup analysis did not show evidence of significant associations (Table 2). The influential analysis for the *ICAM-1* rs5498 polymorphism revealed that there was no single study which significantly influenced the overall results (Fig. 4).

Heterogeneity and publication bias

The present meta-analysis revealed heterogeneity among the included studies (I^2 ranged from 65.3–84.0%). The funnel plot did not demonstrate apparent asymmetry (Fig. 5). Egger's test also did not indicate any evidence of publication bias (Table 3).

Discussion

DR is the most frequent microvascular complication from type 2 diabetes. A large body of clinical and experimental literature has indicates that leucocyte adhesion to the retinal vasculature plays an important role in the pathogenesis of DR. As a central mediator of leukocyte adhesion to and transmigration across the endothelium,

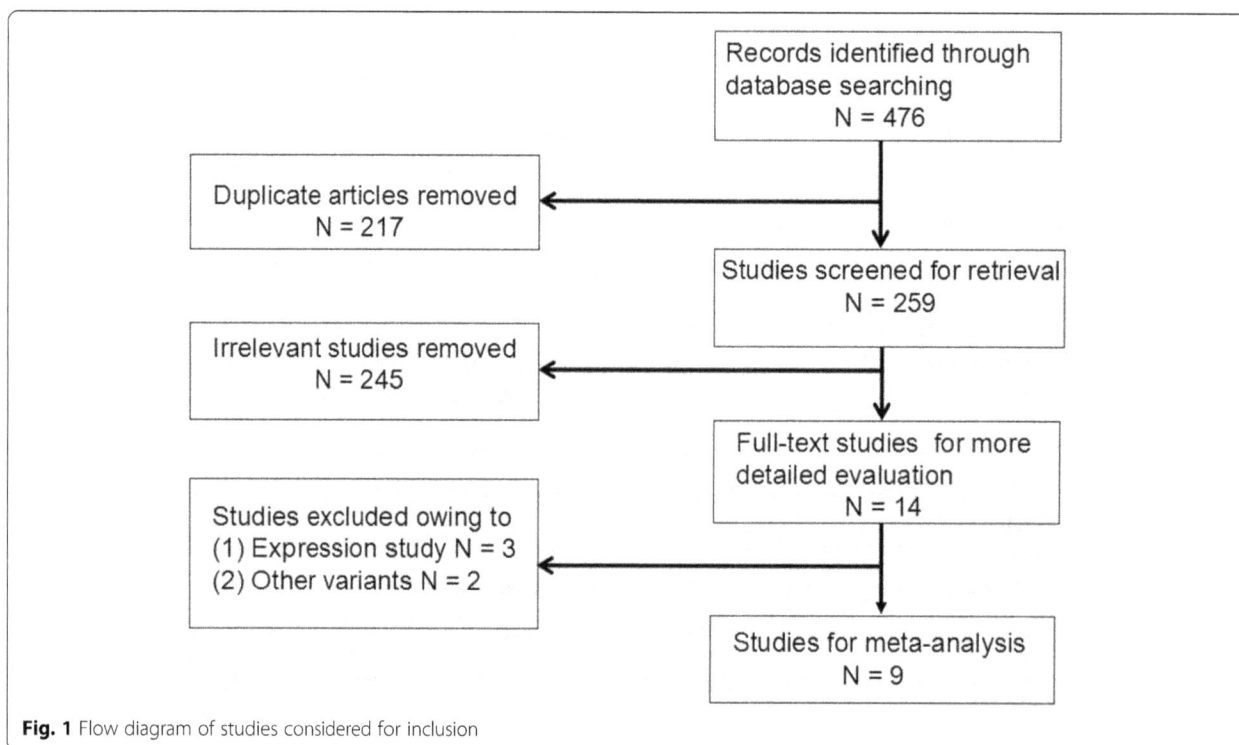

Fig. 1 Flow diagram of studies considered for inclusion

Table 1 Characteristics of the included studies

First author	Year	Country	Ethnicity	Female percentage (%)		HWE	Age		NOS	Method of DR ascertainment	Genotyping method	Cases (n)	Controls (n)	MAF (%)
				Cases	Controls		Cases	Controls						
Kamiuchi	2002	Japan	Asians	52.0	56.8	Yes	64.3 ± 8.9	64.1 ± 9.1	7	Ophthalmoscopy and fluorescein angiography	PCR-RFLP	81	50	50.0
Liu	2006	China	Asians	PDR: 66.3 NPDR: 67.3	50.0	Yes	PDR: 55.0 ± 12.4 NPDR: 63.7 ± 7.9	50.2 ± 10.6	7	NA	DNA sequencing	132	80	38.8
Petrovic	2008	Slovenia	Caucasians	53.3	60.1	Yes	65.2 ± 9.9	66.9 ± 11.5	7	Fundus photographs	Allele-specific PCR	195	143	42.3
Zhou	2010	China	Asians	49.0	48.0	No	55.6 ± 8.8	55.3 ± 8.6	6	Ophthalmoscopy and fluorescein angiography	PCR-RFLP	102	150	33.0
Zhu	2010	China	Asians	NA	NA	Yes	NA	NA	6	Ophthalmoscopy and fluorescein angiography	PCR-RFLP	40	30	16.7
Balasubbu	2010	India	Asians	30.0	42.0	Yes	57 ± 9	59 ± 11	7	Ophthalmoscopy and fundus photographs	SNaPshot PCR	345	359	48.2
Vinita	2012	India	Asians	35.7	37.6	Yes	58.8 ± 8.6	64.3 ± 9.0	8	Fundus photographs	DNA sequencing	199	157	54.8
Lv	2016	China	Asians	56.3	52.6	Yes	62.4 ± 11.9	60.2 ± 11.7	7	Fundus photographs	PCR-LDR	448	344	29.4
Li	2016	China	Asians	PDR: 51.7 NPDR: 46.2	43.8	Yes	PDR: 66.9 ± 6.9 NPDR: 63.1 ± 6.8	54–82	7	NA	DNA sequencing	250	87	41.4

DR diabetic retinopathy, HWE Hardy-Weinberg equilibrium, MAF minor allele frequency, NA not available, NOS Newcastle-Ottawa scale, NPDR non-proliferative diabetic retinopathy, PCR-LDR polymerase chain reaction-ligase detection reaction, PCR-RFLP polymerase chain reaction-restriction fragment length polymorphism, PDR proliferative diabetic retinopathy

Table 2 Meta-analysis of the association between rs5498 and DR in type 2 diabetes

Evaluation	Number of studies	OR (95% CI)	P	P for heterogeneity	I² (%)
GA + GG versus AA					
Total	9	1.00 (0.66–1.50)	0.987	< 0.001	84.0
Asians	8	0.96 (0.61–1.50)	0.843	< 0.001	85.2
Caucasians	1	1.40 (0.86–2.27)	0.173	NA	NA
PDR	4	1.22 (0.61–2.47)	0.577	< 0.001	86.8
NPDR	3	0.60 (0.29–1.21)	0.151	0.007	80.0
GG versus GA + AA					
Total	9	1.24 (0.86–1.77)	0.245	0.003	65.3
Asians	8	1.15 (0.79–1.68)	0.469	0.008	63.2
Caucasians	1	2.00 (1.15–3.48)	0.014	NA	NA
PDR	4	1.90 (0.80–4.50)	0.146	< 0.001	84.2
NPDR	3	0.92 (0.58–1.47)	0.724	0.477	0.0
GG versus AA					
Total	9	1.14 (0.68–1.92)	0.611	< 0.001	78.5
Asians	8	1.04 (0.60–1.81)	0.887	< 0.001	78.1
Caucasians	1	2.21 (1.16–4.22)	0.016	NA	NA
PDR	4	1.91 (0.64–5.73)	0.246	< 0.001	87.6
NPDR	3	0.77 (0.47–1.25)	0.286	0.171	43.5
G allele versus A allele					
Total	9	1.08 (0.81–1.45)	0.592	< 0.001	85.7
Asians	8	1.05 (0.76–1.44)	0.790	< 0.001	86.3
Caucasians	1	1.44 (1.06–1.95)	0.021	NA	NA
PDR	4	1.34 (0.71–2.52)	0.364	< 0.001	82.5
NPDR	3	0.71 (0.43–1.17)	0.180	0.011	77.9

CI confidence interval, *DR* diabetic retinopathy, *NA* not applicable, *NPDR* non-proliferative diabetic retinopathy, *OR* odds ratio, *PDR* proliferative diabetic retinopathy

the gene encoding ICAM-1 is thought to be involved in the development of DR.

The current mete-analytic review was conducted to verify the genetic contribution of a common SNP, rs5498 in the *ICAM-1* gene to retinopathy risk in type 2 diabetes. Our results showed a lack of association between the *ICAM-1* rs5498 polymorphism and risk of retinopathy in type 2 diabetes. Subgroup analysis by ethnicity did not reveal any significant association in Asian populations. In addition, when DR were subdivided into two main stages: non-proliferative and proliferative, we found no association of the *ICAM-1* rs5498 polymorphism with the risk of non-proliferative and proliferative DR.

The *ICAM-1* rs5498 polymorphism results in substitution of an A with a G nucleotide and replaces lysine (K) with a glutamic acid (E). It is thought that the SNP affects mRNA splicing patterns that modify cell-cell interactions and influence inflammatory response [8]. Kamiuchi et al. initially reported a positive association between rs5498 genotypes and retinopathy in type 2 diabetes, using a very small sample size (81 cases and 50 controls) [12]. However, their findings were not replicated by all other studies

on the topic. It was noteworthy that the study by Balasubbu et al. with 704 participants and the study by Lv et al. involving 782 participants were the two having relatively large sample sizes among the included studies, but they did not identify any statistically significant association of rs5498 with DR [17, 19]. We could not exclude the possibility that false-positive findings may be obtained from studies with small sample sizes like one conducted by Kamiuchi et al.

Combining published data from nine studies involving 3192 participants, this is the largest meta-analysis on the relationship between the *ICAM-1* rs5498 polymorphism and retinopathy in type 2 diabetes. Previous meta-analyses on the same topic included fewer studies (Su et al., 2013, n = 5; Sun et al., 2014, n = 7; Fan et al., 2015, n = 7) [21–23]. Results from this meta-analysis differed from those of the meta-analysis by Su et al., which found an association between rs5498 and DR in type 2 diabetes. This was probably because in addition to the five studies included by Su et al. [21], we included four recently published case-control studies and conducted the pooled analyses with a larger sample size [22, 23]. Sun et al. and Fan et al. found no association of

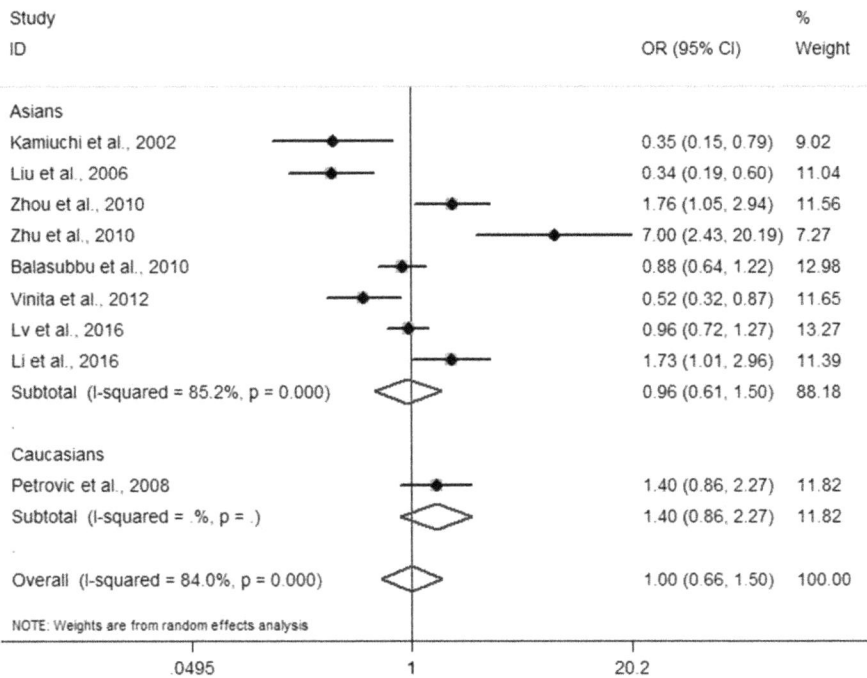

Fig. 2 Forest plot for included studies evaluating the association between the *ICAM-1* rs5498 polymorphism and diabetic retinopathy in type 2 diabetic patients under a dominant model (GG + AG versus AA). OR, oadds ratio; CI, confidence interval

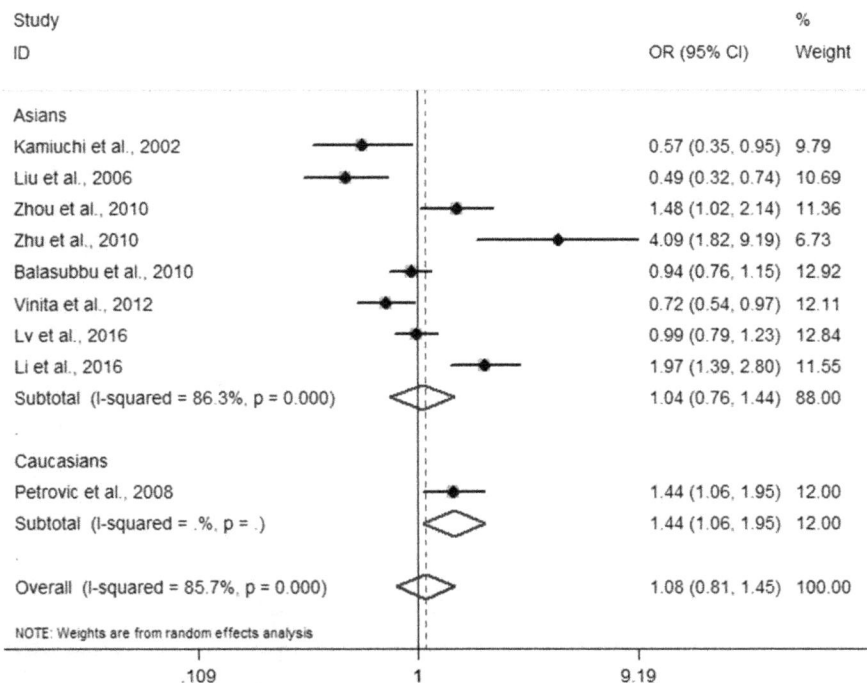

Fig. 3 Forest plot for included studies evaluating the association between the *ICAM-1* rs5498 polymorphism and diabetic retinopathy in type 2 diabetic patients under allele contrast (G allele versus A allele). OR, oadds ratio; CI, confidence interval

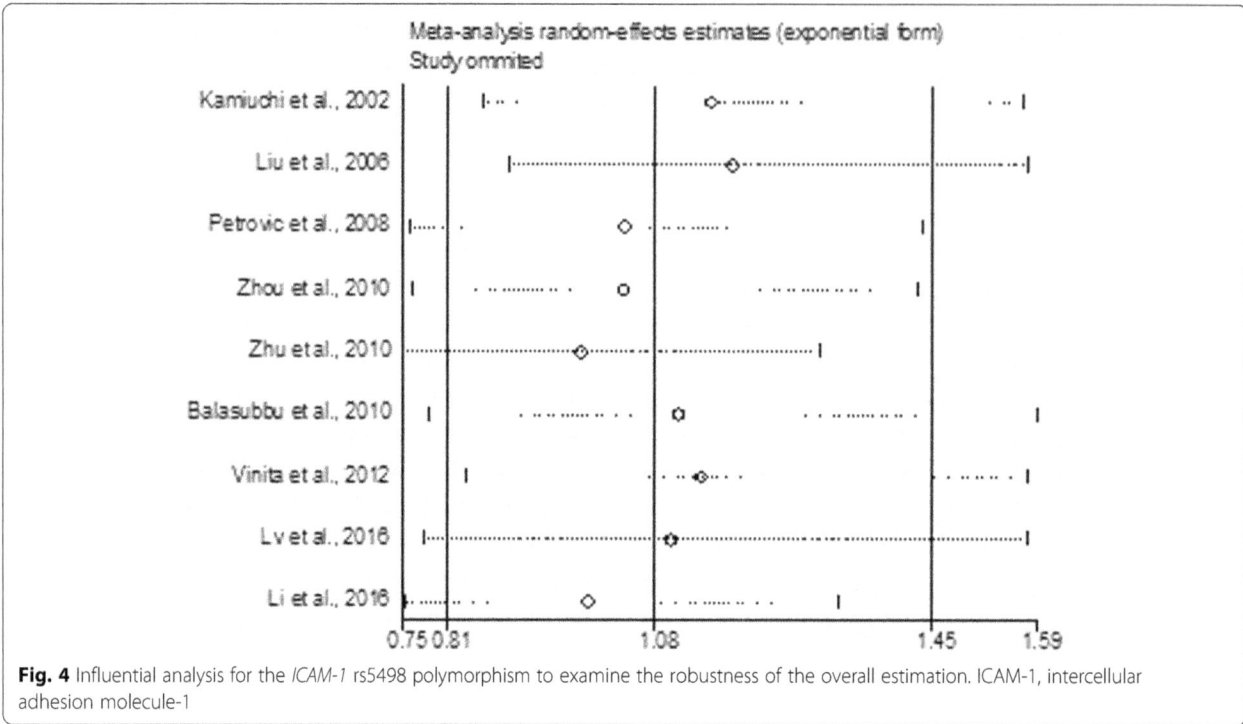

Fig. 4 Influential analysis for the *ICAM-1* rs5498 polymorphism to examine the robustness of the overall estimation. ICAM-1, intercellular adhesion molecule-1

rs5498 with DR; their results were consistent with our calculations. Compared to the previous meta-analyses, our study had several strengths. First, considering that the cause and development of type 1 diabetes and type 2 diabetes were different, we only included retinopathy subjects of type 2 diabetes as cases in our analyses. We did not take into account the results from type 1 diabetes. Second, in addition to subgroup analyses by ethnicity, we performed subtype-specific analyses to evaluate the relation of rs5498 with the risk of non-proliferative and proliferative DR, respectively. Such evaluations were not performed by the previous meta-analyses. Third, we performed influential analysis to ensure the robustness of our combined estimations.

Since most of the included studies were conducted on Asian populations ($n = 8$), it became evident from this meta-analysis that further studies should include larger

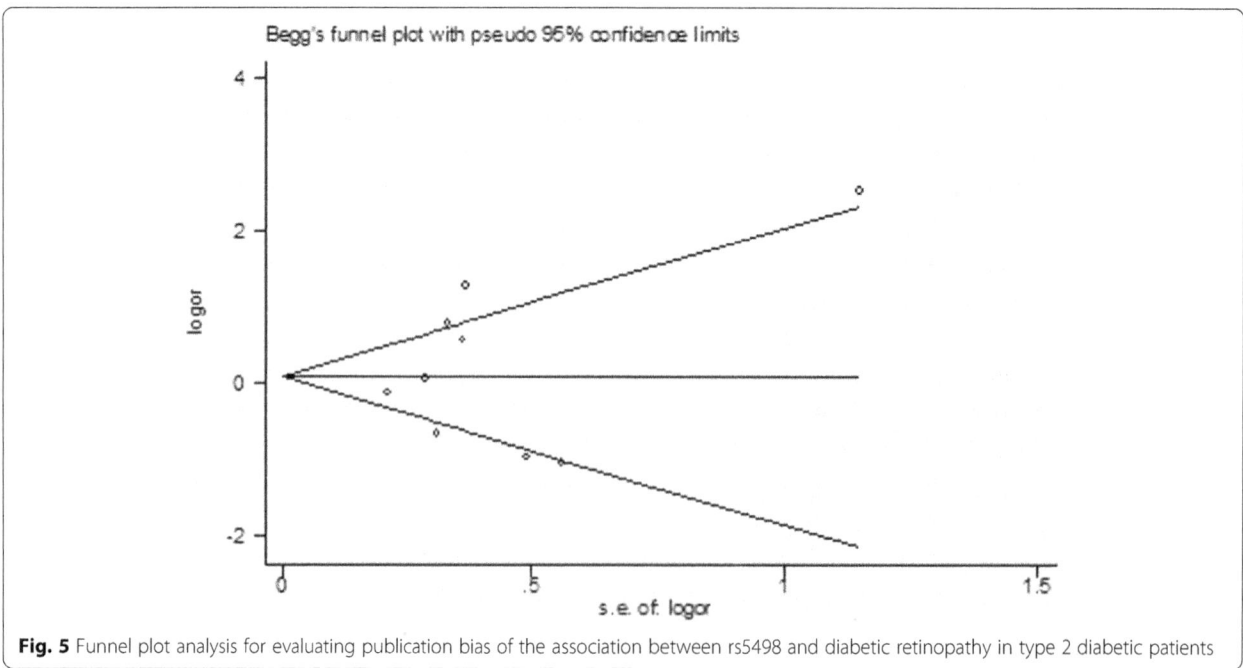

Fig. 5 Funnel plot analysis for evaluating publication bias of the association between rs5498 and diabetic retinopathy in type 2 diabetic patients

Table 3 Assessment of publication bias using Egger's test

	Dominant model	Recessive model	GG versus AA contrast	G allele versus A allele contrast
P value	0.754	0.498	0.641	0.579

non-Asian populations to evaluate race-specific effects of rs5498, such as African and Caucasian populations. The study by Petrovic et al. was the only one performed in Caucasians [14]; their findings should be replicated in other Caucasian populations, including British, German, and French populations. Besides rs5498, more than 200 polymorphisms have been identified in the *ICAM-1* gene. We could not exclude the possibility that other *ICAM-1* polymorphisms played a role in the susceptibility to type 2 DR. The study by Simões et al. identified a significant association between the *ICAM-1* rs1801714 polymorphsim and non-proliferative DR in type 2 diabetes [24]. In addition, a Chinese study assessed the association of DR with the rs1799969 polymorphism which was located in exon 4 of the *ICAM-1* gene [25]. Because the evidence base for other *ICAM-1*polymorphisms was very small at the time of planning our meta-analysis and consequently we chose to focus our analysis only on the rs5498 polymorphism. It would be advisable that in the future attention should be paid to the relationship between other *ICAM-1* polymorphisms and DR in type 2 diabetes.

Several limitations should be considered. First, this study was limited by the unavailability of individual patient data that would allow the identification of potential interactions of rs5498 with specific disease characteristics, including glycemic control, blood pressure control, and hyperlipemia. These factors might have contributed to the lack of success in identifying positive results in association studies for rs5498. Second, like all meta-analyses, the present study was susceptible to reporting biases. Despite the use of comprehensive strategies to identify eligible studies for rs5498, we could not exclude the possibility that some studies might have been erroneously excluded. Third, we did not evaluate the relation of serum soluble ICAM-1 (sICAM-1) levels with DR because of limited published data. There was some evidence suggesting that circulating sICAM levels were positively associated with DR prevalence in type 2 diabetes [14, 26]. It is recommended that future association studies should perform sICAM-1 measurement and evaluate the effects of rs5498 on sICAM levels in DR patients, which could help clarify the role of rs5498 in DR development.

In conclusion, Our meta-analysis has shown that there is no significant association of the *ICAM-1* rs5498 polymorphism with DR in type 2 diabetes. Further investigation involving non-Asian populations is warranted on the association between this polymorphism and DR, particularly studies with larger sample size that adjust for confounding variables.

Abbreviations
BMI: Body mass index; CI: Confidence interval; DR: Diabetic retinopathy; HWE: Hardy-Weinberg equilibrium; ICAM-1: Intercellular adhesion molecule-1; MAF: Minor allele frequency; OR: Odds ratio; SNP: Single-nucleotide polymorphism

Acknowledgements
Not applicable.

Funding
This research receives no funding.

Author's contributions
Conceived and designed the study: ZX and HL; Data acquisition: ZX; Analysis and interpretation: ZX and HL; Drafting the manuscript: ZX; Revising the manuscript critically: ZX and HL. Both authors made substantial contribution to this manuscript meeting authorship criteria, agreed to be accountable for all aspects of the work and have read and approved the final version.

Competing interests
The authors declare that they have no competing interests.

References
1. Eshaq RS, Aldalati AMZ, Alexander JS, Harris NR. Diabetic retinopathy: breaking the barrier. Pathophysiology. 2017;24:229–41.
2. Giloyan A, Harutyunyan T, Petrosyan V. The prevalence of and major risk factors associated with diabetic retinopathy in Gegharkunik province of Armenia: cross-sectional study. BMC Ophthalmol. 2015;15:46.
3. Gu HF, Ma J, Gu KT, Brismar K. Association of intercellular adhesion molecule 1 (ICAM1) with diabetes and diabetic nephropathy. Front Endocrinol (Lausanne). 2013;3:179.
4. Miyamoto K, Khosrof S, Bursell SE, Rohan R, Murata T, Clermont AC, et al. Prevention of leukostasis and vascular leakage in streptozotocin-induced diabetic retinopathy via intercellular adhesion molecule-1 inhibition. Proc Natl Acad Sci U S A. 1999;96:10836–41.
5. Barouch FC, Miyamoto K, Allport JR, Fujita K, Bursell SE, Aiello LP, et al. Integrin-mediated neutrophil adhesion and retinal leukostasis in diabetes. Invest Ophthalmol Vis Sci. 2000;41:1153–8.
6. Matsuoka M, Ogata N, Minamino K, Matsumura M. Leukostasis and pigment epithelium-derived factor in rat models of diabetic retinopathy. Mol Vis. 2007;13:1058–65.
7. Zhang XL, Wen L, Chen YJ, Zhu Y. Vascular endothelial growth factor up-regulates the expression of intracellular adhesion molecule-1 in retinal endothelial cells via reactive oxygen species, but not nitric oxide. Chin Med J. 2009;122:338–43.
8. Joob B, Wiwanitkit V. ICAM-1 K469E polymorphism, increased risk of neurocysticerosis occurrence and immunopathological defect. Arq Neuropsiquiatr. 2017;75:681.
9. Moher D, Liberati A, Tetzlaff J, Altman DG, PRISMA Group. Preferred reporting items for systematic reviews and meta-analyses: the PRISMA statement. Int J Surg. 2010;8:336–41.
10. Stang A. Critical evaluation of the Newcastle-Ottawa scale for the assessment of the quality of nonrandomized studies in meta-analyses. Eur J Epidemiol. 2010;25:603–5.
11. DerSimonian R, Laird N. Meta-analysis in clinical trials. Control Clin Trials. 1986;7:177–88.
12. Kamiuchi K, Hasegawa G, Obayashi H, Kitamura A, Ishii M, Yano M, et al. Intercellular adhesion molecule-1 (ICAM-1) polymorphism is associated with diabetic retinopathy in type 2 diabetes mellitus. Diabet Med. 2002;19:371–6.
13. Liu L, Yu Q, Wang H, Zhang SX, Huang C, Chen X. Association of intercellular adhesion molecule 1 polymorphisms with retinopathy in Chinese patients with type 2 diabetes. Diabet Med. 2006;23:643–8.
14. Petrovic MG, Osredkar J, Saraga-Babić M, Petrovic D. K469E polymorphism of the intracellular adhesion molecule 1 gene is associated with proliferative diabetic retinopathy in Caucasians with type 2 diabetes. Clin Exp Ophthalmol. 2008;36:468–72.
15. Zhou Y, Fu P, Fu X. Study on the gene polymorphism of intercellular adhesion molecule-1 in type 2 diabetes mellitus patients with retinopathy. J Chin Pract Diagn Ther. 2010;10:29–31.

16. Zhu J, Gao S, Chi X, Zhang Y, Lai X, Zhong W. Association between the intercellular adhesion molecule-1 (ICAM-1) K469E polymorphism and diabetic retinopathy. J Fujian Med Univ. 2010;44:190–3.

17. Balasubbu S, Sundaresan P, Rajendran A, Ramasamy K, Govindarajan G, Perumalsamy N, et al. Association analysis of nine candidate gene polymorphisms in Indian patients with type 2 diabetic retinopathy. BMC Med Genet. 2010;11:158.

18. Vinita K, Sripriya S, Prathiba K, Vaitheeswaran K, Sathyabaarathi R, Rajesh M, et al. ICAM-1 K469E polymorphism is a genetic determinant for the clinical risk factors of T2D subjects with retinopathy in Indians: a population-based case-control study. BMJ Open. 2012;2.

19. Lv Z, Li Y, Wu Y, Qu Y. Association of ICAM-1 and HMGA1 gene variants with retinopathy in type 2 diabetes mellitus among Chinese individuals. Curr Eye Res. 2016;41:1118–22.

20. Li L, Yi X, Gu Y, Qian Y, Zheng K. Association of genetic polymorphism of VEGF, ICAM-1 K469E, EPO and TCF7L2 genes with diabetic retinopathy of type 2 diabetes mellitus in Uyghur population in Xinjiang. J Xinjiang Med Univ. 2016;39:1268–71.

21. Su X, Chen X, Liu L, Chang X, Yu X, Sun K. Intracellular adhesion molecule-1 K469E gene polymorphism and risk of diabetic microvascular complications: a meta-analysis. PLoS One. 2013;8:e69940.

22. Sun H, Cong X, Sun R, Wang C, Wang X, Liu Y. Association between the ICAM-1 K469E polymorphism and diabetic retinopathy in type 2 diabetes mellitus: a meta-analysis. Diabetes Res Clin Pract. 2014;104:e46–9.

23. Fan WY, Liu NP. Meta-analysis of association between K469E polymorphism of the ICAM-1 gene and retinopathy in type 2 diabetes. Int J Ophthalmol. 2015;8:603–7.

24. Simões MJ, Lobo C, Egas C, Nunes S, Carmona S, Costa MÂ, et al. Genetic variants in ICAM1, PPARGC1A and MTHFR are potentially associated with different phenotypes of diabetic retinopathy. Ophthalmologica. 2014;232: 156–62.

25. Yang X, Deng Y, Gu H, Ren X, Li N, Lim A, et al. Candidate gene association study for diabetic retinopathy in Chinese patients with type 2 diabetes. Mol Vis. 2014;20:200–14.

26. van Hecke MV, Dekker JM, Nijpels G, Moll AC, Heine RJ, Bouter LM, et al. Inflammation and endothelial dysfunction are associated with retinopathy: the Hoorn study. Diabetologia. 2005;48:1300–6.

Permissions

The contributors of this book come from diverse backgrounds, making this book a truly international effort. This book will bring forth new frontiers with its revolutionizing research information and detailed analysis of the nascent developments around the world.

We would like to thank all the contributing authors for lending their expertise to make the book truly unique. They have played a crucial role in the development of this book. Without their invaluable contributions this book wouldn't have been possible. They have made vital efforts to compile up to date information on the varied aspects of this subject to make this book a valuable addition to the collection of many professionals and students.

This book was conceptualized with the vision of imparting up-to-date information and advanced data in this field. To ensure the same, a matchless editorial board was set up. Every individual on the board went through rigorous rounds of assessment to prove their worth. After which they invested a large part of their time researching and compiling the most relevant data for our readers.

The editorial board has been involved in producing this book since its inception. They have spent rigorous hours researching and exploring the diverse topics which have resulted in the successful publishing of this book. They have passed on their knowledge of decades through this book. To expedite this challenging task, the publisher supported the team at every step. A small team of assistant editors was also appointed to further simplify the editing procedure and attain best results for the readers.

Apart from the editorial board, the designing team has also invested a significant amount of their time in understanding the subject and creating the most relevant covers. They scrutinized every image to scout for the most suitable representation of the subject and create an appropriate cover for the book.

The publishing team has been an ardent support to the editorial, designing and production team. Their endless efforts to recruit the best for this project, has resulted in the accomplishment of this book. They are a veteran in the field of academics and their pool of knowledge is as vast as their experience in printing. Their expertise and guidance has proved useful at every step. Their uncompromising quality standards have made this book an exceptional effort. Their encouragement from time to time has been an inspiration for everyone.

The publisher and the editorial board hope that this book will prove to be a valuable piece of knowledge for researchers, students, practitioners and scholars across the globe.

List of Contributors

Changjun Wang, Qingyao Ning, Kai Jin, Jiajun Xie and Juan Ye
Department of Ophthalmology, the Second Affiliated Hospital of Zhejiang University, College of Medicine, Hangzhou 310009, China

Yeon Woong Chung
Department of Ophthalmology, College of Medicine, St. Vincent's Hospital, The Catholic University of Korea, Suwon, Republic of Korea

Jun Sub Choi and Sun Young Shin
Department of Ophthalmology and Visual Science, College of Medicine, Seoul St. Mary's Hospital, The Catholic University of Korea, Banpo-daero 222, Seocho-gu, Seoul 06591, Republic of Korea

Nohae Park, Byunggun Park and Sunghyuk Moon
Department of Ophthalmology, Busan Paik Hospital, Inje University College of Medicine, 75 Bokji-ro, Busanjin-gu, Busan 47392, Republic of Korea

Minkyung Oh
Department of Pharmacology, Busan Paik Hospital, Inje University College of medicine, Busan, Republic of Korea

Myungmi Kim
Department of Ophthalmology, Yeungnam University College of Medicine, Daegu, Republic of Korea

Lei Xi
Department of Ophthalmology, Peking University International Hospital, Beijing, China

Chen Zhang
Tianjin Medical University Eye hospital, Tianjin Medical University Eye Institute, School of Optometry and Ophthalmology, Tianjin, China

Yanling He
Department of Ophthalmology, Peking University People's Hospital, Beijing, China

Edita Kunceviciene, Margarita Sriubiene, Ilona T. Miceikiene and Alina Smalinskiene
Institute of Biology Systems and Genetic Research, Lithuanian University of Health Sciences, 18 Tilzes St, Kaunas, Lithuania

Rasa Liutkeviciene
Department of Ophthalmology, Lithuanian University of Health Sciences, 2 Eiveniu St, Kaunas, Lithuania

Paula Casas and José A. Cristóbal
Department of Ophthalmology, Hospital Clínico Universitario "Lozano Blesa", San Juan Bosco 15, ES-50009 Zaragoza, Spain

Eugenio Vicente, Gloria Tejero-Garcés and María I. Adiego
Department of Otolaryngology, Hospital Universitario "Miguel Servet", Zaragoza, Spain

Francisco J. Ascaso
Department of Ophthalmology, Hospital Clínico Universitario "Lozano Blesa", San Juan Bosco 15, ES-50009 Zaragoza, Spain
Instituto de Investigación Sanitaria Aragón (IIS Aragón), Zaragoza, Spain

Owen Kim Hee, Zheng-Xian Thng and Hong-Yuan Zhu
National Healthcare Group Eye Institute, Tan Tock Seng Hospital, S308433, Singapore, Singapore

Ecosse Luc Lamoureux
Health Services Research, Singapore Eye Research Institute, Singapore, Singapore

Ceying Shen, Shu Yan, Min Du, Hong Zhao, Ling Shao and Yibo Hu
Department of Zhengzhou Second People Hospital, Ophthalmology, Zhengzhou Eye Hospital, Zhengzhou Ophthalmic Institution, Zhengzhou Hanghai Middle Road No. 90, Zhengzhou 450000, China

Fang Fan, Zhiyang Jia, Kejun Li, Xiaobin Zhao and Qingmin Ma
Department of Ophthalmology, Hebei general hospital, Shijiazhuang, Hebei 050000, People's Republic of China

Yingnan Zhang, Yang Liu and Zhiqiang Pan
Beijing Tongren Eye Center, Beijing Tongren Hospital, Capital Medical University, Beijing Ophthalmology and Visual Science Key Lab, Beijing 100730, China

Qingfeng Liang
Beijing Institute of Ophthalmology, Beijing Tongren Eye Center, Beijing Tongren Hospital, Capital Medical University, Beijing Key Laboratory of Ophthalmology and Visual Sciences, Beijing 100005, China

Christophe Baudouin and Antoine Labbé
Quinze-Vingts National Ophthalmology Hospital, Paris and Versailles Saint-Quentin-en-Yvelines University, Versailles, France
INSERM, U968, Paris, F-75012, France; UPMC Univ Paris 06, UMR_S 968, Institut de la Vision, Paris F-75012, France; CNRS, UMR_7210, Paris F-75012, France, Paris, France

Qingxian Lu
5Department of Ophthalmology and Visual Sciences, University of Louisville,
301 E. Muhammad Ali Blvd, Louisville, KY 40202, USA

Ji Hwan Lee, Christopher Seungkyu Lee and Sung Chul Lee
Department of Ophthalmology, The Institute of Vision Research, Yonsei
University College of Medicine, Yonsei-ro 50-1, Seodaemun-gu, Seoul,
Republic of Korea

Jingjing Liu, Yiye Chen, Shiyuan Wang, Xiang Zhang and Peiquan Zhao
Department of Ophthalmology, Xin Hua Hospital, Shanghai Jiao Tong University School of Medicine, Shanghai 200092, China

Phillip S. Coburn, Austin L. LaGrow, Salai Madhumathi Parkunan, C. Blake Randall and Rachel L. Staats
Department of Ophthalmology, University of Oklahoma Health Sciences Center, DMEI PA-419, 608 Stanton L. Young Blvd, Oklahoma City, OK 73104, USA

Frederick C. Miller
Department of Family and Preventive Medicine, University of Oklahoma Health Sciences Center, Oklahoma City, Oklahoma, USA
Department of Cell Biology, University of Oklahoma Health Sciences Center, Oklahoma City, Oklahoma, USA

Michelle C. Callegan
Department of Ophthalmology, University of Oklahoma Health Sciences Center, DMEI PA-419, 608 Stanton L. Young Blvd, Oklahoma City, OK 73104, USA
Oklahoma Center for Neuroscience, University of Oklahoma Health Sciences Center, Oklahoma City, Oklahoma, USA
Department of Microbiology and Immunology, Dean McGee Eye Institute, University of Oklahoma Health Sciences Center, Oklahoma City, Oklahoma, USA

Seong Jun Park
College of medicine, Soonchunhyang University, 204-ho, 31 Soonchunhyang-6-gil, Dongnam-gu, Cheonan 31151, Choongcheongnam-do, South Korea

Ju Hee Noh and Jong Won Lee
Soo Eye Clinics, 202-13, Miadong, Kangbook-gu, Seoul 01118, South Korea

Ki Bum Park and Sun Young Jang
Department of Ophthalmology, Soonchunhyang University Bucheon Hospital, Soonchunhyang University College of Medicine, 170 Jomaru-ro, Wonmi-gu, Bucheon 14584, Gyeonggi-do, South Korea

Ho Sik Hwang
Department of Ophthalmology, Chuncheon Sacred Heart Hospital, Hallym University, Chuncheon, Korea

Kyong Jin Cho
Department of Ophthalmology, Dankook University College of Medicine, Cheonan, Korea

Gabriel Rand and Roy S. Chuck
Department of Ophthalmology, Montefiore Medical Center, Bronx, New York, USA

Ji Won Kwon
Department of Ophthalmology, Myongji Hospital, Seonam University College of Medicine, 55 Hwasu-Ro 14, Deokyang-Gu, Goyang-Si, Gyeonggi-Do 10475, Korea

Tian Tian, Haiying Jin, Lyu Jiao, Qi Zhang and Peiquan Zhao
Department of Ophthalmology, Xinhua Hospital, Affiliated to Medicine School of Shanghai Jiaotong University, No. 1665, Kongjiang Road, Shanghai 200092, China

Chunli Chen
Department of Ophthalmology, Shengli Oilfield Central Hospital, No.31, Jinan Road, Dong Ying, Shandong, China

Rong Han Wu, Zhong Lin and Qi Hua Liang
The Eye Hospital, School of Ophthalmology and Optometry, Wenzhou Medical University, No. 270 West College Road, Wenzhou 325027, Zhejiang, China

Rui Zhang
Liaocheng People's Hospital of Shandong Province, Liaocheng, Shandong, China

Nived Moonasar
Caribbean Eye Institute, Valsayn, Trinidad and Tobago

Zhaoge Wang, Haixia Zhao, Wenying Guan, Xin Kang, Xue Tai and Ying Shen
Center of Myopia, the Affiliated Hospital of Inner Mongolia Medical
University, 1 Tongdao North Street, Hohhot 010050, China

Laura Hernandez Moreno
Low Vision and Visual Rehabilitation Lab, Department and Center of Physics – Optometry and Vision Science, University of Minho, Braga, Portugal

Pedro Lima Ramos and Antonio Filipe Macedo
Low Vision and Visual Rehabilitation Lab, Department and Center of Physics – Optometry and Vision Science, University of Minho, Braga, Portugal
Department of Medicine and Optometry, Linnaeus University, 39182 Kalmar, Sweden

Rui Santana and Ana Patricia Marques
Centro de Investigação em Saúde Pública, Escola Nacional de Saúde Pública, Universidade NOVA de Lisboa, Lisbon, Portugal

Cristina Freitas
Department of Ophthalmology, Hospital de Braga, Braga, Portugal

Amandio Rocha-Sousa
Department of Surgery and Physiology, Faculty of Medicine, University of Porto, Porto, Portugal

Department of Ophthalmology, Centro Hospitalar São João, Porto, Portugal

Hatem M. Marey, Hesham M. Elmazar, Sameh S. Mandour and Osama A. El Morsy
Department of Ophthalmology, Menoufia Faculty of Medicine, Shebin El Kom, Menoufia, Egypt

Nurgül Örnek, Nesrin Büyüktortop Gökçınar, Tevfik Oğurel, Mehmet Erhan Yumuşak and Zafer Onaran
Department of Ophthalmology, Faculty of Medicine, Kırıkkale University, Kırıkkale, Turkey

Kemal Örnek
Department of Ophthalmology, Kudret Eye Hospital, Ankara, Turkey

Hatice Ayhan Güler
Department of Ophthalmology, Faculty of Medicine, Kırıkkale University, Kırıkkale, Turkey
Department of Ophthalmology, Bayburt State Hospital, Bayburt, Turkey

Ying Li, Ying Cheng and Yi Qu
Department of Geriatrics, Qilu Hospital of Shandong University, No. 107, Wenhuaxi Road, Jinan 250012, Shandong, China

Qian Xu
Department of Geriatrics, Qilu Hospital of Shandong University, No. 107, Wenhuaxi Road, Jinan 250012, Shandong, China
Department of Ophthalmology, The Central Hospital of Taian, Tai'an 271000, Shandong, China

Jacquelyn Daubert, Terrence P. O'Brien and Eldad Adler
Bascom Palmer Eye Institute, University of Miami Miller School of Medicine, Palm Beach Gardens, FL 33418, USA

Oriel Spierer
Bascom Palmer Eye Institute, University of Miami Miller School of Medicine, Palm Beach Gardens, FL 33418, USA
Department of Ophthalmology, Wolfson Medical Center, Sackler Faculty of Medicine, Tel Aviv University, Tel Aviv, Israel

Xiujuan Zhao, Yuxin Zhang, Yan Luo, Xiulan Zhang, Lin Lu and Hui Yang
State Key Laboratory of Ophthalmology, Zhongshan Ophthalmic Center, Sun Yat-Sen University, No. 54 Xianlie South Road, Guangzhou 510060, People's Republic of China

Wei Qiu
Department of Neurology, The Third Affiliated Hospital of Sun Yat-Sen University, Guangzhou, China

Na Yeon Jung, Sung Soon Hwang and Tae-Young Chung
Department of Ophthalmology, Samsung Medical Center, Sungkyunkwan University School of Medicine, #81 Irwon-ro, Gangnam-gu, Seoul 06351, Korea

Dong Hui Lim
Department of Ophthalmology, Samsung Medical Center, Sungkyunkwan University School of Medicine, #81 Irwon-ro, Gangnam-gu, Seoul 06351, Korea
Department of Preventive Medicine, Graduate School, The Catholic University of Korea, Seoul, Korea

Joo Hyun
Department of Ophthalmology, Samsung Medical Center, Sungkyunkwan University School of Medicine, #81 Irwon-ro, Gangnam-gu, Seoul 06351, Korea
Department of Ophthalmology, Saevit Eye Hospital, Goyang, Korea

Bin Wang and Wenwei Li
Department of Ophthalmology, Tongde Hospital of Zhejiang Province, 234 Gucui Road, Hangzhou 310012, China

Minjung Kim, Jong Suk Song and Hyo Myung Kim
Department of Ophthalmology, Korea University College of Medicine, Seoul, South Korea

Youngsub Eom
Department of Ophthalmology, Korea University College of Medicine, Seoul, South Korea
Department of Ophthalmology, Ansan Hospital, Korea University College of Medicine, 123, Jeokgeum-ro, Danwon-gu, Ansan-si, Gyeonggi-do 15355, South Korea

Yi Wang, Ju Liu and Wu Liu
Beijing Tongren Eye Center, Beijing Tongren Hospital, Capital Medical University, Beijng Ophthalmology and Visual Sciences Key Laboratory, Beijing, China

Limei Liu
Beijing Tongren Eye Center, Beijing Tongren Hospital, Capital Medical University, Beijng Ophthalmology and Visual Sciences Key Laboratory, Beijing, China
Department of Ophthalmology, Yantai Yuhuangding Hospital, Affiliated Hospital of Medical College, Qingdao University, Yantai, Shandong, China

An-Lun Wu, Kuan-Jen Chen, Laura Liu, Tun-Lu Chen, Yih-Shiou Hwang, Wei-Chi Wu and Chi-Chun Lai
Department of Ophthalmology, Chang Gung Memorial Hospital, No.5, Fu-Hsin Rd., Fuxing St., Guishan Dist, Taoyuan 33375, Taiwan
College of Medicine, Chang Gung University, No.259, Wenhua 1st Rd., Guishan Dist, Taoyuan 333, Taiwan

Lan-Hsin Chuang and Ling Yeung
College of Medicine, Chang Gung University, No.259, Wenhua 1st Rd., Guishan Dist, Taoyuan 333, Taiwan
Department of Ophthalmology, Chang Gung Memorial Hospital, No.222, Maijin Rd., Anle Dist, Keelung 204, Taiwan

Nan-Kai Wang
Department of Ophthalmology, Chang Gung Memorial Hospital, No.5, Fu-Hsin Rd., Fuxing St., Guishan Dist, Taoyuan 33375, Taiwan
College of Medicine, Chang Gung University, No.259, Wenhua 1st Rd., Guishan Dist, Taoyuan 333, Taiwan
Edward S. Harkness Eye Institute, Department of Ophthalmology, Columbia University, 635 west, 165th street, New York, NY 10032, USA

Barbara Berasategui, Alex Fonollosa and Joseba Artaraz
Department of Ophthalmology, BioCruces Health Research Institute, Cruces Hospital, University of the Basque Country, Cruces square s/n, CP 48903 Baracaldo, Vizcaya, Spain

Ioana Ruiz-Arruza
Autoimmune Diseases Research Unit, Department of Internal Medicine, BioCruces Health Research Institute, Cruces Hospital, University of the Basque Country, Bilbao, Spain

Jose Ríos
Medical Statistics Core Facility, Institut d'Investigacions Biomèdiques August Pi i Sunyer (IDIBAPS), and Hospital Clinic, Barcelona, Spain
Biostatistics Unit, Faculty of Medicine, Universitat Autònoma de Barcelona, Barcelona, Spain

Jessica Matas, Victor Llorenç and Alfredo Adan
Ophthalmology Institute, Hospital Clinic of Barcelona, Barcelona, Spain

David Diaz-Valle, Marina Sastre-Ibañez, Pedro Arriola-Villalobos
Ophthalmology Department and Health Research Institute (IdISSC), Hospital Clinico San Carlos, Madrid, Spain

Laurie Barber
Little Rock Eye Clinic, 203 Executive Court, Suite A, Little Rock, AK 72205, USA

Omid Khodai
Mobile Medical Solutions, Inc., Foothill Ranch, CA, USA

Thomas Croley
Central Florida Eye Institute, Ocala, FL, USA

Christopher Lievens
Southern College of Optometry, Memphis, TN, USA

Stephen Montaquila
West Bay Eye Associates, Warwick, RI, USA

Jillian Ziemanski
School of Optometry, University of Alabama at Birmingham, Birmingham, AL, USA

Melissa McCart and Orsolya Lunacsek
Xcenda, Palm Harbor, FL, USA

Caroline Burk
Health Outcomes Consultant, Laguna Beach, CA, USA

Vaishali Patel
Allergan plc, Irvine, CA, USA

Xinyi Ding, Ruiping Gu, Meng Zhang, Hui Ren, Qinmeng Shu, Gezhi Xu and Haixiang Wu
Department of Ophthalmology, Eye and ENT Hospital of Fudan University, 83 Fen Yang Road, Shanghai 200031, People's Republic of China
Institute of Eye Research, Eye and ENT Hospital of Fudan University, Shanghai, China
Key Laboratory of Myopia of State Health Ministry (Fudan University),
Shanghai, China
Shanghai Key Laboratory of Visual Impairment and Restoration(Fudan University), Shanghai, China

Xiaoming Huang
The School of Medicine, Nankai University, Tianjin 300071, China

Dongrun Tang, Tong Wu and Tianming Jian
Tianjin Medical University Eye Hospital, Tianjin 300384, China
Tianjin Orbital Disease Institute, Tianjin 300384, China

Fengyuan Sun
The School of Medicine, Nankai University, Tianjin 300071, China
Tianjin Medical University Eye Hospital, Tianjin 300384, China
Tianjin Orbital Disease Institute, Tianjin 300384, China

Zikang Xie and Hao Liang
Department of Ophthalmology, First Affiliated Hospital, Guangxi Medical University, Nanning, China

Index

Oxidative Stress, 9-10, 12-13, 112-113, 115, 117-118, 139, 217

P

Pars Plana Vitrectomy, 61, 78, 103, 105-107, 110-111, 178, 193-194, 198

Phacoemulsification, 57, 60-61, 111, 154, 165, 179-180, 183-184

Precizon, 163-171

Pterygium, 94-99, 132, 134

Punctal Stenosis, 90-93

R

Rasgrf1, 29-34

Reactive Oxygen Species, 9, 13, 112, 207, 218, 243

Rectangular Three-snip Punctoplasty, 90-91

Refractory Macular Hole, 78, 193, 196-197

Retinal Capillary, 51-52, 54-56

Retinal Graft, 193-197

Retinal Nerve Fiber Layer, 35, 38, 40, 42-43, 55, 142, 144-148, 155, 159-162

Retinal Pigment Epithelium, 54, 56, 140-148, 161, 200

Retinal Vein Occlusion, 42, 52, 67, 72, 135-139, 188, 195, 206

Retinal-image Quality, 187-191

Retrobulbar Anesthesia, 106-108, 110-111, 194

Rituximab, 1-2, 7-8

Rs5498, 236-238, 240-243

S

Sd-oct, 51, 56, 140-141, 144, 147, 156-157, 196, 199-201, 203, 205-206

Secondary Iol Implantation, 100-101, 103-105

Specular Microscopy, 135-137

Strabismus, 14-15, 18, 20-21, 173, 177, 235

Superficial Retinal Capillary Plexus, 51, 54-55

T

Tecnis, 102, 163-171

Thioredoxin, 9-13

Three Interrupted Sutures, 90-93

Thyroid-associated Ophthalmopathy, 1, 5, 7-8

Tlr4, 79-88, 227

Topical Anesthesia, 106-111

Transepithelial Photorefractive Keratectomy, 22, 24, 27

V

Video-oculography, 14-19, 21

Visual Field, 35-44, 50, 78, 119-120, 173

Vitreoretinal Interface, 72-73, 78, 187